T0073754

Stroke Rehabilitation

Stroke Rehabilitation

RICHARD WILSON, MD, MS
Director
Division of Neurologic Rehabilitation and Stroke Rehabilitation
MetroHealth Rehabilitation Institute
MetroHealth Medical Center
Associate Professor
Case Western Reserve University
Cleveland, OH, United States

PREETI RAGHAVAN, MD
Howard A. Rusk Associate Professor
    of Rehabilitation Research
Vice Chair for Research
Director
Division of Motor Recovery Research
Department of Rehabilitation Medicine
New York University School of Medicine
NYU Langone Health
New York, NY, United States

ELSEVIER

ELSEVIER

3251 Riverport Lane
St. Louis, Missouri 63043

Publisher: Mica Haley
Acquisition Editor: Kayla Wolfe
Editorial Project Manager: Megan Ashdown
Project Manager: Poulouse Joseph
Designer: Alan Studholme

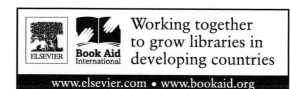

List of Contributors

Bernadette Boden-Albala, MPH, DrPH
Senior Associate Dean of Research and Program
    Development
College of Global Public Health
New York University
New York, NY, United States

Interim Chair
Department of Epidemiology
College of Global Public Health, New York University
New York, NY, United States

Professor
Department of Neurology
New York University Langone Medical Center
New York, NY, United States

Professor
Department of Epidemiology and Health Promotion
New York University College of Dentistry
New York, NY, United States

Li Khim Kwah, BAppSc (Phty), PhD
Senior lecturer
Discipline of Physiotherapy, Graduate School of Health
University of Technology Sydney
Sydney, NSW, Australia

Associate Professor
Health and Social Sciences Cluster
Singapore Institute of Technology
Singapore

Elizabeth E. Galletta, PhD
Clinical Research Specialist
NYU Langone Health
New York, NY, United States

Clinical Assistant Professor
Rehabilitation Medicine
New York University School of Medicine
New York, NY, United States

Adjunct Professor
Communication Sciences and Disorders
New York University Steinhardt School of Culture
Education, and Human Development
New York, NY, United States

Mira Goral, PhD
Professor
Speech Language Hearing Sciences
The Graduate Center and Lehman College, CUNY
Bronx, NY, United States

Adjunct Professor
MultiLing
University of Oslo
Oslo, Norway

Peggy S. Conner, PhD
Assistant Professor
Speech-Language-Hearing Sciences
Lehman College, City University of New York
Bronx, NY, United States

M. Gonzalez-Fernandez, MD, PhD
Associate Professor
Physical Medicine and Rehabilitation
Johns Hopkins University School of Medicine
Baltimore, MD, United States

Managing Director Outpatient Rehabilitation Services
Department of Physical Medicine and Rehabilitation
Johns Hopkins University School of Medicine
Baltimore, MD, United States

Vice-chair for Clinical Operations
Physical Medicine and Rehabilitation
Johns Hopkins University School of Medicine
Baltimore, MD, United States

A.M. Barrett, MD
Director
Stroke Rehabilitation Research
Kessler Foundation
West Orange, NJ, United States

Research Professor
Physical Medicine and Rehabilitation
Rutgers New Jersey Medical School
Newark, NJ, United States

Chief, Neurorehabilitation Program Innovation
Kessler Institute for Rehabilitation
West Orange, NJ, United States

Richard Wilson, MD, MS
Director
Division of Neurologic Rehabilitation and Stroke
   Rehabilitation
MetroHealth Rehabilitation Institute
MetroHealth Medical Center
Associate Professor
Case Western Reserve University
Cleveland, OH, United States

Andrew K. Treister, MD
Fellow, Neurocritical Care
Department of Neurology
Oregon Health and Science University
Portland, OR, United States

Preeti Raghavan, MD
Howard A. Rusk Associate Professor of Rehabilitation
   Research
Vice Chair for Research
Director, Division of Motor Recovery Research
Department of Rehabilitation Medicine
New York University School of Medicine
NYU Langone Health
New York, NY, United States

John J. Lee, MD
PM&R Residency Program Director
Cleveland Clinic
Cleveland, OH, United States

Gerard E. Francisco, MD
Professor and Chair
Department of Physical Medicine and
   Rehabilitation
University of Texas Health Science Center (UTHealth)
McGovern Medical School
Houston, TX, United States

NeuroRecovery Research Center
TIRR Memorial Hermann
Houston, TX, United States

Ricardo E. Jorge, MD
Professor of Psychiatry and Behavioral Sciences
Director
Houston Translational Research Center for TBI and
   Stress Disorders
Acting Director
Beth K. and Stuart C. Yudofsky Division of
   Neuropsychiatry
Michael E DeBakey VA Medical Center
Baylor College of Medicine
Houston, TX, United States

Medical Director of TBI-Related Research
Michael E. DeBakey VA Medical Center
Professor of Psychiatry
Baylor College of Medicine
Houston, TX, United States

John-Ross Rizzo, MD, MSCI
Assistant Professor
Rehabilitation Medicine
NYU Langone Health
New York, NY, United States

Assistant Professor
Neurology
NYU Langone Health
New York, NY, United States

Steven R. Flanagan, MD
Howard A. Rusk Professor and Chair of Rehabilitation
   Medicine
Rehabilitation Medicine
New York University Langone Health
New York, NY, United States

Michael J. Fu, PhD
Research Assistant Professor
Electrical Engineering and Computer Science
Case Western Reserve University
Cleveland, OH, United States

Bioscientific Staff
Physical Medicine & Rehabilitation
MetroHealth System
Cleveland, OH, United States

Jayme S. Knutson, PhD
Department of Physical Medicine & Rehabilitation
Case Western Reserve University
MetroHealth Rehabilitation Institute of Ohio
MetroHealth Medical Center
Cleveland Functional Electrical Stimulation Center
Cleveland, OH, United States

Lena Von Koch, Reg OT, PhD
Professor
Neurobiology, care sciences and society
Karolinska Institutet
Huddinge, Sweden

Gunilla Margareta Eriksson, Reg OT, PhD
Researcher
Department of Neurobiology, Care Sciences
    and Society
Karolinska Institute
Stockholm, Sweden

Researcher
Department of Neuroscience
Uppsala University
Uppsala, Sweden

Ulla Johansson, PhD
Researcher
Department of Occupational Therapy
Neurobiology, Care Sciences and Society
Stockholm, Sweden

Abiodun Akinwuntan, PhD, MPH, MBA
Dean and Professor
School of Health Professions
University of Kansas Medical Center
Kansas City, KS, United States

Joel Stein, MD
Simon Baruch Professor and Chair
Rehabilitation and Regenerative Medicine
Columbia University College of Physicians and
    Surgeons
New York, NY, United States

Professor and Chair
Rehabilitation Medicine
Weill Cornell Medical College
New York, NY, United States

Physiatrist-in-Chief
Rehabilitation Medicine
New York-Presbyterian Hospital
New York, NY, United States

Scott Barbuto, MD, PhD
Neurorehabilitation Research Fellow
Physical Medicine and Rehabilitation
New York Presbyterian Hospital
MetroHealth Rehabilitation Institute of Ohio
MetroHealth Medical Center
Cleveland Functional Electrical Stimulation Center
New York, NY, United States

David A. Cunningham, PhD
Department of Physical Medicine and Rehabilitation
Case Western Reserve University
Cleveland, OH, United States

Lainie K. Holman, MD
Staff Physician
Pediatric Physical Medicine and Rehabilitation
Cleveland Clinic Children's Hospital for Rehabilitation
Cleveland, OH, United States

Clinical Assistant Professor
Pediatrics
Cleveland Clinic Lerner College of Medicine of Case
    Western Reserve University
Cleveland, OH, United States

Matthew A. Plow, PhD
Frances Payne Bolton School of Nursing
Case Western Reserve University
Cleveland, OH, United States

Sheng Li, MD, PhD
Director, NeuroRecovery Research Center
TIRR Memorial Hermann Research Center

Professor
Department of Physical Medicine and Rehabilitation
University of Texas Health Science Center Houston
McGovern Medical School
Houston, TX, United States

Jonathan Oen Thomas, MD
Neurorehabilitation Fellow
Physical Medicine and Rehabilitation
Rutgers New Jersey Medical School
Newark, NJ, United States

Noa Appleton, MPH
Department of Epidemiology
College of Global Public Health
New York University
New York, NY, United States

Benjamin Schram, BS
Department of Epidemiology
College of Global Public Health
New York University
New York, NY, United States

N. Langton-Frost, MA, CCL-SLP, BCS-S
Department of Physical Medicine and Rehabilitation
Johns Hopkins University School of Medicine
Baltimore, MD, United States

M.N. Bahouth, MD
Department of Neurology
Department of Physical Medicine and Rehabilitation
Johns Hopkins University School of Medicine
Baltimore, MD, United States

A.N. Wright, BS
Department of Physical Medicine and Rehabilitation
Johns Hopkins University School of Medicine
Baltimore, MD, United States

E. Karagiorgos, MS, CCC-SLP
Department of Physical Medicine and Rehabilitation
Johns Hopkins University School of Medicine
Baltimore, MD, United States

John Chae, MD, MS
Professor and Chair
MetroHealth Rehabilitation Institute
MetroHealth Medical Center
Department of Physical Medicine and Rehabilitation
Department of Biomedical Engineering
Case Western Reserve University
Cleveland, OH, United States

Melissa Jones, MD
Faculty Psychiatrist
Michael E. DeBakey VA Medical Center
Assistant Professor of Psychiatry
Baylor College of Medicine
Houston, TX, United States

Neera Kapoor, OD, MS, FAAO, FCOVD-A
Clinical Associate Professor
Rehabilitation Medicine
NYU Langone Health
New York, NY, United States

Heidi Fusco, MD
Assistant Professor of Rehab Medicine
RUSK Rehabilitation
Ambulatory Care Center
New York, NY, United States

Hannes Devos, PhD
Assistant Professor
Department of Physical Therapy and Rehabilitation
    Science
University of Kansas Medical Center
Kansas City, KS, United States

Kelsey A. Potter-Baker, PhD
Advanced Platform Technology Center
Louis Stokes Cleveland Department of Veteran's Affairs
Department of Biomedical Engineering
Lerner Research Institute
Cleveland Clinic
Cleveland, OH, United States

Ela B. Plow, PhD, PT
Department of Biomedical Engineering
Lerner Research Institute
Center for Neurological Restoration
Department of Physical Medicine and Rehabilitation
Neurological Institute
Cleveland Clinic
Cleveland, OH, United States

Julia Chang, RN, BSN, SCRN, PhD
Assistant Professor
Frances Payne Bolton School of Nursing
Case Western Reserve University
Cleveland, OH, United States

Eric Y. Chang, MD
Restore Orthopedics & Spine Center
Division of Pain Management
Orange, CA, United States

Yin-Liang Lin, PhD
Department of Biomedical Engineering
Lerner Research Institute
Cleveland Clinic
Cleveland, OH, United States

Gert Kwakkel, PhD
Professor
Department of Rehabilitation Medicine
Amsterdam Movement Sciences
Amsterdam Neuroscience
VU University Medical Center
Amsterdam, The Netherlands

Department of Physical Therapy and Human
   Movement Sciences
Northwestern University
Chicago, IL, United States

Janne M. Veerbeek, PhD
Postdoctoral Research Fellow
Division of Vascular Neurology and Neuro-
   rehabilitation
Department of Neurology
University Hospital and University of Zurich
Zurich, Switzerland

Cereneo
Center for Neurology and Rehabilitation
Vitznau, Switzerland

Mahya Beheshti, MD
Post-Doc Research Fellow, Rehabilitation Medicine,
   RUSK Rehabilitation, New York, NY, United States

Improving the Lives of Stroke Survivors

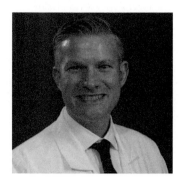

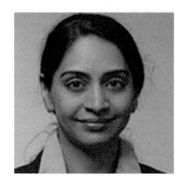

Stroke is a leading cause of serious disability, and the worldwide prevalence of stroke is expected to rise in the coming decades due to an aging population. The genesis of this book is an acknowledgment of the importance of stroke rehabilitation, as a field, in improving the lives of stroke survivors, and in contributing to population health.

The goal of this book is to provide concise and practical guidance on the latest methods and concepts behind stroke rehabilitation necessary for rehabilitation providers to best serve their patients. The intended audience is physiatrists, trainee physiatrists, and other members of the rehabilitation team. Each chapter is authored by topic experts from diverse backgrounds and disciplines. We hope that this collective expertise will provide rehabilitation providers with a clear under-standing of many topic areas to improve the lives of stroke survivors to the highest level of function and quality of life that can be achieved.

We are thankful to all those who contributed to this book. We are grateful to the chapter authors, without whose expertise this book would not have been possible. We appreciate the staff at Elsevier who patiently guided us through the process of editing this book and seeing it through to production.

We hope this text is helpful in the treatment of your patients.

Richard Wilson, MD, MS
*Director, Division of Neurologic Rehabilitation
and Stroke Rehabilitation
MetroHealth Rehabilitation Institute
MetroHealth Medical Center
Associate Professor
Case Western Reserve University
Cleveland, Ohio*

Preeti Raghavan, MD
*Howard A. Rusk Associate Professor
of Rehabilitation Research
Vice Chair for Research
Director, Division of Motor Recovery Research
Department of Rehabilitation Medicine
New York University School of Medicine
NYU Langone Health
New York, New York*

Contents

CHAPTER 1

Stroke Epidemiology and Prevention

BERNADETTE BODEN-ALBALA, MPH, DRPH • NOA APPLETON, MPH •
BENJAMIN SCHRAM, BS

INTRODUCTION

For many years stroke has been recognized as a leading cause of disability and mortality in the United States and other industrialized countries. Stroke is more disabling than fatal: the annual cost of direct and indirect stroke-related healthcare in the United States is estimated to be about 34 billion dollars measured in both healthcare dollars and loss of productivity.[1] Over the last few years stroke has emerged as a major global burden as well, especially with the increase of risk factors such as hypertension, diabetes mellitus, and obesity, and a growing burden in low and middle income countries (LMICs), which are experiencing both chronic and infectious disease.[2] Globally, the burden of stroke and other noncommunicable diseases is on the rise, and projections indicate they will continue to increase in prevalence, reaching epidemic proportions within the next decades.[2]

Awareness of the importance of stroke has led to a vast and accumulating literature on stroke risk factors, stroke etiology, and stroke outcomes. Stroke risk factors have been elucidated and clinical trials have indicated the benefits of treatment for persons with hypertension, atrial fibrillation, hypercholesterolemia, and asymptomatic carotid disease. In 1996, the first approved treatment for acute stroke, recombinant tissue plasminogen activator (rtPA), became available. Additionally, the pharmaceutical industry continues to actively pursue the development of "neuroprotective" agents to be used acutely for enhanced recovery from this disabling disease. Concurrently, over the last decade there has been important research looking at the contribution of devices, especially for clot retrieval, in the acute stroke period.

In the 21st century, technological advancements in the field of brain imaging, genotyping, and medical information systems have begun to facilitate epidemiological study designs that can elucidate stroke risk markers at the molecular level and risk factors at the subclinical level. Such advancements have provided researchers with more precision in stroke diagnosis and classification, including documentation and timing of events through the use of diffusion-weighted brain imaging techniques. Finally, as the relationship between genetic and environmental factors has become clearer, the role of precision medicine in prevention, treatment, and recovery has taken on a more central space.[3]

While improved technology has increased the precision and generalizability of data on stroke, epidemiologists who study stroke still struggle with critical issues. Despite recognition of and treatment modalities for modifiable stroke risk factors such as hypertension and cardiac disease, these risk factors remain highly prevalent. Additionally, overall stroke mortality rates are declining, but differentials continue to be reported between whites and other racial/ethnic groups including African-Americans, Hispanics, Alaska Natives, and Asian Pacific Islanders. In recent decades, the aging of the population and increasing prevalence of certain stroke risk factors have led to an increased absolute number of strokes per year (see Table 1.1), resulting in greater incidence, mortality, morbidity, and cost.[2,4]

CLINICAL DEFINITION OF STROKE

A stroke is clinically defined as a focal neurologic deficit caused by a local disturbance in cerebral circulation—predominantly either an obstruction of cerebral blood (ischemic stroke) or a rupture to a vessel wall supplying blood to either the brain or spinal cord (intracerebral hemorrhage or subarachnoid hemorrhage, respectively). These three distinct etiological groups—ischemic stroke (IS), intracerebral hemorrhage (ICH), and subarachnoid hemorrhage (SAH)—comprise about 87%, 10%, and 3%, respectively, of all strokes annually.[1]

From an epidemiological perspective, the establishment of standardized practical diagnostic criteria for defining stroke is critical. Agreement on a definition

Stroke Rehabilitation. https://doi.org/10.1016/B978-0-323-55381-0.00001-9

TABLE 1.1
Absolute Number of Women and Men With Stroke (in Millions) in the World by Stroke Type in 1990 and 2013 (95% Uncertainty Limits Are in Brackets)

		Women		Men	
		1990	**2013**	**1990**	**2013**
Ischemic stroke	Incident	2.14 (1.96—2.33)	3.28 (3.06—3.52)	2.17 (2.05—2.33)	3.62 (3.43—3.85)
	Prevalent	4.86 (4.56—5.19)	8.66 (8.32—9.00)	5.18 (4.93—5.46)	9.65 (9.27—10.05)
Hemorrhagic stroke	Incident	0.86 (0.79—0.92)	1.53 (1.42—1.63)	1.03 (0.96—1.09)	1.84 (1.72—1.94)
	Prevalent	1.78 (1.67—1.87)	3.36 (3.23—3.51)	2.11 (2.02—2.22)	4.00 (3.81—4.17)

Reprinted with permission from Feigin VL, Norrving B, Mensah GA. Global burden of stroke. *Circ Res.* 2017;120(3):439—448.

for stroke enables comparison of incidence and prevalence rates in studies throughout the world. A number of epidemiological issues arise in the enumeration of stroke cases. Diagnostic criteria for stroke and sensitivity of the diagnosis may differ from study to study. Indeed, early increases in stroke incidence may be attributed to the transition to universal use of CT imaging. Prior to the general use of CT imaging to confirm strokes, underdiagnosis or misclassification of strokes were more likely to occur. With better imaging and the ability to identify abnormalities associated with transient ischemic attack (TIA), we can move toward a more uniform definition of stroke overall.

Over the years, there have emerged a number of different definitions of stroke and TIA. In 2013 the American Heart Association (AHA)/American Stroke Association (ASA) published a consensus statement, *An Updated Definition of Stroke for the 21st Century*, which incorporates clinical and tissue criteria.[5] They defined central nervous system (CNS) infarction as "brain, spinal cord, or retinal cell death attributable to ischemia, based on neuropathological, neuroimaging, and/or clinical evidence of permanent injury."[5] Intracerebral hemorrhage and subarachnoid hemorrhage are also included in the broad definition of stroke. A TIA was originally defined as a neurological deficit lasting less than 24 hours. However, with the increased ability to image lesions with deficits lasting only a few hours, the AHA endorsed a revised, more operational definition of TIA as a "transient episode of neurologic dysfunction caused by focal brain, spinal cord, or retinal ischemia, without acute infarction."[6] After a TIA, risk of stroke is significant, particularly within the first year; 90-day risk estimates are between 9% and 17%.[7,8]

The universal application of computed tomography (CT) brain imaging to confirm the presence of a lesion has been critical for early recognition and diagnosis of stroke. Magnetic resonance imaging (MRI) is also used increasingly in addition to CT to confirm stroke diagnosis. Typically stroke is still confirmed by CT with follow-up MRI often providing more information about the underlying etiology of the disease.

BURDEN OF STROKE

The burden of stroke remains significant: approximately 795,000 people suffer and 130,000 die from either a first or recurrent stroke in the United States annually.[10] Worldwide, there are over 10 million new strokes and 6.5 million stroke deaths each year, making stroke the second leading cause of death.[2] Stroke mortality estimates are typically derived from national or local vital statistics data. Stroke data are obtained from sources that have used standardized classification systems such as the International Code of Diseases.

Mortality rates from stroke have been on the decline in the United States and worldwide. The age-adjusted mortality rate for stroke declined almost 30% between 2004 and 2014 in the United States,[1] although 1-year stroke mortality rates still exceed 20%.[11] In high-income countries, the mortality rate has declined by 37% for ischemic stroke and 38% for hemorrhagic stroke between 1990 and 2010. In LMICs, mortality rates declined by 14% for ischemic and 23% for hemorrhagic stroke in the same time period.[4] Although ischemic stroke accounts for the greatest public health impact because it occurs more frequently, hemorrhagic strokes are more fatal and thus also contribute significantly to the burden of stroke. The mortality rate for hemorrhagic stroke is estimated to be approximately 20% in high income countries and 62% in LMICs.[4]

Stroke mortality rates differ by country and geographic region (Fig. 1.1). According to 2013 data from the Global Burden of Disease Study, Russia and Kazakhstan had the highest reported ischemic stroke mortality rates and Western Europe, North and Central America, Turkmenistan, and Papua New Guinea had the lowest. For hemorrhagic stroke, the highest mortality rates were in Mongolia and Madagascar and the lowest were in North America, most of Western Europe, Australia, New Zealand, Russia, Iran, Saudi Arabia, Morocco, and Japan.[12] There are also significant geographic disparities in stroke mortality within the United States, with an area of the southeast known as the "stroke belt" experiencing death rates approximately 20% higher than the rest of the country.[13,14]

In addition to the decline in stroke mortality, there has also been a steady decline in US age-adjusted stroke incidence rates over the past several decades,[15–17] and globally among high income countries.[4] Recent data from the Greater Cincinnati/Northern Kentucky study showed declining incidence of all strokes driven by a decrease in ischemic stroke in men.[16] However despite these promising trends, there has been a rising incidence of stroke among younger populations, especially individuals 55 years and younger in the United States.[18,19] A 2012 study using data from the US Nationwide Inpatient Sample revealed that although hospitalization rates for acute ischemic stroke decreased overall by 18.4% between 2000 and 2010, they actually increased 43.8% for individuals of ages 25–44 years.[19] This trend is likely a result of the increasing prevalence of stroke risk factors in younger populations, including type 2 diabetes mellitus, hypercholesterolemia, obesity, and alcohol abuse.[19] Younger individuals who suffer from a stroke face the potential of longer-term disability or greater years of potential-life-lost. Implementing early education and early prevention measures are, therefore, crucial in reducing the burden of stroke.

Over the last few decades, a number of important studies have attempted to enumerate the incidence of stroke cases in the United States and other countries each year. Incidence estimates have been indirectly calculated using figures from smaller community samples to project national figures. In the United States, several early population-based studies from Framingham, Massachusetts,[9] Rochester, Minnesota,[20] and the Lehigh Valley, Pennsylvania/New Jersey,[21] have contributed significantly to our knowledge about stroke trends, subtypes, risk factors, and incidence rates in men and women. Extensive stroke surveillance systems were used to ascertain all incident stroke cases within a defined geographical area.

Early incidence figures came from the Framingham Study, a large epidemiological study initiated in 1950 that is following 5000 men and women who were initially free of cardiovascular disease. This study indicated differences in stroke incidence by gender, with greater incidence rates among men than among women.[9] Subsequent studies confirmed this finding, although recent evidence shows a narrowing of this gender gap in the United States.[2,16,22] However, despite some evidence of higher stroke incidence rates in men, women have greater lifetime risk of stroke because they have a longer life expectancy.[23]

Despite the important contributions of these primarily white cohorts, their findings may not be generalizable to multiethnic populations. Studies have reported differences in stroke incidence between racial/ethnic groups, especially stroke incidence rates among blacks. The community-based Northern Manhattan Stroke Study (NOMAS) reported a 2.4-fold higher rate of first stroke among African-Americans and a twofold higher incidence of stroke among Hispanics than that for whites.[24] Various other studies have found similar patterns of increased incidence in these groups.[25,26] In recent years, a number of multiethnic cohort studies in the United States have helped elucidate racial/ethnic disparities in stroke. These studies include the Greater Cincinnati/Northern Kentucky Stroke Study (GCNKSS), the Brain Attack Surveillance in Corpus Christi (BASIC) Project, the Atherosclerosis Risk in Communities (ARIC) study, and the REasons for Geographic and Racial Differences in Stroke (REGARDS) study.[27–30] The 2005–09 Alaska Native Stroke Registry (ANSR) also generated the first estimates of stroke incidence among Alaska Native adults, and found them to be lower or similar to other U.S. racial/ethnic minority groups.[31] Knowledge about incidence differences across racial/ethnic groups may allow for the development of more effective targeted stroke prevention programs.

While there have been major advances in the quality of studies aimed at enumerating stroke incidence and prevalence, a number of epidemiologic issues persist. Difficulty obtaining death certificates and inaccuracy of the diagnosis on death certificates continue to contribute to underreporting of stroke. Assessment of population data such as census data may not be accurate for underserved or minority populations such as blacks or Hispanics because undercounting is considerable. Studies have reported highly variable stroke rates for nonhospitalized cases. This variability in stroke

Age-standardized DALYs rates (per 100,000)

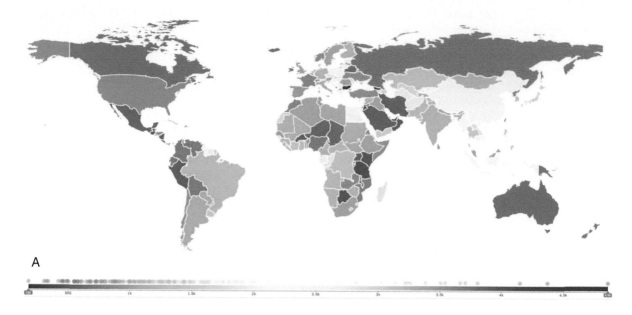

A

Age-standardized mortality rates (per 100,000)

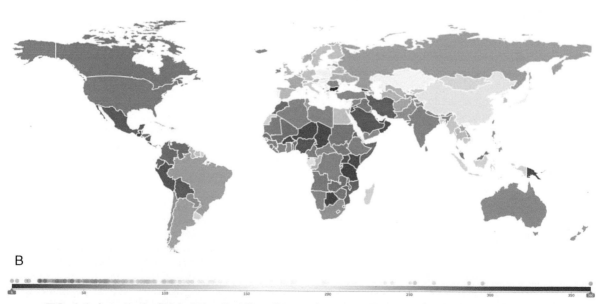

B

FIG. 1.1 Age-standardized stroke disability adjusted life years (DALYs) and mortality rates per 100,000 person-years in various regions of the world in 2013 (both sexes, all ages). (Reprinted with permission from Feigin VL, Norrving B, Mensah GA. Global burden of stroke. *Circ Res.* 2017;120(3):439–448.)

admissions has led to difficulties in obtaining accurate incidence rates using hospital-based cohorts or stroke registries because of underreporting of mild or nonhospitalized cases of stroke. While this problem has decreased, this still contributes somewhat to error in accuracy of reporting.

PREVENTION

In recent years, great strides have been made in understanding the pathophysiology of stroke and in developing treatments that reduce morbidity and mortality after stroke. The most effective way to reduce the burden of stroke, however, is through prevention. Stroke prevention strategies can occur at multiple stages: in the healthy, stroke-free population (primary prevention), among those who have developed recognizable risk factors and may have subclinical disease (late primary or early secondary prevention), and after the development of neurological symptoms of stroke or TIA (late secondary or tertiary prevention).

CLASSIFICATION AND DETERMINATION OF STROKE RISK FACTORS

An understanding of stroke risk factors is essential for effective stroke prevention. Some factors are not modifiable and may be better characterized as risk markers, while others are amenable to behavioral, medical, or surgical modification. Risk markers may include age, gender, race/ethnicity, or heredity. The identification of genetic determinants for stroke would allow early identification of individuals with increased risk of stroke through genetic screening. Social factors have a huge impact on stroke prevention, treatment, and recovery. These include more traditional factors such as education, income/wealth, and access to care, but are not limited to these. Modifiable risk factors, on the other hand, may include environmental or even genetic exposures that, when modified, lead to reductions in the risk of stroke. Factors that may have both environmental and genetic links include hypertension and hyperlipidemia. Various biological and lifestyle risk factors that have been associated with increasing the risk of stroke include hypertension, diabetes, hyperlipidemias, physical inactivity, smoking, diet, sleep and alcohol use, as well as other newer factors. Strategies for effective modification of these factors include risk factor identification, goal attainment for risk control, compliance strategies, and continued follow-up. While each of these lifestyle factors is unique and important, they frequently occur in combination in the same individual and together represent a heavy burden of increased stroke risk.

Stroke risk factors have been identified through both case-control and cohort studies. In case-control studies, selection bias may lead to a collection of cases that do not adequately reflect all individuals with stroke and controls that are not representative of the general population. One solution is to use population-based study designs in which all the cases of stroke within a specific area are included and controls are randomly derived from the same community. In cohort studies, the attributable risk or etiologic fraction—a measure of the proportion of cases explained or attributed to the exposure—can be readily calculated. Prospective cohorts usually require systematic, lengthy follow-up after a baseline assessment. The clear advantage to cohort studies is the measurement of the exposure prestroke and the ability to determine the prevalence of the exposure in the general population; however, these studies are time-consuming and expensive and require large numbers of subjects.

Experimental epidemiological studies such as randomized controlled clinical trials are the mainstay of demonstrating that modification of a risk factor can lead to a reduction in stroke risk. Subjects who exhibit the risk factor of interest are randomly assigned to an intervention or not and then followed for the occurrence of a specific outcome such as stroke. Randomization is used to help ensure that the groups are balanced for known and unknown confounders. While these studies can also be expensive and require large numbers of patients, they are essential to the development of evidence-based guidelines for stroke prevention.

Both the consensus statement "Guidelines for the Prevention of First Stroke" supported by the National Stroke Association (NSA) and the American Heart Association (AHA) scientific statement "Guidelines for the Primary Prevention of Stroke" provide evidence-based recommendations for decreasing stroke risk that act as a template for risk factor reduction (Table 1.2).[32] Lifestyle modifications to reduce stroke risk may present a great challenge in that social, behavioral, and cultural factors increase the complexity of the risk reduction strategy. It must remain the priority of health professionals to define and promote a lifestyle conducive to reducing blood pressure, controlling blood glucose, elevating high-density lipoprotein-cholesterol, increasing physical activity, evaluating alcohol use, and promoting the cessation of cigarette smoking.

TABLE 1.2
Modifiable Risk Factors, Prevalence, Relative Risk, and Management Recommendations for Stroke

Risk Factor	Estimated Prevalence (%)	Estimated Relative Risk	Management Recommendations
Hypertension[32–34]	29	2.0–5.0	Regular BP screening, weight control, limit salt intake, antihypertensive drug treatment, BP self-monitoring
Diabetes[32,34,35]	9.4	1.5–3.0	Tight glucose control through diet, oral hypoglycemics, and insulin. Strict regulation of BP if hypertensive. Statin treatment, especially in those with additional risk factors
Dyslipidemia[32,34]			Lifestyle modification, treatment with statins in patients estimated to have a high 10-year risk for cardiovascular events
Elevated LDL (≥130 mg/dL)[36,37]	30.3	1.2–1.4	
Low HDL[38] (<40 mg/dL)[36]	18.7	1.0–2.2	
Smoking[32,34,39]	15.8	1.5–2.5	Smoking cessation
Physical Inactivity[1,32,34]	21.6	2.0–3.5	Moderate to vigorous intensity aerobic physical activity at least 40 min/day, 3–4 days/week
Excess Alcohol (binge drinking in past 30 days)[32,40,41]	16.9	1.0–2.0	Up to two drinks per day for men and one drink per day for nonpregnant women
Obesity[42,43]	39.6	1.3–2.0	Control of weight through diet and exercise
Sleep Disorders (Obstructive Sleep Apnea)[44,45]	4	1.5–3.2	Screening for sleep apnea and possible treatment using continuous positive airway pressure (CPAP)

BP, blood pressure; *CHD*, coronary heart disease; *HDL*, High-density lipoprotein; *LDL*, low-density lipoprotein.

MODIFIABLE RISK FACTORS

Major reduction in stroke morbidity and mortality are more likely to arise from identification and control of modifiable factors in the stroke-prone individuals. According to data from the Global Burden of Disease Study and the INTERSTROKE study, modifiable risk factors account for up to 90% of the global burden of stroke.[46,47] Modifiable stroke risk factors include hypertension, cardiac diseases (primarily atrial fibrillation), diabetes, dyslipidemia, cigarette use, alcohol abuse, physical inactivity, diet, asymptomatic carotid stenosis, and previous TIAs.

Hypertension. Hypertension is the most powerful and potentially modifiable stroke risk factor, as roughly 75% of stroke victims are hypertensive. Stroke risk rises proportionately with increasing blood pressure.[48] Hypertension is also highly prevalent in the United States, affecting roughly 29% of adults, and is of even greater significance in African-Americans.[33] In

the Northern Manhattan Stroke Study (NOMAS) hypertension was a strong, independent stroke risk factor for whites (OR 1.8), blacks (OR 2.0), and Hispanics (OR 2.1) living in the same community.[34] The REGARDS study, similarly, found that elevated blood pressure had a threefold greater impact on stroke risk in African-Americans compared to whites.[49] Components of blood pressure, such as isolated systolic hypertension, may also contribute to an increased risk of stroke. Isolated systolic hypertension is increasingly prevalent with age and increases the risk of stroke significantly, even after controlling for age and diastolic blood pressure (DBP).[50–52] In the British Regional Heart Study, men with systolic blood pressures (SBPs) between 160 and 180 mmHg were at about four times the risk of stroke compared with men with SBPs below 160 mmHg. Individuals with SBPs above 180 mmHg had a sixfold greater stroke risk.[53] Evidence from the recently completed Systolic Blood Pressure Intervention Trial

(SPRINT) suggests that an SBP target of <120 mmHg leads to significantly greater reductions in cardiovascular events and death compared to a target of <140 mmHg.[54]

Reduction of both systolic and diastolic pressure in hypertensive individuals substantially decreases stroke risk. Pooled results of clinical trials have shown that a 10 mmHg reduction in SBP or 5 mmHg reduction in DBP translates to approximately 40% average reduction in stroke risk, with similar magnitudes of risk reduction regardless of cardiovascular disease history or blood pressure prior to treatment.[55]

Guidelines for treatment of hypertension were recently updated by the Joint National Committee on Prevention, Detection, Evaluation, and Treatment of High Blood Pressure in 2017.[56] Definitions of hypertension have been broadened to include individuals who were once considered borderline hypertensive. Normotensive is now defined as <120/80 mmHg, elevated BP is 120−129/<80, and hypertension is defined as 130/80 and above.[56]

Numerous efficacious treatments exist which reduce BP, and clinical trials have demonstrated that hypertension can be lowered leading to a dramatic reduction in stroke risk. Since the population attributable risk (proportion of strokes explained by hypertension) has been estimated to be as high as 48%, even a slight improvement in the control of hypertension could translate into a substantial reduction in stroke frequency.[46] Despite these facts, the control of blood pressure among different populations is poor; it is estimated that only about 50% of hypertensive patients are controlled.[57] Data suggest that within the United States, hypertension awareness and BP control has improved but remains suboptimal.[58] Much effort is now being focused on the reduction of elevated BP for prevention of stroke. Research has moved beyond treatment modalities to focus on barriers to risk reduction including educational disparities, adherence, access to care, and lack of support services. There are a number of interventions that have been tested with the primary aim of reducing hypertension to decrease the overall burden of stroke.

Cardiac Diseases. Various cardiac conditions have been clearly associated with an increase in the risk of ischemic stroke. Since certain stroke risk factors, such as hypertension may also be determinants of cardiac disease, some cardiac conditions may be viewed as intervening events in the causal chain for stroke. Cardiac factors that independently increase the risk of stroke include atrial fibrillation (AF), valvular heart disease, myocardial infarction, coronary artery disease,

congestive heart failure, and electrocardiographic evidence of left ventricular hypertrophy. Improved cardiac imaging has led to the increased detection of potential stroke risk factors such as mitral annular calcification, patent foramen ovale, aortic arch atherosclerotic disease, atrial septal aneurysms, spontaneous echo contrast (a smoke-like appearance in the left cardiac chambers visualized on transesophageal echocardiography), and valvular strands.

Nonvalvular AF is a potent predictor of stroke, increasing the relative risk of stroke nearly fivefold.[59] It is also associated with greater stroke mortality and recurrence.[60] AF affects more than 5 million Americans, and its prevalence is projected to increase significantly in the coming decades.[61] Early clinical trials as well as more recent metaanalyses have demonstrated evidence of the efficacy of oral anticoagulation for stroke prevention among individuals with nonvalvular AF, although it has also been associated with elevated risk of bleeding. The recommendation from the Ninth American College of Chest Physicians Evidence-Based Clinical Practice Guidelines is that oral anticoagulation be used for patients with AF at high risk of stroke and that patients at lower risk levels receive more individualized consideration.[62]

Stroke risk nearly doubles in those with antecedent coronary artery disease,[59] triples with left ventricular hypertrophy,[63,64] and triples in subjects with cardiac failure.[65] Acute myocardial infarction (AMI) has been associated with stroke, although the risk of stroke following AMI has improved with the increased use of reperfusion treatment with PCI, fibrinolysis, and early revascularization.[66,67] Unrecognized, or silent, myocardial infarction, uncomplicated angina, and non-Q wave infarction were initially identified as stroke risk factors in the Framingham Study cohort,[68] and this was later supported by the Rotterdam Study.[69]

Valvular diseases that can increase the risk of stroke include rheumatic mitral valve disease, endocarditis, and prosthetic heart valves.[32] Atrial septal aneurysm is another important cardiac condition associated with increased stroke risk.[70,71] A number of case-control studies have found significant associations between atrial septal aneurysm and ischemic stroke as well as evidence of a strong synergistic effect for atrial septal aneurysm and PFO, particularly for younger stroke patients.[72] Paradoxical embolism through a PFO has long been recognized as a potential cause of stroke.[73] In 2016 and 2018, the FDA approved the first two PFO closure devices, and their use for reducing risk of recurrent ischemic stroke in certain subgroups of patients is supported by a number of randomized trials.[74–76]

Diabetes Mellitus and Insulin Resistance. Diabetes is a determinant of atherosclerosis and microangiopathy of the coronary, peripheral, and cerebral arteries. Death from stroke is greatly increased among subjects with diabetes.[77] Cohort studies have demonstrated an independent effect of diabetes on stroke risk after controlling for other risk factors, with pooled risk ratios of 2.28 for women and 1.83 for men.[78] The increased risk of stroke among diabetics is more pronounced among women and people under age 65.[78,79] Diabetes is also independently associated with increased risk of recurrent stroke.[80] Insulin resistance has emerged as an important stroke risk factor as well.[81,82]

In the United States, insulin-dependent or type 1 diabetes accounts for about 5%–10% of all diabetic patients.[83] Worldwide, type 2 diabetes is increasing, from an estimated 171 million in 2000 to a predicted 366 million by the year 2030.[84] In a multiethnic community in Northern Manhattan, the prevalence of diabetes is 22% and 20% among elderly African-Americans and Hispanics, respectively, with corresponding attributable risks of stroke of 13% and 20%.[34]

Intensive treatment for both type 1 and type 2 diabetes, aimed at maintaining near-normal levels of blood glucose, can substantially reduce the risk of microvascular complications such as retinopathy, nephropathy, and neuropathy, but has not been conclusively shown to reduce macrovascular complications including stroke. A metaanalysis of four large randomized controlled trials, which included over 27,000 patients followed up for an average of 5.4 years, concluded that intensive glucose control did not lead to decreased incidence of stroke or all-cause mortality.[85] However, much evidence suggests that the aggressive control of hypertension and lipids in patients with diabetes is likely to reduce the risk of stroke.

Dyslipidemias. Abnormalities of serum lipids (triglyceride, cholesterol, low-density lipoprotein [LDL], high-density lipoprotein [HDL]) are clear risk factors for atherosclerotic disease, particularly coronary disease. A number of studies in recent decades have helped clarify the varying relationship between each serum lipid type and stroke risk. Studies utilizing ultrasound technology have established that total cholesterol or LDL cholesterol is directly associated and HDL is inversely associated with extracranial carotid atherosclerosis and intima-media plaque thickness.[86–89] Case control studies have found the concentration of HDL to be lower in stroke cases after controlling for other risk factors.[34,90,91]

Elevated total cholesterol and LDL cholesterol are directly associated with an increased risk of ischemic stroke in most prospective studies. The Asia Pacific Cohort Studies Collaboration conducted a large metaanalysis including 352,033 individuals from Asia and New Zealand and found a 25% increase in ischemic stroke rate for every total cholesterol increase of 1 mmol/L.[92] Total cholesterol levels were also associated with greater risk of ischemic stroke in the Women's Health Study and in the Alpha-Tocopherol Beta Carotene Cancer Prevention Study, a large cohort study of male smokers.[93,94] In contrast, the Eurostroke Project which included over 22,000 subjects did not find a significant relationship between total cholesterol and stroke risk.[63] Serum LDL cholesterol was associated with increased risk of ischemic stroke at 6-year follow-up in the Multiple Risk Factor Intervention Trial (MR FIT), which included over 350,00 men (HR, 1.74; 95% CI, 1.14–2.66; P (trend across quintiles) = 0.003).[95] Lp(a) is an LDL-like particle that has been investigated for its relationship to cardiovascular risk. In a recent metaanalysis, a 3.5-fold higher usual Lp(a) level was associated with an adjusted RR of 1.11 for ischemic stroke.[96]

In contrast to total and LDL cholesterol, HDL cholesterol appears to be associated with a decreased risk of ischemic stroke, although evidence is mixed. The Copenhagen City Heart Study of close to 20,000 adults found a 47% reduction in the risk of nonhemorrhagic stroke for every 1 mmol/L increase in HDL.[97] NOMAS also found an inverse relationship between ischemic stroke and HDL level ≤35 mg/dL (0.91 mmol/L; OR, 0.53; 95% CI, 0.39–0.72).[98] However, ARIC, a large population-based cohort study of middle aged men and women with a mean follow-up of 10 years found no significant relationship between HDL cholesterol and ischemic stroke.[99]

For hemorrhagic stroke, evidence suggests that higher levels of total and LDL cholesterol are associated with decreased risk. MR FIT found a threefold increase in the risk of fatal ICH in patients with total serum cholesterol <4.13 mmol/L when compared with those with values ≥ 4.13 mmol/L.[95] Similarly, the Asia Pacific Cohort Studies Collaboration found that for every 1 mmol/L increase in total cholesterol, there was a 20% reduction in the risk of hemorrhagic stroke. A pooled cohort analysis of the ARIC study and the Cardiovascular Health Study found that LDL cholesterol was inversely associated with hemorrhagic stroke risk (HR for topmost quartile vs. lowest 3 quartiles 0.52; 95% CI, 0.31–0.88).[100] However, a very large metaanalysis from the Emerging Risk Factors Collaboration summarizing 68 prospective studies found no significant association between HDL and ischemic or hemorrhagic stroke.[101]

Clinical trials analyzing the efficacy of lipid-lowering strategies with statins have demonstrated impressive reductions in stroke risk in various high-risk populations with cardiac disease. In these studies, stroke was either a secondary end point or a nonspecified end point determined on the basis of posthoc analyses.[91,102] Metaanalyses of some of these trials have found significant reductions in stroke risk, with each 1 mmol/L decrease in LDL cholesterol translating to a reduction in relative risk for stroke of approximately 21%.[103] Reductions were significant for both primary and secondary prevention.

There is mounting support for the role of lipoproteins as precursors of carotid atherosclerosis and ischemic stroke and for the benefits of cholesterol lowering in stroke reduction. According to current guidelines, statin treatment is recommended for the primary prevention of ischemic stroke in patients estimated to have an elevated 10-year cardiovascular event risk.[104] For secondary prevention, guidelines recommend statin therapy with intensive lipid-lowering effects for patients with ischemic stroke or TIA presumed to be of atherosclerotic origin and an LDL-C level ≥100 mg/dL with or without evidence for other clinical ASCVD and for patients with ischemic stroke or TIA presumed to be of atherosclerotic origin, an LDL-C level <100 mg/dL, and no evidence for other clinical ASCVD.[105]

Cigarette Smoking. Despite the clear evidence that cigarette smoking is an independent determinant of stroke and other diseases, it remains a major modifiable public health threat in every nation. Data from numerous prospective studies suggest that smoking approximately doubles one's risk of stroke, and that a dose-dependent response relationship exists between stroke risk and number of cigarettes smoked per day.[32,106] The stroke risk attributed to smoking is greatest for SAH.[107]

Cigarette smoking is an independent determinant of carotid artery plaque thickness and the strongest predictor of severe extracranial carotid artery atherosclerosis.[108–110] Other biological mechanisms by which cigarettes may predispose to stroke include increased coagulability, blood viscosity, and fibrinogen levels; enhanced platelet aggregation; and elevated blood pressure. Secondhand smoke or passive smoking also contributes to increased stroke risk.[111,112]

There is ample evidence from observational epidemiologic studies that smoking cessation leads to a reduction in stroke risk. The Nurses' Health Study and the Framingham Study both showed that the risk of ischemic stroke is reduced to that of nonsmokers after 2 and 5 years, respectively.[113,114] It has been estimated that smoking accounts for about 20% of the stroke burden globally.[47] The ASA recommends the cessation of smoking as a stroke prevention measure, and suggests counseling combined with drug therapy such as nicotine replacement, bupropion, and varenicline.[32] Public health education programs, economic measures, and individual counseling should be continued and expanded to discourage initial smoking behavior and encourage smoking cessation.

Alcohol Use. The effect of alcohol as a stroke risk factor is controversial and probably dependent on dose. For hemorrhagic stroke, prospective cohort studies have shown that alcohol consumption has a direct dose-dependent effect.[46,115,116] Early case control studies failed to identify a significant association between alcohol and ischemic stroke.[117–119] In northern Manhattan, however, a J-shaped relationship between alcohol use and stroke was found— an elevated stroke risk for heavy alcohol consumption and a protective effect in light to moderate drinkers (2 or fewer drinks per day) when compared with nondrinkers.[40] This J-shaped relationship has also been identified in a cohort and twin study,[120] case cohort,[121] and additional studies.[46,122–124] The combination of the J-shaped relationship for ischemic stroke and graded increased risk for hemorrhagic stroke makes the relationship between alcohol use and stroke complex.

Prospective cohort studies, conducted in predominantly white populations, addressing the relationship of stroke to alcohol intake have found evidence of a protective effect of mild alcohol intake.[120,121,125–127] The Nurses' Health Study found a protective effect of mild alcohol consumption, up to 1.2 drinks per day in women, for ischemic stroke.[125] Several studies looking specifically at ischemic stroke in Japanese subjects failed to show any protective effect of alcohol, suggesting that alcohol's effect as a stroke risk factor may vary by race/ethnicity. The INTERSTROKE 2 study also found significant regional variations in the association between alcohol consumption and stroke.[128] This may be due to regional differences in the patterns and types of alcohol consumption. Spirit or liquor drinkers appear to have increased risk compared to beer or wine drinkers.[129]

The various mechanisms through which alcohol may increase the risk of stroke include hypertension, hypercoagulable states, cardiac arrhythmias, and cerebral blood flow reductions. There is also evidence that light to moderate drinking can increase HDL cholesterol, reduce the risk of coronary artery disease, and increase endogenous tissue plasminogen activator. The combination of deleterious and beneficial effects of alcohol is consistent with the observation of a dose-dependent relationship between alcohol and stroke. Elimination of heavy drinking can reduce incidence of stroke. Since some ingestion of alcohol, perhaps up to 2 drinks per day, may actually help reduce the risk of stroke, drinking in moderation should not be discouraged for most of the public.

Physical Activity. The cardiovascular benefits of physical activity have been broadcast by numerous organizations, including the Centers for Disease Control and Prevention, the National Institutes of Health, and the American Heart Association, based on accumulating data about the effects of physical activity in reducing the risk of heart disease and premature death. Previous studies have shown beneficial effects for physical activity, with varying effects across gender, age, and race/ethnic groups.[34,130–133] The Framingham Study demonstrated the benefits of combined leisure and work physical activity for men, but not for women.[134] Several recent studies, however, have demonstrated a protective effect of moderate physical activity on stroke risk in women as well.[130,131,135,136] In a prospective study of young Swedish men, increased physical activity was related to a reduced stroke incidence and reduced stroke fatality after adjusting for muscle strength.[137] In the ARIC study, increasing physical activity was associated with reduced incidence of stroke among African-Americans,[138] and in REGARDS physical inactivity was associated with a 20% elevated risk of incident stroke.[139] The Nurses' Health Study showed an inverse association between level of physical activity and the incidence of any stroke in women.[140] Finally, in the Northern Manhattan Stroke Study, the benefits of leisure time physical activity were noted for all age, gender, and racial/ethnic subgroups.[40,141]

The optimal amount of exercise needed to prevent stroke is unclear, particularly for the elderly. Vigorous exercise may be no more protective than walking. In the Framingham Study, the strongest protection was detected in medium-tertile physical activity subgroup, with no benefit gained from additional activity.[134] The protective effect of physical activity may be partially mediated through its role in controlling various risk factors such as hypertension, diabetes, and obesity. Other than control of risk factors, biological mechanisms such as increased HDL cholesterol, reduced homocysteine level, reductions in plasma fibrinogen and platelet activity, and elevations in plasma tissue plasminogen

activator activity may also be responsible for the effect of physical activity.[142–146]

Physical activity is a modifiable behavior that requires greater emphasis in stroke prevention campaigns. According to NHANES data from 2011 to 2012, 56% of adults do not achieve the recommended amount of physical activity. Moreover, inactivity is most prevalent in females, older adults, Hispanics, and non-Hispanic blacks.[1] The 2013 AHA/ACC guideline on lifestyle to reduce cardiovascular risk encourages moderate to vigorous aerobic physical activity for at least 40 minutes at a time to be done at least 3–4 days per week in order to reduce BP and improve lipid profile.[147] Increasing physical activity could translate into cost-effective means of decreasing the public health burden of stroke and other cardiovascular diseases among rapidly aging populations.

Dietary Factors and Obesity. While data have suggested that diet may play an important role in stroke risk, few studies have been able to clarify this relationship because of the complex issues associated with dietary intake and nutritional status. Large ecological studies have suggested that excess fat intake associated with migration may lead to increased risk of both coronary heart disease and stroke. High daily dietary intake of fat is associated with obesity and may act independently or may affect risk factors such as hypertension, diabetes, hyperlipidemia, and cardiac disease. A conflicting report from the Framingham Study demonstrated an inverse association between dietary fat and ischemic stroke.[148] Some of the strongest dietary evidence available for stroke is related to sodium and potassium. In prospective studies, lower sodium intake and higher potassium intake have both been associated with reduced risk of stroke, likely at least partially mediated by their effects on hypertension.[149,150]

The effect of broad dietary patterns on stroke risk has been studied as well. The Prevención con Dieta Mediterránea (PREDIMED) study in Spain randomized 7447 adults aged 55–80 to a control group or a Mediterranean diet supplemented with either extra-virgin olive oil or nuts and followed them for a median of 4.8 years. Their results showed that both versions of the Mediterranean diet were significantly associated with a substantially decreased risk of stroke.[151] A recent metaanalysis also found evidence that increased consumption of olive oil, a primary component of the Mediterranean diet, is associated with reduced stroke risk.[152] Another review article focusing on nut consumption found a relationship between nut consumption and stroke mortality.[153] Taken together, these findings provide support for the benefits of a Mediterranean style diet in vascular risk reduction. Another diet that has been associated with lower risks of stroke and cardiovascular disease is known as the DASH diet (Dietary Approaches to Stop Hypertension). The DASH-like eating plan prescribes set daily/weekly intakes of fruits and vegetables, fish, and fiber-rich whole grains and restricts consumption of sodium and sugar sweetened beverages.[154]

Dietary intake of fruits and vegetables may reduce the risk of stroke and contribute to stroke protection by antioxidant mechanisms or by elevating potassium levels.[155–157] Indeed, a number of large prospective studies have found that stroke risk decreases with increasing levels of fruit and vegetable consumption in a dose-response pattern.[158,159] Other dietary factors that have been linked to a reduced risk of stroke include intake of dairy, folate, and fish oils.[160–162] The ASA dietary recommendations for primary prevention of stroke include reduced intake of sodium, increased intake of fruits, vegetables and potassium, and DASH or Mediterranean-style diets.[32]

Obesity is increasing—tripling in children and doubling in adults in the US since 1980.[32] The relationship between obesity and stroke is difficult to disentangle from diabetes, blood pressure, and dietary intake. However, studies have found an independent association between obesity and stroke risk,[43,163] and cardiovascular disease outcomes appear to improve following weight reduction through bariatric surgery[164] or lifestyle changes.[165,166]

Sleep Disorders. Sleep disorders are a group of conditions that affect sleep patterns. Although common, with a growing body of evidence linking sleep disorders (primarily obstructive sleep apnea) to stroke, they remain the most underestimated modifiable risk factor for stroke and their pathophysiology is not fully understood.[167] An estimated 50–70 million US adults have sleep disorders[168] and roughly 4% of Americans have sleep apnea, with men affected more than women.[44]

In the Northern Manhattan Study (NOMAS), daytime sleepiness was associated with an increased risk of ischemic stroke (HR, 2.74, 95% CI, 1.38–5.43), all stroke (3.00 [1.57–5.73]), and all cardiovascular events (2.48 [1.57–3.91]).[169] A number of studies have identified obstructive sleep apnea as an independent risk factor for stroke. The diagnosis and the assessment of the severity of sleep apnea are determined by the apnea-hypopnea index (AHI), measured as the observed number of cessations or reduction of airflow per hour during sleep. Clinically, AHI $\geq$5 is indicative

of sleep apnea.[170] In the Wisconsin Sleep Cohort Study, when compared to those with AHI <5, the adjusted odds of having a stroke was about 4 times higher among participants with AHI >20 (OR, 4.33; 95% CI, 1.32–14.24).[171] In the multicenter Sleep Heart Health Study, more than 5000 participants aged >40 years without a history of stroke and untreated for obstructive sleep apnea were followed up for about 9 years. After controlling for other comorbidities and risk factors, increasing obstructed sleep apnea score was significantly associated with risk of ischemic stroke in men (P-value for linear trend: $P = .016$).[172]

There are several direct and indirect mechanisms that may explain this association, such as recurrent cerebral hypoxia from repetitive blockage of the airway, sympathetic overactivity during sleep, nocturnal hypertension, and inflammation.[173] While sleep disorders may be independent risk factors for stroke, they can also be associated with other vascular pathologies associated with stroke (e.g., hypertension, obesity, and diabetes). In the Sleep Heart Health Study, hypertension significantly increased with increasing measures of obstructive sleep apnea, although some of this association was related to increased body mass index.[174]

The relationship between sleep disorders and stroke could also be bidirectional. Although stroke is a possible outcome of sleep disorders, stroke can be a cause of sleep disorder or exacerbate an existing sleep disorder.[173] After a stroke, sleep apnea is extremely common, affecting more than half of stroke survivors.[175] It is important to evaluate a patient for sleep disorder after a stroke episode because the overall recovery and outcome of a patient with stroke can be affected by a new or preexisting sleep disorder.[176]

Air and Noise Pollution

Air pollution has emerged as an important risk factor for stroke in recent years. According to the Global Burden of Disease Study 2013, air pollution accounts for close to a third of stroke-related Disability Adjusted Life Years (DALYs), making it one of the leading modifiable contributors to the global burden of stroke.[47] The burden of air pollution was also significantly higher in low and middle income countries (33.7%) compared to high income countries (10.2%).[47] Air pollution may impact stroke risk by damaging vascular endothelium or by increasing blood pressure or risk of thrombosis.[177] Different types of air pollution may also have varying effects on vascular risk, with evidence suggesting that fossil fuel emissions may be most dangerous.[178] Strategies aimed at improving air quality could substantially modify the global burden of stroke.

In addition to air pollution, studies have investigated whether noise pollution may similarly impact vascular risk. Noise, particularly at night, can have physiologic consequences, for example, by disrupting sleep or by stimulating the release of stress hormones which can impact heart rate and blood pressure.[179] A large population-based cohort study in Denmark found a strong association between road traffic noise and stroke among people over 64.5 years (IRR: 1.27; 95% CI: 1.13−1.43) after adjusting for air pollution and other potential confounders.[180] Another analysis of this same cohort also found evidence of combined effects of air and noise pollution on ischemic stroke. However, occupational noise exposure was not related to stroke risk in a large Danish cohort study of industrial and financial workers.[181] Current studies are seeking to determine the specific types and levels of noise that lead to adverse cardiovascular effects as well as which other exposures may enhance or diminish these effects.[179,182]

Social Determinants: Research over the past few decades has yielded a number of important insights regarding the impact of social support, education, and socioeconomic status (SES) on stroke. In NOMAS prestroke social isolation was significantly associated with recurrent ischemic stroke and vascular outcomes (OR: 1.4, 95% CI: 1.1−1.8).[183] Similarly, in ARIC, small social networks were predictive of incident stroke, after adjusting for key socio-demographic and clinical factors.[184] Social isolation may contribute to worse poststroke outcomes by increasing the likelihood of poor medical adherence, depression, and stress. Various stroke risk factors are also associated with social isolation and lack of social support. In NOMAS social isolation was related to elevated blood pressure 1 year post stroke (OR 1.9, $P < .06$)[185] and was also significantly associated with physical inactivity.[186] In response to these findings, stroke interventions have begun to actively incorporate social support and social network involvement into their design.[187]

Low education level and low SES are also noted risk factors for stroke. A metaanalysis based on 79 studies reported that having less than 11 years of education was associated with about a one-third increased relative risk of stroke.[188] SES, similarly, has a major impact on stroke risk and stroke mortality with up to a 30% higher stroke incidence in lower socioeconomic groups, even after adjusting for classic vascular risk factors.[189,190] To address these stark disparities, prevention strategies must specifically target vulnerable groups and tailor interventions to their unique needs.

INTERVENTIONS AND EDUCATIONAL APPROACHES

Focus on clinical treatment alone will not reduce the burden of stroke. There needs to be a shift toward acknowledging the importance of behavioral change science and population level interventions. The science of behavioral change is a complex endeavor, and addressing the changes throughout the life course needed to reduce the burden of stroke remains a significant challenge. Critical is identifying and testing mechanisms for changing vascular risk behaviors; supporting the maintenance of healthy behaviors; and choosing the appropriate level for behavioral change (i.e., individual change vs. population level or structural change). Behavioral theory used in the design of interventions allows us to make predictions about why people behave the way they do. An accompanying theoretical platform, such as the Transtheoretical Model, Social Cognitive Theory, or the Health Belief Model provides the framework for the type of strategy or process needed to guide individual or system level interventions.

Literature exists to suggest individual level behavioral change is possible and that different modalities for change (i.e., in-person, web-based remote delivery) are successful. Even the most intractable behaviors, such as weight loss, have been successfully addressed with individual interventions.[194] For cerebrovascular disease, further consideration is needed about specific types of behaviors and what types of strategies optimally achieve change. Key areas of behavior modification include stroke preparedness, prevention (primary and secondary), and recovery.

With the emergence of tissue-type tPA in 1996, there has been an emphasis on reducing stroke morbidity and mortality through increased action during acute stroke.[195] Being prepared to take action requires individuals to be able to recall and recognize stroke warning signs, call 911, facilitate a dialogue about stroke, and navigate the emergency department so appropriate stroke codes are activated.

Several interventions have actively addressed preparedness with mixed success in different populations. One study reported that widespread acute stroke education in the US "Stroke Belt" was associated with a 10% decrease in the proportion of stroke patients presenting within 3 h of symptom onset, prompting a revision of public stroke-related educational programs.[196] Some educational interventions have successfully targeted improving children's intent to call 911 for stroke.[197−199] The Kids Identifying and Defeating Stroke (KIDS) was a pilot, randomized controlled trial to encourage calling 911 for witnessed stroke among middle-school children and their parents in Corpus Christi, Texas.[198] While the children's knowledge improved significantly after the educational intervention, the authors were not able to determine dissemination to parents due to poor response rates. Another school-based stroke literacy program, the Hip Hop Stroke intervention, was recently tested in a randomized trial in New York City and resulted in 14% more parents and 22% more children retaining perfect scores on a stroke knowledge/preparedness test at 3-month follow-up.[200] The community placed health-literate beauty shop intervention in African-American women improved knowledge of stroke warning signs and calling 911, and this knowledge was sustained for ≥5 months.[192]

Although these studies have focused on increased knowledge and behavioral intent (i.e., will call 911), data from the Stroke Warning and Information and Faster Treatment Study (SWIFT) specifically measured preparedness outcomes in a randomized cohort of 1193 multiethnic stroke and TIA survivors.[201] SWIFT found that in pre and post analysis, there was a 49% increase in the proportion arriving <3 h ($P = .001$); the intervention group also had greater stroke knowledge at 1 month and preparedness capacity at 1 and 12 months.[201] The Acute Stroke Program of Interventions Addressing Racial and Ethnic Disparities (ASPIRE) study is a multilevel program, which aims to decrease acute stroke presentation times and increase intravenous tPA utilization among black communities in the DC metro area.[202]

Behavioral strategies focused on both primary and secondary preventions may be more complex. Indeed, prevention requires a different set of skills and actions taken during the life course. Primary prevention programs targeting hypertension, diabetes mellitus, and improving healthy behaviors are relevant for reduction of all cardiovascular risk and will not be addressed here in detail. However, a few recent behavioral interventions with notable results are highlighted below. The "Shake, Rattle and Roll" trial in Kaiser Permanente Northern California (KPNC) randomized primary care providers and their panels of black patients to (1) usual care, (2) enhanced monitoring of current KPNC BP management protocol, or (3) culturally tailored diet and lifestyle coaching focused on the DASH eating plan. At 15-month follow-up, BP control rates were 69% in the enhanced monitoring group and 71% in the lifestyle coaching group compared to 53% in usual care, $P < .001$.[203] Another recent study enrolled 319 black male barbershop patrons with uncontrolled hypertension to a pharmacist-led intervention at their barbershop or to an active control group (which included lifestyle coaching from barbers). Mean systolic blood pressure reduction was 21.6 mmHg greater in the intervention group compared to the active control at 6-month follow-up ($P < .001$).[204] The Stroke Health and Risk Education (SHARE) study was a cluster-randomized, church-based educational intervention study aimed at primary stroke prevention for Mexican Americans and non-Hispanic whites using a community-based participatory research approach. SHARE was successful in increasing fruit and vegetable intake and decreasing sodium intake, but not in increasing physical activity.[205,206]

Vascular risk reduction is a critical target in the prevention of secondary stroke, as demonstrated in the evidence-based guidelines. Strategies include modification of lifestyle behaviors and medication adherence targets. Motivation and reinforcement may be two key components for successful and sustainable lifelong interventions. With regard to intervention design, two distinctly different approaches to secondary prevention of stroke have emerged: (1) community engaged, and (2) structural. Behavioral economics suggests that we can compel action through structure. A focus on structural interventions include the integration of behavioral strategies, such as medication adherence into existing structures or systems allowing for process evaluations and use of quality indicators to test success of implementation.

As a structural intervention, the Preventing Recurrence of Thromboembolic Events through Coordinated Treatment (PROTECT) study included integration of a quality initiative program, which mandated documentation of discharge medications among stroke/TIA patients.[207] This discharge intervention demonstrated success in increasing adherence to stroke discharge medications during the first year after stroke and reported 90-day adherence rates of 100% antithrombotics, 99% statins, 92% angiotensin-converting enzyme, 99% statins, 80% thiazides. The primary aim of the Integrated Care for the Reduction of Secondary Stroke (ICARUSS) study was to promote the management of vascular risk factors through ongoing patient contact and education via an integrated care model, involving collaboration between a specialist stroke service, a hospital coordinator, and a patient's general practitioner.[208] At 12 months post stroke, systolic blood pressure decreased in the integrated care group and increased in controls ($P = .04$).[209]

There is an ongoing concern that vascular risk reduction programs have not been widely implemented or successful in reducing risk factors outside of a trial setting because interventions have not included community infrastructure or addressed behavioral barriers to vascular risk factor reduction, including health literacy. There are numerous ongoing studies that have integrated components of community engagement into secondary stroke prevention. PROTECT DC piloted the use of community health workers as vehicles for reducing disparities in risk control after stroke.[209] Prevent Recurrence of All Inner-City Strokes through Education (PRAISE), a community-based peer education workshop versus usual care among self-identified stroke survivors, demonstrated significant improvements in BP control in intervention versus control groups at 6 months.[193] The recently completed Discharge Educational Strategies for Reduction of Vascular Events (DESERVE) study in multiethnic stroke/TIA patients incorporates a chronic care model of vascular risk management strategies with emphasis on integration of skills related to risk perception, medication adherence and patient/physician communication.[210] At 12 months post discharge, DESERVE found a nonsignificant 2.5 mmHg greater reduction in systolic blood pressure in the intervention arm compared to usual care, and over 9 mmHg greater reduction among Hispanic participants.[211]

This is an exciting time for behavioral interventions in stroke. There are a substantial number of interventions currently underway. Each of these trials will add unique information and ultimately inform optimal strategies for both stroke prevention and stroke preparedness. Key issues surrounding intervention design that still need to be resolved include cost, optimal reinforcement strategies, and the appropriate use of usual care for testing behavioral interventions because even educational brochures systematically distributed can be considered an intervention. Furthermore, given stark disparities in stroke incidence, recurrence, and mortality, it may be that although some interventions prove efficacious overall, the disparities gradient persists. Indeed, designing efficacious interventions is a good first step but not enough, and continued work identifying mechanisms and designing strategies addressing disparities will be critical. Finally, dissemination and implementation of successful intervention strategies must be prioritized so that what is successful in a few communities can be disseminated to all.

FUTURE DIRECTIONS AND CONCLUSIONS

Based on the prevalence of risk factors and their attributable risk of stroke in the United States and worldwide, it is estimated that a significant proportion of strokes could be prevented through the control of modifiable risk factors.[128] Despite the wealth of data on the importance of stroke risk factors, population level control and prevention remains a challenge. The process requires changes in national health policy directed at public health practices to promote healthy lifestyles, recognition of who is at increased risk of stroke, and modification of this risk. Lifestyle changes require continued support and encouragement. Strategies such as goal attainment while utilizing broader social and political interventions may be effective in changing certain behaviors. Employing surveillance to identify where gaps in the healthcare service persist is an epidemiological approach to evaluate improvement. Developing diverse interventions to engage community members in order to enhance community-clinical connections helps to promote healthier choices and results in better health outcomes. Despite the obstacles to modification of lifestyle factors, health professionals should be encouraged to continue to identify such factors to help prevent stroke.

REFERENCES

1. Benjamin EJ, Blaha MJ, Chiuve SE, et al. Heart disease and stroke Statistics-2017 update: a report from the american heart association. *Circulation*. 2017;135(10): e146—e603.
2. Feigin VL, Norrving B, Mensah GA. Global burden of stroke. *Circulation Res*. 2017;120(3):439—448.
3. Hinman JD, Rost NS, Leung TW, et al. Principles of precision medicine in stroke. *J Neurol Neurosurg Psychiatry*. 2017;88(1):54—61.
4. Krishnamurthi RV, Feigin VL, Forouzanfar MH, et al. Global and regional burden of first-ever ischaemic and haemorrhagic stroke during 1990-2010: findings from the Global Burden of Disease Study 2010. *Lancet Glob Health*. 2013;1(5):e259—281.
5. Sacco RL, Kasner SE, Broderick JP, et al. An updated definition of stroke for the 21st century: a statement for healthcare professionals from the American Heart Association/American Stroke Association. *Stroke*. 2013;44(7): 2064—2089.
6. Easton JD, Saver JL, Albers GW, et al. Definition and evaluation of transient ischemic attack: a scientific statement for healthcare professionals from the American Heart Association/American Stroke Association Stroke Council; Council on Cardiovascular Surgery and Anesthesia; Council on Cardiovascular Radiology and Intervention; Council on Cardiovascular Nursing; and The Interdisciplinary Council on Peripheral Vascular Disease. The American Academy of Neurology affirms the value of this statement as an educational tool for neurologists. *Stroke*. 2009;40(6):2276—2293.

7. Himmelstein DU, Wright A, Woolhandler S. Hospital computing and the costs and quality of care: a national study. *Am J Med*. 2010;123(1):40−46.

8. Al-Khatib SM, Hellkamp A, Curtis J, et al. Non-evidence-based ICD implantations in the United States. *JAMA*. 2011;305(1):43−49.

9. Wolf PA, D'Agostino RB, O'Neal MA, et al. Secular trends in stroke incidence and mortality. The Framingham Study. *Stroke*. 1992;23(11):1551−1555.

10. Mozaffarian D, Benjamin EJ, Go AS, et al. Heart disease and stroke statistics-2016 update: a report from the American heart association. *Circulation*. 2016;133.

11. Koton S, Schneider AL, Rosamond WD, et al. Stroke incidence and mortality trends in US communities, 1987 to 2011. *JAMA*. 2014;312(3):259−268.

12. Feigin VL, Krishnamurthi RV, Parmar P, et al. Update on the global burden of ischemic and hemorrhagic stroke in 1990-2013: the GBD 2013 study. *Neuroepidemiology*. 2015;45(3):161−176.

13. Howard G, Anderson R, Johnson NJ, Sorlie P, Russell G, Howard VJ. Evaluation of social status as a contributing factor to the stroke belt region of the United States. *Stroke*. 1997;28(5):936−940.

14. Howard VJ, Kleindorfer DO, Judd SE, et al. Disparities in stroke incidence contributing to disparities in stroke mortality. *Ann Neurol*. 2011;69(4):619−627.

15. Carandang R, Seshadri S, Beiser A, et al. Trends in incidence, lifetime risk, severity, and 30-day mortality of stroke over the past 50 years. *JAMA*. 2006;296(24): 2939−2946.

16. Madsen TE, Khoury J, Alwell K, et al. Sex-specific stroke incidence over time in the Greater Cincinnati/Northern Kentucky Stroke Study. *Neurology*. 2017;89(10): 990−996.

17. Fang MC, Coca Perraillon M, Ghosh K, Cutler DM, Rosen AB. Trends in stroke rates, risk, and outcomes in the United States, 1988 to 2008. *Am J Med*. 2014; 127(7):608−615.

18. Kissela BM, Khoury JC, Alwell K, et al. Age at stroke: temporal trends in stroke incidence in a large, biracial population. *Neurology*. 2012;79(17):1781−1787.

19. Ramirez L, Kim-Tenser MA, Sanossian N, et al. Trends in acute ischemic stroke hospitalizations in the United States. *J Am Heart Assoc*. 2016;5(5).

20. Brown RD, Whisnant JP, Sicks JD, O'Fallon WM, Wiebers DO. Stroke incidence, prevalence, and survival: secular trends in Rochester, Minnesota, through 1989. *Stroke*. 1996;27(3):373−380.

21. Friday G, Lai SM, Alter M, et al. Stroke in the Lehigh Valley: racial/ethnic differences. *Neurology*. 1989;39(9): 1165−1168.

22. Reeves MJ, Bushnell CD, Howard G, et al. Sex differences in stroke: epidemiology, clinical presentation, medical care, and outcomes. *Lancet Neurol*. 2008; 7(10):915−926.

23. Seshadri S, Beiser A, Kelly-Hayes M, et al. The lifetime risk of stroke. *Estim Fram Study*. 2006;37(2):345−350.

24. Sacco RL, Boden-Albala B, Gan R, et al. Stroke incidence among white, black, and Hispanic residents of an urban community: the Northern Manhattan Stroke Study. *Am J Epidemiol*. 1998;147(3):259−268.

25. Kissela B, Schneider A, Kleindorfer D, et al. Stroke in a biracial population: the excess burden of stroke among blacks. *Stroke*. 2004;35(2):426−431.

26. Morgenstern LB, Smith MA, Lisabeth LD, et al. Excess stroke in Mexican Americans compared with non-Hispanic whites: the brain attack surveillance in Corpus Christi Project. *Am J Epidemiol*. 2004;160(4): 376−383.

27. Howard VJ, Cushman M, Pulley L, et al. The reasons for geographic and racial differences in stroke study: objectives and design. *Neuroepidemiology*. 2005;25(3): 135−143.

28. Smith MA, Risser JM, Moye LA, et al. Designing multi-ethnic stroke studies: the brain attack surveillance in Corpus Christi (BASIC) project. *Ethn Dis*. 2004;14(4): 520−526.

29. Broderick J, Brott T, Kothari R, et al. The Greater Cincinnati/Northern Kentucky Stroke Study. Preliminary first-ever and total incidence rates of stroke among blacks. *Stroke*. 1998;29(2):415−421.

30. The Atherosclerosis Risk in Communities (ARIC) Study. Design and objectives. The ARIC investigators. *Am J Epidemiol*. 1989;129(4):687−702.

31. Boden-Albala B, Allen J, Roberts ET, Bulkow L, Trimble B. Ascertainment of Alaska native stroke incidence, 2005-2009: lessons for assessing the global burden of stroke. *J Stroke Cerebrovasc Dis*. 2017;26(9):2019−2026.

32. Meschia JF, Bushnell C, Boden-Albala B, et al. Guidelines for the primary prevention of stroke. A statement for healthcare professionals from the American Heart Association/American Stroke Association. *Stroke*. 2014;45(12): 3754−3832.

33. Yoon SS, Carroll MD, Fryar CD. Hypertension prevalence and control among adults: United States, 2011-2014. *NCHS Data Brief*. 2015;(220):1−8.

34. Sacco RL, Boden-Albala B, Abel G, et al. Race-ethnic disparities in the impact of stroke risk factors: the northern Manhattan stroke study. *Stroke*. 2001;32(8):1725−1731.

35. *National Diabetes Statistics Report*. Atlanta, GA: Centers for Disease Control and Prevention, US Department of Health and Human Services; 2017.

36. CDC C. National health and nutrition examination survey. In: NCFHS (NCHS), ed. Hyattsville, MD: US Department of Health and Human Services, Centers for Disease Control and Prevention; 2005.

37. Silverman MG, Ference BA, Im K, et al. Association between lowering ldl-c and cardiovascular risk reduction among different therapeutic interventions: a systematic review and meta-analysis. *JAMA*. 2016;316(12):1289−1297.

38. Wannamethee SG, Shaper AG, Ebrahim S. HDL-cholesterol, total cholesterol, and the risk of stroke in middle-aged British men. *Stroke.* 2000;31(8):1882–1888.

39. Ward B, Clarke T, Nugent C, Schiller J. *Early Release of Selected Estimates Based on Data from the 2015 National Health Interview Survey.* Center for Disease Control and Prevention, U.S. Department of Health and Human Services; 2016.

40. Sacco RL, Elkind M, Boden-Albala B, et al. The protective effect of moderate alcohol consumption on ischemic stroke. *JAMA.* 1999;281(1):53–60.

41. Organization W.H., Unit WHOMoSA. *Global Status Report on Alcohol and Health.* World Health Organization; 2014.

42. Hales CM, Fryar CD, Carroll MD, Freedman DS, Ogden CL. Trends in obesity and severe obesity prevalence in us youth and adults by sex and age, 2007-2008 to 2015-2016. *JAMA.* 2018;319(16):1723–1725.

43. Strazzullo P, D'elia L, Cairella G, Garbagnati F, Cappuccio FP, Scalfi L. Excess body weight and incidence of stroke: meta-analysis of prospective studies with 2 million participants. *Stroke.* 2010;41(5):e418–e426.

44. Lee W, Nagubadi S, Kryger MH, Mokhlesi B. Epidemiology of obstructive sleep apnea: a population-based perspective. *Expert Rev Respir Med.* 2008;2(3):349–364.

45. Loke YK, Brown JWL, Kwok CS, Niruban A, Myint PK. Association of obstructive sleep apnea with risk of serious cardiovascular events. Systematic review and meta-analysis. *Circ Cardiovasc Qual Outcomes.* 2012;5(5):720–728.

46. O'Donnell MJ, Xavier D, Liu L, et al. Risk factors for ischaemic and intracerebral haemorrhagic stroke in 22 countries (the INTERSTROKE study): a case-control study. *Lancet.* 2010;376(9735):112–123.

47. Feigin VL, Roth GA, Naghavi M, et al. Global burden of stroke and risk factors in 188 countries, during 1990-2013: a systematic analysis for the Global Burden of Disease Study 2013. *Lancet Neurol.* 2016;15(9):913–924.

48. Katsanos AH, Filippatou A, Manios E, et al. Blood pressure reduction and secondary stroke prevention: a systematic review and metaregression analysis of randomized clinical trials. *Hypertension.* 2017;69(1):171–179.

49. Howard G, Lackland DT, Kleindorfer DO, et al. Racial differences in the impact of elevated systolic blood pressure on stroke risk. *JAMA Intern Med.* 2013;173(1):46–51.

50. Davis PH, Dambrosia JM, Schoenberg BS, et al. Risk factors for ischemic stroke: a prospective study in Rochester, Minnesota. *Ann Neurol.* 1987;22(3):319–327.

51. MacMahon S, Rodgers A. Blood pressure, antihypertensive treatment and stroke risk. *J Hypertens Suppl.* 1994;12(10):S5–S14.

52. Kurl S, Laukkanen JA, Rauramaa R, Lakka TA, Sivenius J, Salonen JT. Systolic blood pressure response to exercise stress test and risk of stroke. *Stroke.* 2001;32(9):2036–2041.

53. Shaper AG, Phillips AN, Pocock SJ, Walker M, Macfarlane PW. Risk factors for stroke in middle aged British men. *BMJ.* 1991;302(6785):1111–1115.

54. Group SR, Wright Jr JT, Williamson JD, et al. A randomized trial of intensive versus standard blood-pressure control. *N Engl J Med.* 2015;373(22):2103–2116.

55. Law MR, Morris JK, Wald NJ. Use of blood pressure lowering drugs in the prevention of cardiovascular disease: meta-analysis of 147 randomised trials in the context of expectations from prospective epidemiological studies. *BMJ.* 2009;338:b1665.

56. Whelton PK, Carey RM, Aronow WS, et al. 2017 ACC/AHA/AAPA/ABC/ACPM/AGS/APhA/ASH/ASPC/NMA/PCNA guideline for the prevention, detection, evaluation, and management of high blood pressure in adults. A report of the American College Cardiology/American Heart Association Task Force on Clinical Practice Guidelines. *J Am Coll Cardiol.* 2018;71(19):e127–e248. https://doi.org/10.1016/j.jacc.2017.11.006.

57. Gillespie CD, Hurvitz KA, Centers for Disease Control and Prevention. Prevalence of hypertension and controlled hypertension - United States, 2007-2010. *MMWR Suppl.* 2013;62(3):144–148.

58. Egan BM, Zhao Y, Axon RN. US trends in prevalence, awareness, treatment, and control of hypertension, 1988-2008. *JAMA.* 2010;303(20):2043–2050.

59. Wolf PA, Abbott RD, Kannel WB. Atrial fibrillation as an independent risk factor for stroke: the Framingham Study. *Stroke.* 1991;22(8):983–988.

60. Marini C, De Santis F, Sacco S, et al. Contribution of atrial fibrillation to incidence and outcome of ischemic stroke. Results from a population-based study. *Stroke.* 2005;36(6):1115–1119.

61. Colilla S, Crow A, Petkun W, Singer DE, Simon T, Liu X. Estimates of current and future incidence and prevalence of atrial fibrillation in the U.S. Adult population. *Am J Cardiol.* 2013;112(8):1142–1147.

62. You JJ, Singer DE, Howard PA, et al. Antithrombotic therapy for atrial fibrillation: antithrombotic therapy and prevention of thrombosis, 9th ed: American College of Chest Physicians Evidence-Based Clinical Practice Guidelines. *Chest.* 2012;141(2 suppl):e531S–e575S.

63. Bots M, Elwood P, Nikitin Y, et al. Total and HDL cholesterol and risk of stroke. EUROSTROKE: a collaborative study among research centres in Europe. *J Epidemiol Community Health.* 2002;56(suppl 1):i19–i24.

64. Di Tullio MR, Sacco RL, Sciacca RR, Homma S. Left atrial size and the risk of ischemic stroke in an ethnically mixed population. *Stroke.* 1999;30(10):2019–2024.

65. Witt BJ, Brown Jr RD, Jacobsen SJ, et al. Ischemic stroke after heart failure: a community-based study. *Am Heart Journal.* 2006;152(1):102–109.

66. Van De Graaff E, Dutta M, Das P, et al. Early coronary revascularization diminishes the risk of ischemic stroke with acute myocardial infarction. *Stroke.* 2006;37(10):2546–2551.

67. Ulvenstam A, Kajermo U, Modica A, Jernberg T, Söderström L, Mooe T. Incidence, trends, and predictors of ischemic stroke 1 year after an acute myocardial infarction. *Stroke.* 2014;45(11):3263–3268.

68. Kannel WB, Abbott RD. Incidence and prognosis of unrecognized myocardial infarction. *New Engl J Med.* 1984;311(18):1144–1147.

69. Ikram MA, Hollander M, Bos MJ, et al. Unrecognized myocardial infarction and the risk of stroke the Rotterdam Study. *Neurology.* 2006;67(9):1635–1639.

70. Lucas C, Goullard L, Marchau M, et al. Higher prevalence of atrial septal aneurysms in patients with ischemic stroke of unknown cause. *Acta Neurol Scand.* 1994;89(3):210–213.

71. Mas JL, Arquizan C, Lamy C, et al. Recurrent cerebrovascular events associated with patent foramen ovale, atrial septal aneurysm, or both. *N Engl J Med.* 2001;345(24): 1740–1746.

72. Overell JR, Bone I, Lees KR. Interatrial septal abnormalities and stroke: a meta-analysis of case-control studies. *Neurology.* 2000;55(8):1172–1179.

73. Lechat P, Mas JL, Lascault G, et al. Prevalence of patent foramen ovale in patients with stroke. *N Engl J Med.* 1988;318(18):1148–1152.

74. Mas JL, Derumeaux G, Guillon B, et al. Patent foramen ovale closure or anticoagulation vs. Antiplatelets after stroke. *N Engl J Med.* 2017;377(11):1011–1021.

75. Sondergaard L, Kasner SE, Rhodes JF, et al. Patent foramen ovale closure or antiplatelet therapy for cryptogenic stroke. *N Engl J Med.* 2017;377(11):1033–1042.

76. Lee PH, Song J-K, Kim JS, et al. Cryptogenic stroke and high-risk patent foramen ovale. The DEFENSE-PFO trial. *J Am Coll Cardiol.* 2018;71(20):2335–2342.

77. Eriksson M, Carlberg B, Eliasson M. The disparity in long-term survival after a first stroke in patients with and without diabetes persists: the northern Sweden MONICA study. *Cerebrovasc Dis.* 2012;34(2):153–160.

78. Peters SA, Huxley RR, Woodward M. Diabetes as a risk factor for stroke in women compared with men: a systematic review and meta-analysis of 64 cohorts, including 775,385 individuals and 12,539 strokes. *Lancet.* 2014; 383(9933):1973–1980.

79. Khoury JC, Kleindorfer D, Alwell K, et al. Diabetes mellitus: a risk factor for ischemic stroke in a large biracial population. *Stroke.* 2013;44(6):1500–1504.

80. Shou J, Zhou L, Zhu S, Zhang X. Diabetes is an independent risk factor for stroke recurrence in stroke patients: a meta-analysis. *J Stroke Cerebrovasc Dis.* 2015;24(9): 1961–1968.

81. Adachi H, Hirai Y, Tsuruta M, Fujiura Y, Imaizuml T. Is insulin resistance or diabetes mellitus associated with stroke? An 18-year follow-up study. *Diabetes Res Clin Pract.* 2001;51(3):215–223.

82. Rundek T, Gardener H, Xu Q, et al. Insulin resistance and risk of ischemic stroke among nondiabetic individuals from the northern Manhattan study. *Arch Neurol.* 2010; 67(10):1195–1200.

83. Redberg RF, Greenland P, Fuster V, et al. Prevention conference VI: diabetes and cardiovascular disease: writing group III: risk assessment in persons with diabetes. *Circulation.* 2002;105(18):e144–e152.

84. Wild S, Roglic G, Green A, Sicree R, King H. Global prevalence of diabetes: estimates for the year 2000 and projections for 2030. *Diabetes Care.* 2004;27(5): 1047–1053.

85. Marso SP, Kennedy KF, House JA, McGuire DK. The effect of intensive glucose control on all-cause and cardiovascular mortality, myocardial infarction and stroke in persons with type 2 diabetes mellitus: a systematic review and meta-analysis. *Diabetes Vasc Dis Res.* 2010;7(2): 119–130.

86. Heiss G, Sharrett AR, Barnes R, Chambless LE, Szklo M, Alzola C. Carotid atherosclerosis measured by B-mode ultrasound in populations: associations with cardiovascular risk factors in the ARIC study. *Am J Epidemiol.* 1991;134(3):250–256.

87. O'Leary D. Distribution and correlates of sonographically detected carotid artery disease in the Cardiovascular Health Study. *Stroke.* 1992;23(12):1752–1760.

88. Fine-Edelstein JS, Wolf PA, O'Leary DH, et al. Precursors of extracranial carotid atherosclerosis in the Framingham Study. *Neurology.* 1994;44(6):1046–1050.

89. Ansell BJ. Cholesterol, stroke risk, and stroke prevention. *Curr Atheroscler Rep.* 2000;2(2):92–96.

90. Qizilbash N, Jones L, Warlow C, Mann J. Fibrinogen and lipid concentrations as risk factors for transient ischaemic attacks and minor ischaemic strokes. *BMJ.* 1991; 303(6803):605–609.

91. Group SSSS. Randomized trail of cholesterol lowering in 4444 patients with coronary heart disease: the Scandinavian Simvastatin Study (4S). *Lancet.* 1994; 344(1383–1389).

92. Zhang X, Patel A, Horibe H, et al. Cholesterol, coronary heart disease, and stroke in the Asia Pacific region. *Int J Epidemiol.* 2003;32(4):563–572.

93. Leppala JM, Virtamo J, Fogelholm R, Albanes D, Heinonen OP. Different risk factors for different stroke subtypes: association of blood pressure, cholesterol, and antioxidants. *Stroke.* 1999;30(12):2535–2540.

94. Kurth T, Everett BM, Buring JE, Kase CS, Ridker PM, Gaziano JM. Lipid levels and the risk of ischemic stroke in women. *Neurology.* 2007;68(8):556–562.

95. Iso H, Jacobs DR, Wentworth D, Neaton JD, Cohen JD. Serum cholesterol levels and six-year mortality from stroke in 350,977 men screened for the multiple risk factor intervention trial. *N Engl J Med.* 1989;320(14):904–910.

96. Collaboration ERF. Lipoprotein (a) concentration and the risk of coronary heart disease, stroke, and nonvascular mortality. *JAMA.* 2009;302(4):412.

97. Lindenstrom E, Boysen G, Nyboe J. Influence of total cholesterol, high density lipoprotein cholesterol, and triglycerides on risk of cerebrovascular disease: the Copenhagen City Heart Study. *BMJ.* 1994;309(6946):11–15.

98. Sacco RL, Benson RT, Kargman DE, et al. High-density lipoprotein cholesterol and ischemic stroke in the elderly: the northern manhattan stroke study. *JAMA.* 2001; 285(21):2729–2735.

99. Shahar E, Chambless LE, Rosamond WD, et al. Plasma lipid profile and incident ischemic stroke: the Atherosclerosis Risk in Communities (ARIC) study. *Stroke*. 2003; 34(3):623−631.

100. Sturgeon JD, Folsom AR, Longstreth WT, Shahar E, Rosamond WD, Cushman M. Risk factors for intracerebral hemorrhage in a pooled prospective study. *Stroke*. 2007;38(10):2718−2725.

101. Di Angelantonio E, Sarwar N, Perry P, et al. Major lipids, apolipoproteins, and risk of vascular disease. *JAMA*. 2009;302(18):1993−2000.

102. Group TLL-TIwPiIDS. Prevention of cardiovascular events and death with pravastatin in patients with coronary heart disease and a broad range of initial cholesterol levels. *Natl Engl J Med*. 1998;339(1349−1357).

103. Amarenco P, Labreuche J. Lipid management in the prevention of stroke: review and updated meta-analysis of statins for stroke prevention. *Lancet Neurol*. 2009;8(5): 453−463.

104. Stone NJ, Robinson JG, Lichtenstein AH, et al. 2013 ACC/AHA guideline on the treatment of blood cholesterol to reduce atherosclerotic cardiovascular risk in adults: a report of the American College of Cardiology/American Heart Association Task Force on Practice Guidelines. *J Am Coll Cardiol*. 2014;63(25 pt B):2889−2934.

105. Kernan WN, Ovbiagele B, Black HR, et al. Guidelines for the prevention of stroke in patients with stroke and transient ischemic attack. A guideline for healthcare professionals from the American Heart Association/American Stroke Association. *Stroke*. 2014;45(7):2160−2236.

106. Bhat VM, Cole JW, Sorkin JD, et al. Dose-response relationship between cigarette smoking and risk of ischemic stroke in young women. *Stroke*. 2008;39(9):2439−2443.

107. Kissela BM, Sauerbeck L, Woo D, et al. Subarachnoid hemorrhage: a preventable disease with a heritable component. *Stroke*. 2002;33(5):1321−1326.

108. Mast H, Thompson JL, Lin IF, et al. Cigarette smoking as a determinant of high-grade carotid artery stenosis in Hispanic, black, and white patients with stroke or transient ischemic attack. *Stroke*. 1998;29(5):908−912.

109. Sacco RL, Roberts JK, Boden-Albala B, et al. Race-ethnicity and determinants of carotid atherosclerosis in a multiethnic population. The Northern Manhattan Stroke Study. *Stroke*. 1997;28(5):929−935.

110. O'Leary DH, Polak JF, Kronmal RA, et al. Distribution and correlates of sonographically detected carotid artery disease in the cardiovascular health study. The CHS collaborative research group. *Stroke*. 1992;23(12):1752−1760.

111. Oono IP, Mackay DF, Pell JP. Meta-analysis of the association between secondhand smoke exposure and stroke. *J Public Health (Oxf)*. 2011;33(4):496−502.

112. Lee PN, Thornton AJ, Forey BA, Hamling JS. Environmental tobacco smoke exposure and risk of stroke in never smokers: an updated review with meta-analysis. *J Stroke Cerebrovasc Dis*. 2017;26(1):204−216.

113. Wolf PA, D'Agostino RB, Kannel WB, Bonita R, Belanger AJ. Cigarette smoking as a risk factor for stroke. The Framingham Study. *JAMA*. 1988;259(7):1025−1029.

114. Kawachi I, Colditz GA, Stampfer MJ, et al. Smoking cessation in relation to total mortality rates in women. A prospective cohort study. *Ann Intern Med*. 1993;119(10):992−1000.

115. Donahue RP, Abbott RD, Reed DM, Yano K. Alcohol and hemorrhagic stroke. The Honolulu Heart Program. *JAMA*. 1986;255(17):2311−2314.

116. Tanaka H, Ueda Y, Hayashi M, et al. Risk factors for cerebral hemorrhage and cerebral infarction in a Japanese rural community. *Stroke*. 1982;13(1):62−73.

117. Ben-Shlomo Y, Markowe H, Shipley M, Marmot MG. Stroke risk from alcohol consumption using different control groups. *Stroke*. 1992;23(8):1093−1098.

118. Beghi E, Boglium G, Cosso P, et al. Stroke and alcohol intake in a hospital population. A case-control study. *Stroke*. 1995;26(9):1691−1696.

119. Gorelick PB. Stroke prevention: windows of opportunity and failed expectations? A discussion of modifiable cardiovascular risk factors and a prevention proposal. *Neuroepidemiology*. 1997;16(4):163−173.

120. Kadlecová P, Andel R, Mikulík R, Handing EP, Pedersen NL. Alcohol consumption at midlife and risk of stroke during 43 years of follow-up. Cohort twin analyses. *Stroke*. 2015;46(3):627−633.

121. Ricci C, Wood A, Muller D, et al. Alcohol intake in relation to non-fatal and fatal coronary heart disease and stroke: EPIC-CVD case-cohort study. *BMJ*. 2018:361.

122. Reynolds K, Lewis B, Nolen JL, Kinney GL, Sathya B, He J. Alcohol consumption and risk of stroke: a meta-analysis. *JAMA*. 2003;289(5):579−588.

123. Larsson SC, Wallin A, Wolk A, Markus HS. Differing association of alcohol consumption with different stroke types: a systematic review and meta-analysis. *BMC Med*. 2016;14(1):178.

124. Zhang C, Qin Y-Y, Chen Q, et al. Alcohol intake and risk of stroke: a dose−response meta-analysis of prospective studies. *Int J Cardiol*. 2014;174(3):669−677.

125. Stampfer MJ, Colditz GA, Willett WC, et al. A prospective study of moderate alcohol drinking and risk of diabetes in women. *Am J Epidemiol*. 1988;128(3):549−558.

126. Truelsen T, Gronbaek M, Schnohr P, Boysen G. Intake of beer, wine, and spirits and risk of stroke: the copenhagen city heart study. *Stroke*. 1998;29(12):2467−2472.

127. Klatsky AL, Armstrong MA, Friedman GD, Sidney S. Alcohol drinking and risk of hospitalization for ischemic stroke. *Am J Cardiol*. 2001;88(6):703−706.

128. O'Donnell MJ, Chin SL, Rangarajan S, et al. Global and regional effects of potentially modifiable risk factors associated with acute stroke in 32 countries (INTERSTROKE): a case-control study. *Lancet*. 2016;388(10046):761−775.

129. Smyth A, Teo KK, Rangarajan S, et al. Alcohol consumption and cardiovascular disease, cancer, injury, admission to hospital, and mortality: a prospective cohort study. *Lancet*. 2015;386(10007):1945−1954.

130. Tikk K, Sookthai D, Monni S, et al. Primary preventive potential for stroke by avoidance of major lifestyle risk factors. The European Prospective Investigation into Cancer and Nutrition-Heidelberg Cohort. 2014;45(7):2041−2046.

131. Armstrong MEG, Green J, Reeves GK, Beral V, Cairns BJ. Frequent physical activity may not reduce vascular disease risk as much as moderate activity: large prospective study of UK women. *Circulation.* 2015;131(8):721−729.

132. Willey JZ, Moon YP, Sacco RL, et al. *Physical Inactivity Is a Strong Risk Factor for Stroke in the Oldest Old: Findings from a Multi-ethnic Population (The Northern Manhattan Study).* London, England: SAGE Publications Sage; 2017.

133. Pandey A, Patel MR, Willis B, et al. Association between midlife cardiorespiratory fitness and risk of stroke. The Cooper Center Longitudinal Study. 2016;47(7):1720−1726.

134. Kiely DK, Wolf PA, Cupples LA, Beiser AS, Kannel WB. Physical activity and stroke risk: the Framingham Study. *Am J Epidemiol.* 1994;140(7):608−620.

135. Blomstrand A, Blomstrand C, Ariai N, Bengtsson C, Björkelund C. Stroke incidence and association with risk factors in women: a 32-year follow-up of the Prospective Population Study of Women in Gothenburg. *BMJ Open.* 2014;4(10):e005173.

136. Willey JZ, Voutsinas J, Sherzai A, et al. Trajectories in leisure-time physical activity and risk of stroke in women in the California teachers study. *Stroke.* 2017;48(9):2346−2352.

137. Åberg ND, Kuhn HG, Nyberg J, et al. Influence of cardiovascular fitness and muscle strength in early adulthood on long-term risk of stroke in Swedish men. *Stroke.* 2015;46(7):1769−1776.

138. Bell EJ, Lutsey PL, Windham BG, Folsom AR. Physical activity and cardiovascular disease in African Americans in atherosclerosis risk in communities. *Med Sci Sports Exerc.* 2013;45(5):901−907.

139. McDonnell MN, Hillier SL, Hooker SP, Le A, Judd SE, Howard VJ. Physical activity frequency and risk of incident stroke in a national US study of blacks and whites. *Stroke.* 2013;44(9):2519−2524.

140. Hu FB, Stampfer MJ, Colditz GA, et al. Physical activity and risk of stroke in women. *JAMA.* 2000;283(22):2961−2967.

141. Sacco RL, Gan R, Boden-Albala B, et al. Leisure-time physical activity and ischemic stroke risk. *Stroke.* 1998;29(2):380.

142. Nygård O, Vollset SE, Refsum H, et al. Total plasma homocysteine and cardiovascular risk profile. The Hordaland Homocysteine Study. *JAMA.* 1995;274(19):1526−1533.

143. Lee IM. Exercise and risk of stroke in male physicians. In: Hennekens CH, ed. *Stroke.* Vol. 30. 1999:1−6.

144. Refsum H, Nurk E, Smith AD, et al. The Hordaland homocysteine study: a community-based study of homocysteine, its determinants, and associations with disease. *J Nutr.* 2006;136(6):1731S−1740S.

145. Panagiotakos DB, Pitsavos C, Chrysohoou C, Kavouras S, Stefanadis C. The associations between leisure-time physical activity and inflammatory and coagulation markers related to cardiovascular disease: the ATTICA Study. *Prev Med.* 2005;40(4):432−437.

146. Goldstein LB, Adams R, Alberts MJ, et al. Primary prevention of ischemic stroke: a guideline from the American heart association/American stroke association stroke council: cosponsored by the atherosclerotic peripheral vascular disease interdisciplinary working group; cardiovascular nursing council; clinical cardiology council; nutrition, physical activity, and metabolism council; and the quality of care and outcomes research interdisciplinary working group: the American academy of neurology affirms the value of this guideline. *Stroke.* 2006;37(6):1583−1633.

147. Eckel RH, Jakicic JM, Ard JD, et al. 2013 AHA/ACC guideline on lifestyle management to reduce cardiovascular risk: a report of the American College of cardiology/American heart association task force on practice guidelines. *J Am Coll Cardiol.* 2014;63(25 part B):2960−2984.

148. Gillman MW, Cupples LA, Gagnon D, Millen BE, Ellison RC, Castelli WP. Margarine intake and subsequent coronary heart disease in men. *Epidemiology.* 1997;8(2):144−149.

149. Aaron KJ, Sanders PW. Role of dietary salt and potassium intake in cardiovascular health and disease: a review of the evidence. *Mayo Clin Proc.* 2013;88(9). https://doi.org/10.1016/j.mayocp.2013.1006.1005.

150. Larsson SC, Orsini N, Wolk A. Dietary potassium intake and risk of stroke: a dose-response meta-analysis of prospective studies. *Stroke.* 2011;42(10):2746−2750.

151. Estruch R, Ros E, Salas-Salvado J, et al. Primary prevention of cardiovascular disease with a Mediterranean diet. *N Engl J Med.* 2013;368(14):1279−1290.

152. Martinez-Gonzalez MA, Dominguez LJ, Delgado-Rodriguez M. Olive oil consumption and risk of CHD and/or stroke: a meta-analysis of case-control, cohort and intervention studies. *Br J Nutr.* 2014;112(2):248−259.

153. Mayhew AJ, de Souza RJ, Meyre D, Anand SS, Mente A. A systematic review and meta-analysis of nut consumption and incident risk of CVD and all-cause mortality. *Br J Nutr.* 2016;115(2):212−225.

154. Sacks FM, Obarzanek E, Windhauser MM, et al. Rationale and design of the Dietary Approaches to Stop Hypertension trial (DASH). A multicenter controlled-feeding study of dietary patterns to lower blood pressure. *Ann Epidemiol.* 1995;5(2):108−118.

155. Gillman MW, Cupples LA, Gagnon D, et al. Protective effect of fruits and vegetables on development of stroke in men. *JAMA.* 1995;273(14):1113−1117.

156. Boden-Albala B, Sacco RL. Lifestyle factors and stroke risk: exercise, alcohol, diet, obesity, smoking, drug use, and stress. *Curr Atheroscler Rep.* 2000;2(2):160−166.

157. Larsson SC, Virtamo J, Wolk A. Total and specific fruit and vegetable consumption and risk of stroke: a prospective study. *Atherosclerosis*. 2013;227(1):147−152.

158. He FJ, Nowson CA, MacGregor GA. Fruit and vegetable consumption and stroke: meta-analysis of cohort studies. *Lancet*. 2006;367(9507):320−326.

159. Joshipura KJ, Ascherio A, Manson JE, et al. Fruit and vegetable intake in relation to risk of ischemic stroke. *JAMA*. 1999;282(13):1233−1239.

160. Chowdhury R, Stevens S, Gorman D, et al. Association between fish consumption, long chain omega 3 fatty acids, and risk of cerebrovascular disease: systematic review and meta-analysis. *BMJ*. 2012;345:e6698.

161. Alexander DD, Bylsma LC, Vargas AJ, et al. Dairy consumption and CVD: a systematic review and meta-analysis. *Br J Nutr*. 2016;115(4):737−750.

162. Huo Y, Li J, Qin X, et al. Efficacy of folic acid therapy in primary prevention of stroke among adults with hypertension in China: the CSPPT randomized clinical trial. *JAMA*. 2015;313(13):1325−1335.

163. Prospective Studies C. Body-mass index and cause-specific mortality in 900 000 adults: collaborative analyses of 57 prospective studies. *Lancet*. 2009;373(9669):1083−1096.

164. Sjöström L. Review of the key results from the Swedish Obese Subjects (SOS) trial − a prospective controlled intervention study of bariatric surgery. *J Intern Med*. 2013;273(3):219−234.

165. Zhang Y, Tuomilehto J, Jousilahti P, Wang Y, Antikainen R, Hu G. Lifestyle factors and antihypertensive treatment on the risks of ischemic and hemorrhagic stroke. *Hypertension*. 2012;60(4):906−912.

166. Caterson I, Finer N, Coutinho W, et al. Maintained intentional weight loss reduces cardiovascular outcomes: results from the Sibutramine Cardiovascular OUTcomes (SCOUT) trial. *Diabetes Obes Metab*. 2012;14(6):523−530.

167. Hermann DM, Bassetti CL. Sleep-related breathing and sleep-wake disturbances in ischemic stroke. *Neurology*. 2009;73(16):1313−1322.

168. Somers VK, White DP, Amin R, et al. Sleep apnea and cardiovascular disease: an American Heart Association/American College of Cardiology Foundation Scientific Statement from the American Heart Association Council for High Blood Pressure Research Professional Education Committee, Council on Clinical Cardiology, Stroke Council, and Council on Cardiovascular Nursing. In collaboration with the National Heart, Lung, and Blood Institute National Center on Sleep Disorders Research (National Institutes of Health). *Circulation*. 2008;118(10):1080−1111.

169. Boden-Albala B, Roberts ET, Bazil C, et al. Daytime sleepiness and risk of stroke and vascular disease. Findings from the Northern Manhattan Study (NOMAS). *Circ Cardiovasc Qual Outcomes*. 2012;5(4):500−507.

170. Epstein LJ, Kristo D, Strollo Jr PJ, et al. Clinical guideline for the evaluation, management and long-term care of obstructive sleep apnea in adults. *J Clin Sleep Med*. 2009;5(3):263−276.

171. Arzt M, Young T, Finn L, Skatrud JB, Bradley TD. Association of sleep-disordered breathing and the occurrence of stroke. *Am J Respir Crit Care Med*. 2005;172(11):1447−1451.

172. Redline S, Yenokyan G, Gottlieb DJ, et al. Obstructive sleep apnea-hypopnea and incident stroke: the sleep heart health study. *Am J Respir Crit Care Med*. 2010;182(2):269−277.

173. Wallace DM, Ramos AR, Rundek T. Sleep disorders and stroke. *Int J Stroke*. 2012;7(3):231−242.

174. Nieto FJ, Young TB, Lind BK, et al. Association of sleep-disordered breathing, sleep apnea, and hypertension in a large community-based study. Sleep Heart Health Study. *JAMA*. 2000;283(14):1829−1836.

175. Johnson KG, Johnson DC. Frequency of sleep apnea in stroke and TIA patients: a meta-analysis. *J Clin Sleep Med*. 2010;6(2):131−137.

176. Hermann DM, Bassetti CL. Role of sleep-disordered breathing and sleep-wake disturbances for stroke and stroke recovery. *Neurology*. 2016;87(13):1407−1416.

177. Shah ASV, Lee KK, McAllister DA, et al. Short term exposure to air pollution and stroke: systematic review and meta-analysis. *BMJ*. 2015:350.

178. Ostro B, Hu J, Goldberg D, et al. Associations of mortality with long-term exposures to fine and ultrafine particles, species and sources: results from the California Teachers Study Cohort. *Environ Health Perspect*. 2015;123(6):549−556.

179. Münzel T, Gori T, Babisch W, Basner M. Cardiovascular effects of environmental noise exposure. *Eur Heart J*. 2014;35(13):829−836.

180. Sørensen M, Hvidberg M, Andersen ZJ, et al. Road traffic noise and stroke: a prospective cohort study. *Eur Heart J*. 2011;32(6):737−744.

181. Stokholm ZA, Bonde JP, Christensen KL, Hansen ÅM, Kolstad HA. Occupational noise exposure and the risk of stroke. *Stroke*. 2013;44(11):3214−3216.

182. Davies H, Kamp IV. Noise and cardiovascular disease: a review of the literature 2008-2011. *Noise Health*. 2012;14(61):287−291.

183. Boden-Albala B, Litwak E, Elkind MS, Rundek T, Sacco RL. Social isolation and outcomes post stroke. *Neurology*. 2005;64(11):1888−1892.

184. Nagayoshi M, Everson-Rose SA, Iso H, Mosley Jr TH, Rose KM, Lutsey PL. Social network, social support, and risk of incident stroke: atherosclerosis Risk in Communities study. *Stroke*. 2014;45(10):2868−2873.

185. Boden-Albala B, Evers S, Elkind M, Chen J, Sacco R. Blood pressure status one year post-stroke: findings from the northern manhattan stroke study. *Stroke*. 2001;32:322.

186. Willey JZ, Paik MC, Sacco R, Elkind MS, Boden-Albala B. Social determinants of physical inactivity in the Northern Manhattan Study (NOMAS). *J Community Health*. 2010;35(6):602−608.

187. Bakas T, Clark PC, Kelly-Hayes M, King RB, Lutz BJ, Miller EL. Evidence for stroke family caregiver and dyad interventions: a statement for healthcare professionals from the American Heart Association and American Stroke Association. *Stroke*. 2014;45(9):2836−2852.

188. McHutchison CA, Backhouse EV, Cvoro V, Shenkin SD, Wardlaw JM. Education, socioeconomic status, and intelligence in childhood and stroke risk in later life: a meta-analysis. *Epidemiology*. 2017;28(4):608−618.

189. Kerr GD, Slavin H, Clark D, Coupar F, Langhorne P, Stott DJ. Do vascular risk factors explain the association between socioeconomic status and stroke incidence: a meta-analysis. *Cerebrovasc Dis*. 2011;31(1):57−63.

190. Addo J, Ayerbe L, Mohan KM, et al. Socioeconomic status and stroke. *An Updat Rev*. 2012;43(4):1186−1191.

191. Horowitz CR, Brenner BL, Lachapelle S, Amara DA, Arniella G. Effective recruitment of minority populations through community-led strategies. *Am J Prev Med*. 2009; 37(6 suppl 1):S195−S200.

192. Kleindorfer D, Miller R, Sailor-Smith S, Moomaw CJ, Khoury J, Frankel M. The challenges of community-based research: the beauty shop stroke education project. *Stroke*. 2008;39(8):2331−2335.

193. Kronish IM, Goldfinger JZ, Negron R, et al. Effect of peer education on stroke prevention: the prevent recurrence of all inner-city strokes through education randomized controlled trial. *Stroke*. 2014;45(11):3330−3336.

194. Appel LJ, Champagne CM, Harsha DW, et al. Effects of comprehensive lifestyle modification on blood pressure control: main results of the PREMIER clinical trial. *JAMA*. 2003;289(16):2083−2093.

195. Boden-Albala B, Tehranifar P, Stillman J, Paik MC. Social network types and acute stroke preparedness behavior. *Cerebrovasc Dis Extra*. 2011;1(1):75−83.

196. Goldstein LB, Edwards MG, Wood DP. Delay between stroke onset and emergency department evaluation. *Neuroepidemiology*. 2001;20(3):196−200.

197. Miller ET, King KA, Miller R, Kleindorfer D. FAST stroke prevention educational program for middle school students: pilot study results. *J Neurosci Nurs*. 2007;39(4): 236−242.

198. Morgenstern LB, Gonzales NR, Maddox KE, et al. A randomized, controlled trial to teach middle school children to recognize stroke and call 911: the kids identifying and defeating stroke project. *Stroke*. 2007;38(11): 2972−2978.

199. Williams O, Noble JM. 'Hip-hop' stroke: a stroke educational program for elementary school children living in a high-risk community. *Stroke*. 2008;39(10):2809−2816.

200. Williams O, Leighton-Herrmann Quinn E, Teresi J, et al. Improving community stroke preparedness in the HHS (Hip-Hop stroke) randomized clinical trial. *Stroke*. 2018;49(4):972−979.

201. Boden-Albala B, Stillman J, Roberts ET, et al. Comparison of acute stroke preparedness strategies to decrease emergency department arrival time in a multiethnic cohort: the stroke warning information and faster treatment study. *Stroke*. 2015;46(7):1806−1812.

202. Boden-Albala B, Edwards DF, St Clair S, et al. Methodology for a community-based stroke preparedness intervention: the acute stroke program of interventions addressing racial and ethnic disparities study. *Stroke*. 2014;45(7):2047−2052.

203. Nguyen-Huynh MN, Young JD, Chin TA, et al. Abstract WMP52: Shake, Rattle & Roll trial - effects on blood pressure control and therapy. *Stroke*. 2016;47(suppl 1): AWMP52.

204. Victor RG, Lynch K, Li N, et al. A cluster-randomized trial of blood-pressure reduction in black barbershops. *N Engl J Med*. 2018;378(14):1291−1301.

205. Brown DL, Conley KM, Resnicow K, et al. Stroke Health and Risk Education (SHARE): design, methods, and theoretical basis. *Contemp Clin Trials*. 2012;33(4): 721−729.

206. Brown DL, Conley KM, Sánchez BN, et al. A multicomponent behavioral intervention to reduce stroke risk factor behaviors. The Stroke Health and Risk Education Cluster-Randomized Controlled Trial. *Stroke*. 2015;46(10):2861−2867.

207. Ovbiagele O. In-hospital initiation of secondary stroke prevention therapies yields high rates of adherence at follow-up. In: JL Saver, ed. *Stroke*. Vol. 35. 2004:2879−2883.

208. Joubert J, Reid C, Barton D, et al. Integrated care improves risk-factor modification after stroke: initial results of the integrated care for the reduction of secondary stroke model. *J Neurol Neurosurg Psychiatry*. 2009;80(3):279−284.

209. Dromerick AW, Gibbons MC, Edwards DF, et al. Preventing recurrence of thromboembolic events through coordinated treatment in the District of Columbia. *Int J Stroke*. 2011;6(5):454−460.

210. Lord AS, Carman HM, Roberts ET, et al. Discharge educational strategies for reduction of vascular events (DESERVE): design and methods. *Int J Stroke*. 2015; 10(suppl A100):151−154.

211. Boden-Albala B, Goldmann E, Parikh NS, et al. Discharge educational strategies for reduction of vascular events (DESERVE): a randomized clinical trial. *JAMA Neurol*. 2018 [in Press].

212. Boden-Albala B, Goldmann E, Parikh NS, et al. Efficacy of a Discharge Educational Strategy vs Standard Discharge Care on Reduction of Vascular Risk in Patients With Stroke and Transient Ischemic Attack:The DESERVE Randomized Clinical Trial. *JAMA Neurol*. Published online October 08, 2018. https://doi.org/10.1001/jamaneurol.2018.2926.

CHAPTER 2

Prediction of Motor Recovery and Outcomes After Stroke

LI KHIM KWAH, BAPPSC (PHTY), PHD • GERT KWAKKEL, PHD •
JANNE M. VEERBEEK, PHD

INTRODUCTION

Imagine you are a clinician working in an acute stroke unit. You are seeing an 80-year-old gentleman Mr. B who has just sustained a severe right middle cerebral artery stroke. Based on Mr. B's age, premorbid function, and presenting problems (e.g., weakness and sensory deficits in his left leg, and inability to sit without assistance), you might predict that Mr. B has a low probability of walking independently at 6 months. His family has informed you that they wish to care for him at home and are willing to provide physical help if needed. Based on your prediction, your team, Mr. B, and Mr. B's family might work toward a discharge goal of safe transfers and assisted walking, rather than independent walking. Therapy might focus more on carer training and equipment prescription, rather than intensive gait training (with or without devices). You and your team might also start organizing community services and home modifications to support Mr. B and his family at home. As a result, Mr. B does not stay in acute or rehabilitation care longer than needed and is discharged home in less than 6 weeks. As part of stroke management, clinicians often have to make predictions on the recovery and outcomes of individual patients. These predictions allow clinicians to inform patients and their families about expected recovery and outcomes; consequently, better decisions can be made regarding therapy goals and discharge planning,[1,2] which invariably lead to a more efficient use of stroke care resources,[3] as illustrated in the example above.

In this chapter, we focus on the prediction of motor recovery and motor outcomes after stroke, as these are important to patients, caregivers, and clinicians.[4] Measures of motor recovery and outcomes refer to measures of arm motor function, arm activity, leg motor function, leg activity, and global disability (see Box 2.1 for definitions in relation to the International Classification of Functioning, Disability and Health (ICF) framework). The terms "recovery" and "outcomes" are slightly distinct from each other, in that "recovery" refers to a change score in function or activity measured between two or more time points after stroke, while "outcome" refers to a score of function or activity measured at one time point after stroke. Due to this distinction, we have used both terms to describe what we are predicting in this chapter.

Our chapter has three aims. First, we outline the integration of clinical experience and research evidence in guiding predictions in clinical practice. Second, we help readers identify if a prediction model of motor recovery or outcome is ready for use in clinical practice by considering four criteria: (1) recruitment of representative cohort, (2) standardized measurement of predictors, (3) standardized measurement of outcome, and

---

BOX 2.1
Definitions of Motor Recovery and Outcomes

Arm motor function: measured on the body function and structure level of the ICF framework. Includes measures of arm muscle strength and movement (e.g., Fugl–Meyer Assessment–Upper Extremity subscale).

Arm activity: measured on the activity level of the ICF framework. Includes measures of arm and hand capacity (e.g., Action Research Arm Test, Motor Assessment Scale).

Leg motor function: measured on the body function and structure level of the ICF framework. Includes measures of leg muscle strength and movement (e.g., Fugl–Meyer Assessment–Lower Extremity subscale).

Leg activity: measured on the activity level of the ICF framework. Includes measures of walking (e.g., Functional Ambulation Category).

Global disability: measured on the activity level of the ICF framework. Include measures of activities of daily living, such as a combination of toileting, dressing, and showering (e.g., modified Rankin Scale, Barthel Index).

ICF, International Classification of Functioning, Disability and Health.

Stroke Rehabilitation. https://doi.org/10.1016/B978-0-323-55381-0.00002-0

(4) external validation of model. Third, we highlight prediction models of motor recovery and outcomes that have fulfilled these four criteria and are potentially ready for use by stroke clinicians.

WHAT CAN CLINICIANS USE TO GUIDE PREDICTIONS IN CLINICAL PRACTICE?

In general, clinicians rely on clinical experience and research evidence to guide their predictions of patients' recovery and outcomes. Clinicians assess and treat many patients on a daily basis. It is therefore not surprising that experienced clinicians start to recognize patterns in characteristics of patients who recover (or, achieve a certain outcome) and those who do not. These clinicians inherently learn to predict a patient's recovery and outcomes accurately.[5] However, studies have shown that the accuracy of clinicians' predictions vary greatly from 33% to 88% when neurologists and therapists were asked to make early predictions of 6-month functional outcomes in patients after a neurologic illness.[6-8] (Note: Accuracy was calculated as proportion of good and bad outcomes correctly predicted divided by total number of predictions in the studies.) Clinicians also tend to be more pessimistic about stroke outcomes. That is, they were less accurate in predicting favorable outcomes than unfavorable outcomes,[6,7] or they gave patients lower predicted scores on functional scales than what patients actually achieved.[8] This is of concern, because appropriate care might be withdrawn too early, before the patient has reached his or her maximum abilities. Contrary to popular belief, experienced clinicians did not necessarily make more accurate predictions than less experienced clinicians.[8] Therefore, it appears that clinical experience—though intuitively useful—cannot be relied upon solely to guide our prognoses on patients' recovery and outcomes.

The next best source of information that clinicians can rely on to make accurate predictions is research evidence.[5] Here, research evidence refers to multivariable prediction models developed from prognostic studies or prediction modeling studies.[9,10] (Note: In this chapter, we equate prognostic studies to prediction modeling studies, as both types of studies are longitudinal, and measure the occurrence of an outcome in the future. However, readers should note that there is often a greater emphasis on variable/predictor selection and model presentation in prediction modeling studies than in prognostic studies. These two type of studies also have different statements to guide the report and conduct of studies. For example, the STROBE[11] and the QUIPS[12] statements guide the report and conduct of prognostic studies; while the TRIPOD[13] and the

CHARMS[10] statements guide the report and conduct of prediction modeling studies. Multivariable prediction models are mathematical equations that calculate probabilities of recovery or outcomes based on the input of two or more predictors.[14] An example of an equation for outcome prediction is shown here:

Probability of walking independently at 6 months

$$= 1/(1 + \exp^{-11.02852 - 0.1053\ \text{age} - 0.2436\ \text{NIHSS}})^{15}$$

NIHSS refers to the National Institutes of Health Stroke Scale measured at 4 weeks after stroke; it measures stroke severity.

Prediction modeling studies aim to identify the probability of a patient having a certain recovery or outcome in the future.[9,10] It is necessary to consider multiple predictors, since a single predictor is unlikely to result in accurate predictions compared to the combination of multiple predictors. Data collected in prediction modeling studies typically include potential predictors collected at onset of disease and outcome collected at a later time point after disease.[9] (For the prediction of motor recovery and motor outcomes after stroke, outcomes are collected at two or more time points in motor recovery studies, while motor outcome studies collect outcomes at one time point after stroke.) In the example of the equation above, predictors are age and NIHSS, while the outcome is independent walking. To build the multivariable prediction model, potential predictors undergo a variable selection procedure[9,10] to identify the predictors that are most strongly associated with recovery or outcomes after stroke.

Three types of studies are associated with multivariable prognostic research: *development study*, *validation study*, and *impact study* (see Box 2.2 for definitions of these studies). There is wide consensus that a prediction model should *not* be used in clinical practice, unless development and external validation studies have been conducted on the prediction model.[9,19,20,21] In the next section, we consider some factors that might help readers determine if a prediction model for motor recovery or outcome is ready for use in clinical practice.

IS THIS PREDICTION MODEL OF MOTOR RECOVERY OR OUTCOME READY FOR USE IN CLINICAL PRACTICE?

Prior to the use of research evidence in clinical practice, clinicians often consider two questions: "Can we trust the results of the research study?" and "Can we apply the results of the research study to our patients?" To answer these questions and determine if the results of prediction modeling studies are valid and applicable in clinical practice, we consider four common criteria used in checklists to rate the quality of prediction modeling studies.[10,12] These four criteria are: (1) recruitment of representative cohort, (2) standardized measurement of predictors, (3) standardized measurement of outcome, and (4) external validation of model.

Did the Development Study Recruit a Representative Cohort?

If prediction models of motor recovery and outcomes are to be used by clinicians early after stroke, it is important that models are developed on cohorts that are representative of the patients seen by clinicians early after stroke. In other words, a representative cohort for the prediction of motor recovery and motor

outcomes is that of an acute stroke cohort. To determine if a cohort is representative of an acute stroke cohort, we consider two factors: the time point of recruitment (i.e., *when* patients entered the study) and the method of sampling (i.e., *how* patients entered the study). For the time point of recruitment, it is ideal if patients are recruited in the first few days after stroke. Such a cohort is often termed an inception cohort, and refers to a group of patients recruited at an early and uniform time point in the course of their disease.[5,22] The recruitment of an inception cohort is important to ensure accurate estimates of prognosis, since the prognosis of a patient with an acute stroke ($\leq$7 days post stroke)[23] is likely to differ from the prognosis of a patient with subacute (7 days–6 months post stroke)[23] or chronic stroke (>6 months post stroke).[23] Regarding the method of sampling, aspects of an ideal sampling method include a prospective cohort study design (to minimize missing data), recruitment of consecutive cases (to ensure patients are not selectively recruited), and a broad inclusion criteria (to ensure patients recruited are generalizable to the patients seen by clinicians early after stroke).[10]

Several prediction modeling studies of arm and leg motor function and activities have fulfilled most of these criteria (i.e., three out of four criteria), by recruiting inception cohorts, collecting data prospectively, enrolling consecutive cases, and/or including patients with minimal restrictions on inclusion criteria.[15,24–31] In addition, some studies have also recruited patients from multiple hospitals[26,27] or registries,[32] which increase the generalizability of the cohorts to a wider stroke population. It should be noted that sometimes prediction models of arm and leg motor function and activities are developed on a select group of patients included in trials[33–40] or referred for rehabilitation.[41–62] These two cohorts are less representative of acute stroke cohorts because trial cohorts are sometimes recruited at different time points post stroke, and enrolment is based on strict inclusion criteria, while rehabilitation cohorts may have atypically good prognoses. Use of these samples in the development of models may therefore produce biased predictions that cannot be applied to the wider stroke population. Other than the time point of recruitment and method of sampling, clinicians should also check that the demographics and baseline clinical characteristics of the study cohort are similar to that of patients seen in their practice to determine representativeness of the cohort.

Did the Development Study Standardize Measurement of Predictors?

For models to be accurate in predicting motor recovery and outcomes, predictors have to be standardized in their definitions, measurement methods, and timing of measurement.[9,10,12] Standardization of definitions and measurement methods of predictors are important because heterogeneity in the definition and measurement of predictors might influence the strength of the predictors, thus affecting their inclusion in the final model.[10] With regards to the timing of measurement, it is ideal if predictors can be collected at a similar time point to when the model might be used in clinical practice.[9,10] Therefore, if a model is to be used early after stroke, predictors should be collected shortly after stroke onset (e.g., first few days after stroke), or before the outcome of interest has occurred. It is also necessary to ensure that the predictors can be obtained at the time of measurement.[9,10] Therefore, standardized predictors are often data that are routinely collected at stroke admission to acute stroke units, such as age, premorbid dependency, and neurological impairments. This makes it easier for clinicians to use the final prediction model in clinical practice.[1,9,17,63]

Standardization of the definitions and measurement methods of predictors can be achieved by using measurement tools that have been shown to be reliable and valid,[12] such as the National Institutes of Health Stroke Scale (NIHSS). The NIHSS is a 15-item impairment scale that measures stroke severity, with a final score ranging from 0 to 42. The higher the score, the more severe the stroke.[64] The NIHSS has demonstrated moderate to high reliability ($\kappa = 0.66$ to 0.77)[65] and moderate concurrent validity when compared to computed tomography (CT) and magnetic resonance imaging (MRI) data on infarct size and volume ($r = 0.61$ and 0.68).[65,66] In some prediction models of arm motor outcomes, predictors such as active range of motion, muscle strength, and sensation of the affected arm have been identified.[39,67,68] These predictors were measured with equipment such as a 3D tracking system,[67] a handheld dynamometer,[39] and a two-point discriminator,[68] respectively. The issues with these measurement tools are that their reliability and validity have not been tested (or reported in original studies), and that they are less readily available in stroke units. Scales that measure a combination of impairments such as the Orpington Prognostic Score and the Orgogozo Score have also been identified as predictors of arm and leg motor outcomes.[31,51] but these scales are less commonly used than the NIHSS.[64] Therapy intensity or length of stay has also been

identified to predict the recovery of walking.[24,46,69] However, it is not possible to obtain these predictors early after stroke since therapy has not commenced and length of hospital stay is not known. The biggest problem perhaps with the measurement of predictors is the timing of measurements after stroke onset. We have mentioned that clinicians often need to make predictions of motor outcomes early after stroke and hence, predictors should ideally be collected in the first few days after stroke. However, a number of prediction modeling studies of arm and leg motor outcomes have measured predictors in a time frame that extends beyond 7 days of stroke onset (i.e., within 2−4 weeks after stroke).[15,33,34,38,44,54,61,70] Some clinicians might therefore consider these prediction models less applicable to their acute patient cohorts.

Did the Development Study Standardize Measurement of Outcomes?

The reasons for standardizing outcomes in terms of definitions, measurement methods, and timing of measurement are similar to the reasons for standardizing predictors.[10] If outcome definitions and methods are not consistently measured across studies, it is likely that reported outcomes might not reflect the actual outcomes achieved by patients, resulting in biased predictions from the model.[10] In terms of timing of outcome assessment, it is important that outcome assessments are performed at a fixed time point after stroke onset when recovery of motor outcomes has more or less plateaued.[71] This is important for two reasons. First, a fixed time point (e.g., 6 months after stroke) as opposed to a variable time point (e.g., discharge) will reduce the heterogeneity in outcomes achieved by patients. Second, outcomes collected at a fixed time point when recovery has plateaued (e.g., 3 months after stroke) are likely to reflect a patient's optimum physical capacity.[71] In fact, studies have shown that the recovery pattern of stroke follows a nonlinear pathway, with patients showing a steep and then gradual improvement in their motor function and activities in the first few weeks after stroke, followed by a plateau around 3−6 months after stroke[34,38,57,72−76] (see Fig. 2.1 for a hypothetical pattern of stroke recovery; similar figures of recovery pattern can also be found in studies that have measured recovery of motor function and activities in patients after stroke[34,38,57,72−76]).

For the most part, prediction modeling studies on arm and leg motor function and activities have used reliable and valid outcome measures. Common outcome measures used in prediction modeling studies

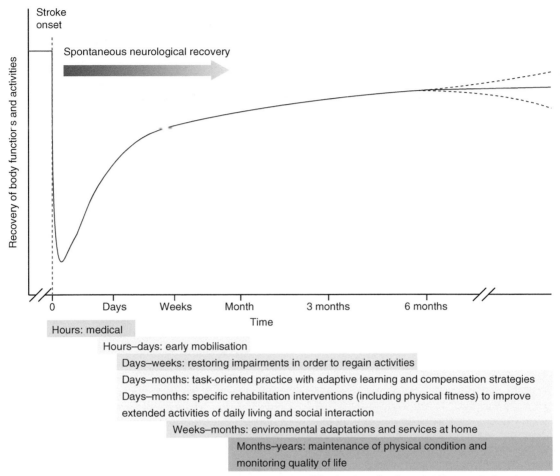

FIG. 2.1 Hypothetical pattern of recovery after stroke. (Obtained and adapted with permission from Langhorne P, Bernhardt J, Kwakkel G. Stroke rehabilitation. *Lancet*. May 14, 2011;377(9778):1693—1702.)

of arm and leg motor function include the Fugl—Meyer Assessment—Upper Extremity subscale (FMA-UE)[25,78] and Fugl—Meyer Assessment—Lower Extremity subscale (FMA-LE).[79] For measures of arm activities, common measurement instruments include the Action Research Arm Test (ARAT),[27,37,59,68,80] the Nine Hole Peg Test (NHPT),[25,31,38] and upper limb subscale of the Motor Assessment Scale (MAS),[15,81—83] while measurement instruments selected for leg activities (i.e., walking) include the Functional Ambulation Classification (FAC),[26,33,44,47,52] the Rivermead Mobility Index,[50,54] walking items of the MAS,[15] the Barthel Index (BI),[30,46,82,84] and the Functional Independence Measure (FIM).[43,45,53,70,85] Data regarding the reliability and validity of these outcome measures can

be found on the Rehabilitation Measures Database: http://www.rehabmeasures.org/default.aspx or Stroke Engine Database: https://www.strokengine.ca/find-assessment/. However, standardization of the timing of outcome assessment can be improved, as a substantial number of prediction modeling studies measure arm and leg motor function and activities at discharge,[29,30,32,43,46,47,50,53,69,82,83,85] which is highly variable in terms of timing post stroke and can vary significantly across stroke and rehabilitation units in different countries. Outcomes should preferably be measured at a fixed time point when recovery has plateaued (e.g., 3 months or 6 months after stroke).[71]

Due to poor standardization of predictor and/or outcome measurements, many prediction models of arm and leg motor function and activities may be susceptible to overfitting and predictor selection bias. It is likely that some of the predictors in these models will have spurious associations with the outcomes and that the models will inevitably produce inaccurate predictions when applied to new cohorts of patients.[10,17,20] Ultimately, the strongest protection against these problems comes from external validation of the models prior to their use in clinical practice.

Did the Validation Study Conduct External Validation?

If a prediction model is to be used in clinical practice, it must not only perform well in the original cohort on which it was developed, but also in new cohorts—preferably from other centers.[9,20,21] To allow comparisons between the model's performance in the development cohort and in the validation cohort, certain statistical measures have to be reported. Here, we briefly cover the most common statistical measures reported in prediction modeling studies of arm and leg motor function and activities so that readers can interpret the results from development and validation studies.

The two most common regression approaches used in prediction modeling studies of arm and leg motor recovery and outcomes are linear regression and logistic regression.[17] Linear regression is used when the outcome is considered to be continuous,[17] such as arm and leg motor function measured with the FMA.[78,79] The statistical measure that represents performance of a linear regression model is R^2—the variance in outcomes explained by the model. The higher the variance, the better the model is at predicting stroke recovery or outcome. Logistic regression is used when the endpoint is dichotomous,[17] such as ability to walk independently ("yes" or "no") measured with the FAC (score ≥ 4 vs. score <4)[26] or item 5 of the MAS (score ≥ 3 vs. score <3).[15] For logistic regression, performance of the model is usually reported in terms of discrimination and calibration.[10] Discrimination refers to how well the model can distinguish between patients with good and bad outcomes and is often quantified with the concordance statistic (C-stat) or the area under the receiver operating characteristic curve (AUC).[10] A perfect model will have a C-stat or AUC of 1[17]; this means that a model with a C-stat or AUC of 0.5 does no better than chance in predicting a patient's recovery or outcome. Calibration refers to how well-observed probabilities agree with predicted probabilities. These probabilities are often plotted against each other

so that, with perfect predictions (i.e., observed probabilities matching predicted probabilities) the observations fall along a line.[17] Other measures of model performance such as sensitivity and specificity (for discrimination) and the Hosmer–Lemeshow test (for calibration) are widely used but are less useful for quantifying model performance.[10,17]

To date, none of the prediction models of arm and leg motor function and activities is ready for use in clinical practice. The models have either not been externally validated, or there have been methodological issues with the external validation studies. We consider these problems in turn. Despite being reasonably well developed, some prediction models of arm and leg motor function and activities have not been externally validated.[15,25–28] In Tables 2.1 and 2.2, we present models of arm and leg motor function and activities that have fulfilled three of the four criteria (i.e., recruited representative cohorts, standardized measurements of predictors and outcomes, and conducted external validation of models). Several reasons may explain why most of the models are not externally validated. Researchers might not have access to new datasets from other centers, or lack the resources to repeat the study in the same center.[17] In addition, the model may require certain predictor and outcome measurements that are not available in other datasets, reducing the chances of external validation. For example, prediction modeling studies of walking have included predictors such as sitting balance measured with the Trunk Control Test, and muscle strength measured with the Motricity Index,[26] while outcome measurements have included the MAS[15] and FAC.[26] These measurements might be commonly performed by therapists in certain parts of the world, but data are not routinely collected as part of a national stroke registry or data bank.

For the prediction models of arm motor function and activities, two models—the Proportional Recovery (PR) model [78] (for recovery of arm motor function) and the Predict Recovery Potential (PREP) algorithm[80] (for outcome of arm activity)—have been externally validated.[40,86–88] However, there were three issues with the methods and the reporting of results in the external validation studies that question the generalizability of the models. First, in one of the validation studies for the PR model, the validation cohort included 14 out of the 30 participants who had been in the development cohort.[86] Second, the predictive accuracy of the PR model was often inflated by the exclusion of outliers in the development and validation studies. The development study reported high predictive accuracy

TABLE 2.1
Development and Validation Studies That Predict Arm Motor Function and Activities

Prediction Model; Authors (Year)	Sample Size, Type of Stroke; Source of Data	Timing of Predictors	Timing of Outcomes	Predictors in Multivariable Model (Measurement Tool)	Outcomes (Measurement Tool)	Results from Development Study	Results from External Validation Studies
PR; Prabhakaran (2008)[78]	N = 41 Ischemic; Hospital (one site)	≤ 3 days	6 months	• Arm motor function (FMA-UE)	Arm motor function (FMA-UE)	R^2 = 47% R^2 = 90% (excluding outliers)	SPE = 96% (excluding outliers)[§,86] SPE = 16% (including outliers)[§,86] R^2 = 0.94 (excluding outliers)[87] R^2 = 0.68 to 0.95 (in subgroups of patients)[§,40]
Persson (2015)[28]	N = 112 Ischemic and haemorrhagic; Hospital (one site)	3 days	10 days 1 month 12 months	• Arm activity (ARAT – two items: "pour water from glass to glass" and "place hand on top of head")	Arm motor function (FMA-UE ≥ 32)	AUC = 0.91 to 0.99	–
Kwah (2013)[15]	N = 51 Ischemic and haemorrhagic; Hospital (one site)	≤ 30 days (Median 6 days)	6 months (Median 6.1 months)	• Age • Severity of stroke (NIHSS)	Arm activity – Hand movements (MAS item 7 ≥ 5)	AUC = 0.73	–
	N = 56 Ischemic and haemorrhagic; Hospital (one site)	≤ 30 days (Median 6 days)	6 months (Median 6.1 months)	• Severity of stroke (NIHSS)	Arm activity – Advanced hand activities (MAS item 8 ≥ 5)	AUC = 0.82	–
Nijland (2010)[27]	N = 156 Ischemic; Hospitals (nine sites)	≤ 3 days 5 days 9 days	6 months	• Movement of finger extension (FMA-FE) • Movement of shoulder abduction (MI-SA)	Arm activity – Hand function (ARAT ≥ 10)	Sens = 0.89 to 0.95 Spec = 0.83 to 0.83	–

Continued

TABLE 2.1
Development and Validation Studies That Predict Arm Motor Function and Activities—cont'd

Prediction Model; Authors (Year)	Sample Size, Type of Stroke; Source of Data	Timing of Predictors	Timing of Outcomes	Predictors in Multivariable Model (Measurement Tool)	Outcomes (Measurement Tool)	Results from Development Study	Results from External Validation Studies
PREP; Stinear (2012)[80]	N = 40 Ischemic; Hospital (one site)	3 days	3 months	• Muscle strength of finger extension (MRC) • Muscle strength of shoulder abduction (MRC) • Presence of MEP (TMS) • Asymmetry index of FA (DW-MRI)	Arm activity – Excellent recovery (ARAT 51-57); Good recovery (ARAT 34-50); Limited recovery (ARAT 13-33); No recovery (ARAT 0-12)[88]	Sens = 0.73 Spec = 0.88 (for Excellent recovery)	Accuracy (% of correct predictions) = 80%[88]
Smania (2007)[25]	N = 48 Ischemic; Hospital (one site)	1 week	2 weeks 1 month 3 months 6 months	• Muscle strength of finger extension (MRC) • Presence/absence of shoulder shrug • Range of shoulder abduction • Hand movement scale	Arm motor function (FMA-UE, MI-arm); Arm activity (NHPT)	R² = 38 to 84%	-

ARAT, Action Research Arm Test; *AUC*, Area Under Curve; *DW-MRI*, Diffusion-Weighted Magnetic Resonance Imaging; *FA*, Fractional Anisotropy in the posterior limbs of the internal capsules; *FMA-UE*, Fugl-Meyer Assessment – Upper Extremity subscale; *FMA-FE*, Fugl-Meyer Assessment - Finger Extension; *MAS*, Motor Assessment Scale; *MEP*, Motor Evoked Potentials; *MI-arm*, Motricity Index – arm subscale; *MI-SA*, Motricity Index item - Shoulder Abduction; *MRC*, Medical Research Council; *NIHSS*, National Institutes of Health Stroke Scale; *NHPT*, Nine Hole Peg Test; *PREP*, Predicting Recovery Potential model; *PR*, Proportional Recovery model; R^2, Variance explained by linear regression model; *SPE*, Squared Prediction Error; *Sens*, Sensitivity; *Spec*, Specificity; *TMS*, Transcranial Magnetic Stimulation.

§Time point of outcome measure differs from time point used in original model.[86,40]

TABLE 2.2
Development Studies That Predict Leg Motor Function and Activities

Prediction Model; Authors (Year)	Sample Size, Type of Stroke; Source of Data	Timing of Predictors	Timing of Outcomes	Predictors in Multivariable Model (Measurement Tool)	Outcomes (Measurement Tool)	Results from Development Study	Results from External Validation Studies
PR; Smith (2017)[79]	N = 32 Ischemic and haemorrhagic; Hospital (one site)	3 days	3 months	• Leg motor function (FMA-LE)	Leg motor function (FMA-LE)	R^2 = 93%	-
Kwah (2013)[15]	N = 114 Ischemic and haemorrhagic; Hospital (one site)	≤ 30 days (Median 6 days)	6 months (Median 6.1 months)	• Age • Severity of stroke (NIHSS)	Leg activity – Independent walking (MAS item 5 ≥ 3)	AUC = 0.84	-
Veerbeek (2011)[26]	N = 154 Ischemic; Hospitals (nine sites)	≤ 3 days 5 days 9 days	6 months (Median 6.1 months)	• Sitting (TCT) • Muscle strength of leg (MI-leg)	Leg activity – Independent walking (FAC ≥ 4)	Sens = 0.93 to 0.94 Spec = 0.63 to 0.83	-

AUC, Area Under Curve; *FAC*, Functional Ambulation Category; *FMA-LE*, Fugl-Meyer Assessment – Lower Extremity; *MAS*, Motor Assessment Scale; *MI-leg*, Motricity Index of leg; *NIHSS*, National Institutes of Health Stroke Scale; *PR*, Proportional Recovery model; *TCT*, Trunk Control Test; R^2, Variance explained by linear regression model; *Sens*, Sensitivity; *Spec*, Specificity.

($r^2 = 0.90$) after excluding 7 of 41 patients with severe initial impairment on the grounds that they were "outliers."[78] With the outliers included, the original adjusted r^2 was only 0.47.[78] The same issue arose in the validation studies, which reported high predictive accuracy after excluding 65 of 211 patients[87] and 7 of 30 patients.[86] In the third validation study of the PR model, the performance of the PR model was only reported in subgroups of patients (i.e., patients with motor evoked potentials or patients with an FMA score of >10) rather than the whole cohort.[40] Third, the performance of the PREP model in the validation cohort has yet to be presented in full.[88] Authors have stated that the PREP model correctly predicted arm recovery in 80% of patients in the validation cohort.[88] However, without the presentation of discrimination and calibration results, it is hard to make direct comparisons of the model's performance between the development and the validation cohorts. In addition, some of the predictors in the PREP model require the use of neurophysiology and neuroimaging data, such as the presence of motor evoked potentials measured with Transcranial Magnetic Stimulation (TMS) and the asymmetry index of fractional anisotropy (FA) measured with Diffusion-Weighted Magnetic Resonance Imaging (DW-MRI).[80] These measurement tools might not be readily available in acute stroke units, or trained personnel might not be available to operate the equipment and interpret the results. For these reasons, it might be more difficult for clinicians to use the PREP model compared to models that only require clinical data.

WHICH PREDICTION MODEL OF MOTOR RECOVERY OR OUTCOME MIGHT BE READY FOR USE IN CLINICAL PRACTICE?

In the previous section, we covered four main criteria that clinicians can use to determine if the results of a prediction model are valid and applicable in clinical practice. We learned that prediction models of arm and leg motor function and activities are not ready for clinical implementation due to the lack of external validation or presence of methodological issues with external validation studies. Most prediction models of global disability, on the other hand, might be ready for use in clinical practice.

In a simple search of the literature, we identified 17 prediction models of global disability,[89–103] all of which have been externally validated with about half already tested in more than three different cohorts. Most of the models have performed well in these

external validation cohorts, with 14 models scoring an AUC or C-statistic greater than or equal to 0.80.[89–96,98–103] Most of the models recruited representative acute stroke cohorts, with 12 models developed on studies that recruited cohorts from prospective cohort studies,[89–91,93–103] registries,[89,91,93,94,96,103] or consecutive cohorts from hospitals.[89–92,96,98–101,103] For the most part, predictors were standardized in their definitions and measurement methods. Common predictors in the ischemic stroke models included age, severity of stroke (NIHSS), and presence of comorbidities (e.g., cancer, atrial fibrillation), while common predictors in the hemorrhagic stroke models included age, level of consciousness (Glasgow Coma Scale), and volume and location of hemorrhage (CT). The timing of predictors was also standardized, with most studies measuring predictors early after stroke onset (i.e., admission to 3 days).[89–93,95–103] All studies used standardized outcome measures such as the BI, modified Rankin Scale (mRS), Oxford Handicap Scale (OHS), and the Glasgow Outcome Scale (GOS). Most studies carried out measurement of outcomes at fixed and late time points after stroke (i.e., 3–12 months),[89,90,92–98,100,101] with only two studies measuring global disability at discharge[91,103] and two studies measuring global disability at 1 month.[99,102] Further details of the prediction models of global disability can be found in Table 2.3.

Here, we highlight two models of global disability that stand out above the rest. One model predicts outcome of global disability in ischemic strokes,[90] while the other model predicts outcome of global disability in hemorrhagic strokes.[104] These models have been developed on representative cohorts and have standardized their predictors and outcomes. In addition, both models have performed well in three or more external validation cohorts, and are presented in a simple user-friendly format. For these reasons, the ASTRAL model and the ESSEN ICH model might be more appealing for clinicians to use in clinical practice.

The ASTRAL Model

The ASTRAL model was developed on a consecutive cohort of 1645 patients who were admitted to a hospital in Lausanne, Switzerland, between January 1, 2003 and July 24, 2010.[90] The dataset was named the Acute Stroke Registry and Analysis of Lausanne (ASTRAL) and was designed to prospectively collect epidemiological, clinical, laboratory, and brain imaging data of patients with acute ischemic stroke within 24 hours after symptom onset.[105] The predictors in

TABLE 2.3
Development and Validation Studies That Predict Global Disability

Prediction Model; Authors (Year)	Sample Size, Type of Stroke; Source of Data	Timing of Predictors	Timing of Outcomes	Predictors in Multivariable Model (Measurement Tool)	Outcomes (Measurement Tool)	Results from Development Study	Results from External Validation Studies
DFS-AIS; Ji (2014)[89]	N = 7215 Ischemic; Registry	Admission	Discharge 3 months 6 months 12 months	• Age • Gender • Co-morbidities (DM, Stroke TIA) • Current smoking status • AF • Pre-stroke dependence • Pre-stroke statins • Severity of stroke (NIHSS) • BGL	Survival with no disability or mild disability (mRS 0-2)	AUC = 0.84 to 0.85[†]	AUC = 0.84[89]
ASTRAL; Ntaios (2012)[90]	N = 1645 Ischemic; Hospital (one site)	≤ 24 hours	3 months	• Age • Severity of stroke (NIHSS) • Time from onset to admission • Visual field deficit (item 3 of NIHSS) • BGL • LOC	Survival with moderate-severe disability or death (mRS 3-6)	AUC = 0.85	AUC = 0.80 to 0.81[†,‡,89] AUC = 0.77 and 0.93 (or combined = 0.90)[†,90] AUC = 0.78 and 0.79[†,108] AUC = 0.79[106] AUC = 0.81 and 0.82[†,107]
PLAN; O'Connell (2012)[103]	N = 4943 Ischemic; Registry	Admission	Discharge	• Pre-admission co-morbidities (Dependence, Ca, CHF, AF) • LOC • Age • Neurological deficits (Arm weakness, leg weakness, neglect or aphasia)	Survival with no disability or mild disability (mRS 0-2); Survival with severe disability or death (mRS 5-6)	AUC = 0.77 and 0.89[†]	AUC = 0.75 to 0.77[†,‡,89] AUC = 0.74 and 0.76[†,108] AUC = 0.80 and 0.88[†,103] AUC = 0.82 and 0.86[†,122]

Continued

TABLE 2.3
Development and Validation Studies That Predict Global Disability—cont'd

Prediction Model; Authors (Year)	Sample Size, Type of Stroke; Source of Data	Timing of Predictors	Timing of Outcomes	Predictors in Multivariable Model (Measurement Tool)	Outcomes (Measurement Tool)	Results from Development Study	Results from External Validation Studies
iScore*; Saposnik (2011)[109]	N = 3818 Ischemic; Registry	Admission	Discharge	• Age • Gender • Severity of stroke (CNS) • Stroke subtype • Risk factor (AF, CHF) • Co-morbidities (Ca, renal dialysis) • Pre-admission disability • BGL	Survival with moderate-severe disability (mRS 3-5) or death at 30 days; Institutionalization or death at 30 days	C-stat = 0.79 and 0.33[†]	AUC = 0.70 to 0.72[†,‡,89] AUC = 0.66 and 0.68[†,108] C-stat = 0.68 and 0.74[†,109] C-stat = 0.82[§,123]
FSV; Reid (2010)[92]	N = 538 Ischemic and haemorrhagic; Hospital (one site)	Admission	6 months	• Age • Independent pre-stroke • Normal verbal score (GCS) • Able to lift both arms • Able to walk	Survival with no disability or mild disability (mRS 0-2)	AUC = 0.88	AUC = 0.83 and 0.85[†,122] AUC = 0.77 and 0.79[†,92] AUC = 0.87[‡,124] AUC = 0.88 and 0.90[†,‡,§,125] ORC = 0.75[‡,126]
Weimar (2004)[93]	N = 1079 Ischemic; Registry	≤ 6 hours	100 days	• Age • Severity of stroke (NIHSS)	Dependence in daily activities (BI < 95) or death	AUC = 0.86 R² = 51%	AUC = 0.80 to 0.82[†,‡,§,89] ORC = 0.73[‡,§,126] R² = 44%[93] AUC = 0.81[§,127] C-stat = 0.73[‡,§,128]

Study	Population	Timing	Timepoint	Predictors	Outcome	AUC	AUC
SSV; Counsell (2002)[94]	N = 530 Ischemic and haemorrhagic; Registry	≤ 30 days (Median 4 days)	6 months	• Age • Living alone • Independent pre-stroke • Normal verbal score (GCS) • Able to lift both arms • Able to walk	Survival with no disability or mild disability (OHS 0-2)	AUC = not reported	AUC = 0.84 to 0.90[†,‡,§,125]; ORC = 0.72[‡,126]; C-stat = 0.73 and 0.74[†,‡,§,128]; AUC = 0.84[94]; AUC = 0.79[†,129]; AUC = 0.82[130]; C-stat = 0.77[†,‡,131]
ICHOP[87] and ICHOP,[26] Gupta (2017)[95]	N = 365 and 321[†] Haemorrhagic; Hospital (one site)	Admission	3 months 12 months	• LOC (GCS) • Severity of stroke (NIHSS) • Severity of disease (APACHE II$_{Phys}$) • Pre-morbid function (mRS) • Hematoma volume	Survival with no disability or mild-moderate disability (mRS 0-3); Survival with moderately severe-severe disability or death (mRS 4-6)	AUC = 0.89 and 0.87[†]	AUC = 0.75 and 0.84[†,95]
ICH-FOS; Ji (2013)[96]	N = 1953 Haemorrhagic; Registry	Admission	12 months	• Age • Severity of stroke (NIHSS) • LOC (GCS) • BGL • ICH location • Haematoma volume • IVH	Survival with moderate-severe disability or death (mRS 3-6); Survival with moderately severe-severe disability or death (mRS 4-6); Survival with severe disability or death (mRS 5-6)	AUC = 0.83 to 0.85[†]	AUC = 0.83 to 0.84[†,96]
s-ICH*; Bruce (2011)[97]	N = 84 Haemorrhagic; Hospital (one site)	Admission	3 months	• Age • LOC (GCS) • History of HT • BGL • Dialysis dependency	Survival with moderate-severe disability or death (mRS 3-6)	AUC = 0.89	AUC = 0.73 to 0.74[†,‡,96]

Continued

TABLE 2.3
Development and Validation Studies That Predict Global Disability—cont'd

Prediction Model; Authors (Year)	Sample Size, Type of Stroke; Source of Data	Timing of Predictors	Timing of Outcomes	Predictors in Multivariable Model (Measurement Tool)	Outcomes (Measurement Tool)	Results from Development Study	Results from External Validation Studies
FUNC; Rost (2008)[98]	N = 418 Haemorrhagic; Hospital (one site)	Admission	3 months	• Age • ICH volume • ICH location • LOC (GCS) • Pre-ICH cognition	Survival with no disability or mild-moderate disability (GOS 4-5)	C-stat = 0.88	AUC = 0.76 to 0.77[†,‡,96] C-stat = 0.82[98]
ICH-GS; Ruiz-Sandoval (2007)[99]	N = 310 Haemorrhagic; Hospital (one site)	Admission	1 month	• Age • LOC (GCS) • ICH location • ICH volume (supratentorial) • ICH volume (infratentorial) • IVH	Survival with no disability or mild-moderate disability (GOS 4-5)	AUC = 0.86	AUC = 0.77 to 0.78[‡,‡,96] AUC = 0.88[‡,§,97] AUC = 0.69[‡,§,111] AUC = 0.71 to 0.81[‡,‡,112]
Essen ICH; Weimar (2006)[100]	N = 340 Haemorrhagic; Hospitals (30 sites)	≤ 24 hours	100 days	• Age • Severity of stroke (NIHSS) • LOC (NIHSS item)	Independence in daily activities (BI ≥ 95)	AUC = 0.91	AUC = 0.81 to 0.84[‡,‡,§,96] AUC = 0.93[‡,§,97] AUC = 0.88[100] AUC = 0.79[§,132]
mICH-A and mICH-B; Godoy (2006)[101]	N = 153 Haemorrhagic; Hospitals (two sites)	≤ 24 hours	6 months	• Age • LOC (GCS) • ICH volume • IVH • Co-morbidities (APACHE II)	Survival with no disability or mild-moderate disability (GOS 4-5)	AUC for mICH-A = 0.89 AUC for mICH-B = 0.90	AUC for mICH-A = 0.91[‡,§,97] AUC for mICH-B = 0.90[‡,97]
New ICH; Cheung (2003)[102]	N = 141 Haemorrhagic; Hospital (one site)	Admission	1 month	• Severity of stroke (NIHSS) • Temperature • IVH • Pulse pressure • SAH	Survival with no disability or mild disability (mRS 0-2)	Sens = 0.70 Spec = 0.92 PPV = 0.85 NPV = 0.82 YI = 0.62	AUC = 0.74[‡,§,97]

				Outcome measure	Statistics	AUC/C-stat
Modified ICH; Cheung (2003)[102]	N = 141 Haemorrhagic; Hospital (one site)	Admission	1 month	Survival with no disability or mild disability (mRS 0-2)	Sens = 0.86 Spec = 0.78 PPV = 0.71 NPV = 0.90 YI = 0.64	AUC = 0.79 to 0.81[†,‡,96] AUC = 0.85[†,§,97] AUC = 0.75[†,‡,111] AUC = 0.81[†,§,100] AUC = 0.69 and 0.77[†,‡,§,113]
	Predictors: Age; Severity of stroke (NIHSS); ICH location; ICH volume; IVH					
Original ICH*; Cheung (2003)[102]	N = 141 Haemorrhagic; Hospital (one site)	Admission	1 month	Survival with no disability or mild disability (mRS 0-2)	Sens = 0.94 Spec = 0.61 PPV = 0.59 NPV = 0.94 YI = 0.54	AUC = 0.66 to 0.84[†,‡,95] AUC = 0.75 to 0.76[†,‡,96] AUC = 0.86[†,§,97] AUC = 0.82[†,§,99] AUC = 0.78[†,§,100] AUC = 0.84[†,§,101] AUC = 0.68[†,§,111] AUC = 0.72 to 0.79[†,‡,§,112] AUC = 0.72 and 0.79[†,‡,§,113] C-stat = 0.80 to 0.84[†,§,114]
	Predictors: Age; LOC (GCS); ICH location; ICH volume; IVH					

AF, Atrial Fibrillation; *APACHE II*, Acute Physiology and Chronic Health Evaluation II; *APACHE II$_{Phys}$*, Physiologic component of Acute Physiology and Chronic Health Evaluation II (excludes GCS); *ASTRAL*, Acute Stroke Registry and Analysis of Lausanne; *AUC*, Area Under Curve; *BGL*, Blood Glucose Levels; *BI*, Barthel Index; *Ca*, Cancer; *CHF*, Congestive Heart Failure; *CNS*, Canadian Neurological Scale; *C-stat*, C-statistic; *DFS-AIS*, Dynamic Functional Status after Acute Ischemic Stroke; *DM*, Diabetes Mellitus; *FSV*, Five Simple Variables; *FUNC*, Functional Independence score; *GCS*, Glasgow Coma Scale; *GOS*, Glasgow Outcome Scale; *HT*, Hypertension; *ICH*, Intracerebral Haemorrhage score; *ICH-3S*, Intracerebral Haemorrhage Grading Scale; *ICHOP*, Intracerebral Haemorrhage Outcomes Project; *ICH-FOS*, Intracerebral Haemorrhage-Functional Outcome Score; *iSCORE*, Ischemic Stroke Predictive Risk Score; *IVH*, Intraventricular Haemorrhage/extension; *LOC*, Level of Consciousness; *mICH-A and m-ICH-B*, modified Intracerebral Haemorrhage-A and modified Intracerebral Haemorrhage-B scores (similar to original ICH score except removal of localization as a variable, and use of different cut-off values for other variables); *mRS*, modified Rankin Scale; *NPV*, Negative Predictive Value; *NIHSS*, National Institutes of Health Stroke Scale; *OHS*, Oxford Handicap Scale; *ORC*, Ordinal equivalent to the AUC; *PPV*, Positive Predictive Value; *PLAN*, Preadmission comorbidities, Level of consciousness, Age, and Neurologic deficit; *R²*, Variance explained by linear regression model; *SAH*, Subarachnoid Haemorrhage/extension; *Sens*, Sensitivity; *s-ICH*, simplified ICH score; *Spec*, Specificity; *SSV*, Six Simple Variables; *TIA*, Transient Ischemic Attack; *YI*, Youden's Index.

*The iScore, ICH score and s-ICH score were originally developed to predict mortality.[109,133,134]

†Numbers relate to two or more groups of patients; groups of patients differ either in terms of outcome measures,[109] cut-off points used for outcome measures; (i.e., two or more than two cut-off points using the same outcome measure were reported in studies),[19,96,103,112,114] time points of outcome measures,[89,95,96,107,112,113,122,125,128] type of cohort (e.g. two different validation cohorts,[90,92,95] two different data analyses,[108,128] or two different types of treatment/care that patients received).[113]

‡Outcome measure differs from outcome measure used in original model; either a different scale or a different cut-off point was used[89,95–97,99–101,111–113,124–126,128,129,131]

§Time point of outcome measure differs from time point used in original model[41,95–97,99–101,111–114,123,125–128]

Definition of outcomes in table were classified as follows: "Survival with no disability or mild disability" if mRS = 0-2 or OHS = 0-2; "Survival with no disability" or mild-moderate disability" if mRS = 0-3 or GOS = 4-5; "Survival with moderate-severe disability or death" if mRS = 3-6; "Survival with moderately severe-severe disability or death" if mRS = 4-6; "Survival with severe disability or death" if mRS = 5-6; "Independence in daily activities" if BI ≥ 95; "Dependence in daily activities" if BI < 95.

the final model included age, severity of stroke (NIHSS), stroke onset to admission time, visual field deficit (item 3 of NIHSS), blood glucose levels, and level of consciousness. All are data that are easily obtained in acute stroke units. The endpoint was unfavorable outcome (moderate to severe disability or death), defined as a score of >2 on the mRS at 3 months. Not only did the ASTRAL model perform well in the development cohort (AUC = 0.85), it also performed well in five external validation cohorts (range of AUC = 0.77 to 0.93).[89,90,106–108] In addition, the ASTRAL model outperformed most of the other prediction models of global disability when applied to a large independent cohort of patients (N = 4811) from the China National Stroke Registry (see Fig. 2.2).

A prediction model may be well developed and perform well in external validation cohorts, but still may not be used by busy clinicians if the model is presented in its raw format of a mathematical equation with its regression coefficients.[1,2] To present the ASTRAL model in a user-friendly format, Ntaios and colleagues have used a color chart to present probabilities of an

unfavorable outcome of global disability in a patient (see Fig. 2.3).

As an example, an 85-year-old gentleman arrives at the hospital 4 h (240 min) after acute stroke onset with a blood glucose level of 9.0 mmol/L and an NIHSS score of 15. The patient is alert and oriented and has no visual field deficits. Based on the color chart, the patient has an 80%–89% probability of moderate to severe disability or death at 3 months.

The ESSEN ICH Model

In general, ischemic strokes and hemorrhagic strokes are believed to have different prognoses due to different stroke mechanisms and risk factors.[109,110] This explains why most prediction models are either developed on patients with ischemic strokes or hemorrhagic strokes (see Table 2.3). The ESSEN ICH model was developed on data obtained from the German Stroke Data Bank.[104] The cohort included 340 patients recruited consecutively from 30 hospital sites between 1998 and 1999 in Essen, Germany.[100] Predictors in the ESSEN ICH model included age, severity of stroke

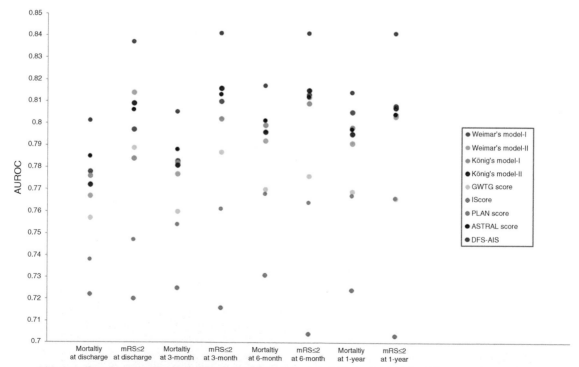

FIG. 2.2 Comparison of model performance in predicting mortality and global disability in a registry cohort of patients with ischemic stroke. (Obtained with permission from Ji R, Du W, Shen H, et al. Web-based tool for dynamic functional outcome after acute ischemic stroke and comparison with existing models. *BMC Neurol.* 2014;14:214.)

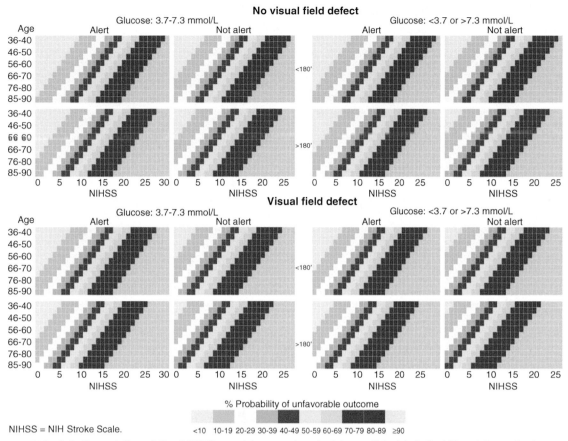

FIG. 2.3 Presentation of the ASTRAL model as a color chart to predict global disability at 3 months in ischemic strokes. (Obtained with permission from Ntaios G, Faouzi M, Ferrari J, Lang W, Vemmos K, Michel P. An integer-based score to predict functional outcome in acute ischemic stroke: the ASTRAL score. *Neurology*. June 12, 2012;78(24):1916–1922.)

(NIHSS), and level of consciousness (item 1 of NIHSS). Endpoint in the ESSEN ICH model was outcome of functional independence in activities of daily living (e.g., a combination of feeding, dressing, walking, grooming, toileting, and bathing) measured with the 100-point version of the BI. Functional independency was defined as a score of ≥95 on the BI. Out of the 10 prediction models developed on hemorrhagic strokes, the ESSEN model[100] had the best performance in its external validation cohorts (AUC range 0.79−0.93) compared to other models such as the ICH-GS (Intracerebral Haemorrhage Grading Scale) model[99] (AUC range 0.69 to 0.88[96,97,111,112]) and the original ICH (Intracerebral Haemorrhage) model[102] (AUC and C-statistic range 0.66 to 0.86[95−97,99,101,111−114]) (see Table 2.3). Furthermore,

the ESSEN ICH model outperformed most of the other prediction models of global disability outcome when applied to a large independent cohort of patients (N = 3255) from the China National Stroke Registry (see Fig. 2.4).

The ESSEN ICH model is presented as a score chart ranging from 0 to 10 (see Fig. 2.5). Using the same patient as seen earlier for the ASTRAL model, an 85-year-old gentleman with an NIHSS score of 15 and who is alert and orientated will score an ESSEN ICH score of 5. The score indicates to users that the patient is unlikely to die, but also unlikely to achieve functional independence. However, the caveat with the ESSEN ICH score is that, unlike the ASTRAL score, it does not inform the user regarding the specific probability of outcomes.

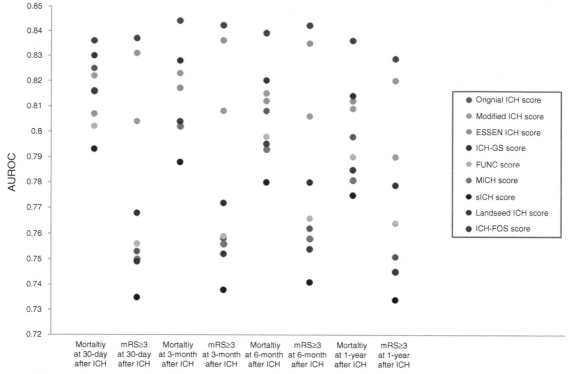

FIG. 2.4 Comparison of model performance in predicting mortality and global disability in a registry cohort of patients with hemorrhagic stroke. (Obtained with permission from Ji R, Shen H, Pan Y, et al. A novel risk score to predict 1-year functional outcome after intracerebral hemorrhage and comparison with existing scores. *Crit Care.* November 29, 2013;17(6):R275.)

CONCLUSIONS: SUMMARY AND IMPLICATIONS FOR CLINICIANS AND RESEARCHERS

In the preceding chapter, we learned that clinical experience and research evidence (i.e., prediction models) are the two best sources of information to guide our predictions of motor recovery and outcomes after stroke. To determine if the results of a prediction model are valid and applicable in clinical practice, we consider four main criteria [see Box 2.3 for summary of four criteria].

It is important for readers to note that there are other criteria that might influence the risk of bias and applicability of a prediction model (e.g., handling of continuous predictors and missing data, sample size, ratio of predictors to outcomes, and type of selection method for predictors during multivariable analysis).[10,12] Readers can refer to the QUIPS (Quality In Prognostic Studies) tool[12] and CHARMS (CHecklist for critical Appraisal and data extraction for systematic

Reviews of prediction Modelling Studies) checklist[10] for a more in-depth read of these criteria. In this chapter, we have also provided an overview of prediction models of motor outcomes in stroke. While many models predicting global disability after stroke appear well developed and externally validated, few models for predicting arm and leg motor function and activities have been well developed and none have been fully externally validated. Hence, models of global disability might potentially be more ready for use in clinical practice than models of arm and leg motor function and activities. We conclude the chapter with recommendations for clinicians and researchers.

Implications for clinicians: We recommend clinicians to use both clinical experience and research evidence to guide predictions of motor recovery and outcomes after stroke. These predictions are needed for organizing and delivering ongoing appropriate care to patients with stroke. We recommend clinicians to reassess patients regularly to optimize predictions,

Table 1 Prognostic scores for complete recovery and death following intracerebral haemorrhage

Predictors	Essen ICH score	ICH score[8]	Modified ICH score[7]
Age	<60 = 0 60–69 = 1 70–79 = 2 ≥80 = 3	<80 = 0 ≥80 = 1	<80 = 0 ≥80 = 1
NIH-SS	0–5 = 0 6–10 = 1 11–15 = 2 16–20 = 3 >20 or coma = 4		0–10 = 0 11–20 = 1 21–40 = 2
NIH-SS level of consciousness	Alert = 0 Drowsy = 1 Stupor = 2 Coma = 3		
Glasgow coma scale (GCS)		3–4 = 2 5–12 = 1 13–15 = 0	
Haemorrhage volume (cm^3)		≥30 = 1 <30 = 0	≥30 = 1 <30 = 0
Infratentorial origin		Yes = 1 No = 0	Yes = 1 No = 0
Intraventricular haemorrhage		Yes = 1 No = 0	Yes = 1 No = 0
Maximum score	10	6	6
Death predicted	>7	≥3	≥3
Good outcome predicted	<3	<3	<3
Definition of good outcome	Barthel index ≥95	Rankin scale ≤2	Rankin scale ≤2
Follow up (days)	100	30	30

ICH, intracerebral haemorrhage; NIH-SS, National Institutes of Health stroke scale.

FIG. 2.5 Presentation of the ESSEN ICH model as a scoring chart to predict global disability at 100 days in hemorrhagic strokes. (Obtained with permission from Weimar C, Benemann J, Diener HC, German Stroke Study C. Development and validation of the Essen intracerebral haemorrhage score. *J Neurol Neurosurg Psychiatry*. May 2006;77(5):601–605.)

and with that care. Reassessment is particularly important for patients who might be expected to have unfavorable outcomes but achieve favorable outcomes instead. Frequency of reassessments should be done in a fading manner; more frequent reevaluation early after stroke (e.g., every week in the first few weeks), followed by less frequent reevaluation later after stroke (e.g., monthly till 6 months).[115] Prior to using a prediction model in clinical practice, check that the model has been well developed (i.e., recruited representative cohort, standardized measurement of predictors and outcomes) and externally validated with good performance. In addition, select the prediction model based on the motor function or activity you wish to predict and the predictors available to you in your practice.

BOX 2.3
Four Criteria to Determine if a Prediction Model is Ready for Use in Clinical Practice

1. **Did the development study recruit representative cohorts?** Cohorts have to be similar to the patients seen by clinicians in the acute stage after stroke. Cohorts are considered to be representative of acute stroke cohorts, if they meet most of these criteria, that is, recruited inception cohorts, collected data prospectively, enrolled consecutive cases, and included patients based on a broad inclusion criteria.
2. **Did the development study standardize measurement of predictors?** Predictors have to be standardized in terms of definition, measurement methods, and timing of assessment. Measurements are considered to be standardized if measured with reliable and valid measurement tools at fixed and early time points after stroke (e.g., first few days after stroke).
3. **Did the development study standardize measurement of outcomes?** Outcomes have to be standardized in terms of definition, measurement methods, and timing of assessment. Measurements are considered to be standardized if measured with reliable and valid measurement tools at fixed and late time points after stroke (e.g., ≥3 months after stroke).
4. **Did the validation study conduct external validation?** External validation requires testing the performance of the prediction model on a new cohort of patients (i.e., patients that were not in the development study). New patients can be recruited from the same center or different centers.

Implications for researchers: In this chapter, we have highlighted eight models of arm and leg motor function and activities that are well developed. However, these models require external validation. Models of global disability have progressed to the stage where impact studies are needed, particularly if clinicians wish for more evidence that using these models will lead to improvement in patients' recovery and outcomes, and cost-effectiveness of care.

Most models presented in this chapter have measured outcomes at one time point. These models only provide insight into the prediction of outcomes, but not the prediction of *recovery patterns*. In order to predict recovery patterns, there is a need for the development of patient-specific (dynamic) models that have the ability to predict the time course of recovery after stroke.[71] As these dynamic models measure predictors and outcomes at multiple time points after disease, they allow clinicians to predict recovery patterns, rather than the presence or absence of an outcome measured

at one time point after stroke.[73,74] These dynamic models may therefore be useful in identifying patients that do not follow the expected time-course of recovery within the first 3 months after stroke. It should be noted however that the development of dynamic models requires intensive repeated measurement of clinical predictors and outcomes after stroke. Therefore, the challenge for the future is to develop and externally validate these dynamic and patient-specific models,[73,74] so that stroke care can be better tailored and reevaluated over time. Acknowledging that the time-course of stroke recovery is mainly driven by processes of poorly understood reactive neurobiological recovery, recent studies have introduced the proportional recovery rule for estimating the impact of expected change on the body function level of the ICF framework. This rule suggests that patients regain 70% of their maximum potential recovery in arm motor function,[78,87] language function,[116] and perceptual cognitive function[117] within the first 3 months. Lastly, we recommend researchers of future development studies to refer to the consensus-based core recommendations recently published by the Stroke Recovery and Rehabilitation Roundtable (SRRR) taskforce.[23,118−121] This series of landmark papers include recommendations for standardized definitions, measurement tools, and time points to be included in future studies on stroke recovery, and are significant in moving stroke recovery research forward.

REFERENCES

1. Counsell C, Dennis M. Systematic review of prognostic models in patients with acute stroke. *Cerebrovasc Dis.* 2001;12(3):159−170.
2. Veerbeek JM, Kwakkel G, van Wegen EE, Ket JC, Heymans MW. Early prediction of outcome of activities of daily living after stroke: a systematic review. *Stroke.* 2011;42(5):1482−1488.
3. Stinear C. Prediction of recovery of motor function after stroke. *Lancet Neurol.* 2010;9(12):1228−1232.
4. Pollock A, St George B, Fenton M, Firkins L. Top 10 research priorities relating to life after stroke—consensus from stroke survivors, caregivers, and health professionals. *Int J Stroke.* 2014;9(3):313−320.
5. Herbert R, Jamtvedt G, Mead J, Hagen K. *Practical Evidence-based Physiotherapy.* 2nd ed. United Kingdom: Elsevier Butterworth Heinemann; 2011.
6. Navi BB, Kamel H, McCulloch CE, et al. Accuracy of neurovascular fellows' prognostication of outcome after subarachnoid hemorrhage. *Stroke.* 2012;43(3):702−707.
7. Finley Caulfield A, Gabler L, Lansberg MG, et al. Outcome prediction in mechanically ventilated neurologic patients by junior neurointensivists. *Neurology.* 2010;74(14):1096−1101.

8. Kwakkel G, van Dijk GM, Wagenaar RC. Accuracy of physical and occupational therapists' early predictions of recovery after severe middle cerebral artery stroke. *Clin Rehabil.* 2000;14(1):28–41.

9. Moons KG, Royston P, Vergouwe Y, Grobbee DE, Altman DG. Prognosis and prognostic research: what, why, and how? *BMJ Clin Res Ed.* 2009;338:b375.

10. Moons KG, de Groot JA, Bouwmeester W, et al. Critical appraisal and data extraction for systematic reviews of prediction modelling studies: the CHARMS checklist. *PLoS Med.* 2014;11(10):e1001744.

11. von Elm E, Altman DG, Egger M, Pocock SJ, Gotzsche PC, Vandenbroucke JP. The strengthening the reporting of observational studies in epidemiology (STROBE) statement: guidelines for reporting observational studies. *J Clin Epidemiol.* 2008;61(4):344–349.

12. Hayden JA, van der Windt DA, Cartwright JL, Cote P, Bombardier C. Assessing bias in studies of prognostic factors. *Ann Intern Med.* 2013;158(4):280–286.

13. Collins GS, Reitsma JB, Altman DG, Moons KG. Transparent reporting of a multivariable prediction model for individual prognosis or diagnosis (TRIPOD): the TRIPOD statement. *BMJ.* 2015;350:g7594.

14. Moons KG, Altman DG, Reitsma JB, et al. Transparent reporting of a multivariable prediction model for individual prognosis or diagnosis (TRIPOD): explanation and elaboration. *Ann Intern Med.* 2015;162(1):W1–W73.

15. Kwah LK, Harvey LA, Diong J, Herbert RD. Models containing age and NIHSS predict recovery of ambulation and upper limb function six months after stroke: an observational study. *J Physiother.* 2013;59(3):189–197.

16. Altman DG, Vergouwe Y, Royston P, Moons KG. Prognosis and prognostic research: validating a prognostic model. *BMJ Clin Res Ed.* 2009;338:b605.

17. Steyerberg E. *Clinical Prediction Models: A Practical Approach to Development, Validation, and Updating.* Rotterdam, The Netherlands: Springer; 2010.

18. Moons KG, Altman DG, Vergouwe Y, Royston P. Prognosis and prognostic research: application and impact of prognostic models in clinical practice. *BMJ Clin Res Ed.* 2009;338:b606.

19. Steyerberg EW, Moons KGM, van der Windt DA, et al. Prognosis research strategy (PROGRESS) 3: prognostic model research. *PLoS Med.* 2013;10(2).

20. Harrell FE Jr, Lee KL, Mark DB. Multivariable prognostic models: issues in developing models, evaluating assumptions and adequacy, and measuring and reducing errors. *Statistics Med.* 1996;15(4):361–387.

21. Altman DG, Royston P. What do we mean by validating a prognostic model? *Statistics Med.* 2000;19(4):453–473.

22. Fletcher RH, Fletcher SW. *Clinical Epidemiology: The Essentials.* 4th ed. Philadelphia, Pennsylvania, USA: Lippincott Williams & Wilkins; 2005.

23. Bernhardt J, Hayward KS, Kwakkel G, et al. Agreed definitions and a shared vision for new standards in stroke recovery research: the stroker recovery and rehabilitation roundtable taskforce. *Int J Stroke.* 2017;12(5):444–450.

24. Scrivener K, Sherrington C, Schurr K. Amount of exercise in the first week after stroke predicts walking speed and unassisted walking. *Neurorehabil Neural Repair.* 2012; 26(8):932–938.

25. Smania N, Paolucci S, Tinazzi M, et al. Active finger extension: a simple movement predicting recovery of arm function in patients with acute stroke. *Stroke.* 2007; 38(3):1088–1090.

26. Veerbeek JM, Van Wegen EE, Harmeling-Van der Wel BC, Kwakkel G. Is accurate prediction of gait in nonambulatory stroke patients possible within 72 hours poststroke? The EPOS study. *Neurorehabil Neural Repair.* 2011;25(3): 268–274.

27. Nijland RHM, van Wegen EEH, Harmeling-van der Wel BC, Kwakkel G, Investigators E. Presence of finger extension and shoulder abduction within 72 hours after stroke predicts functional recovery. Early prediction of functional outcome after stroke: the EPOS cohort study. *Stroke.* 2010;41(4):745–750.

28. Persson HC, Alt Murphy M, Danielsson A, Lundgren-Nilsson A, Sunnerhagen KS. A cohort study investigating a simple, early assessment to predict upper extremity function after stroke – a part of the SALGOT study. *BMC Neurol.* 2015;15(1):92.

29. Wandel A, Jorgensen HS, Nakayama H, Raaschou HO, Olsen TS. Prediction of walking function in stroke patients with initial lower extremity paralysis: the Copenhagen stroke study. *Arch Phys Med Rehabil.* 2000;81(6): 736–738.

30. Jorgensen HS, Nakayama H, Raaschou HO, Olsen TS. Recovery of walking function in stroke patients – the Copenhagen stroke study. *Arch Phys Med Rehabil.* 1995; 76(1):27–32.

31. Meldrum D, Pittock SJ, Hardiman O, Ni Dhuill C, O'Regan M. Recovery of the upper limb post ischaemic stroke and the predictive value of the Orpington prognostic score. *Clin Rehabil.* 2004;18(6):694–702.

32. Dallas MI, Rone-Adams S, Echternach JL, Brass LM, Bravata DM. Dependence in prestroke mobility predicts adverse outcomes among patients with acute ischemic stroke. *Stroke.* 2008;39(8):2298–2303.

33. Kollen B, Kwakkel G, Lindeman E. Longitudinal robustness of variables predicting independent gait following severe middle cerebral artery stroke: a prospective cohort study. *Clin Rehabil.* 2006;20(3):262–268.

34. Kollen B, van de Port I, Lindeman E, Twisk J, Kwakkel G. Predicting improvement in gait after stroke: a longitudinal prospective study. *Stroke.* 2005;36(12):2676–2680.

35. Prescott RJ, Garraway WM, Akhtar AJ. Predicting functional outcome following acute stroke using a standard clinical examination. *Stroke.* 1982;13(5):641–647.

36. Kwakkel G, Kollen B. Predicting improvement in the upper paretic limb after stroke: a longitudinal prospective study. *Restor Neurol Neurosci.* 2007;25(5–6):453–460.

37. Kwakkel G, Kollen BJ, van der Grond J, Prevo AJH. Probability of regaining dexterity in the flaccid upper limb – impact of severity of paresis and time since onset in acute stroke. *Stroke*. 2003;34(9):2181–2186.

38. Sunderland A, Tinson D, Bradley L, Hewer RL. Arm function after stroke - an evaluation of grip strength as a measure of recovery and a prognostic indicator. *J Neurol Neurosurg Psychiatry*. 1989;52(11):1267–1272.

39. Wagner JM, Lang CE, Sahrmann SA, Edwards DF, Dromerick AW. Sensorimotor impairments and reaching performance in subjects with poststroke hemiparesis during the first few months of recovery. *Phys Ther*. 2007; 87(6):751–765.

40. Byblow WD, Stinear CM, Barber PA, Petoe MA, Ackerley SJ. Proportional recovery after stroke depends on corticomotor integrity. *Ann Neurol*. 2015;78(6): 848–859.

41. Feys H, De Weerdt W, Nuyens G, van de Winckel A, Selz B, Kiekens C. Predicting motor recovery of the upper limb after stroke rehabilitation: value of a clinical examination. *Physiother Res Int*. 2000;5(1):1–18.

42. Feys H, Van Hees J, Bruyninckx F, Mercelis R, De Weerdt W. Value of somatosensory and motor evoked potentials in predicting arm recovery after a stroke. *J Neurol Neurosurg Psychiatry*. 2000;68(3):323–331.

43. Chae J, Johnston M, Kim H, Zorowitz R. Admission motor impairment as a predictor of physical disability after stroke rehabilitation. *Am J Phys Med Rehabil*. 1995; 74(3):218–223.

44. Duarte E, Marco E, Muniesa JM, Belmonte R, Aguilar JJ, Escalada F. Early detection of non-ambulatory survivors six months after stroke. *NeuroRehabilitation*. 2010;26(4): 317–323.

45. Hellstrom K, Lindmark B, Wahlberg B, Fugl-Meyer AR. Self-efficacy in relation to impairments and activities of daily living disability in elderly patients with stroke: a prospective investigation. *J Rehabil Med*. 2003;35(5): 202–207.

46. Hu MH, Hsu SS, Yip PK, Jeng JS, Wang YH. Early and intensive rehabilitation predicts good functional outcomes in patients admitted to the stroke intensive care unit. *Disabil Rehabil*. 2010;32(15):1251–1259.

47. Masiero S, Avesani R, Armani M, Verena P, Ermani M. Predictive factors for ambulation in stroke patients in the rehabilitation setting: a multivariate analysis. *Clin Neurol Neurosurg*. 2007;109(9):763–769.

48. Mayo NE, Korner-Bitensky NA, Becker R. Recovery time of independent function post-stroke. *Am J Phys Med Rehabil*. 1991;70(1):5–12.

49. Olsen TS. Arm and leg paresis as outcome predictors in stroke rehabilitation. *Stroke*. 1990;21(2):247–251.

50. Paolucci S, Bragoni M, Coiro P, et al. Quantification of the probability of reaching mobility independence at discharge from a rehabilitation hospital in nonwalking early ischemic stroke patients: a multivariate study. *Cerebrovasc Dis*. 2008;26(1):16–22.

51. Petrilli S, Durufle A, Nicolas B, Pinel JF, Kerdoncuff V, Gallien P. Prognostic factors in the recovery of the ability to walk after stroke. *J Stroke Cerebrovasc Dis*. 2002;11(6): 330–335.

52. Sanchez-Blanco I, Ochoa-Sangrador C, Lopez-Munain L, Izquierdo-Sanchez M, Fermoso-Garcia J. Predictive model of functional independence in stroke patients admitted to a rehabilitation programme. *Clin Rehabil*. 1999;13(6):464–475.

53. Singh R, Hunter J, Philip A, Todd I. Predicting those who will walk after rehabilitation in a specialist stroke unit. *Clin Rehabil*. 2006;20(2):149–152.

54. van de Port IG, Kwakkel G, Schepers VP, Lindeman E. Predicting mobility outcome one year after stroke: a prospective cohort study. *J Rehabil Med*. 2006;38(4): 218–223.

55. Hatakenaka M, Miyai I, Sakoda S, Yanagihara T. Proximal paresis of the upper extremity in patients with stroke. *Neurology*. 2007;69(4):348–355.

56. Katrak P, Bowring G, Conroy P, Chilvers M, Poulos R, McNeil D. Predicting upper limb recovery after stroke: the place of early shoulder and hand movement. *Arch Phys Med Rehabil*. 1998;79(7):758–761.

57. Wade DT, Langton-Hewer R, Wood VA, Skilbeck CE, Ismail HM. The hemiplegic arm after stroke: measurement and recovery. *J Neurol Neurosurg Psychiatry*. 1983; 46(6):521–524.

58. Paolucci S, Grasso MG, Antonucci G, et al. Mobility status after inpatient stroke rehabilitation: 1-year follow-up and prognostic factors. *Arch Phys Med Rehabil*. 2001;82(1): 2–8.

59. Broeks JG, Lankhorst GJ, Rumping K, Prevo AJH. The long-term outcome of arm function after stroke: results of a follow-up study. *Disabil Rehabil*. 1999;21(8): 357–364.

60. Mirbagheri MM, Rymer WZ. Time-course of changes in arm impairment after stroke: variables predicting motor recovery over 12 months. *Arch Phys Med Rehabil*. 2008; 89(8):1507–1513.

61. Canning CG, Ada L, Adams R, O'Dwyer NJ. Loss of strength contributes more to physical disability after stroke than loss of dexterity. *Clin Rehabil*. 2004;18(3): 300–308.

62. Koh CL, Pan SL, Jeng JS, et al. Predicting recovery of voluntary upper extremity movement in subacute stroke patients with severe upper extremity paresis. *PLoS One*. 2015;10(5):e0126857.

63. Whiteley W, Chong WL, Sengupta A, Sandercock P. Blood markers for the prognosis of ischemic stroke: a systematic review. *Stroke*. 2009;40(5):e380–389.

64. Kasner SE. Clinical interpretation and use of stroke scales. *Lancet Neurol*. 2006;5(7):603–612.

65. Brott T, Adams HP, Olinger CP, et al. Measurements of acute cerebral infarction - a clinical examination scale. *Stroke*. 1989;20(7):864–870.

66. Schiemanck SK, Post MW, Witkamp TD, Kappelle LJ, Prevo AJ. Relationship between ischemic lesion volume and functional status in the 2nd week after middle cerebral artery stroke. *Neurorehabil Neural Repair*. 2005; 19(2):133–138.

67. Beebe JA, Lang CE. Active range of motion predicts upper extremity function 3 months after stroke. *Stroke*. 2009; 40(5):1772−1779.
68. Au-Yeung SS, Hui-Chan CW. Predicting recovery of dextrous hand function in acute stroke. *Disabil Rehabil*. 2009;31(5):394−401.
69. Bohannon RW, Ahlquist M, Lee N, Maljanian R. Functional gains during acute hospitalization for stroke. *Neurorehabil Neural Repair*. 2003;17(3):192−195.
70. Patel AT, Duncan PW, Lai SM, Studenski S. The relation between impairments and functional outcomes poststroke. *Arch Phys Med Rehabil*. 2000;81(10): 1357−1363.
71. Kwakkel G, Kollen BJ. Predicting activities after stroke: what is clinically relevant? *Int J Stroke*. 2013;8(1):25−32.
72. Jorgensen HS, Nakayama H, Raaschou HO, Vive-Larsen J, Stoier M, Olsen TS. Outcome and time course of recovery in stroke. Part II: time course of recovery. The Copenhagen stroke study. *Arch Phys Med Rehabil*. 1995;76(5): 406−412.
73. Tilling K, Sterne JA, Rudd AG, Glass TA, Wityk RJ, Wolfe CD. A new method for predicting recovery after stroke. *Stroke*. 2001;32(12):2867−2873.
74. Douiri A, Grace J, Sarker SJ, et al. Patient-specific prediction of functional recovery after stroke. *Int J Stroke*. 2017. https://doi.org/10.1177/1747493017706241.
75. Nakayama H, Jorgensen HS, Raaschou HO, Olsen TS. Recovery of upper extremity function in stroke patients: the Copenhagen stroke study. *Arch Phys Med Rehabil*. 1994; 75(4):394−398.
76. Kwakkel G, Kollen B, Twisk J. Impact of time on improvement of outcome after stroke. *Stroke*. 2006;37(9): 2348−2353.
77. Langhorne P, Bernhardt J, Kwakkel G. Stroke rehabilitation. *Lancet*. 2011;377(9778):1693−1702.
78. Prabhakaran S, Zarahn E, Riley C, et al. Inter-individual variability in the capacity for motor recovery after ischemic stroke. *Neurorehabil Neural Repair*. 2008;22(1): 64−71.
79. Smith MC, Byblow WD, Barber PA, Stinear CM. Proportional recovery from lower limb motor impairment after stroke. *Stroke*. 2017;48(5):1400−1403.
80. Stinear CM, Barber PA, Petoe M, Anwar S, Byblow WD. The PREP algorithm predicts potential for upper limb recovery after stroke. *Brain*. 2012;135(Pt 8):2527−2535.
81. Kong KH, Chua KS, Lee J. Recovery of upper limb dexterity in patients more than 1 year after stroke: frequency, clinical correlates and predictors. *NeuroRehabil*. 2011; 28(2):105−111.
82. Loewen SC, Anderson BA. Predictors of stroke outcome using objective measurement scales. *Stroke*. 1990;21(1): 78−81.
83. Williams BK, Galea MP, Winter AT. What is the functional outcome for the upper limb after stroke? *Aust J Physiother*. 2001;47(1):19−27.
84. Wade DT, Hewer RL. Functional abilities after stroke: measurement, natural history and prognosis. *J Neurol Neurosurg Psychiatry*. 1987;50(2):177−182.
85. Shelton FD, Volpe BT, Reding M. Motor impairment as a predictor of functional recovery and guide to rehabilitation treatment after stroke. *Neurorehabil Neural Repair*. 2001;15(3):229−237.
86. Zarahn E, Alon L, Ryan SL, et al. Prediction of motor recovery using initial impairment and fMRI 48 h poststroke. *Cereb Cortex*. 2011;21(12):2712−2721.
87. Winters C, van Wegen EE, Daffertshofer A, Kwakkel G. Generalizability of the proportional recovery model for the upper extremity after an ischemic stroke. *Neurorehabil Neural Repair*. 2015;29(7):614−622.
88. Stinear CM, Byblow WD, Ackerley SJ, Barber PA, Smith MC. Predicting recovery potential for individual stroke patients increases rehabilitation efficiency. *Stroke*. 2017;48(4):1011−1019.
89. Ji R, Du W, Shen H, et al. Web-based tool for dynamic functional outcome after acute ischemic stroke and comparison with existing models. *BMC Neurol*. 2014; 14:214.
90. Ntaios G, Faouzi M, Ferrari J, Lang W, Vemmos K, Michel P. An integer-based score to predict functional outcome in acute ischemic stroke: the ASTRAL score. *Neurology*. 2012;78(24):1916−1922.
91. Saposnik G, Raptis S, Kapral MK, et al. The iScore predicts poor functional outcomes early after hospitalization for an acute ischemic stroke. *Stroke*. 2011;42(12): 3421−3428.
92. Reid JM, Gubitz GJ, Dai D, et al. Predicting functional outcome after stroke by modelling baseline clinical and CT variables. *Age Ageing*. 2010;39(3):360−366.
93. Weimar C, Konig IR, Kraywinkel K, Ziegler A, Diener HC. Age and National Institutes of Health Stroke Scale Score within 6 hours after onset are accurate predictors of outcome after cerebral ischemia: development and external validation of prognostic models. *Stroke*. 2004; 35(1):158−162.
94. Counsell C, Dennis M, McDowall M, Warlow C. Predicting outcome after acute and subacute stroke: development and validation of new prognostic models. *Stroke*. 2002;33(4):1041−1047.
95. Gupta VP, Garton ALA, Sisti JA, et al. Prognosticating functional outcome after intracerebral hemorrhage: the ICHOP score. *World Neurosurg*. 2017;101:577−583.
96. Ji R, Shen H, Pan Y, et al. A novel risk score to predict 1-year functional outcome after intracerebral hemorrhage and comparison with existing scores. *Crit Care*. 2013; 17(6):R275.
97. Bruce SS, Appelboom G, Piazza M, et al. A comparative evaluation of existing grading scales in intracerebral hemorrhage. *Neurocrit Care*. 2011;15(3):498−505.
98. Rost NS, Smith EE, Chang Y, et al. Prediction of functional outcome in patients with primary intracerebral hemorrhage: the FUNC score. *Stroke*. 2008;39(8): 2304−2309.
99. Ruiz-Sandoval JL, Chiquete E, Romero-Vargas S, Padilla-Martinez JJ, Gonzalez-Cornejo S. Grading scale for prediction of outcome in primary intracerebral hemorrhages. *Stroke*. 2007;38(5):1641−1644.

100. Weimar C, Benemann J, Diener HC. German stroke study C. Development and validation of the Essen intracerebral haemorrhage score. *J Neurol Neurosurg Psychiatry*. 2006; 77(5):601–605.

101. Godoy DA, Pinero G, Di Napoli M. Predicting mortality in spontaneous intracerebral hemorrhage: can modification to original score improve the prediction? *Stroke*. 2006;37(4):1038–1044.

102. Cheung RT, Zou LY. Use of the original, modified, or new intracerebral hemorrhage score to predict mortality and morbidity after intracerebral hemorrhage. *Stroke*. 2003; 34(7):1717–1722.

103. O'Donnell MJ, Fang J, D'Uva C, et al. The PLAN score: a bedside prediction rule for death and severe disability following acute ischemic stroke. *Arch Intern Med*. 2012: 1–9.

104. Weimar C, Weber C, Wagner M, et al. Management patterns and health care use after intracerebral hemorrhage. a cost-of-illness study from a societal perspective in Germany. *Cerebrovasc Dis*. 2003;15(1–2):29–36.

105. Michel P, Odier C, Rutgers M, et al. The Acute STroke Registry and Analysis of Lausanne (ASTRAL): design and baseline analysis of an ischemic stroke registry including acute multimodal imaging. *Stroke*. 2010;41(11): 2491–2498.

106. Cooray C, Mazya M, Bottai M, et al. External validation of the ASTRAL and DRAGON scores for prediction of functional outcome in stroke. *Stroke*. 2016.

107. Liu G, Ntaios G, Zheng H, et al. External validation of the ASTRAL score to predict 3- and 12-month functional outcome in the China National Stroke Registry. *Stroke*. 2013;44(5):1443–1445.

108. Quinn TJ, Singh S, Lees KR, Bath PM, Myint PK. Validating and comparing stroke prognosis scales. *Neurology*. 2017.

109. Saposnik G, Kapral MK, Liu Y, et al. IScore: a risk score to predict death early after hospitalization for an acute ischemic stroke. *Circulation*. 2011;123(7):739–749.

110. Dierick F, Dehas M, Isambert JL, et al. Hemorrhagic versus ischemic stroke: who can best benefit from blended conventional physiotherapy with robotic-assisted gait therapy? *PLoS One*. 2017;12(6):e0178636.

111. Heeley E, Anderson CS, Woodward M, et al. Poor utility of grading scales in acute intracerebral hemorrhage: results from the INTERACT2 trial. *Int J Stroke*. 2015;10(7): 1101–1107.

112. Wang W, Lu J, Wang C, et al. Prognostic value of ICH score and ICH-GS score in Chinese intracerebral hemorrhage patients: analysis from the China National Stroke Registry (CNSR). *PLoS One*. 2013; 8(10):e77421.

113. Sembill JA, Gerner ST, Volbers B, et al. Severity assessment in maximally treated ICH patients: the max-ICH score. *Neurology*. 2017;89(5):423–431.

114. Hemphill 3rd JC, Farrant M, Neill Jr TA. Prospective validation of the ICH Score for 12-month functional outcome. *Neurology*. 2009;73(14):1088–1094.

115. KNGF. *Clinical Practice Guideline for Physical Therapy in Patients with Stroke*; 2014. https://www.fysionet-evidencebased.nl/images/pdfs/guidelines_in_english/stroke_practice_guidelines_2014.pdf.

116. Lazar RM, Minzer B, Antoniello D, Festa JR, Krakauer JW, Marshall RS. Improvement in aphasia scores after stroke is well predicted by initial severity. *Stroke*. 2010;41(7): 1485–1488.

117. Winters C, van Wegen EE, Daffertshofer A, Kwakkel G. Generalizability of the maximum proportional recovery rule to visuospatial neglect early poststroke. *Neurorehabil Neural Repair*. 2017;31(4):334–342.

118. Kwakkel G, Lannin NA, Borschmann K, et al. Standardized measurement of sensorimotor recovery in stroke trials: consensus-based core recommendations from the stroke recovery and rehabilitation roundtable. *Int J Stroke*. 2017;12(5):451–461.

119. Walker MF, Hoffmann TC, Brady MC, et al. Improving the development, monitoring and reporting of stroke rehabilitation research: consensus-based core recommendations from the stroke recovery and rehabilitation roundtable. *Int J Stroke*. 2017;12(5):472–479.

120. Corbett D, Carmichael ST, Murphy TH, et al. Enhancing the alignment of the preclinical and clinical stroke recovery research pipeline: consensus-based core recommendations from the stroke recovery and rehabilitation roundtable translational working group. *Int J Stroke*. 2017;12(5):462–471.

121. Boyd LA, Hayward KS, Ward NS, et al. Biomarkers of stroke recovery: consensus-based core recommendations from the stroke recovery and rehabilitation roundtable. *Int J Stroke*. 2017;12(5):480–493.

122. Reid JM, Dai D, Delmonte S, Counsell C, Phillips SJ, MacLeod MJ. Simple prediction scores predict good and devastating outcomes after stroke more accurately than physicians. *Age Ageing*. 2016;0:1–6.

123. Park TH, Saposnik G, Bae HJ, et al. The iScore predicts functional outcome in Korean patients with ischemic stroke. *Stroke*. 2013;44(5):1440–1442.

124. Reid JM, Dai D, Christian C, et al. Developing predictive models of excellent and devastating outcome after stroke. *Age Ageing*. 2012.

125. Ayis SA, Coker B, Rudd AG, Dennis MS, Wolfe CD. Predicting independent survival after stroke: a European study for the development and validation of standardised stroke scales and prediction models of outcome. *J Neurol Neurosurg Psychiatry*. 2013;84(3):288–296.

126. Thompson DD, Murray GD, Sudlow CL, Dennis M, Whiteley WN. Comparison of statistical and clinical predictions of functional outcome after ischemic stroke. *PLoS One*. 2014;9(10):e110189.

127. Konig IR, Ziegler A, Bluhmki E, et al. Predicting long-term outcome after acute ischemic stroke: a simple index works in patients from controlled clinical trials. *Stroke.* 2008;39(6):1821–1826.

128. Sim J, Teece L, Dennis MS, Roffe C, Team SOSS. Validation and recalibration of two multivariable prognostic models for survival and independence in acute stroke. *PLoS One.* 2016;11(5):e0153527.

129. Reid JM, Gubitz GJ, Dai D, et al. External validation of a six simple variable model of stroke outcome and verification in hyper-acute stroke. *J Neurol Neurosurg Psychiatry.* 2007;78(12):1390–1391.

130. Lewis SC, Sandercock PA, Dennis MS. Predicting outcome in hyper-acute stroke: validation of a prognostic model in the Third International Stroke Trial (IST3). *J Neurol Neurosurg Psychiatry.* 2008;79(4):397–400.

131. Teale E, Young J, Dennis M, Sheldon T. Predicting patient-reported stroke outcomes: a validation of the six simple variable prognostic model. *Cerebrovasc Dis Extra.* 2013;3(1):97–102.

132. Weimar C, Ziegler A, Sacco RL, Diener HC, Konig IR, investigators V. Predicting recovery after intracerebral hemorrhage–an external validation in patients from controlled clinical trials. *J Neurol.* 2009;256(3):464–469.

133. Hemphill 3rd JC, Bonovich DC, Besmertis L, Manley GT, Johnston SC. The ICH score: a simple, reliable grading scale for intracerebral hemorrhage. *Stroke.* 2001;32(4):891–897.

134. Chuang YC, Chen YM, Peng SK, Peng SY. Risk stratification for predicting 30-day mortality of intracerebral hemorrhage. *Int J Qual Health Care.* 2009;21(6):441–447.

CHAPTER 3

Aphasia Rehabilitation

ELIZABETH E. GALLETTA, PhD • MIRA GORAL, PhD • PEGGY S. CONNER, PhD

DEFINITION

Aphasia is a language disorder secondary to an acquired brain injury, most commonly due to stroke. Memory and other cognitive abilities are generally spared, yet aphasia is sometimes referred to as a cognitive language disorder as it can be defined based on the cognitive processes that underlie language use.[1] Nonlinguistic executive function skills, often impaired post stroke, can affect language and communication and therefore impact persons with aphasia (PWA). In addition to stroke, other acquired brain injuries such as traumatic brain injury, tumor, and neurologic disease can also cause aphasia. In this chapter we describe post-stroke aphasia and language rehabilitation approaches for PWA.

Aphasia post stroke results from focal brain damage to regions in the language-dominant hemisphere (left in most people), including cortical (e.g., Broca and Wernicke areas) and subcortical areas, and/or damage to the white matter tracks connecting these regions. Oral language impairment can include oral expressive and/or auditory comprehension deficits. Both oral expressive and oral receptive language impairment may be evidenced in any of the linguistic domains of phonology, semantics, morphology, or syntax (although pragmatic skills are often preserved). In addition, language impairment in the visual language domain may be evidenced in reading (*alexia*) and/or writing (*agraphia*); manual language (sign language) and gesture can also be affected. In essence, all modalities of language: oral expressive, oral receptive, reading, writing, and manual/gesture can be impaired after stroke, resulting in aphasia, alexia, and agraphia.

CLASSIFICATION AND TYPES OF APHASIA

There have been numerous classification systems proposed for describing aphasia (as many as 30, see Ref. 2). A current widely used aphasia classification system among aphasiologists is the Boston classification system[3] that reflects the classical associative connectionist model based on the Wernicke/Lichtheim model with some modifications by Geschwind.[4,5] The commonly used Boston Diagnostic Aphasia Examination (BDAE) originally published by Goodglass and Kaplan,[6] with its most recent publication in 2001 (Goodglass, Kaplan, and Barresi) classifies aphasia based on a neurolinguistic system.

Depending upon the location of the brain damage, and the relative degree of impairment and sparing of language skills, classic subtypes of aphasia have been defined.[3] While individuals with Broca and transcortical motor aphasia are associated with anterior brain damage, those with posterior brain damage present with Wernicke, transcortical sensory, conduction, or anomic aphasia. Individuals with global aphasia have both anterior and posterior brain damage. Aphasia is referred to as nonfluent or fluent, based on the degree of fluency in oral expressive language. Fluency only describes the degree to which oral language is expressed in connected speech and is defined by the number of connected words expressed. When there are at least five to eight connected words in an utterance (e.g., The boy and girl are eating breakfast), the utterance is described as an example of *fluent* speech. When there are less than five connected words in an utterance (e.g., boy girl breakfast), the utterance is described as an example of *nonfluent* speech. Degree of fluency immediately suggests whether the lesion is anterior or posterior to the central sulcus. The characteristics of each of these classic subtypes of aphasia are described below.

- Broca aphasia—anterior brain damage, nonfluent speech, auditory comprehension is a relative strength. Repetition is impaired.
- Transcortical motor aphasia—anterior brain damage, nonfluent speech, auditory comprehension is a relative strength. Repetition is a strength.
- Wernicke aphasia—posterior brain damage, fluent speech, poor auditory comprehension, repetition is impaired.
- Transcortical sensory aphasia—posterior brain damage, fluent speech, poor auditory comprehension, repetition is a strength.

Stroke Rehabilitation. https://doi.org/10.1016/B978-0-323-55381-0.00003-2

49

- Conduction aphasia—damage to the arcuate fasciculus (the white matter track connecting Broca and Wernicke areas), fluent speech, poor auditory comprehension, severely impaired repetition.
- Anomic aphasia—variable brain damage, fluent speech, auditory comprehension is intact, repetition is a strength. The salient characteristic of this aphasia is word retrieval impairment.
- Global aphasia—both anterior and posterior brain damage to the language areas (Broca and Wernicke areas), severe nonfluent speech, poor auditory comprehension, and impaired repetition.

While these classic aphasia syndromes are often referred to in clinical descriptions of individuals with aphasia, in reality, individuals with post-stroke aphasia rarely fit into these specific classic subtypes. Rather than labeling the aphasia as one of these subtypes, a description of the effect of the stroke on the five language modalities (oral expressive, oral receptive, reading, writing, manual/gesture) may more accurately reflect the aphasia presentation. It is important to note that the manifestation of aphasia in any two individuals is not identical. Yet one feature that is present in everyone with aphasia is difficulty retrieving words or a word finding problem (termed anomia). Therefore, the presentation of anomia does not add specific information to the classification of aphasia type.

Alternative classification approaches to aphasia have also been in use. The psycholinguistic approach identifies the linguistic domains that appear impaired (e.g., morphology, semantics) and localizes the impairment within a cognitive neuropsychological processing model rather than within specific brain regions.[1] Thus, for example, a PWA may experience difficulty in comprehending a spoken word but possess the intact ability to comprehend the same word when presented in writing, due to deficit along the link between spoken language and the semantic representation. In contrast, another PWA may have deficit in semantic representation and processing resulting in difficulty comprehending words, whether they are presented auditorily or visually.

As well, social functional approaches to aphasia classification identify breakdown in communication and in life participation with less emphasis on the linguistic impairment.[7] Such approaches assess the effects of interlocutors, settings, and context on the degree of communication success.

APHASIA REHABILITATION IN THE UNITED STATES

The history of aphasia rehabilitation in the United States is linked to the history of the medical specialty of Physical Medicine and Rehabilitation, which became a recognized medical specialty by the American Medical Association in 1947 (http://www.aapmr.org/about-physiatry/history-of-the-specialty). PWA are treated by speech language pathologists as inpatients in acute and subacute facilities in the earlier stages post stroke and in outpatient clinics in the chronic phase, after 1 year post stroke. In the acute stages, patients often receive short therapy sessions daily; for outpatients, treatment is often administered twice weekly and a therapy session's duration is typically 30—45 minutes. Recent research, however, suggests that a more intense therapy schedule may yield better results, although the ideal dosage is yet to be determined.[8,9]

Recovery from aphasia varies among individuals. Most adults who acquire aphasia live with the impairment and never regain their pre-stroke abilities. Nevertheless, most PWA experience continual improvement in their language and communication abilities, especially following intervention. While in the acute stages post stroke, aphasia may be severe, during the initial period of days and weeks after the stroke, some language can recover spontaneously. It is not clear what factors are responsible for the variable recovery experienced by PWA.[10] However, research studies have documented that aphasia therapy is beneficial and promotes language recovery compared to spontaneous language improvements without therapy.[11] In the chronic phase, language recovery can continue and individuals with aphasia have demonstrated language improvement with therapy several years post stroke (e.g., Ref. 12). The notion that language recovery plateaus after the first year post stroke is a myth, which should be extinguished.

APHASIA TREATMENT PRINCIPLES

Aphasia treatments can be broadly categorized as restitutive impairment-focused or vicariative compensatory-focused approaches. While restitutive therapies are mechanistic approaches that aim to improve linguistic function, vicariative aphasia rehabilitation techniques are more focused on compensating for the aphasia language deficits and include functionally oriented treatments.

Research on the principles of neuroplasticity has supported the development of restitutive approaches to aphasia rehabilitation that aim to promote neuroplastic changes in the brain. Neuroscientists have documented that behavioral training influences brain cells and promotes neuroplasticity, and that this process allows the brain to relearn behaviors lost secondary to brain damage.[13] Ten principles of neuroplasticity have been described by Kleim and Jones. These are: use it or lose it, use it and improve it, specificity, repetition matters, intensity matters, time matters, salience matters, age matters, transference, interference. In Table 3.1 we provide a description of each principle, as well as an example of its application to aphasia rehabilitation. When constraint-induced (CI) therapy is applied to aphasia rehabilitation the focus is on oral language production and therapy includes massed-practice of activities, in line with principle 4 in Table 3.1.

A fundamental consideration for the efficacy of aphasia treatment is how generalizable the effects are to everyday conversation. This has been measured by improved performance on untrained items or tasks following treatment, as well as by the length of time this improvement can be sustained. Many factors appear to influence generalization of treatment for PWA in the chronic stage, such as treatment type, schedule, duration, and intensity, as well as client-specific considerations. A complete description of these factors should include elicitation methods, linguistic levels, treatment focus, and other methodological and person-specific considerations that are beyond the scope of this chapter.[13a] Moreover, the variable nature of aphasia makes systematic exploration of these factors on a large-scale basis untenable, and much of what we know about effective interventions is based on small-group or single-subject research.

TABLE 3.1
Principles of Experience-Dependent Neuroplasticity Applied to Aphasia Rehabilitation

Principle	Description	Application to Aphasia Therapy Techniques
1. Use it or lose it	Failure to drive specific brain functions can lead to functional degradation.	Active engagement in specific language production or comprehension tasks.
2. Use it and improve it	Training that drives a specific brain function can enhance that function.	Active engagement in the act of speaking, comprehending, and using language.
3. Specificity	The nature of the training experience dictates the nature of the plasticity.	Training a specific function such as oral production of sentences will promote oral sentence production.
4. Repetition matters	Induction of plasticity requires sufficient repetition.	Training numerous trials of the same target during a therapy session.
5. Intensity matters	Induction of plasticity requires sufficient training intensity.	Defined by number of hours of treatment in a period of time (e.g., an Intensive Comprehensive Aphasia Program is defined as at least 9 hours of therapy weekly).
6. Time matters	Different forms of plasticity occur at different times during training.	Training during the early recovery period post stroke interacts with spontaneous recovery.
7. Salience matters	The training experience must be explicitly salient to induce plasticity.	The language materials must be interesting and relevant to the PWA.
8. Age matters	Training induced plasticity occurs more readily in younger brains.	Younger adults may respond to aphasia treatment more readily than older adults.
9. Transference	Plasticity in response to one training experience can enhance the acquisition of similar experiences.	For example, practicing verb production can facilitate the production of unpracticed verbs.
10. Interference	Plasticity in response to one experience can interfere with the acquisition of other behaviors.	Therapy that benefits one skill (e.g., use of a tablet to type lists to use to support short-term memory) may interfere with response to another skill (e.g., mechanics of writing since typing rather than writing is practiced).

Adapted from Kleim JA, Jones TA. Principles of experience-dependent neural plasticity: implications for rehabilitation after brain damage. *J Speech Lang Hear Res.* 2008;51(1):S225–S239.

IMPAIRMENT-BASED TREATMENT APPROACHES

Here we discuss examples of impairment-focused verbal production therapies that employ phonological and semantic approaches to word retrieval, as well as syntactic impairment, and highlight recent evidence for generalization of treatment effects. We also briefly discuss treatment for the reading and writing difficulties that can result from a brain lesion. This is not intended to be a comprehensive review of these treatment types. Rather we provide examples of the various ways clinicians provide impairment-based treatment, with the understanding that most treatment is highly individualized and within a given individual, deficits may be domain-specific or, more commonly, apparent in multiple domains. For a review of aphasia therapy research, see Brady et al.[14] In addition, several books focus specifically on aphasia rehabilitation (e.g., Refs. 7,15,16); these are excellent sources for further reading. In these publications, both impairment-focused and social-focused treatments for aphasia are described.

In impairment-focused treatment, the overall goal of therapy is to regain or relearn an impaired process, and promote a successful outcome, evidenced by generalization to novel items or tasks. For example, if the individual experiences difficulty producing complete sentences that contain conjugated verbs, the treatment can target complete-sentence production with the aim of generalization to unpracticed sentences. Generalization is thought to result from functional reorganization of the damaged brain (e.g., Refs. 17–20). Treatment can be implicit and focus on the practice of language production and comprehension, and can be explicit in its instruction and interaction, bringing into play metalinguistic processes.

VERBAL PRODUCTION TREATMENT
Phonological-Based Treatment

Impairment-focused treatment of phonology targets the retrieval of the speech sounds within a word to facilitate oral naming. In one form of this treatment, a hierarchical cueing strategy has been used to elicit picture naming. For example, an initial cue may consist of a spoken word or nonword that rhymes with the target word; a subsequent cue would be the first sound of the target word and then, if needed, repetition of the target word is elicited (e.g., Refs. 21,22). Orthographic as well as phonologic cues have been used successfully to improve picture naming for targeted words (e.g., Ref. 23), and there is evidence that a combination of both written and verbal cueing may yield greater generalization effects to untrained words and connected speech.[24]

In a recent investigation, Kendall, Oelke, Brookshire, and Nadeau[25] employed a phonologic and multimodal approach consisting of articulatory-motor, tactile-kinesthetic, visual, conceptual, orthographic, and auditory training. Sixty hours of this treatment, named Phonomotor Treatment, was given in an intensive schedule over 5 weeks to 26 adults with aphasia. The outcome was improvement in confrontation naming 3 months post treatment on untrained nouns, and the reported 5% post-treatment increase in confrontation naming was significant. In this well-designed study, the authors' use of a staggered treatment schedule and repeated testing averaged over 3 days for each baseline provided the necessary control for possible improvement due to the passage of time and repeated testing, and for the characteristic interindividual variability in performance.

Semantic-Based Treatment

A semantic-based aphasia treatment aims to improve verbal production focused on word meaning. Activities are designed to strengthen the semantic network and facilitate word production in confrontation naming and in the context of sentences. Semantic therapy can be either specific to a grammatical class at the word level (e.g., Refs. 26,27) or broader, targeting phrase structures, such as using verb argument structure as a basis for generating verb schemas and related semantic networks.[28,29] The potential for these methods to generalize to untrained items or connected speech is dependent upon the complexity of the items used and the challenge of evoking broad changes to a vast semantic network within the confines of specific treatment items.[26,30] At the word level, efforts to develop semantic treatment paradigms that generalize to unpracticed conditions have had mixed results. In one approach, Kiran and colleagues have found that training atypical items of a given category (e.g., pelican) facilitates naming of untrained typical items (robin) but no effect for generalization of typical to atypical has been observed.[19,27,31,32] In another approach named Semantic Feature Analysis (SFA), improvement in trained items has not generalized consistently to untrained items or tasks. In SFA treatment a set of target words is selected and different features of each word's conceptual network are systematically practiced.[32a] The PWA produces words for a set of semantic features for each target word (i.e., related action, descriptor, category, etc.); for example, for the word *water* the features *drinking*, *transparent*, *liquid* could be elicited. Then, through repetition, the feature generation is theorized to strengthen the semantic network and increase the likelihood of word retrieval and production. Although generalization to untreated words has been observed in many studies (e.g., Boyle and Coelho, 1995; Refs. 33–37), it has not been noted in others (e.g., Refs. 38,39; see Ref. 40 for a review; Ref. 41).

To evoke broader changes to the semantic network and improve generalization to connected speech of individuals with aphasia, Edmonds and colleagues have conducted a series of studies on an approach called Verb Network Strengthening Treatment (VNeST).[28,29,42] In this method which utilizes the thematic roles of the verb, the clinician elicits from the PWA several target actions, as well as various options for the agent (the doer) and the patient (the recipient) of each action. The investigators posit that the action of generating the selected event schemas not only strengthens the various dimensions in the meaning of each verb but also activates related verbs as well as related agents and patients.[28,29] Therefore, for the verb *measure* the agent-patient pairs of *chef-sugar* or *designer-room* might also activate related verbs *weigh* or *draw* and related agents and patients such as *cook-flour* or *architect-house*. The generative focus of VNeST is further reinforced because the treated verbs are presented without pictures that might bias the participants' responses.[29] Across these VNeST studies, although not every participant improved on every measure, the findings supported significant improvement on lexical retrieval and on several measures of generalization including untreated items and connected speech.[28,29,42,43]

Syntax Treatment

Syntax, a third area of impairment-based treatment, is a principle target for the recovery of verbal production in people with agrammatism, a subtype of aphasia in which grammar is the main level of affected language. In an example that demonstrates generalization within linguistic levels, Thompson and colleagues have developed an approach known as Treatment of Underlying Forms (TUF), whereby verb production is treated within the argument structure in sentences.[44,45] As is suggested by the name, the active or underlying form of the verb is used for training comprehension and production, for example, *Mark is cooking soup*. Thematic roles are reviewed and movement operations (i.e., affecting word order) are presented as the clinician demonstrates how to derive the surface form of the target sentence, for example, *What is Mark cooking?*.[46] The method is designed to promote generalization of movement operations from trained to untrained constructions most notably for those sentences that share similar linguistic

properties.[47] Moreover, generalization appears to be greater from more complex to less complex structures, a parallel finding to the typicality treatment discussed above (Kiran and colleagues). Thus, this generalization effect renders the treatment more effective.

In a related finding, Thompson found that the training of more complex three-argument verbs, for example, *The girl gave the apple to the teacher* affects improvement of untrained one-argument sentences, such as *The boy is swimming*, and two-argument verbs, *The boy is eating candy*. Consistently, generalization occurs if the information regarding the simpler form is contained within the more complex form.[48] Moreover, recent neuroimaging findings have provided evidence of functional reorganization of neural structures in individuals with aphasia following verb argument treatment with posttreatment activation noted in areas that are involved in processing verb argument in healthy individuals.[48]

READING AND WRITING TREATMENT

The disruption of verbal language processes that we define as aphasia usually impedes written language as well. Often individuals with aphasia demonstrate analogous deficits in written language skills. However, reading and writing skills can be differentially impaired and alexia and agraphia can occur independent of oral language impairments. The modular yet connected nature of the processes that underlie reading and their anatomical correlates give rise to the types of disruption we see post stroke.

Alexia, an acquired breakdown in the process of reading, can occur centrally—in conjunction with aphasia—or peripherally—without a general language disorder. Central alexias are classified by the reading route that is disrupted. In English, for example, we read by sounding out words via a phonological route, one that is heavily relied upon during reading acquisition. Damage to this route results in *phonological alexia*, characterized by a reliance on whole word recognition and difficulty reading unfamiliar words or nonwords. In contrast, *surface alexia* is the result of damage to the direct lexical route for reading, whole word recognition. As skilled readers, rather than sounding out words, we rely on instant visual recognition of whole words with immediate access to their meaning. Surface alexia is characterized by preserved ability to sound out words, but difficulty with recognition of whole words, chiefly those that are irregularly spelled such as "yacht" or "knowledge." Deep alexia is commonly defined as damage to both routes resulting in more global reading difficulties. Deficits in grapheme-to-phoneme conversion are accompanied by reading errors that are visual (*cool* for *cook*) or semantic (*banana* for *apple*).

Peripheral alexias are typically classified by the presence or absence of agraphia, visual field deficits, and visual neglect. Pure alexia most commonly occurs following a stroke involving the left posterior cerebral artery with damage to the occipitotemporal cortex.[49] Behaviorally, alexia without agraphia is characterized by a spared ability to write, but an inability to read what one has written. A common comorbid condition is right hemianopsia (right visual field deficit). Alexia with agraphia is often seen after a parietotemporal lesion and is characterized by parallel difficulties with reading and writing. Pure agraphia without alexia is markedly less common but has been documented.[50–52]

Similar to treatment of oral language, therapy approaches for alexia and agraphia often combine aspects of impairment-based treatment and compensatory strategies. Treatment selection is dependent upon an individual's specific reading and writing deficits and functional communication needs.

Change in reading ability may result from techniques to further develop existing communication strengths, as well as remediate areas of impairment. As an example, for individuals with deep alexia working on matching written synonyms may capitalize on their ability to derive partially preserved semantic information from the text and practice accessing finer-grained semantic knowledge.[16 (p. 343)] Similarly, specific training on relearning letter-sound correspondence has been successful with some clients to sound out and identify problematic function words (e.g., articles, prepositions) that have little or no semantic content.[16 (p. 343)]

Of particular interest are methods that may benefit oral as well as written language. One such method, Oral Reading for Language in Aphasia (ORLA), uses choral and repeated reading and paced practice to enhance reading fluency, natural intonation and prosody. Significant improvement has been found on reading comprehension and oral reading rate for individuals with aphasia and alexia, as well as on measures of verbal language production.[53,54]

In the case of agraphia, treatment to enhance writing may facilitate word retrieval in verbal production or serve as an independent form of communication for writing notes, emails, or texts. In severe aphasia, several treatment methods use repetitive practice on a limited set of items in an effort to reactivate key words essential for functional communication.[55 (p. 297)] The Copy and Recall Treatment or CART is an example of a method that trains the spelling of highly functional words through repeated copying and written confrontation naming of pictures.[56,57] This treatment has not been shown to generalize to untrained items, but has been successful in helping PWA with severe nonfluent aphasia and agraphia; they learn to write a small subset of words for everyday use. Beeson, Higginson, and Rising[58] adapted this method (T-CART) to provide practice with text messaging for a 31-year-old man with severe Broca aphasia. Prior to T-CART, the client received 6 weeks of standard CART and demonstrated significant gains in writing with his nondominant left hand (from 11% to 90% spelling accuracy on trained words over 6 weeks) as well as gains in oral production. During the T-CART treatment, the client repeatedly copied the target words on his cell phone keypad saying the word each time he typed it. Marked improvement in spelling and oral naming suggested that this treatment for agraphia facilitated lexical access in both the oral and written language domains.

In sum, the objective of treatment for alexia and agraphia may be limited to rehabilitation of written language processes or more commonly may target both oral and written communication. As in aphasia treatment, significant improvement with generalization offers the PWA greater functionality of skills acquired. Although some treatments result in improvement in reading and writing without generalization, better functional language output for the PWA can significantly enhance day-to-day communication and quality of life.

Summary of Impairment Treatment-Related Progress in Research Studies

As in other types of post-stroke rehabilitation, impaired communication skills in people with aphasia, alexia, and agraphia require a multifaceted approach. Consideration of the PWA's current communication strengths and pattern and severity of deficits can inform the selection of treatment objectives and methods. PWA typically experience asymmetrical difficulties in comprehension and expression, and may have differential impairment in linguistic domains such as phonology, semantics, and morpho-syntax. Generalization of treatment effects for these areas has been mixed and dependent upon task complexity, the typicality of items, the generative focus of treatment, and the multimodal nature of the approach. Of course, the breakdown in communication for PWA occurs in the context of their community. This has promoted an increased interest in treatment approaches that focus on social-functional communication.

SOCIAL-COMMUNICATION TREATMENT APPROACHES

The World Health Organization[59] proposed the International Classification of Functioning Disability and Health, referred to as the ICF model, for characterizing a health condition among three domains: impairment, activities, and participation. The restitutive verbal production therapy approaches to aphasia rehabilitation we have described reflect the impairment domain of the ICF model. Some alexia and agraphia treatments reflect the impairment domain as well. The example of a writing treatment noted above, T-CART, in which the participant copied specific functional words for text messaging, is considered a functional treatment approach.[58] Several social-communication treatment approaches have been developed for the treatment of aphasia, and these reflect the activities and participation domains of the ICF model. Such approaches to aphasia treatment focus on the ability of the individuals with aphasia to communicate their needs and thoughts and to continue their participation in life interaction, without targeting the PWA's impaired linguistic skills. Within such frameworks, intervention targets communicative situations and aims to train and educate the interlocutors (e.g., caregivers and family members), not only the PWA. This philosophy and model of service delivery is known as the Life Participation Approach to Aphasia (LPAA).[7] Aphasia Access, an alliance of life participation providers (http://www.aphasiaaccess.org/), lists centers in the United States and Canada where the LPAA approach is practiced. Within this philosophy and model of aphasia rehabilitation, reengagement in social interactions in life is emphasized rather than focusing on impaired linguistic forms. In addition to centers dedicated broadly to this approach, specific social/functional communication treatments for aphasia can considered to be a part of the LPAA. An example of a social therapeutic approach to aphasia rehabilitation is the supported conversation approach, developed by Kagan and colleagues. This intervention focuses on maximizing the communication success of PWA by training skilled conversation partners.[60] Accordingly, the outcome measures used to assess efficacy focus on communication and participation, not on accuracy of language production. Furthermore, social conversation therapy administered in groups, rather than individually, has proven highly beneficial for PWA. The group sessions promote communication and social interaction, and allow for interindividual exchanges in a more natural setting (e.g., Ref. 61).

BIOLOGICAL TREATMENT APPROACHES

Neural remediation and reorganization is the direct target of biological interventions for aphasia. Biological aphasia treatments include pharmacological therapy and noninvasive cortical stimulation used in conjunction with speech language therapy to promote language recovery. It is known that biological interventions to promote behavioral change do not act in isolation and require interaction with the behavior in order to promote recovery. For example, drug treatments administered for stroke rehabilitation have demonstrated positive results when the pharmacologic therapy is accompanied by behavioral practice.[62]

Pharmacology for aphasia rehabilitation has involved administration of several different medications; yet, no one agent is currently recommended for the promotion of aphasia recovery. While Small and Llano[63] report on studies of pharmacologic agents (e.g., bromocriptine, memantine) that have been investigated for use in aphasia therapy trials, optimal study design to establish that a specific drug treatment promotes brain reorganization for the promotion of language recovery post stroke has not been employed in most studies. Drug studies for aphasia are still at the initial stages along the continuum of levels of research. The study of the use of pharmacotherapy for aphasia requires further research in order for the possibility of identifying and implementing medication as a part of the standard of care for aphasia rehabilitation in the future.

Noninvasive brain stimulation for aphasia rehabilitation is another type of a biological treatment approach that is gaining attention in the field of aphasia rehabilitation. The noninvasive brain stimulation techniques that have been administered for aphasia rehabilitation include transcranial magnetic stimulation (TMS) and transcranial direct current stimulation (tDCS). Similar to pharmacologic agents, noninvasive brain stimulation does not act in isolation and is administered concomitantly with speech language therapy. While the first TMS study for PWA administered TMS over the contralateral homologue of Broca's area, hypothesizing that suppressing the right hemisphere may promote language recovery,[64] the first tDCS aphasia research study applied tDCS over Broca area as well as over the right Broca's homologue.[65] In both of these early studies, brain stimulation was not combined with behavioral therapy. More recently, and now consistently, noninvasive brain stimulation in the form of tDCS is combined with behavioral speech language therapy to investigate the effect of using this method to promote aphasia language recovery (see Ref. 66 for a review). In this literature, researchers have generally employed tDCS in two different montages, either aiming to downregulate the right hemisphere or upregulate the left hemisphere with the suggestion that within subject variables affect optimal montage (e.g., see Ref. 67). Generally the tDCS aphasia rehabilitation studies published have been small, within-subject crossover designs. While larger, between-subject studies are needed to better evaluate this treatment method, the review by Elsner and his coauthors reports several studies that noted language improvement when behavioral speech language therapy is combined with tDCS. Although many of the tDCS aphasia studies do not describe the behavioral intervention that is combined with tDCS, it is thought that the combination of tDCS and behavioral intervention interacts for the promotion of language recovery in post-stroke aphasia. For a review of the types of behavioral interventions implemented in tDCS aphasia rehabilitation research, see Galletta et al.[68] Both impairment-based and social-communication treatment approaches have been employed.

TREATMENT WITH MULTILINGUAL AND MULTICULTURAL INDIVIDUALS AND WORK WITH INTERPRETERS

Multilingual individuals, those who speak more than one language prior to the aphasia onset, often experience comparable impairment in all their languages. However, variables including language proficiency and frequency of use, among others, may yield differential levels of impairment and recovery in two or more languages, and language-specific characteristics may yield differential types of impairment in two or more languages.[69] Treatment studies have demonstrated that multilingual individuals with aphasia improve following treatment, whether the treatment is provided in their first acquired or more dominant language, or in another language.[70] Mixed results have been reported regarding cross-language generalization, that is, whether treatment in one language of a multilingual individual with aphasia yields improvement also in the nontreated language(s). Studies have demonstrated that cross-language generalization may depend on the relative preonset proficiency of the languages and on their relative degree of postaphasia impairment, their relative structural similarity, the focus of the treatment, and the linguistic context of the environment.[71–73] Multilingual individuals with aphasia, like neurologically intact multilingual people, may mix their languages

within and between sentences when communicating with multilingual interlocutors. Failure to inhibit the nontarget language and a faulty language control mechanism may lead to inappropriate or unintentional language mixing.

When the PWA do not speak the majority language, the SLP may need to administer treatment with the help of interpreters. Interpreters must be trained in how to best communicate with a person with aphasia. The American Speech Language Hearing Association[74] outlines specific suggestions for speech language clinicians working with patients who are in need of interpreters (www.asha.org). These include recommendations to implement before, during, and after the therapy session and are focused on ensuring that the interpreter and therapist understand their roles in supporting the patient and promoting the provision of language therapy to the PWA. In therapy sessions, an interpreter relies on the clinician to take the lead and determine the input needed from the interpreter. At times the interpreter translates each and every word, and at times an interpreter is used as needed. Nonetheless, the interpreter provides an important and necessary skill for the provision of therapy to multilingual and multicultural individuals with aphasia.

CONCLUSIONS

Aphasia rehabilitation can involve a variety of treatments that are generally described as either restitutive or vicariative treatment approaches. Therapy can be provided in a number of settings and under a wide range of intensities. It can target specific linguistic elements or underlying processes, and it can offer strategies to improve communication. Many speech language pathologists employ a variety of approaches and techniques and tailor the therapy they provide to the individual patient. Research evidence confirms that PWA benefit from speech language therapy and continue to improve their language and communication skills. Treatment-related gains are small at times, especially in the chronic stages, but an upward trajectory can be observed in all aphasia types and degrees of severity. Recent neuroimaging studies have begun to associate aphasia recovery with neuronal reorganization. Data to date suggest that reorganization processes within the language-dominant hemisphere are associated with language improvement.[75,76]

Future clinical research studies are warranted to better harness neuroplasticity in the administration of aphasia therapy to increase language and communication recovery following brain damage.

REFERENCES

1. Hillis AE, Newport M. Cognitive neuropsychological approaches to treatment of language disorders: Introduction. In: Chapey R, ed. *Language Intervention Strategies in Aphasia and Related Neurogenic Communication Disorders*. Philadelphia: Walters Kluer; 2008.

2. McNeil MR. The nature of aphasia in adults. In: Lass N, McReynolds L, Northern J, Yoder D, eds. *Speech, Language, and Hearing*. Vol. II. 1982:692–740.

3. Goodglass H, Kaplan E, Barresi B. *Boston Diagnostic Aphasia Examination*. Philadelphia, PA: Lippincott Williams & Wilkins; 2001.

4. Geshwind N. Disconnection syndromes in animals and man. I. *Brain*. 1965;88:237–294.

5. Geshwind N. Disconnection syndromes in animals and man. II. *Brain*. 1965;88:585–644.

6. Goodglass H, Kaplan E. *The Assessment of Aphasia and Related Disorders*. Philadelphia: Lea & Febiger; 1972.

7. Chapey R, ed. *Language Intervention Strategies in Aphasia and Related Neurogenic Communication Disorders*. Baltimore: Lippincott Williams & Wilkins; 2008.

8. Bhogal SK, Teasell R, Speechley M. Intensity of aphasia therapy, impact on recovery. *Stroke*. 2003;34(4):987–993.

9. Cherney LR, Patterson JP, Raymer AM. Intensity of aphasia therapy: evidence and efficacy. *Curr Neurol Neurosci Rep*. 2011;11(6):560–569.

10. Lazar RM, Minzer B, Antoniello D, Festa JR, Krakauer JW, Marshall RS. Improvement in aphasia scores after stroke is well predicted by initial severity. *Stroke*. 2010:1485–1488.

11. Raymer A, Beeson P, Holland A, et al. Translational research in aphasia: from neuroscience to neurorehabilitation. *J Speech Lang Hear Res*. 2008;51:S259–S275.

12. Smania N, Gandolfi M, Aglioti SM, Girardi P, Fiaschi A, Girardi F. How long is the recovery of global aphasia? Twenty-five years of follow-up in a patient with left hemisphere stroke. *Neurorehabil Neural Repair*. 2010;24(9):871–875.

13. Kleim JA, Jones TA. Principles of experience-dependent neural plasticity: implications for rehabilitation after brain damage. *J Speech Lang Hear Res*. 2008;51(1):S225–S239.

13a. Webster J, Whitworth A, Morris J. Is it time to stop "fishing"? A review of generalisation following aphasia intervention. *Aphasiology*; 2015. https://doi.org/10.1080/02687038.2015.1027169.

14. Brady MC, Kelly H, Godwin G, Enderby P, Campbell P. Speech and language therapy for aphasia following stroke. *Cochrane Database Syst Rev*. 2016;5:1–45. https://doi.org/10.1002/14651858.CD000425.pub4.

15. Coppens P, Patterson J. *Aphasia Rehabilitation: Clinical Challenges*. Burlington: Jones & Bartlett Learning; 2017.

16. Helm-Estabrooks N, Albert ML, Nicholas M. *Manual of Aphasia and Aphasia Therapy*. Austin, TX: Pro-ed; 2014.

17. Abel S, Weiller C, Huber W, Willmes K. Neural underpinnings for model-oriented therapy of aphasic word production. *Neuropsychologia*. 2014;57:154–165.

18. Abel S, Weiller C, Huber W, Willmes K, Specht K. Therapy-induced brain reorganization patterns in aphasia. *Brain A J Neurol*. 2015;138(Pt 4):1097–1112.

19. Kiran S, Bassetto G. Evaluating the effectiveness of semantic-based treatment for naming deficits in aphasia: what works? *Semin Speech Lang*. 2008;29(1):71–82.

20. Meinzer M, Harnish S, Conway T, Crosson B. Recent developments in functional and structural imaging of aphasia recovery after stroke. *Aphasiology*. 2011;25(3):271–290.

21. Raymer AM, Thompson CK, Jacobs B, Le Grand H. Phonological treatment of naming deficits in aphasia: model-based generalization analysis. *Aphasiology*. 1993;7(1):27–53.

22. Wambaugh JL, Linebaugh CW, Doyle PJ, Martinez AL, Kalinyak-Fliszar M, Spencer KA. Effects of two cueing treatments on lexical retrieval in aphasic speakers with different levels of deficit. *Aphasiology*. 2001;15(10–11):933–950.

23. Hickin J, Best W, Herbert R, Howard D, Osborne F. Phonological therapy for word-finding difficulties: a re-evaluation. *Aphasiology*. 2002;16(10–11):981–999.

24. Greenwood A, Grassly J, Hickin J, Best W. Phonological and orthographic cueing therapy: a case of generalised improvement. *Aphasiology*. 2010;24(9):991–1016.

25. Kendall DL, Oelke M, Brookshire CE, Nadeau SE. The influence of phonomotor treatment on word retrieval abilities in 26 individuals with chronic aphasia: an open trial. *J Speech, Lang Hear Res*. 2015;58(3):798–812.

26. Boyle M. Semantic feature analysis treatment for aphasic word retrieval impairments: what's in a name? *Top Stroke Rehabilitation*. 2010;17(6):411–422.

27. Kiran S, Thompson CK. The role of semantic complexity in treatment of naming DeficitsTraining semantic categories in fluent aphasia by controlling exemplar typicality. *J Speech Lang Hear Res*. 2003;46(4):773–787.

28. Edmonds LA, Nadeau SE, Kiran S. Effect of verb network strengthening treatment (VNeST) on lexical retrieval of content words in sentences in persons with aphasia. *Aphasiology*. 2009;23(3):402–424.

29. Edmonds LA, Mammino K, Ojeda J. Effect of verb network strengthening treatment (VNeST) in persons with aphasia: extension and replication of previous findings. *Am J Speech Lang Pathol*. 2014;23(2):S312–S329.

30. Webster J, Whitworth A. Treating verbs in aphasia: exploring the impact of therapy at the single word and sentence levels. *Int J Lang Commun Disord*. 2012;47(6):619–636.

31. Kiran S, Ntourou K, Eubanks M, Shamapant S. Typicality of inanimate category exemplars in aphasia: further evidence for the semantic complexity effect. *Brain Lang*. 2005;95(1):178–180.

32. Kiran S, Shamapant S, DeLyria SK. Typicality within well defined categories in aphasia. *Brain Lang*. 2006;99(1–2):159–161.

32a. Boyle M, Coelho CA. Application of semantic feature analysis as a treatment for aphasic dysnomia. *American Journal of Speech Language Pathology*. 1995;4:94–98.

33. Boyle M. Semantic feature analysis treatment for anomia in two fluent aphasia syndromes. *Am J Speech Lang Pathol*. 2004;13(3):236–249.

34. Davis LA, Stanton ST. Semantic feature analysis as a functional therapy tool. *Contemp Issues Commun Sci Disord.* 2005;32:85−92.

35. Lowell S, Beeson PM, Holland AL. The efficacy of a semantic cueing procedure on naming performance of adults with aphasia. *Am J Speech Lang Pathol.* 1995;4(4):109−114.

36. Marcotte K, Adrover-Roig D, Damien B, et al. Therapy-induced neuroplasticity in chronic aphasia. *Neuropsychologia.* 2012;50(8):1776−1786.

37. Peach RK, Reuter KA. A discourse-based approach to semantic feature analysis for the treatment of aphasic word retrieval failures. *Aphasiology.* 2010;24(9):971−990.

38. Kristensson J, Behrns I, Saldert C. Effects on communication from intensive treatment with semantic feature analysis in aphasia. *Aphasiology.* 2015;29(4):466−487.

39. Wambaugh JL, Ferguson M. Application of semantic feature analysis to retrieval of action names in aphasia. *J Rehabil Res Dev.* 2007;44(3):381−394.

40. Maddy KM, Capilouto GJ, McComas KL. The effectiveness of semantic feature analysis: an evidence-based systematic review. *Ann Phys Rehabil Med.* 2014;57(4):254−267.

41. Rider JD, Wright HH, Marshall RC, Page JL. Using semantic feature analysis to improve contextual discourse in adults with aphasia. *Am J Speech Lang Pathol.* 2008;17(2):161−172.

42. Edmonds LA, Babb M. Effect of verb network strengthening treatment in moderate-to-severe aphasia. *Am J Speech Lang Pathol.* 2011;20(2):131−145.

43. Edmonds LA. Tutorial for verb network strengthening treatment (VNeST): detailed description of the treatment protocol with corresponding theoretical rationale. *Perspect Neurophysiol Neurogen Speech Lang Disord.* 2014;24(3):78−88.

44. Ballard KJ, Thompson CK. Treatment and generalization of complex sentence production in agrammatism. *J Speech Lang Hear Res.* 1999;42(3):690−707.

45. Jacobs BJ, Thompson CK. Cross-modal generalization effects of training noncanonical sentence comprehension and production in agrammatic aphasia. *J Speech Lang Hear Res.* 2000;43(1):5−20.

46. Thompson CK, Shapiro LP. Complexity in treatment of syntactic deficits. *Am J Speech Lang Pathol.* 2007;16(1):30−42.

47. Thompson CK, Shapiro LP, Kiran S, Sobecks J. The role of syntactic complexity in treatment of sentence deficits in agrammatic Aphasia: the complexity account of treatment efficacy (CATE). *J Speech Lang Hear Res.* 2003;46(3):591−607.

48. Thompson CK, Riley EA, den Ouden D-B, Meltzer-Asscher A, Lukic S. Training verb argument structure production in agrammatic aphasia: behavioral and neural recovery patterns. *Cortex.* 2013;49(9):2358−2376.

49. Cohen L, Martinaud O, Lemer C, et al. Visual word recognition in the left and right hemispheres: anatomical and functional correlates of peripheral alexias. *Cereb Cortex.* 2003;13(12):1313−1333.

50. Laine T, Marttila RJ. Pure agraphia: a case study. *Neuropsychologia.* 1981;19(2):311−316. (study).

51. Rosati G, De Bastiani P. Pure agraphia: a discrete form of aphasia. *J Neurol Neurosurg Psychiatry.* 1979;42(3):266−269.

52. Sakurai Y, Matsumura K, Iwatsubo T, Momose T. Frontal pure agraphia for kanji or kana: dissociation between morphology and phonology. *Neurology.* 1997;49(4):946−952.

53. Cherney L. Aphasia, alexia, and oral reading. *Top Stroke Rehabil.* 2004;11(1):22−36.

54. Cherney LR. Oral reading for language in aphasia (ORLA): evaluating the efficacy of computer-delivered therapy in chronic nonfluent aphasia. *Top Stroke Rehabil.* 2010;17(6):423−431.

55. Whitworth A, Webster J, Howard D. *A Cognitive Neuropsychological Approach to Assessment and Intervention in Aphasia: A Clinician's Guide.* Psychology Press; 2014.

56. Beeson PM. Treating acquired writing impairment: strengthening graphemic representations. *Aphasiology.* 1999;13(9−11):767−785.

57. Beeson PM, Rising K, Volk J. Writing treatment for severe aphasia: who benefits? *J Speech Lang Hear Res.* 2003;46(5):1038−1060.

58. Beeson PM, Higginson K, Rising K. Writing treatment for aphasia: a texting approach. *J Speech Lang Hear Res.* 2013;56(3):945−955.

59. World Health Organization. *International Classification of Functioning, Disability, and Health.* Geneva: ICF; 2001.

60. Kagan A. Supported conversation for adults with aphasia: methods and resources for training conversation partners. *Aphasiology.* 1988;12:816−830.

61. Elman R. The importance of aphasia group treatment for rebuilding community and health. *Top Lang Disord.* 2007;27(4):300−308.

62. Small SL. Biological approaches to the treatment of aphasia. In: Hillis A, ed. *Handbook on Adult Language Disorders: Integrating Cognitive Neuropsychology, Neurology, and Rehabilitation.* Philadelphia: Psychology Press; 2001: 397−411.

63. Small SL, Llano DA. Biological approaches to aphasia treatment. *Curr Neurol Neurosci Rep.* 2009;9:443−450.

64. Martin PI, Naeser MA, Theoret H, et al. Transcranial magnetic stimulation as a complementary treatment of aphasia. *Semin Speech Lang.* 2004;25(2):181−191.

65. Monti A, Cogiamanian F, Marceglia S, et al. Improved naming after transcranial direct current stimulation in aphasia. *J Neurol Neurosurg Psychiatry.* 2008;79(4):451−453.

66. Elsner B, Kugler J, Pohl M, Mehrholz J. Transcranial direct current stimulation (tDCS) for improving aphasia in patients after stroke (Art. No. CD009760). *Cochrane Data- Base Syst Rev.* 2015. https://doi.org/10.1002/14651858.CD009760.pub2.

67. Shah-Basak PP, Norise C, Torres J, Faseyitan O, Hamilton R. Individualized treatment with transcranial direct current stimulation in patients with chronic non-fluent aphasia due to stroke. *Front Hum Neurosci.* 2015;9:201.

68. Galletta EE, Conner P, Vogel-Eyny A, Marangolo P. Use of tDCS in aphasia rehabilitation: a systematic review of the

behavioral interventions implemented with noninvasive brain stimulation for language recovery. *Am J Speech Lang Pathol.* 2016;25(4S):S854. https://doi.org/10.1044/2016_AJSLP-15-0133.

69. Ansaldo A, Saidi L. Aphasia therapy in the age of globalization: cross-linguistic therapy effects in bilingual aphasia. *Behav Neurol.* 2014:603085.

70. Faroqi-Shah Y, Frymark T, Mullen R, Wang B. Effect of treatment for bilingual individuals with aphasia: a systematic review of the evidence. *J Neurolinguistics.* 2010;23:319–341. https://doi.org/10.1016/j.jneuroling.2010.01.002.

71. Goral M, Levy ES, Obler LK, Cohen E. Lexical connections in the multilingual lexicon. *Brain Lang.* 2006;98:235–247.

72. Goral M, Rosas J, Conner PS, Maul KK, Obler LK. Effects of language proficiency and language of the environment on aphasia therapy in a multilingual. *J Neurolinguistics.* 2012;25:538–551.

73. Knoph M, Lind M, Simonsen H. Semantic feature analysis targeting verbs in a quadrilingual speaker with aphasia. *Aphasiology.* 2015;29:1473–1496.

74. American Speech Language Hearing Association. Collaborating with interpreters. http://www.asha.org/Practice-Portal/Professional-Issues/Collaborating-With-Interpreters/.

75. Cappa S. The neural basis of aphasia rehabilitation: evidence from neuroimaging and neurostimulation. *Neuropsychol Rehabil.* 2011;21(5):742–754.

76. Crinion JT. Using functional imaging to understand therapeutic effects in poststroke aphasia. *Curr Opin Neurol.* 2015;28(4):330–337.

CHAPTER 4

Swallowing Disorders After Stroke

M. GONZALEZ-FERNANDEZ, MD, PHD • N. LANGTON-FROST, MA, CCC-SLP, BCS-S • A.N. WRIGHT, BS • E. KARAGIORGOS, MS, CCC-SLP • M.N. BAHOUTH, MD

SWALLOWING EPIDEMIOLOGY

Swallowing dysfunction, or dysphagia, is common after stroke. Estimates on the prevalence are variable based on the type of stroke and method of dysphagia evaluation. Estimates suggest that about half of the stroke patients have acute swallowing problems.[1] Fortunately dysphagia resolves within 2 weeks for half of the patients affected. Approximately 15% of stroke patients have long-standing swallowing problems (lasting 6 months or more). Malnutrition, dehydration, airway obstruction, and aspiration pneumonia are among the most feared consequences of dysphagia.

Malnutrition has been associated with poor stroke outcomes. This includes longer length of stay and increased risk of other complications such as infections and falls.[2] Dysphagia after stroke is an important risk factor for malnutrition, increasing the odds of malnutrition after stroke by 2.6 times.[3] Dysphagia has also been associated with dehydration after stroke at hospital admission and discharge based on BUN/creatinine levels.[4] Oral intake of fluids is limited in people with dysphagia, particularly those for whom treatment recommendations include thickened liquids.[5,6] The risk of aspiration pneumonia is markedly increased for stroke patients with dysphagia.[7] Ho et al. reported an incidence of aspiration pneumonia of 19% in a large 4-year stroke cohort.[8] Mortality in this cohort was significantly increased for people with dysphagia (10.45% of those with dysphagia vs. 4.77% in those without dysphagia). Stroke subjects' risk of aspiration pneumonia increases up to 20 times when videofluoroscopy-confirmed aspiration is present.[9] Silent aspiration, aspiration without a cough, is also common after stroke occurring in about 65% of stroke patients.[10]

NEURAL CONTROL OF SWALLOWING

Swallowing is a complex process that needs to be performed accurately hundreds of times a day. It requires a tightly orchestrated sequence of events to protect the airway while transport of the bolus occurs in close proximity. The contractions of more than 20 muscles have to be tightly orchestrated for a normal swallow to occur.

Swallowing physiology is elegantly coordinated via a series of neural control centers. The neural control of swallowing involves afferent and efferent communication between cortical, subcortical, and brainstem structures. Brain stem dysfunction often leads to swallowing problems when lower motor neurons are involved. However supramedullary lesions resulting in motor dysfunction or attention deficits also play an important role in dysphagia. The most frequent brain hemisphere areas associated with dysphagia include the insula, frontal operculum, internal capsule, thalamus, precentral gyrus, and postcentral gyrus. Discrete lesions in any of these regions result in specific dysfunction and unique clinical presentations of dysphagia.

Brainstem

The brainstem is a densely populated region of the brain containing cranial nerve nuclei and decussating fibers, as they travel from the cortex to the spinal cord. Thus lesions in this area can often contribute to dysphagia through a variety of mechanisms. The central pattern generator, located in the lateral medulla bilaterally, is thought to be the primary swallowing center. Damage to the rostral and/or dorsolateral medulla may result in weakness of the pharynx, larynx, and soft palate, as well as the ability to initiate and coordinate a swallow.[11] Dysphagia was a key finding in Wallenberg syndrome caused by a lateral medullary

Stroke Rehabilitation. https://doi.org/10.1016/B978-0-323-55381-0.00004-4

lesion. Stroke patients with lateral medullary syndromes are at high risk for dysphagia and aspiration.[12]

Oropharyngeal sensation

In order to initiate an effective swallow, a bolus must be sensed in the oropharyngeal cavity. Afferent fibers from the maxillary branch of the trigeminal nerve, chorda tympani branch of the facial nerve (taste), the glossopharyngeal nerve, and superior laryngeal branch of the vagus nerve transmit sensory information from the sensory receptors of the oral cavity (CN V), the dorsum of the tongue (CN XI), laryngeal surface of the epiglottis, the plexus of the pharynx, and the larynx (CN IX, X) to the solitary tract and terminates in the nucleus tractus solitarius (NTS) located in the medulla.[13,14] Damage to the afferent fibers or NTS may affect the oral and pharyngeal phases of swallow by disrupting the sensory input from a bolus in the oral, oropharyngeal, or pharyngeal cavities. This in turn can affect the timing or the sequence of events required for a normal swallow, most prominently, swallow initiation.

Dorsal swallow group (DSG)

Interneurons within the NTS and adjacent reticular formation receive and integrate the sensory information from the cortical and peripheral nerve system. The DSG assists with initiating the swallow, determining the force required to propel the bolus into the pharynx, and facilitates normal timing of the oropharyngeal swallow. This integration is essential in modulating the needed swallow response based on the size and texture of the bolus received. Interneurons from the DSG communicate with the ventral swallow group.[11]

Ventral swallow group (VSG)

The ventral swallow group (VSG) contains interneurons that are located in the ventrolateral medulla above the nucleus ambiguus. The trigeminal (CN V) and hypoglossal (CN XII) motor nuclei synapses lie in the ventral medulla. The VSG sends efferent signals to the trigeminal nerve (CN V), the facial nerve (CN VII), the glossopharyngeal nerve (CN IX), the vagus nerve (CN X), and the hypoglossal nerve (XII) to initiate motor movement of oropharyngeal muscles. These peripheral connections modulate and coordinate different phases of deglutition.[11]

Supramedullary Control

A large body of swallowing neurophysiology research has focused on the brainstem for localization of swallow dysfunction. More recently, attention has shifted to include the contribution of supratentorial lesions. Damage to cortical and subcortical areas along the corticobulbar, corticospinal, and extrapyramidal tracts have been found to be important in disrupting normal swallowing function.

Corticobulbar and extrapyramidal tracts

The corticobulbar tract originates in the precentral gyrus (primary motor cortex) sending fibers that pass through the operculum, the corona radiata, and the internal capsule before reaching the brain stem's central pattern generator. The central pattern generator, in turn, sends efferent signals to the muscles involved in swallowing. This tract may also receive input from the supplemental motor area and premotor cortex. Damage to the corticobulbar tract may result in delayed swallow initiation, prolonged anterior to posterior oral transit, and reduced swallow coordination.[15,16] In addition, the extrapyramidal tract, assists with initiation of movement, and more specifically, the rate or force required for movement. This tract begins at the primary motor strip, passing through the basal ganglia to the thalamus. The thalamus then sends and receives messages to and from the central pattern generator and relays that information to the premotor and motor cortex.[17–20]

Insula

Research suggests that the insula is activated early during deglutition. Tasting of food activates the insula to prepare the circuit for effective swallowing. The insula also plays a vital role in swallow function predominantly in the area of sensorimotor control.[14,20,21] It receives sensory information from the oral cavity and communicates sensory information to the NTS via the ventroposterior medial nucleus of the thalamus. Additionally, the insula connects to the primary motor cortex, which suggests that the insula plays a role in sensorimotor integration. Finally, damage to the insula often results in issues with speech and auditory processes, which may play an important role in rehabilitation of dysphagia after a lesion occurs in this region.

Lesion laterality

The effect of dominant versus nondominant (left vs. right) hemispheric lesions on swallowing function is unclear.[22,23] With the use of functional MRI, Mihai P described activation bilaterally in the primary motor cortex, primary somatosensory cortex, supplemental motor area, primary motor area, anterior and posterior insula, cerebellum, and thalamus when swallowing water.[24] This suggests that both the left and right hemispheres are involved in swallow function. Discrete lesions in either hemisphere could contribute to attention, motor control in the oropharynx, and sensory feedback of bolus control during swallow.

A summary of the brain areas associated with swallowing is presented in Table 4.1.

SCREENING FOR DYSPHAGIA IN ACUTE STROKE PATIENTS

Early identification of dysphagia by screening acute stroke patients allows for timely delivery of treatment interventions and improves outcomes.[27] The evidence suggests that dysphagia screening can reduce mortality, morbidity, length of hospital stay, healthcare costs, and burden of swallowing impairment.[27] Early identification of dysphagia after stroke has been shown to significantly decrease the incidence of pneumonia and improve patient outcomes after stroke.[28] An effective screening aims to identify signs of dysphagia and aspiration and determine the need for further evaluation and testing by a licensed Speech-Language Pathologist (SLP).

As nurses are often the first to interact with the patient in the hospital setting, they are positioned to identify possible swallowing difficulties, initiate dysphagia screening, and advise the interdisciplinary team accordingly.[27]

Several screening tests are available for evaluating patients after stroke with varying sensitivity and specificity. Most dysphagia screening tests include a clinical evaluation followed by a water swallowing trial. In a recent metaanalysis including 22 studies, Brodsky and colleagues formally evaluated the screening accuracy for aspiration using bedside water swallowing tests. The analysis concluded that currently used bedside swallowing screening tests are sufficient for screening for aspiration.[29]

ASSESSMENT OF DYSPHAGIA AFTER STROKE

Clinical Evaluation

The clinical bedside assessment of swallowing encompasses clinical history and examinations of the oral, pharyngeal, and laryngeal anatomy.[30] In patients with stroke, a comprehensive neurologic evaluation including assessment of sensory and motor function, cognition, and language abilities is recommended. Trial feeding can be performed as part of the evaluation. Several factors have been associated with increased aspiration risk including: (1) dysphonia, (2) dysarthria,

(3) abnormal gag reflex, (4) cough and cough abnormalities, and (5) voice changes.[31,32] The presence of silent aspiration in a large proportion of stroke patients limits the information that a clinician may obtain during a bedside assessment. Instrumental assessment is needed in cases where silent aspiration is a concern or when the pathophysiology of dysphagia needs to be evaluated to design a training plan.

Instrumental Assessment

Instrumental examination allows for direct evaluation of swallowing physiology. The two most common tools are the videofluoroscopic swallowing study (VFSS) and fiberoptic endoscopic evaluation of swallowing (FEES). Both tools allow for examination of anatomic structures and physiologic functioning, as well as assessing the utility of compensatory techniques in facilitating airway protection and bolus flow.

VFSS is the most commonly used tool to evaluate swallowing. Using lateral or anteroposterior fluoroscopy, the patient is observed drinking barium contrast or eating barium-coated food of various consistencies to assess bolus flow and airway protection. One of the goals of the VFSS is to determine the presence or absence of aspiration. Equally important is to characterize the physiologic deficits that are resulting in dysphagia in order to design a treatment plan that addresses those directly. Radiation exposure is a concern when performing this test and appropriate exposure mitigation strategies such as collimation and avoidance of magnification should be used.

FEES involves the use of a transnasal fiberoptic endoscope to view the pharynx superiorly. Aspiration cannot be appreciated in real time as there is a "white out" during laryngeal vestibule closure. However, aspiration can be observed immediately before the swallow or inferred after the swallow based on telltale residue in the trachea after the swallow or spontaneous ejection of material from the trachea. FEES does not allow for visualization of the oral cavity or the esophagus, thus limiting the information being obtained. One advantage of FEES is that it allows a clinician to monitor feeding during a longer period of time and without the need for contrast.

Other instrumental assessments are available including: ultrasound, pharyngeal high-resolution manometry, and 320 detector-row computerized tomography. These assessments are beneficial and can be used when additional information is needed on the anatomy, pharyngeal or esophageal contraction, or pressure dynamics and when a detailed evaluation of areas not clearly visualized in VFSS or FEES is needed.

TABLE 4.1
Neural Regions Associated With Swallowing Function

Region	Localization	Symptom/Clinical Correlate
Cortical	Lateral precentral gyrus[14,22,24]	• Control tongue and face • Initiation of swallowing sequence
	Supplementary motor area (SMA)[9,25]	• Motor planning and sequential movements • Oral preparatory phase
	Anterior cingulate cortex (primary motor cortex)[17,22,24]	• Attention component of swallowing • Complex motor planning • Aspiration on videofluoroscopy
	Insula/Operculum[11,18–22,26]	• Sensorimotor integration • Taste • Swallow initiation • Confluence of the most caudal parts of the pre- and postcentral gyri • Necessary for structural aspects of bolus and timing of consecutive states of deglutition
	Somatosensory and parietal cortex[22]	• Sensory input may be linked to modulation of motor activity via connectivity with precentral cortex and insula
	Temporal cortex[23]	• Works with the prefrontal cortex. May play a supplementary role in the regulation of swallowing and feeding • Taste recognition
	Posterior central gyrus (primary sensory cortex)[24,27,28]	• Oropharyngeal sensory processing
	Precuneus[22]	• Sensory integration with thalamus

	Location	Symptoms/Details
Subcortical	Internal capsule[29]	• Disconnect between cortex and central pattern generator. Motor control
	Basal ganglia[9]	• Assists with motor control and sets up motor plans
	Thalamus[30,31]	• A communication station receiving sensory information from the cortex • Swallow initiation

TREATMENT APPROACHES FOR THE PATIENT WITH DYSPHAGIA

Dysphagia Treatment: External Factors

Foundational to dysphagia treatment is starting with the appropriate environment and posture. An environment devoid of distractions is needed to ensure that the instructions can be carefully followed and understood. Compensatory strategies may be effective for some patients but require practice and consistent use. Patients should be sitting upright and support should be provided to reduce the energy expenditure of maintaining an upright position for patients with hemiparesis or poor trunk control.

Principles of Dysphagia Therapy

Treatment of dysphagia after stroke includes multiple interventions that can be classified as compensatory, restorative, or both. Compensatory maneuvers seek to maintain safe oral feeding, in spite of physiologic impairments, and without attempting to improve the underlying pathophysiology. Some therapies can be considered both compensatory and restorative, as they not only ameliorate symptoms but can also result in changes that restore lost function (usually through strengthening). Restorative interventions are used to impact swallowing physiology with the goal of restoring function. Common treatment strategies include postural maneuvers, bolus modifications, and exercises.[33] Generally speaking, postural maneuvers and bolus modifications are compensatory while exercises are restorative. Some postural maneuvers are also restorative: effortful swallow, supraglottic swallow, super-supraglottic swallow, and Mendelsohn maneuver. Treatment strategies should be trialed during instrumental evaluation of swallowing (VFSS or FEES) to determine their effectiveness in reducing aspiration and improving the patient's ability to meet his or her nutritional and hydration needs.

Liquids or Food Texture Modification

One of the most common treatment strategies for dysphagia management is liquid and food modifications. The viscosity and volume of liquids can be modified to reduce the risk of aspiration. Increasing the viscosity of liquids is used primarily to slow bolus transit and prevent aspiration. Food texture modifications may be used when patients are at high risk for choking, have poor dentition or inability to chew, or when tongue weakness may limit the person's ability to transport the bolus to the oropharynx. Diet modifications should be reserved for those patients at risk of aspiration when other treatment options are

unsuccessful in reducing aspiration, as the palatability of altered liquids or foods may decrease overall consumption potentially compromising nutrition and hydration.

Maneuvers

Chin tuck

Chin tuck is one of the most commonly used tools for people with dysphagia. For this maneuver, patients are asked to "bring their chin to their chest" for the duration of the swallow.[32a] This posture helps liquids remain proximal in the oral cavity and may be helpful when swallow initiation is delayed. This position approximates the tongue base and the pharyngeal wall thus being useful in cases when tongue base retraction is impaired.

Head turn and tilt

Head turn and tilt maneuvers can be very useful in people with unilateral weakness. The maneuvers are used to redirect the bolus away from the weak side. The head turn (rotation) maneuver is accomplished by the following command: "turn your head to the side as if you are looking over your shoulder."[33] The head is rotated to the impaired side closing it and redirecting the bolus to the opposite and stronger side of the pharynx.[34] The head tilt maneuver is performed by instructing the patient to "tilt your head like you're trying to touch your ear to your shoulder."[33] The head is tilted to the strong side in order to redirect the bolus toward the unimpaired side of the oral cavity thus allowing better oral control.

Effortful swallow

The effortful swallow requires the person to volitionally attempt to increase the strength of muscle contraction while swallowing. The patient is asked to squeeze the throat muscles as hard as he or she can when swallowing.[34a] The process of volitionally enhancing muscle contraction can compensate for a weak swallow but also strengthens the muscles used.

Supraglottic and super-supraglottic swallow

The supraglottic and super-supraglottic swallowing maneuvers are designed to increase airway protection by using a person's ability to voluntarily hold their breath. To perform the supraglottic swallow, patients are asked to take a deep breath, hold their breath; followed by swallowing while continuing to hold their breath and end by coughing immediately after the swallow (before the next inhalation).[35] The super-supraglottic swallow adds increased effort or bearing down during the breath hold. The effort required for the super-supraglottic swallow may result in Valsalva. In stroke patients, clinicians should be cautious as these maneuvers have been associated with self-limiting arrhythmias.[36]

Mendelsohn maneuver

The Mendelsohn maneuver requires the patient to voluntarily maintain the hyolaryngeal elevation occurring at the peak of the swallow. By increasing the duration of the anterior-superior movement, the larynx traction on the anterior wall of the UES is maintained, delaying sphincter closure.[37] This maneuver may be particularly useful for patients who have aspiration or residue above the UES placing the person at risk for aspiration after the swallow.

Restorative Approaches
Tongue hold

The tongue hold maneuver (also referred to as the Masako maneuver) is performed by holding the anterior tongue between the teeth while swallowing to increase bulging of the posterior pharyngeal wall.[38,39] The maneuver can strengthen the posterior pharyngeal wall, thus improving bolus flow.

Shaker exercises

Shaker exercises were designed to improve strength of the anterior neck muscles and upper esophageal sphincter opening. The protocol requires the person to lay supine and perform three sustained head lifts for 1 min each followed by 30 head lifts of 2 s duration. The exercise is to be performed three times a day for 6 weeks.[40]

Other Treatment Approaches

Neuromuscular electrical stimulation (NMES) is a treatment modality that directs electrical currents to the muscle of the anterior neck to produce muscle contraction. Research both for and against the use of NMES for dysphagia treatment has been published.[41–45] One of the most recent studies on the topic suggests that NMES as an adjuvant to traditional therapy may be beneficial for people with long standing dysphagia unresponsive to traditional therapy alone.[46] Conversely, NMES did not add benefit to traditional dysphagia treatment (exercises) in a randomized controlled trial of patients with head and neck cancer.[25]

Oral exercises (lips and tongue) and oral sensory stimulation have also been potential treatments for dysphagia. Ice massage was used in one study reporting shortened latency for swallow initiation.[26] Other studies evaluating thermal application for the treatment of dysphagia after stroke failed to reveal improvements

in swallowing function.[47] Evidence to date as to the effectiveness of lingual strengthening to improve swallowing is conflicting. In stroke patients, lingual exercises increased lingual strength, swallowing pressures, airway protection, and lingual volume.[48] A recent systematic review reported that the current literature on isometric lingual strength training is too variable to confidently report specific therapeutic benefits.[49]

Brain-based therapies such as transcranial magnetic stimulation (TMS) and transcranial direct current stimulation (tDCS) have been studied in the context of dysphagia. A systematic review in 2016 found evidence for the efficacy of noninvasive brain stimulation on poststroke dysphagia.[50]

Oral Versus Nonoral Feeding in Neurologic Dysphagia

Dysphagia often improves quickly over the first 2 weeks after stroke; however, it may persist for weeks or months. Current recommendations for stroke patients with dysphagia may include alternate, nonoral strategies for nutrition. There are a variety of options including temporary enteral access (e.g., tube feed via nasogastric tube), parenteral forms (e.g., PPN peripheral parenteral nutrition), and semipermanent approaches (e.g., tube feeding via percutaneous endoscopic gastrostomy tube).

In the United States, the most frequently used enteral tube feeding modalities for acute stroke patients are nasogastric tube (NGT) and percutaneous endoscopic gastrostomy (PEG) tubes.

Nasogastric tubes

NGT are widely used to provide enteral nutrition to patients with dysphagia, especially in the early period after stroke when rapid recovery is expected. Temporary use, no longer than 3–4 weeks, is recommended due to risk of mucosal injury and infection. Complications related to shortterm NGT use (under 2 weeks) are typically not serious and include discomfort, dislodgment, or gastrointestinal complications such as nausea or abdominal distention.[51] Some controversy exists regarding the impact of NGT on swallow function, airway protection, and swallow rehabilitation.[52,53] However, Leder SB and Suiter DM found no significant difference in airway protection for thin liquids or pureed solids with or without NGT.[54]

Percutaneous endoscopic gastrostomy tubes

PEG tubes are a semipermanent option for patients with prolonged dysphagia. Approximately 5% of all acute stroke patients have a PEG tube inserted during initial hospitalization in the United States.[55] Typically this tube is placed before hospital discharge. A variety of complications from PEG tube placement has been reported and includes leakage of gastric contents around the tube, persistent abdominal pain, or dislodgment. More notable complications related to PEG include gastric bleeding, necrotizing fasciitis, development of a fistula, or injury to internal organs.[56] For patients where dysphagia is likely to persist for greater than 2–3 weeks, PEG tubes are a common alternative to maintain adequate nutrition while swallowing rehabilitation continues. While PEG tube placement is a relatively safe and reasonable option for patients with prolonged dysphagia, there have been mixed reports about the impact of PEG tube use on stroke outcome.

A multicenter randomized control trial compared outcomes for acute stroke patients who received enteral tube feeding via PEG versus NGT.[57] In this cohort, subjects with PEGs were more likely to be living in institutions, reported a lower quality of life, demonstrated clinically significant poorer functional outcomes (modified Rankin score), and higher death rates when compared to patients with NGT 1 year post stroke. They concluded that PEG tube placement should only be considered if enteral tube feeding is suspected to be required for more than 14–21 days unless a practical reason prevents the use of NGT. Nutritional guidelines updated within the past 10 years have cited the FOOD trial when provided recommendations for enteral nutrition (Table 4.2).[57]

In the acute stroke population, when a patient is determined to be at high risk of aspiration or choking, nonoral nutrition is recommended in an attempt to prevent possible complications related to aspiration such as pneumonia. Although the risk of aspiration and related complications may be reduced with the placement of enteral tube feeding, it is not eliminated.

Oral care

Aspiration of secretions or reflux aspiration may still occur with the presence of nonoral nutrition. Therefore diligent oral care is an important component of managing a patient with dysphagia following standard aspiration precautions. Multiple factors in addition to the presence of dysphagia led to increased risk of pneumonia in the acute care patient including limited mobility and poor oral hygiene.[58] A study has shown that implementation of an oral hygiene protocol reduced the risk of pneumonia.[59]

Dysphagia and nonoral feeding

Wilmskoetter and George et al. evaluated the timing of semipermanent feeding access after stroke.[55,60] A retrospective study of all acute stroke patients found that a PEG was typically placed on day 7.[55] Further, a retrospective study of acute ischemic stroke patients across the United States found that 53% of patients received PEG before or on day 7, thereby suggesting that current practice is not in line with recommended guidelines. Additionally, PEG tube placement, specifically before

TABLE 4.2 Post-Stroke PEG Guidelines			
Association	**Country**	**Year**	**Recommended Timeline for PEG Placement**
American Heart Association/ American Stroke Association[46]	US	2013	PEG if indicated after 14–21 days
American Gastroenterological Association	US	1995	PEG if indicated after 30 days
National Collaborating Centre for Acute Care	UK	2006	PEG if indicated after 14–28 days
German Society for Clinical Nutrition	Germany	2013	PEG if indicated after 14–28 days
Scottish Intercollegiate Guidelines Network	Scotland	2010	PEG if indicated after 28 days
European Society for Clinical Nutrition and Metabolism	UK	2005	PEG if indicated after 14 days
British Society for Gastroenterology	UK	2008	PEG if indicated after 14 days

day 11 of hospital admission, was found to be an independent predictor of 30 day readmissions for acute stroke patients.[61] Alternative feeding approaches including continued use of NGT during the early recovery period may benefit the patient long term.

CONCLUSION

Dysphagia is common after stroke and contributes to morbidity and mortality. Swallowing is a complex task that requires cortical, subcortical, and brainstem sensory and motor input. A multidisciplinary team approach is necessary to assess the type of swallow dysfunction and develop an individualized, goal-directed treatment plan to assist with the recovery from dysphagia after stroke.

REFERENCES

1. Rofes L, Muriana D, Palomeras E, et al. Prevalence, risk factors and complications of oropharyngeal dysphagia in stroke patients: a cohort study. *Neurogastroenterol Motil.* 2018:e13338.
2. Martineau J, Bauer JD, Isenring E, Cohen S. Malnutrition determined by the patient-generated subjective global assessment is associated with poor outcomes in acute stroke patients. *Clin Nutr.* 2005;24(6):1073–1077.
3. Chen N, Li Y, Fang J, Lu Q, He L. Risk factors for malnutrition in stroke patients: a meta-analysis. *Clin Nutr.* 2017. https://doi.org/10.1016/j.clnu.2017.12.014.
4. Crary MA, Humphrey JL, Carnaby-Mann G, Sambandam R, Miller L, Silliman S. Dysphagia, nutrition, and hydration in ischemic stroke patients at admission and discharge from acute care. *Dysphagia.* 2013;28(1): 69–76.
5. Finestone HM, Foley NC, Woodbury MG, Greene-Finestone L. Quantifying fluid intake in dysphagic stroke patients: a preliminary comparison of oral and nonoral strategies. *Arch Phys Med Rehabil.* 2001;82(12): 1744–1746.
6. Murray J, Miller M, Doeltgen S, Scholten I. Intake of thickened liquids by hospitalized adults with dysphagia after stroke. *Int J Speech Lang Pathol.* 2014;16(5):486–494.
7. Martino R, Foley N, Bhogal S, Diamant N, Speechley M, Teasell R. Dysphagia after stroke: incidence, diagnosis, and pulmonary complications. *Stroke.* 2005;36(12): 2756–2763.
8. Ho CH, Lin WC, Hsu YF, Lee IH, Hung YC. One-year risk of pneumonia and mortality in patients with poststroke dysphagia: a nationwide population-based study. *J Stroke Cerebrovasc Dis.* 2018;27(5):1311–1317.
9. Teasell RW, McRae M, Marchuk Y, Finestone HM. Pneumonia associated with aspiration following stroke. *Arch Phys Med Rehabil.* 1996;77(7):707–709.
10. Holas MA, DePippo KL, Reding MJ. Aspiration and relative risk of medical complications following stroke. *Arch Neurol.* 1994;51(10):1051–1053.
11. Ertekin C, Aydogdu I. Neurophysiology of swallowing. *Clin Neurophysiol.* 2003;114(12):2226–2244.
12. Aydogdu I, Ertekin C, Tarlaci S, Turman B, Kiylioglu N, Secil Y. Dysphagia in lateral medullary infarction (Wallenberg's syndrome): an acute disconnection syndrome in premotor neurons related to swallowing activity? *Stroke.* 2001;32(9):2081–2087.
13. Leonard R, Kendall K. *Dysphagia Assessment and Treatment Planning: A Team Approach.* Cengage Learning; 1997.
14. Steele CM, Miller AJ. Sensory input pathways and mechanisms in swallowing: a review. *Dysphagia.* 2010;25(4): 323–333.
15. Teismann IK, Dziewas R, Steinstraeter O, Pantev C. Time-dependent hemispheric shift of the cortical control of volitional swallowing. *Hum Brain Mapp.* 2009;30(1):92–100.
16. Jean A. Brain stem control of swallowing: neuronal network and cellular mechanisms. *Physiol Rev.* 2001; 81(2):929–969.
17. Michou E, Hamdy S. Cortical input in control of swallowing. *Curr Opin Otolaryngol Head Neck Surg.* 2009; 17(3):166–171.
18. Leopold NA, Daniels SK. Supranuclear control of swallowing. *Dysphagia.* 2010;25(3):250–257.
19. Mosier KM, Liu WC, Maldjian JA, Shah R, Modi B. Lateralization of cortical function in swallowing: a functional MR imaging study. *AJNR Am J Neuroradiol.* 1999;20(8): 1520–1526.
20. Daniels SK, Foundas AL. Lesion localization in acute stroke. *J Neuroimaging.* 1999;9(2):91–98.
21. Hamdy S, Mikulis DJ, Crawley A, et al. Cortical activation during human volitional swallowing: an event-related fMRI study. *Am J Physiol Gastrointest Liver Physiol.* 1999; 277(1):G219–G225.
22. May NH, Pisegna JM, Marchina S, Langmore SE, Kumar S, Pearson Jr WG. Pharyngeal swallowing mechanics secondary to hemispheric stroke. *J Stroke Cerebrovasc Dis.* 2017; 26(5):952–961.
23. Somasundaram S, Henke C, Neumann-Haefelin T, et al. Dysphagia risk assessment in acute left-hemispheric middle cerebral artery stroke. *Cerebrovasc Dis.* 2014;37(3): 217–222.
24. Mihai PG, Otto M, Domin M, Platz T, Hamdy S, Lotze M. Brain imaging correlates of recovered swallowing after dysphagic stroke: a fMRI and DWI study. *Neuroimage Clin.* 2016;12:1013–1021.
25. Langmore SE, McCulloch TM, Krisciunas GP, et al. Efficacy of electrical stimulation and exercise for dysphagia in patients with head and neck cancer: a randomized clinical trial. *Head Neck.* 2016;38(suppl 1):E1221–E1231.
26. Parker C, Power M, Hamdy S, Bowen A, Tyrrell P, Thompson DG. Awareness of dysphagia by patients following stroke predicts swallowing performance. *Dysphagia.* 2004;19(1):28–35.

27. Barnard SL. Nursing dysphagia screening for acute stroke patients in the emergency department. *J Emerg Nurs.* 2011;37(1):64–67.

28. Yeh SJ, Huang KY, Wang TG, et al. Dysphagia screening decreases pneumonia in acute stroke patients admitted to the stroke intensive care unit. *J Neurol Sci.* 2011;306(1–2):38–41.

29. Brodsky MB, Suiter DM, Gonzalez-Fernandez M, et al. Screening accuracy for aspiration using bedside water swallow tests: a systematic review and meta-analysis. *Chest.* 2016;150(1):148–163.

30. Carnaby-Mann G, Lenius K. The bedside examination in dysphagia. *Phys Med Rehabil Clin N Am.* 2008;19(4): 747–768, viii.

31. Ramsey DJ, Smithard DG, Kalra L. Early assessments of dysphagia and aspiration risk in acute stroke patients. *Stroke.* 2003;34(5):1252–1257.

32. Daniels SK, Brailey K, Priestly DH, Herrington LR, Weisberg LA, Foundas AL. Aspiration in patients with acute stroke. *Arch Phys Med Rehabil.* 1998;79(1):14–19.

32a. Welch MV, Logemann JA, Rademaker AW, Kahrilas PJ. Changes in pharyngeal dimensions effected by chin tuck. *Arch Phys Med Rehabil.* 1993;74(2):178–181.

33. Vose A, Nonnenmacher J, Singer ML, Gonzalez-Fernandez M. Dysphagia management in acute and subacute stroke. *Curr Phys Med Rehabil Rep.* 2014;2(4): 197–206.

34. Logemann JA, Kahrilas PJ, Kobara M, Vakil NB. The benefit of head rotation on pharyngoesophageal dysphagia. *Arch Phys Med Rehabil.* 1989;70(10):767–771.

34a. Kahrilas PJ, Logemann JA, Krugler C, Flanagan E. Volitional augmentation of upper esophageal sphincter opening during swallowing. *Am J Physiol Gastrointest Liver Physiol.* 1991;260(3):G450–G456.

35. Martin BJ, Logemann JA, Shaker R, Dodds WJ. Normal laryngeal valving patterns during three breath-hold maneuvers: a pilot investigation. *Dysphagia.* 1993;8(1): 11–20.

36. Chaudhuri G, Hildner CD, Brady S, Hutchins B, Aliga N, Abadilla E. Cardiovascular effects of the supraglottic and super-supraglottic swallowing maneuvers in stroke patients with dysphagia. *Dysphagia.* 2002;17(1):19–23.

37. Kahrilas PJ, Logemann JA, Krugler C, Flanagan E. Volitional augmentation of upper esophageal sphincter opening during swallowing. *Am J Physiol.* 1991;260(3 pt 1): G450–G456.

38. Fujiu M, Logemann JA, Pauloski BR. Increased postoperative posterior pharyngeal wall movement in patients with anterior oral cancer: preliminary findings and possible implications for treatment. *Am J Speech Lang Pathol.* 1995; 4(2):24–30.

39. Fujiu-Kurachi M, Fujiwara S, Tamine K, et al. Tongue pressure generation during tongue-hold swallows in young healthy adults measured with different tongue positions. *Dysphagia.* 2014;29(1):17–24.

40. Shaker R, Kern M, Bardan E, et al. Augmentation of deglutitive upper esophageal sphincter opening in the elderly by exercise. *Am J Physiol.* 1997;272(6 pt 1): G1518–G1522.

41. Bulow M, Speyer R, Baijens L, Woisard V, Ekberg O. Neuromuscular electrical stimulation (NMES) in stroke patients with oral and pharyngeal dysfunction. *Dysphagia.* 2008; 23(3):302–309.

42. Kushner DS, Peters K, Eroglu ST, Perless-Carroll M, Johnson-Greene D. Neuromuscular electrical stimulation efficacy in acute stroke feeding tube-dependent dysphagia during inpatient rehabilitation. *Am J Phys Med Rehabil.* 2013;92(6):486–495.

43. Xia W, Zheng C, Lei Q, et al. Treatment of post-stroke dysphagia by vitalstim therapy coupled with conventional swallowing training. *J Huazhong Univ Sci Technolog Med Sci.* 2011;31(1):73–76.

44. Ludlow CL, Humbert I, Saxon K, Poletto C, Sonies B, Crujido L. Effects of surface electrical stimulation both at rest and during swallowing in chronic pharyngeal dysphagia. *Dysphagia.* 2007;22(1):1–10.

45. Ludlow CL. Electrical neuromuscular stimulation in dysphagia: current status. *Curr Opin Otolaryngol Head Neck Surg.* 2010;18(3):159–164.

46. Frost J, Robinson HF, Hibberd J. A comparison of neuromuscular electrical stimulation and traditional therapy, versus traditional therapy in patients with longstanding dysphagia. *Curr Opin Otolaryngol Head Neck Surg.* 2018; 26(3):167–173.

47. Rosenbek JC, Robbins J, Fishback B, Levine RL. Effects of thermal application on dysphagia after stroke. *J Speech Hear Res.* 1991;34(6):1257–1268.

48. Robbins J, Kays SA, Gangnon RE, et al. The effects of lingual exercise in stroke patients with dysphagia. *Arch Phys Med Rehabil.* 2007;88(2):150–158.

49. Kern MK, Jaradeh S, Arndorfer RC, Shaker R. Cerebral cortical representation of reflexive and volitional swallowing in humans. *Am J Physiol Gastrointest Liver Physiol.* 2001; 280(3):G354–G360.

50. Pisegna JM, Kaneoka A, Pearson Jr WG, Kumar S, Langmore SE. Effects of non-invasive brain stimulation on post-stroke dysphagia: a systematic review and meta-analysis of randomized controlled trials. *Clin Neurophysiol.* 2016;127(1):956–968.

51. Dharmarajan TS, Unnikrishnan D. Tube feeding in the elderly. the technique, complications, and outcome. *Postgrad Med.* 2004;115(2):51–54, 58–61.

52. Dziewas R, Warnecke T, Hamacher C, et al. Do nasogastric tubes worsen dysphagia in patients with acute stroke? *BMC Neurol.* 2008;8:28. https://doi.org/10.1186/1471-2377-8-28.

53. Huggins PS, Tuomi SK, Young C. Effects of nasogastric tubes on the young, normal swallowing mechanism. *Dysphagia.* 1999;14(3):157–161.

54. Leder SB, Suiter DM. Effect of nasogastric tubes on incidence of aspiration. *Arch Phys Med Rehabil.* 2008;89(4): 648–651.

55. Wilmskoetter J, Simpson AN, Simpson KN, Bonilha HS. Practice patterns of percutaneous endoscopic gastrostomy tube placement in acute stroke: are the guidelines achievable? *J Stroke Cerebrovasc Dis.* 2016;25(11): 2694–2700.

56. Blumenstein I, Shastri YM, Stein J. Gastroenteric tube feeding: techniques, problems and solutions. *World J Gastroenterol.* 2014;20(26):8505–8524.

57. Dennis MS, Lewis SC, Warlow C, FOOD Trial Collaboration. Effect of timing and method of enteral tube feeding for dysphagic stroke patients (FOOD): a multicentre randomised controlled trial. *Lancet.* 2005; 365(9461):764–772.

58. Langmore SE, Terpenning MS, Schork A, et al. Predictors of aspiration pneumonia: how important is dysphagia? *Dysphagia.* 1998;13(2):69–81.

59. Wagner C, Marchina S, Deveau JA, Frayne C, Sulmonte K, Kumar S. Risk of stroke-associated pneumonia and oral hygiene. *Cerebrovasc Dis.* 2016;41(1–2):35–39.

60. George BP, Kelly AG, Albert GP, Hwang DY, Holloway RG. Timing of percutaneous endoscopic gastrostomy for acute ischemic stroke: an observational study from the US nation-wide inpatient sample. *Stroke.* 2017;48(2):420–427.

61. Wilmskoetter J, Simpson KN, Bonilha HS. Hospital read-missions of stroke patients with percutaneous endoscopic gastrostomy feeding tubes. *J Stroke Cerebrovasc Dis.* 2016; 25(10):2535–2542.

CHAPTER 5

Right Brain Stroke Syndromes

JONATHAN OEN THOMAS, MD • A.M. BARRETT, MD

INTRODUCTION

The right hemisphere of the brain critically supports multiple functions including spatial cognition, self-awareness, and emotional cognitive processing. Because it manages these activities that are fundamental to function and freedom, it is ironic that the right brain is sometimes called the "nondominant" hemisphere. In general, the domains for which the right brain is dominant could be said to involve the "how" rather than the "what" of mental abilities. Our understanding of many of these cognitive domains is in evolution, and continues to be further defined.

In this chapter, we will review information about the right brain, right brain function, and rehabilitation of right brain deficits after stroke. Much of the information we have about cognitive processes managed by the right hemisphere comes from classical neurologic observations in lesion studies. Increasingly, however, we learn about the function of the healthy brain with techniques such as functional magnetic resonance imaging (fMRI), and these methods of tracking patterns of brain activation help us understand complex neural processes that the right brain orchestrates.

Right brain disorders adversely affect stroke care outcomes,[1] and it is possible that underidentification and undertreatment of right brain–related symptoms[2] may be partly responsible for this health disparity. Unfortunately, the impact and disability associated with right brain deficits are not regularly reviewed as part of medical and neurological education. This suggests that, despite the key role the right hemisphere plays in numerous neurologic and systemic processes, there is a bias within the medical infrastructure and society at large in recognizing and treating right hemisphere strokes. This is a public health problem, as there is strong evidence of disability associated with right brain disorders.

Lateralization of Function in the Cerebral Hemispheres

The functions of the cerebral hemispheres can be described as shared, lateralized, or dominant. Shared functions are those which receive equal input from each hemisphere. These are somewhat rare throughout the nervous system, but include systems responsible for axial strength and stability.[3] In general, human brain functions are specialized or lateralized between hemispheres. This may improve speed and efficiency of brain processing. A brain region is considered lateralized if a lesion to the opposite corresponding region of brain does not produce the same deficit. A simple example is motor control of the left arm in the right precentral gyrus. A lesion to the left precentral gyrus does not produce this effect; rather it produces motor abnormalities in the right arm.

A brain region is considered dominant if dysfunction in this region produces bilateral symptoms. An example would be language dominance; aphasia occurs after left brain lesions.[4] Brain hemispheric dominance is cognitive domain-specific. In this chapter, we will focus on those cognitive domains for which the right brain is dominant. As we noted above, many physicians are unaware of decades of mounting evidence that right hemispheric stroke is a significant source of disability, because of the right brain's dominant functions.

Stroke is a common and disabling clinical entity. It is a leading cause of disability and death in the United States and worldwide,[5] and there are approximately 7.2 million stroke survivors in the United States.[6] While there may not be a difference in overall incidence of left and right brain stroke,[7,8] there is considerable inequality in management and outcomes between strokes based on lateralization. Symptoms following right hemispheric stroke are disabling, yet frequently underdiagnosed and undertreated.[9,10] Acutely, right

Stroke Rehabilitation. https://doi.org/10.1016/B978-0-323-55381-0.00005-6

hemispheric strokes are less likely to receive thrombolysis,[11] are less likely to benefit from thrombolysis compared to left hemispheric strokes,[12] and are more slowly transferred to acute stroke care centers.[13]

Healthcare disparities affecting people with right brain stroke are likely due to a combination of factors. These include difficulty that patients and their families have in identifying the signs and symptoms associated with right hemisphere injury compared to more overt symptoms such as paralysis. This effect may be a result of the cognitive syndrome of unawareness of deficit (anosognosia), commonly complicating right brain stroke.[14] Another factor which likely contributes to the discrepancy between right and left stroke care is difficulty that clinicians have with identifying right brain stroke symptoms, and suboptimal sensitivity of diagnostic instruments. For example, the National Institutes of Health Stroke Scale (NIHSS)[15] is a widely utilized standardized clinical tool for the acute assessment of ischemic stroke. Out of 42 possible NIHSS points, only 2 points for extinction/inattention specifically assess a component of spatial neglect and right brain function. This is compared to up to 7 points for left-brain-specific symptoms (verbal communication, dysarthria, and language comprehension).[9] Thus, the NIHSS overweights left versus right-brain-associated symptoms,[16] and this instrument underestimates stroke volumes in right brain stoke compared to left brain stroke, and may be insensitive to right brain stroke symptoms in general.[17] The insensitivity of the NIHSS may be partly related to differences in specificity of instructions for right versus left-stroke-related items, as well as areas of right brain function omitted from the NIHSS. See Table 5.1 for outline.

Better identification and treatment of right brain stroke may reduce the significant longterm disability following right brain events. Right brain stroke is associated with longer length of stay in rehabilitation, lower functional independence measure (FIM) scores, and worse functional outcomes.[18]

In this chapter, we will describe core syndromes associated with right brain stroke that cause functional disability. These include spatial neglect, anosognosia, and emotional processing disorders, such as emotional aprosodia. In each section, we will define the disorder, discuss its neuroanatomy and mechanisms, and review its clinical presentation. Lastly, we will discuss what has been reported about rehabilitation of each syndrome. We will end this chapter discussing lesser-known syndromes associated with right brain stroke, and emerging areas of research. Our goal is to provide information useful to plan and tailor rehabilitation to manage and rehabilitate the specific effects of these deficits on functional activity and participation.

TABLE 5.1

Symptoms With Unilateral Hemispheric Dominance (Left vs. Right Hemisphere) and Indication If Tested on NIHSS (National Institutes of Health Stroke Scale)[15]

Left Stroke Symptom	Tested on NIHSS?	Right Stroke Symptom	Tested on NIHSS
Aphasia	Yes-7 points Items: 1b. patient is asked the month and his/her age (2 pts) 1c. patient is asked to open and close eyes, and grip and release nonparetic hand (2 pts) 9. describe picture, name pictured items, read sentences (3 pts)	Spatial neglect	Yes-2 points Item 11 Instructions state that information from testing previous items can be used to assess visual, tactile, auditory, or personal inattention. Specific testing of auditory or personal spatial cognition is not specified, however. How to test for extinction in the presence of sensory deficits is not specified.
		Anosognosia for hemiparesis	No
		Emotional processing deficit	No

SPATIAL NEGLECT
Definitions/History

Spatial neglect is defined as pathologically asymmetric spatial performance in a patient with a brain lesion, associated with functional disability.[19] Spatial bias in this syndrome[20] takes the form of asymmetric reporting or response to stimuli, and asymmetric orienting/movement. Because accuracy in the interaction of our bodies with the 3D environment is basic to all of our self-care, adaptive activity, and independence, derangement of spatial function in spatial neglect causes falls, accidents, increased disability, and increased care costs in these patients.[21,22]

Early descriptions of the spatial neglect syndrome in people emphasized asymmetric sensory, perceptual, and visual organization functions of the right brain.[23-26] However, asymmetric movement, orienting, and posture are part of the spatial neglect syndrome in animals,[27] and these behaviors were also part of early descriptions of human spatial neglect.[28]

Pathophysiology/Neuroanatomy

During medical training, many of us learned that damage to the right parietal and temporal lobes causes spatial neglect. This simple formula is inadequate. Damage to other brain regions results in spatial neglect, including the thalamus, striatum, superior colliculus, dorsolateral frontal regions, and cingulate cortex.[29] Animal literature and studies of brains in patients are a major source of information about the pathophysiology of the spatial neglect syndrome. Behavioral and neurophysiologic assessments of rodents, cats, monkeys[30] and people with brain lesions[31] as well as healthy controls suggest that a number of brain sites contribute to a coordinated network of cortical and subcortical brain regions active in functional, adaptive spatial cognition.

Although multiple brain regions work together in functional networks to support spatial function, the treatment relevance of a theory of spatial neglect based on functional neuroanatomic networks is still limited. For example, there is still debate about which regions, among the brain regions that participate in spatial function, are critical—in other words, which regions, when damaged, will always be associated with clinical impairment. Models proposed by different theorists do not exactly overlap.[29,32-34] Within and between previous studies, neuroradiological analyses from different kinds of subjects (for example, stroke survivors at different stages of recovery) have been grouped. A significant challenge to validity of a distributed network hypothesis for spatial neglect, for example, is that averaged data

used to generate a network model may not represent the brain anatomy of any of the individuals contributing to the dataset. Thus, such a network model may never be able to reflect the biological basis of spatial neglect symptoms in an individual patient.

There is also reason to conclude that both "hubs" of the spatial cognitive networks (specific brain regions) and the quality of their connection (white matter integrity, interhemispheric balance of interaction[25,31,35,36]) are needed to maintain healthy spatial function. The treatment relevance of a theory of spatial neglect based on white matter integrity, however, is also unclear at this point. Thus, although the distributed network hypothesis of spatial neglect is fascinating, at this point how network theories of spatial cognitive function should be applied to plan biological or behavioral approaches to rehabilitation is unknown. This will likely be clarified as we collect more information about how patients with different lesion sites respond to therapies, especially if the therapies can be linked to specific brain processes.

Clinical Presentation

Below, we briefly describe symptoms of spatial neglect observed at the bedside. For a more comprehensive presentation and discussion of spatial neglect symptoms, please see reviews on this topic.[37,38]

Where perceptual-attentional spatial neglect symptoms. Two major input-associated symptoms occur as part of spatial neglect after right brain stroke, including unawareness of left-sided stimuli and extinction to double simultaneous stimulation.

Unawareness of left-sided stimuli. When ecologically relevant events occur in the body space on the opposite side to a brain lesion (contralesional body space), the patient with spatial neglect after right brain stroke may be unaware of those events. For example, such a patient may walk up to a sink with separate hot and cold water faucets, and put her hands under a running hot water faucet, unaware of the water pouring out on the left side. As a result, she may burn herself. Another patient with spatial Where neglect might sit quietly looking out the window on the right, completely unaware that someone sitting on her left side is speaking to her, and completely failing to respond to that person's questions. The auditory information was never perceived or detected.

Extinction to double simultaneous stimulation. Because spatial neglect is a cognitive disorder, like the cognitive disorder aphasia, it can be associated with input, storage, or output stages of processing. Perceptual-attentional symptoms in spatial neglect include extinction of perceptual stimuli in the visual, tactile, or auditory modalities to double simultaneous stimulation. This symptom is observed when a single stimulus can be detected on the neglected side of space (for example, a patient with a right brain stroke can see the examiner moving a finger on his left side), however that same stimulus (a left-sided visual stimulus) cannot be detected when it is presented simultaneously with a stimulus on the right side. Thus, when the examiner moves a finger on the left side of the patient, the patient correctly responds that there is a stimulus "on the left"; however, when the examiner moves a finger on both the left and the right side, the patient responds to the stimulus "on the right" only. The ability to detect a single stimulus on the left distinguishes extinction to double simultaneous stimulation from left-sided visual field deficit.

Extinction to double simultaneous stimulation is, like unawareness, an input-associated symptom. It can be demonstrated to be directly related to perceptual-attentional capacity: for example, it occurs for left-sided stimuli even when both stimuli are in the "good" right body space.[39]

Representational symptoms. Spatial neglect affects representations, which are usually also regarded as dependent on Where cognitive processing. By definition, when a patient with spatial neglect after right brain stroke has this kind of symptom, he is not actively taking in information about the external world, but rather he is using information about the 3D world in his mind. An example of representational spatial neglect would be a patient who when asked what state is west of Nevada responds "Iowa." Another example of representational neglect would be a patient who when asked to spell the word "world" responds "rld." Lastly, a patient with representational neglect after right brain stroke might be asked "what number is halfway between 60 and 20?" and might respond "50." In all of these examples, the patient is not actually referring to a physical stimulus, but is rather using an internal image or memory to respond. Representational neglect affected the internal image, so that it was either missing left-sided information, or left-sided information was distorted and less available than right-sided information.

Aiming motor-intentional spatial neglect symptoms. Pathologically asymmetric movements in 3D space are part of the spatial neglect syndrome, and can include any of the following spatial-motor symptoms. Spatial Aiming neglect can include directional hypokinesia (problems moving leftward with the eyes, head, limbs, or axial body[40]), asymmetric motor response inhibition,[41,42] asymmetric ability to move the left versus right side of the body, not accounted for by corticospinal tract

involvement and paralysis alone,[43] and smaller or weaker movements in contralesional space, as compared to movements executed in ipsilesional space, with any part of the body (hemispatial hypokinesia[44]).

Directional hypokinesia after right brain stroke in patients with neglect was demonstrated in multiple studies by Barrett and colleagues.[19,45,46] We identified patients who specifically fail at making leftward movements because of spatial neglect, independent of left-sided perceptual-attentional abilities. Barrett and colleagues used a video line bisection apparatus similar to those invented by Na et al.[47] and Bisiach et al.[48] These methods dissociate the direction that a patient moves the right hand (which is usually unaffected by left brain stroke) from the left-right-viewed side of space. Barrett and colleagues demonstrated that directional hypokinesia is specifically improved by prism adaptation, a highly effective treatment for spatial neglect,[49] and that people with directional hypokinesia as part of Aiming spatial neglect better to prism adaptation training than do patients who lack directional hypokinesia.[50]

Aiming spatial neglect at the bedside can be identified when we see patients with marked leaning, veering,

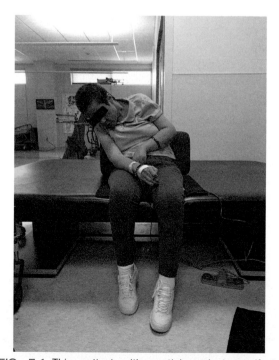

FIG. 5.1 This patient with spatial neglect manifests rightward rotation and leaning of her torso. This postural disturbance is the human analog of pathologically asymmetric motor behaviors seen in animal models of the spatial neglect syndrome. Photo credit: Dr. Peii Chen

or postural rotation to the ipsilesional side (Fig. 5.1), although contralesional leaning can sometimes be observed. To assess disability-relevant Aiming components of spatial neglect in rehabilitation settings, we recommend that the clinician use an assessment that captures asymmetric movement[51] and predict functional disability related to spatial neglect. The most feasible for inpatient care is a test based on observed asymmetry of functional performance, the Catherine Bergego Scale.[52] Like the NIH Stroke Scale, this assessment requires the examiner to be reliability trained, and patients must actually be observed performing daily life tasks.

Rehabilitation of Spatial Neglect

Two recent sets of consensus recommendations, from the American Heart Association (AHA) and from the American Occupational Therapy Association, included guidelines for the treatment of spatial neglect.[53,54] Unfortunately, these recommendations are not exactly overlapping. We reviewed the problem of conflicting consensus recommendations in recent publications.[21,55]

Three approaches stand out on the basis of (1) strong evidence supporting efficacy to improve functional performance at daily life tasks from multiple controlled, systematic studies (2) feasibility with respect to accessibility: cost of equipment, time required for treatment, therapist training required to administer treatment. These include prism adaptation,[56,57] limb activation,[58,59] and visual scanning training.[60,61]

Prism adaptation is a treatment technique having patients with spatial neglect after right brain stroke wear yoked optical wedge prisms that shift what they see 11.4 degrees rightward. An occluder blocks the first part of their arm and hand movement from view[50,62] and patients complete 20-min sessions of visually guided movement practice. In the protocol used in our program, patients mark lines and circles in left, central, and right space. Prisms are worn only for 20-min sessions; the entire protocol of treatment is 10 sessions over 14 days. Both the AHA and the American Occupational Therapy Association recommend this treatment for spatial neglect; the AHA categorized the recommendation for cognitive rehabilitation treatment of spatial neglect as Class IIa, Level A (reasonable to recommend treatment, supported by multiple randomized clinical trials), although other spatial neglect treatments, including the two described below, were included in the recommendation as a generic list. Champod et al.[56] reviewed more than 20 controlled studies that demonstrated improvement in functional disability

during daily activities with prism adaptation treatment. Because the treatment is not yet widely used despite strong evidence supporting its efficacy, we (Barrett et al.[55]) described the problem as a classic implementation and translation block, needing to be improved in order to address the large healthcare disparity right brain stroke and spatial neglect patients face.

Limb activation is a treatment technique which requires patients with left neglect after right brain stroke to activate the left side of the body as they do other tasks such as perceptual search tasks, walking, or functional activity training.[58,59] Directing movements of the left body would be expected to enhance left limb kinesia, a form of spatial motor Aiming.[38] However, existing studies of limb activation examined spatial neglect improvement generically, without specifically examining spatial Aiming or related mechanisms of spatial cognitive processing.

The most commonly used approach to treating spatial neglect in the United States is not in itself evidence-based, but is a modification of an evidence-based treatment approach—visual scanning training. Nevertheless, it is regarded as a practice standard.[63] Visual scanning training was pioneered in the United States in a rehabilitation setting where stroke patients came to be hospitalized for rehabilitation after weeks or even months of acute care hospitalization.[60,61] Patients received 3 h of visual scanning training daily, and in the New York University randomized controlled trials of Weinberg and colleagues, their leftward orienting was promoted with a light scanning device. Subsequent studies cited in consensus recommendations[64,65] were performed in Europe, where patients received long periods of treatment (40 or more sessions, over as long as 2 months). Unlike prism adaptation training, which has a defined protocol used similarly across multiple studies, the protocol originally evaluated in randomized controlled trials for visual scanning training is very different from that being used in the United States during inpatient and outpatient rehabilitation as part of clinical practice. Current practice in US rehabilitation may involve using components of visual scanning training (for example, a red "anchor" strip of paper placed on the left side of a workspace) to train patients in strategic self-cuing ("look to the left") during short sessions given, at most, 8–15 times over a period of inpatient rehabilitation. This particular regimen has not been rigorously evaluated in a randomized, controlled trial. Further, such a study which closely replicated the original visual scanning training protocol did not find generalization of visual scanning training to untrained tasks or motor skills.[66]

Compensatory manipulation of the environment, such as placing the stroke survivor's bed on the good side of the room so that she or he will "need to look" to the neglected side, or standing on the stroke survivor's bad side, so as to "draw attention" to that direction, have been examined only in an inpatient study of bed placement, which found no beneficial effect.[67] In our opinion, these manipulations may not be useful. If they are helpful, they may benefit only some patients. For example, it is possible that a patient with a mild, primary spatial Aiming (motor-intentional) neglect may orient leftward after searching extensively for her telephone on the right side and finding only a blank wall. However, a patient with spatial neglect whose primary deficit is "Where" perceptual-attentional neglect, may become disoriented in the same situation, due to sensory deprivation.

ANOSOGNOSIA OR UNAWARENESS OF DEFICIT

Definitions/History

Anosognosia is defined as a condition in which brain-injured patients deny or fail to acknowledge their deficits.[68] Babinski originated this term to describe patients who were unaware of hemiparesis.[69] Anosognosia can occur in association with many cognitive and physical symptoms; however, anosognosia for hemiparesis has been strongly associated with right brain stroke for more than 30 years,[70] especially when it is moderate to severe.[71,72]

Pathophysiology/Neuroanatomy

Powerful evidence for the association of anosognosia for hemiparesis with right brain lesions comes from experimentally induced hemiplegia during intracarotid barbiturate injection (the Wada paradigm[73–76]). Intracarotid barbiturate injection studies are often done in the clinical setting to assist with analyzing hemispheric lateralization for language and memory, for example, so that a clinical team can plan epilepsy surgery. In the prior research studies, patients received infusion of anesthetic to one carotid artery, selectively affecting one side of the brain. After the anesthetic injection, patients manifest hemispherically associated deficits, including weakness on the contralateral side, for several minutes. In these experiments, shortly after recovering from anesthetic, patients were asked if they had arm weakness after the injection. After left carotid injection, even though both aphasia and hemiparesis usually resulted from the anesthetic injection, patients recovered from anesthesia and were able to report that they had right arm and hand weakness. However, even

though patients had left arm and hand weakness during right carotid anesthetic injection, after they recovered from the anesthetic they denied that this had happened.

It is unclear exactly what brain systems are responsible for awareness of hemiparesis, and what brain systems are dysfunctional in anosognosia for hemiparesis. However, studies indicate that right subcortical as well as cortical stroke are associated with anosognosia for hemiparesis (caudate,[77] thalamic,[78] and even pontine[79] stroke). Previously, Levine[80] suggested that anosognosia is due to global cognitive impairment, reducing the capacity for multiple parallel cognitive operations needed in self-appraisal. However, association of anosognosia for hemiparesis with focal subcortical lesions is not consistent with a global cognitive deficit hypothesis. A modular cognitive processing hypothesis proposes that a person able to detect weakness in her arm assesses whether anticipated and observed movements match; a mismatch triggers awareness of the deficit.[68,81] However, neuroanatomic and neurophysiologic correlates to the matching and comparing functions have so far been elusive. Other authors proposed that brain systems supporting perspective-taking associated with lesions affecting the right inferior and middle frontal gyrus and right superior temporal gyrus may account for anosognosia.[82] These authors argued that body function is normally mentalized from third-person perspectives. However, it is unclear whether external perspective-taking really does alter fundamental self-assessment of body function. This idea is counterintuitive from a survival/evolutionary perspective, since self-assessment of body function would seem to be critically important in many daily life circumstances, and might have developed relatively early in the evolution of human cognition. Theory of mind requires a relatively advanced cognitive set of skills, which might be expected to have arisen at a later stage.

Clinical Presentation

In some instances, clinicians may find it easy to identify anosognosia for hemiparesis. Asked to tell the story of his acute illness and hospitalization for stroke, a patient may claim that he came to the hospital because other people insisted, or because of vague, nonspecific problems (weakness all over the body). Some patients are unaware of all of their other deficits, in addition to hemiparesis. A patient who is anosognosic for several deficits, for example, may not be aware that she has left hemiparesis, and may state that the arm is "strong, but resting." She may also be unaware of right ptosis, stating that both eyes are open. Lastly, she may state that her memory is normal, even right after demonstration that it is impaired, and she is unable to remember three words after 2 min of distraction.

However, it is definitely true that patients can be unaware of hemiplegia, despite being aware of other deficits such as hemianopia.[83] Such "double dissociations" (unawareness of one deficit but awareness of another) regularly occur between anosognosia for hemiparesis and awareness of hemianesthesia.[70] Thus, the clinician needs to be aware that anosognosia can occur even in patients who do not obviously have unawareness. In particular, it may be present in patients who are aware of some other deficits. It is also easy to miss anosognosia for hemiparesis when patients have a conative disorder (amotivational or generative deficit or abulia), decreased overall activity, or decreased engagement. Because of the possibility of missing anosognosia in patients who are aware of other symptoms, or who have problems generating spontaneous behaviors, awareness of hemiparesis should be formally and regularly assessed as part of stroke rehabilitation.

Formal screening for anosognosia for hemiparesis can be completed in just a few seconds. In the past, we presented patients with a simple vertical line on an otherwise blank page. Immediately after identifying a deficit on exam—for example, immediately after testing for shoulder and arm strength to confrontation, identifying significant weakness—we show the patient the vertical line, and ask her to mark the line, placing a pen in her other hand. We instruct the patient as follows:

Show me on this line, how you just performed on the strength testing in your left arm and shoulder. Point to the top of the line (examiner indicates top end of the line) if your strength is at 100%, completely normal. Point to the bottom of the line if you were unable to move at all (examiner indicates bottom end of the line). Your performance may have been somewhere in between. (Examiner sweeps the hand up and down the line). Can you show me where you would rate your performance?

Although with this quick formal screening it is not possible to identify anosognosia that causes relatively small magnitude overestimation of self-performance, large-magnitude inconsistencies between self-rating and performance are regularly identified using this method. The vertical line rating also provides a convenient way to communicate with others on the care team—by showing nurses, therapists, and family caregivers that a patient who is plegic marked her strength above the halfway mark on the vertical line; we can communicate the patient's impaired awareness quickly.

If more detailed assessment is required, a semiquantitative scale is also available to rate anosognosia for hemiparesis in research settings, somewhat analogous to the NIH Stroke Scale.[70]

A second, very important, point for clinicians to remember about anosognosia is that it is not the same as psychological denial, and does not protect the individual from the emotional impact of having had a stroke. Although patients with anosognosia may show signs of psychological denial,[53] there are several key differences between anosognosia and psychological denial. An ego defense like psychological denial protects against perceived ego threat by reducing the impact/disability of a deficit. Thus, when patients near the time of hospital discharge and face the realities of a home transition, we expect to see psychological denial increase. In contrast, anosognosia is usually worst immediately after a stroke, and improves rapidly over weeks or even days.[68] Further evidence of dissociation between denial and anosognosia comes from studies of experimentally induced anosognosia for hemiparesis after right hemispheric anesthesia, as summarized above.[84] Patients who had been weak after a right-versus left-sided intracarotid anesthesia injection were asked about whether their arms were weak, after they had completely recovered. These patients had the same disability-related motivation in both cases; they had recovered from anesthesia and had no disability when they were asked. However, the same patients stated that their left hand was not weak after right brain anesthesia, while admitting that the right hand was weak after left brain anesthesia. This is consistent with a neuropsychological deficit localized to the right brain, rather than a psychologically motivated ego defense.

Patients with right brain stroke and anosognosia for hemiparesis experience the same range of emotions as control subjects.[85] It is likely that they are aware of the disabling consequences of their stroke and hemiparesis; however, their awareness may be implicit. This means they may not be able to articulate the awareness or their distress.[86] Thus, they may even be at higher risk of depression than other patients with right brain stroke and hemiparesis. Researchers specifically examining whether anosognosia protects patients from depression found no evidence that anosognosia is protective.[87] We are further concerned that, if the clinical care team views anosognosia as protective, they may not focus on the maladaptive effects of anosognosia. This may impair patients' acquisition of emotional and cognitive approaches to manage physical limitation,[88] and thus increase their disability.

Rehabilitation of Anosognosia for Hemiparesis

Experts in rehabilitation of anosognosia and anosognosia for hemiparesis have published on this topic in patients with both stroke[72] and traumatic brain injury.[89-91] Although not all available treatments have been demonstrated to be effective in controlled randomized studies in stroke patients with unawareness of hemiparesis, the most important point to recognize is that there are treatments for anosognosia, and most treatments are straightforward and feasible. We encourage clinicians to work on specific anosognosia treatment with their therapy teams, encouraging cross-application of techniques the team may be accustomed to using in traumatic brain injury settings.

Also very importantly, patients with anosognosia benefit from inpatient rehabilitation. In the past, some authorities felt that unawareness was an insurmountable obstacle to undergoing 3 h of daily therapy delivered in postacute, inpatient rehabilitation. Hartman-Maier and colleagues[72] reported strong evidence supporting inpatient rehabilitation for poststroke anosognosia. In 60 stroke patients, inpatient multidisciplinary rehabilitation was associated with reduction in overestimation errors (from 53% overestimation to 27% upon discharge, an improvement of about 50%). Awareness at admission did not contribute to the prediction of functional activity level at 1 year, beyond admission level of disability. However, at discharge from inpatient rehabilitation, 27% of the right brain stroke survivors still overestimated their total competency at activities of daily living and unawareness at discharge was an independent predictor of impaired functional activities at 1 year. In recent years, patients with unawareness of deficit have not been systematically limited from admission to inpatient rehabilitation. However, if patient-reported outcomes become the main path of entry to rehabilitation care, access to inpatient rehabilitation and other forms of intensive therapy may again become limited.[92] We urge our colleagues who practice in the acute care setting to help people working in healthcare delivery to understand that most patients with anosognosia for hemiparesis can still experience the substantial benefit of inpatient rehabilitation after stroke.[93]

Beyond the techniques that all practitioners in speech-language pathology, occupational therapy, and physical therapy use during rehabilitation, researchers have examined improving awareness of hemiplegia by using a variety of specific protocols. Protocols to improve anosognosia include self-awareness training[90,94] and spatial neglect interventions such as vestibular stimulation[95] and self-observation via video feedback.[96,97] Improved self-awareness has been linked to goal attainment in rehabilitation.[98] Treatment of anosognosia may be helpful for some, but not all, self-judgments: a report of behavioral modification in one patient for anosognosia after traumatic brain injury noted that self-error detection improved, but overall overestimation of abilities persisted.[99] However, even partial improvement in self-monitoring, such as improving self-error detection, may still help patients reach their functional goals.

EMOTIONAL PROCESSING DEFICITS, INCLUDING EMOTIONAL APROSODIA
Definitions/History

Emotions are a central element of the human experience. Emotional and social interaction, motivation, and cognition are key to daily activities and participation in community life.

Because of this importance, scientists have attempted for well over a century to empiricize emotions and their biological substrates. More than 35 years ago, classic studies demonstrated the primary aspects and universality of emotions.[100] More recently, advanced imaging and anatomic techniques have been used to study emotional processing deficits after stroke, and emotional processing disorders have been clearly linked to right brain deficits.[101]

Emotion can be defined as perception, experience, physiologic change, or manifest behavior (display) related to affective information, including primary (happy, sad, fearful) and social (embarrassed) feelings.[102,103] In healthy people, many years ago behavioral studies demonstrated right brain dominance for emotional facial recognition,[104,105] recall of emotional faces,[106] recognition of emotional prosody in others' vocalizations,[107] and production of emotional facial expressions.[108]

Since the 1980s and 1990s, studies demonstrated emotional processing deficits in patients with right brain lesions.[109,110] Although able to recognize the identity of people by their facial appearance, people with right brain damage have difficulty recognizing emotional facial expressions. At about this time, it was also demonstrated that stroke survivors with right brain injury had difficulty identifying affect conveyed vocally (e.g., an angry tone of voice) despite being able to hear and recognize the words spoken.[111] Such patients could identify features of the spoken information such as the identity or gender of the speaker, but not the emotion communicated by vocal inflection. Bowers and Heilman[112] suggested that the right brain stores knowledge of emotional facial configuration, and similarly the right brain might be assumed to store knowledge about vocal emotional prosodic cues and emotionally expressive body posture.

In these studies, right brain deficits in emotional cognitive processing were potentially independent of perceptual problems that might affect visuospatial or acoustic material. Rather, right brain-damaged patients could be shown to have trouble with using stored knowledge, or emotional representations.[113] Experimenters asked patients to evaluate meaningful information described verbally (e.g., "She shook her fist,") and identify the emotion matched to this information. The emotional descriptions were more easily matched to an emotion by patients with intact right brain structures, as compared with patients with right brain damage after stroke. This supports right brain dominance in maintaining emotional cognitive representations. Further, right brain stroke patients had more difficulty than did left brain stroke patients answering yes/no questions correctly, as they imagined an emotional face (e.g., "Are the eyes opened wide?" for surprise).[114] The "emotional experience and communication lexicon" or stored knowledge that patients draw upon when emotional questions were asked is analogous to the store of words available for verbal expression during speech and language processing. Emotional cognition can thus be considered in separate information processing stages (Fig. 5.2).

Our emotional states may directly drive autonomic activity, resistant to changes from internal stimuli.[115] Emotion networks are likely proactive, rather than reactive, in creating our emotion states.[115] By creating predictions of impending autonomic changes, emotional representations are bound to autonomic states. These representations can thus interact with other cognitive systems. Therefore, emotional processing can be considered an element of cognition in the same way as processing speed or memory (Fig. 5.3).

With regard to output stages for emotional cognitive information processing, reports more than 40 years ago of abnormal emotional expression after right brain stroke came from Gainotti,[117] Heilman and colleagues,[118] and Buck and Duffy.[119] Gainotti noted "indifference" of emotional responses as common after right brain stroke, suggesting a reduced range and frequency of emotional facial affect as well as verbal emotional prosodic expression. Heilman and colleagues linked this indifference to hypoarousal. Patients with right brain stroke had reduced galvanic skin response to painful stimuli, compared with left brain stroke patients and controls. Buck and Duffy reported that spontaneous facial expressions when viewing emotional slides were much less marked. Borod and colleagues demonstrated that this was true for voluntarily produced emotional facial expressions, as well.[120,121]

In the 1990s, Ross[122] suggested that although the right brain is dominant for cognitive processing of primary emotions, the left brain may play a role in processing and expressing "social" emotions such as embarrassment, shame, and guilt. Unfortunately, although these social, emotional, perceptual, representational, and expressive functions are tremendously important to activities like working and participating in meaningful roles in religious, family, and social contexts, studies examining the functional impact of these problems have not yet been performed. Even studies examining the impact of changes in cognitive processing of primary emotional states like anger or fear do not yet show clear correlated changes in reported daily life activities.

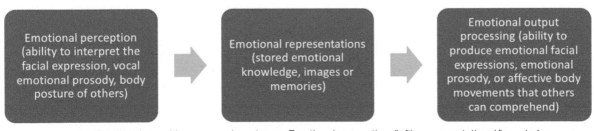

FIG. 5.2 Emotional cognitive processing stages. Emotional perception (left), representational/knowledge, and emotional output (right) can be dissociably impaired after right brain injury (Heilman et al.[101]). In different patients one or more than one modality of communication may be affected.

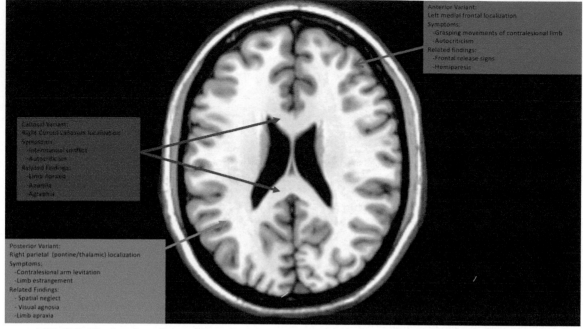

FIG. 5.3 Alien hand syndrome variants by brain anatomic localizations. Right side of brain appears on left side of image. Background image from MRIcron (Rorden and Brett[116]).

Pathophysiology/Neuroanatomy

Recent neurophysiologic studies of brain activation suggest that not right cortical dominance but bilateral subcortical processing in the basal ganglia and limbic system can be observed during emotional perceptual tasks.[123–126] However, as Heilman and colleagues have pointed out,[101] physiologic changes in subcortical structures such as the hypothalamus and amygdala[127,128] that have long been known to correlate with affective states (rage, fear) do not constitute the whole of interpretation or integration of complex stimuli, as happens in typical emotional perceptual situations in daily life. Also, these structures are unlikely to store complex memory representations or generate subtle behaviors, which again are critical to social function and freedom. We agree with Heilman and colleagues that modular information processing obviously takes place in emotional thinking, and that the complexity of this activity implicates right cortical networks. Emotional cortical networks include both multimodal perceptual regions and movement-related systems.

However, it is interesting that there may be cortical hemispheric differences in processing basic physiologic somatic input. More than 25 years ago, serotonergic binding was found to be reduced, associated with depression, after left brain stroke, by Robinson and Starkstein.[129] As noted above, right brain-damaged patients have reduced galvanic skin responses to emotional stimuli, suggesting that sympathetic response to arousing stimuli depends critically on right cortical networks.[117,130] De Raedt and colleagues,[131] reviewing literature on the role of right versus left cortical networks in brain-autonomic interaction, suggested that the right brain may establish sympathetic homeostasis, while the left brain modulates parasympathetic activity.

The right temporal, insular, and amygdalar regions are particularly critical in processing autonomic information[132] and are potentially hubs for network processing of emotional perception, emotional experience, and producing emotional behaviors, including facial expressions,[132–134] vocal prosody,[4,135] and even comprehension of body gestures.[134,136] Other frontal and parietal right brain regions also contribute to these functions.[137,138]

Clinical Presentation

Identifying emotional processing deficits requires critical observation and, usually, a brief cognitive examination. The clinician may observe patients with emotional processing deficits to have deficits in production of facial emotional expression—appearing consistently impassive, or voices that lack prosodic line, sounding flat and robotic. Deficient ability to produce emotional facial expressions or deficient ability to inflect spoken language with appropriate emotional prosody may initially appear to represent a restricted range of affect or depression.

A lack of expressed emotion in facial expression and vocal prosody can be distinguished from affective disorders by accompanying emotional perceptual deficits. Thus, if a patient with unemotional facial expression or vocal tone is unable to distinguish 2 or 3 facial expressions made by an examiner, this supports an emotional processing disorder. The examiner could say, "In a few minutes I am going to make an expression on my face. I want you to tell me if the way my face looks is the expression I would have on my face if I were feeling happy, sad, angry, frightened, or if I were not feeling anything. Ready? Here is the expression." If a patient has difficulty identifying basic emotions pantomimed on the face very broadly such as happiness or sadness, this is definitely abnormal.

Assessing the ability to perceive emotional prosody in spoken language may feel like it is more complicated, because the melody of speech can express more than just emotion. For example, the melodic line of a sentence goes up in pitch if we are asking a question versus making a statement. This does not express an emotion, but rather is a grammatical mark. It is useful to distinguish linguistic prosody (variation in pitch and tone that occurs in speech in order to express grammar, word meaning, etc.) from emotional prosody by using a technique introduced by Tucker and colleagues.[139] The examiner says a sentence that is neutral in linguistic content such as "The boy went to the store" after instructing the patient as follows: "In a minute I am going to say the sentence 'The boy went to the store.' I am going to say the sentence as though I am having an emotional feeling, however. The feeling could be happy, sad, angry, frightened, or I might not be feeling anything. What feeling am I expressing now?" Importantly, the examiner should use a piece of paper or similar-sized object to cover her face as she emotionally intones the sentence so that the patient is using the auditory information and not an emotional facial expression that might "leak" out. If an attentive patient cannot identify emotions such as happiness, sadness, or anger, this is abnormal performance.

An even more straightforward way to demonstrate that emotional processing disorder is responsible for impassive facial expressions or flat, unemotional prosody is to ask patients to produce emotional facial expressions or emotional prosody on command. This testing approach has the advantage of targeting the problem if patients have an isolated disorder of production affecting either emotional facial expressions or emotional vocal prosody. In other words, some patients may be able to identify facial expressions made by the examiner, or sentences emotionally intoned by the examiner, but cannot make the same facial expressions or emotional prosodic inflection that they just heard. Interestingly, patients with deficits in producing emotional facial expressions who attempt to make facial expressions on command may not change an impassive facial expression at all. However, if asked whether they did a good job, these patients may state "yes" reflecting unawareness of deficit (anosognosia). Patients asked to emotionally intone a sentence may elaborate the sentence content as they repeat it. So, if asked to intone the sentence "The boy went to the store" in a sad tone of voice, a patient with an emotional processing deficit may say, "The boy went to the store, he was sad." Again, if asked, such a patient may report that he did "a good job," reflecting conscious unawareness of deficit.

Lastly, patients with emotional processing disorder should be directly asked if they feel depressed, sad, hopeless, or helpless, and asked about other symptoms of depression, anxiety, or anhedonia. Although depression and emotional processing deficit can cooccur, if these symptoms are absent, and patients report euthymic mood, then restricted range of emotional facial expression or emotional vocal prosody is more likely due to emotional processing deficit after right brain stroke.

In spontaneous social behaviors with family or loved ones, emotional processing disorders can also be suspected when the clinician observes impaired empathy (an implicit understanding of the emotional states of others)[140] or an altered expression of a sense of humor.[141] These symptoms may also be reported by family; they are relatively uncommon in left brain stroke, despite the problems left brain stroke survivors can have with linguistic communication.

Although, as noted above, understanding the emotional body postures and body gestures of others and producing emotional body gestures are probably also symptoms of emotional processing deficit, unfortunately there are not yet established clinical approaches for identifying these problems at the bedside.

Rehabilitation of Emotional Processing Deficits

Management and education is the current care standard for emotional processing deficits; explaining changes in behavior to patients, families, and informal caregivers is very important. Family members and informal caregivers can be urged to "use words"—when communicating with the right stroke survivors and to explain emotional reactions verbally whenever possible. This makes the emotional component of communication accessible for the patient, who is no longer able to hear or see that information. For example, a spouse can tell the patient, "I am feeling sad right now since my mom passed away. I miss her very much." In the same way, family members can be educated about asking the patient what his or her feelings are, because the patient may not be able to express them on the face, or in spoken words.

Brain stimulation, medications, or other biological treatments could be expected to alter patterns of cortical and subcortical activation in emotional processing. However, at this point we lack specific information about the influence on emotional processing of medications, hormonal manipulation, or noninvasive electrical or magnetic brain stimulation.

A method of restitutive training restoring function of neural networks normally supporting emotional processing has been used to improve perception of emotional facial expressions. In patients with traumatic brain injury, Radice-Neumann and colleagues[142,143] used Facial Affect Recognition (FARS) training, focusing attention on facial feature configurations, and also examined the impact of interventions on social and emotional perceptual behaviors. In an initial study of 19 people with right brain injury, and later in a randomized controlled trial in 203 patients, they demonstrated that training face recognition consistently improved emotional perception of facial expressions on impairment tasks. Effects persisted at 6 months in the randomized controlled trial. In the initial study, investigators also examined a vicariative approach. With the vicariative approach, they had patients infer the emotional content of situational information in potentially emotional situations (e.g., being fired). This approach improved ability to perceive emotional facial expression in the pilot study; however, the vicariative treatment effect was not confirmed in the randomized controlled trial. In addition, emotional vocal prosody did not improve with FARS.

However, in these studies, the team did not assess any impact on emotional production deficits, and unfortunately their work did not demonstrate whether the intervention had any effect on functional performance in everyday life. Although the initial study and randomized controlled trial were performed in traumatic brain injury, further trials of this approach to improve facial expression recognition after stroke are appropriate. Such studies need to evaluate whether there is an impact on functional activity in daily life of emotional processing intervention. Because we lack other evidence-based approaches, however, it is justifiable for speech language pathologists, occupational therapists, or psychologists involved in cognitive rehabilitation to attempt FARS implementation. Specific information about how to implement this approach in clinical practice is not yet available; however, it is low-risk and low cost, except for time and labor.

Based on previous pilot work,[144] Rosenbek and colleagues[145] found that 12 patients with emotional prosodic production deficits after stroke improved their performance on impairment tasks after receiving either imitative (drills) or cognitive-linguistic training (strategic instruction on how to vary their vocal pitch to express emotion). Although no functional impact was assessed, reduction in impairment persisted at 3 months. Other researchers have not been able to demonstrate persistent reduction of emotional prosodic production impairment or functional impact after emotional prosody training, however.[146] Therefore, training emotional prosody outside research settings is probably not yet justifiable.

ALIEN HAND SYNDROME
Definitions/History

This important, but rare cognitive-motor is defined by involuntary movement in a limb, together with the sense of loss of limb ownership, and was first described in 1908 by Goldstein.[147] A 57-year-old woman developed uncontrollable movements of the left hand; it would act as if under its own agency, and actually tried to grasp and choke her. Autopsy later revealed strokes of the right brain and corpus callosum. In the 1940s, Akelaitis observed opposing actions between the hands of patients who had undergone corpus callosotomy which he termed "diagnostic dyspraxia,"[148] and in 1972 Brion and Jedynak coined the term "le signe de la main etrangere" (the sign of the foreign hand) to describe patients with tumors of the corpus callosum who were unable to recognize their own left arms without visual input.[149] Bogen later borrowed the term, converting it to "alien hand" to describe "intermanual conflict," when the affected limb directly opposes the actions of the unaffected limb.[150]

Pathophysiology/Neuroanatomy

There are three major forms of alien hand syndrome (AHS): anterior, callosal, or posterior, based on the location of the causative lesion (Figure 5.3).[151,152] Right brain stroke is associated with the callosal or posterior form; the anterior or frontal form[153] is more commonly associated with left brain dysfunction and affects the right hand. The other two forms, callosal and posterior, are right brain syndromes and exclusively affect the left limbs in right-handed patients. Because mesial structures are damaged in all three forms of AHS, there are also mixed forms of AHS with both frontal and callosal features; the leg can also be affected.[154]

In the callosal and posterior forms associated with right brain stroke, AHS is associated with anterior cerebral artery and posterior cerebral artery territory infarctions.[155] The anterior cerebral artery feeds the medial frontal lobes and anterior corpus callosum, while the posterior cerebral artery feeds the parietooccipital junction, thalamus, and the posterior corpus callosum, respectively. The posterior variant, or sensory AHS,[156] is typically seen in association with lesions of the right parietal lobe, often extending to the splenium of the corpus callosum.[157] Intriguingly, this subtype has also been observed secondary to lesions of the right thalamus and pons.[158–160] It is thought that in the posterior variant, because the right parietal lobe plays a pivotal role in self and environmental perception, disruption of the tracts leading to and from this region could lead to an impaired sense of body awareness.[161] One group utilizing functional magnetic resonance imaging in a patient with AHS after a right parietal stroke found that volitional motor activity resulted in extensive activation of bilateral cortices. In this study, activation included primary motor, inferior frontal, and parietal regions, while involuntary motor activity produced activation of the contralateral primary motor cortex alone.[162] Other studies utilized techniques such as diffusion tensor tractography to demonstrate callosal lesions in patients with AHS.[163–165]

Anterior variant AHS is typically observed in lesions of the frontal lobe, particularly the medial frontal lobes. This variant is more commonly observed in the setting of left brain stroke.[166]

Clinical Presentation

Callosal variant AHS accompanies lesions of the corpus callosum and is more common after right brain stroke. Intermanual conflict may be the predominant symptom. When a patient initiates an action with the "good" hand/arm, the contralesional arm might directly oppose the action.[167] This bizarre phenomenon has been reported as the affected hand pulling away a block of wood just as the other tries to hammer a nail into it, the affected hand pulling away a candle as the other

tries to light it, and the affected hand unbuttoning a piece of clothing as the other arm tries to button it while dressing.[168,169] This variant is often accompanied by autocriticism (negative expressed feelings toward the affected limb), as well as features of callosal disconnection including apraxia, tactile and visual anomia, and agraphia.[170] In the posterior variant, patients may report a sense of estrangement from the contralesional limb, a sense that the limb is not theirs despite evidence to the contrary, and nonpurposeful movements of the contralesional arm, such as arm levitation.[171] Patients can continue to feel a sense of estrangement even when symptoms are successfully treated through rehabilitative intervention.[172]

Anterior variant AHS after left brain stroke[166] is defined by the presence of grasping movements of the contralesional limb, reported by the patient as unintentional. In the anterior variant, patients again typically experience intensely negative feelings toward the affected limb (autocriticism, or misoplegia, if the limb is weak). Comorbid conditions frequently encountered in this variant are those seen in frontal lobe lesions including frontal release signs (grasp reflex, glabellar sign, palmomental reflex, etc.), hemiparesis, and nonfluent aphasia.[170]

Rehabilitation of Alien Hand Syndrome

Until recently, much of our understanding of AHS has been relegated to single case studies or case series, limiting what could be concluded about its management and treatment. With the rise of electronic health records and large-scale data collection, it has become possible to summarize information about larger groups of patients with AHS. Graff-Radford and colleagues conducted a retrospective analysis of 150 patients with AHS at a single tertiary care center over a 15-year period.[173]

Rehabilitation of right brain stroke–related AHS is supported in a review summarizing 18 prior studies.[174] In these 18 studies, 25 patients, 18 right brain stroke patients, and 7 left brain stroke patients were reported. The authors stated that while 15 patients (68%) had improvement in their symptoms over time, 10 (32%) had persistent symptoms up to 1 year later. They suggested that AHS after right brain stroke may have a better overall prognosis than the same symptoms following left stroke.

Specific rehabilitation techniques utilized in AHS include mirror box therapy, distraction of the affected limb (e.g., with a ball or other object), visualizing a given task, and compensatory strategies.[172,175] Pharmacologic therapies attempted with some success for AHS include clonazepam, carbamazepine, and onabotulinum toxin A injections to the affected arm.[158,176] Unfortunately, studies with randomized assignment or appropriate controls have not yet been performed to examine these techniques.

Treatment of limb apraxia, disordered skilled learned purposive limb movements after stroke and brain injury,[177] is appropriate for crossapplication in AHS. For limb apraxia, two treatment approaches are suggested in guidelines from the American Occupational Therapy Association.[54] It would be appropriate to try both of these approaches: as noted above, strategy training as a compensatory strategy is effective. Secondly, gesture training using a method of successive cuing[178,179] has been shown to improve activities of daily living in stroke survivors, with improved daily life function persisting 2 months later.

CONCLUSIONS AND FUTURE DIRECTIONS

Spatial neglect, anosognosia for hemiparesis, emotional processing deficits, and AHS are not the only cognitive deficits associated with disability after right brain stroke. There are, of course, other cognitive and behavioral problems that occur in patients with right brain stroke. However, we feel these clinical topics present major opportunities for rehabilitation clinicians to gain knowledge for assessment and treatment planning in the inpatient rehabilitation setting, and in the first phases of outpatient care.

In each of these syndromes—spatial neglect, anosognosia, emotional processing disorder, and AHS—a key step in successful rehabilitation is prompt identification of symptoms for the treatment. As we note above, it is ideal for clinicians to use assessments with demonstrated validity to predict functional disability[22] in routine screening of all right brain stroke patients. Otherwise, patients who have more severe deficits or certain subsets of symptoms may only be referred for assessment.

A number of interesting approaches for rehabilitation of right brain disorders are at this point still under development. These include personalized treatment with biological approaches such as noninvasive brain stimulation[180] or basing stroke rehabilitation treatment on genetic factors,[181] and using combined protocols of cognitive and motor training tailored to right brain disorders.[182] The chapter includes pragmatic choices for assessment and treatment among low-risk or well-demonstrated choices. However, new, higher-risk biological approaches will definitely become available, and the responsible clinician continues to follow the literature for new guidelines and consensus recommendations from scientific and professional associations.

ACKNOWLEDGMENTS

The authors' work on this chapter was supported by the Kessler Foundation, the Wallerstein Foundation for Geriatric Improvement, and the Charles and Ann Serraino Foundation, as well as the National Institute for Disability, Independent Living, and Rehabilitation Research (901F0037, PI Barrett) and the National Institutes of Health (K24HD062647, PI Barrett).

REFERENCES

1. Gillen R, Tennen H, McKee T. Unilateral spatial neglect: relation to rehabilitation outcomes in patients with right hemisphere stroke. *Arch Phys Med Rehabil.* 2005;86(4): 763–767.
2. Chen P, McKenna C, Kutlik AM, Frisina PG. Interdisciplinary communication in inpatient rehabilitation facility: evidence of under-documentation of spatial neglect after stroke. *Disabil Rehabil.* 2013;35(12):1033–1038.
3. Blumenfeld H. *Neuroanatomy through Clinical Cases.* 2nd ed. Sunderland, MA: Sinauer Associates; 2010.
4. Ross ED, Monnot M. Neurology of affective prosody and its functional-anatomic organization in right hemisphere. *Brain Lang.* 2008;104(1):51–74.
5. Mendis S, Norrving B. Organizational update: World Health Organization. *Stroke.* 2014;45(2):e22–e23.
6. Stuntz M, Busko K, Irshad S, Paige T, Razhkova V, Coan T. Nationwide trends of clinical characteristics and economic burden of emergency department visits due to acute ischemic stroke. *Open Access Emerg Med.* 2017;9: 89–96.
7. Agis D, Goggins MB, Oishi K, et al. Picturing the size and site of stroke with an expanded National Institutes of Health stroke scale. *Stroke.* 2016;47(6):1459–1465.
8. Wei N, Yong W, Li X, et al. Post-stroke depression and lesion location: a systematic review. *J Neurol.* 2015; 262(1):81–90.
9. Jordan LC, Hillis AE. Aphasia and right hemisphere syndromes in stroke. *Curr Neurol Neurosci Rep.* 2005;5(6): 458–464.
10. Suhr JA, Grace J. Brief cognitive screening of right hemisphere stroke: relation to functional outcome. *Arch Phys Med Rehabil.* 1999;80(7):773–776.
11. Palmerini F, Bogousslavsky J. Right hemisphere syndromes. *Front Neurol Neurosci.* 2012;30:61–64.
12. Losoi H, Kettunen JE, Laihosalo M, et al. Predictors of functional outcome after right hemisphere stroke in patients with or without thrombolytic treatment. *Neurocase.* 2012;18(5):377–385.
13. McCluskey G, Wade C, McKee J, McCarron P, McVerry F, McCarron MO. Stroke laterality bias in the management of acute ischemic stroke. *J Stroke Cerebrovasc Dis.* 2016; 25(11):2701–2707.
14. Cherney LR. Ethical issues involving the right hemisphere stroke patient: to treat or not to treat? *Top Stroke Rehabil.* 2006;13(4):47–53.

15. Brott T, Adams Jr HP, Olinger CP, et al. Measurements of acute cerebral infarction: a clinical examination scale. *Stroke*. 1989;20(7):864–870.
16. Woo D, Broderick JP, Kothari RU, et al. Does the National Institutes of Health stroke scale favor left hemisphere strokes? NINDS t-PA stroke study group. *Stroke*. 1999; 30(11):2355–2359.
17. Glymour MM, Berkman LF, Ertel KA, Fay ME, Glass TA, Furie KL. Lesion characteristics, NIH stroke scale, and functional recovery after stroke. *Am J Phys Med Rehabil*. 2007;86(9):725–733.
18. Cherney LR, Halper AS, Kwasnica CM, Harvey RL, Zhang M. Recovery of functional status after right hemisphere stroke: relationship with unilateral neglect. *Arch Phys Med Rehabil*. 2001;82(3):322–328.
19. Barrett AM, Burkholder S. Monocular patching in subjects with right-hemisphere stroke affects perceptual-attentional bias. *J Rehabil Res Dev*. 2006;43(3):337–345.
20. Heilman KM, Valenstein E. Mechanisms underlying hemispatial neglect. *Ann Neurology*. 1979;5(2):166–170.
21. Riestra AR, Barrett AM. Rehabilitation of spatial neglect. *Handb Clin Neurol*. 2013;110:347–355.
22. Chen P, Chen CC, Hreha K, Goedert KM, Barrett AM. Kessler Foundation Neglect Assessment Process uniquely measures spatial neglect during activities of daily living. *Arch Phys Med Rehabil*. 2015;96(5):869–876.e1.
23. Brain WR. Visual disorientation with special reference to lesions of the right cerebral hemisphere. *Brain*. 1941; 64(4):244–272.
24. Battersby WS, Bender MB, Pollack M, Kahn RL. Unilateral "spatial agnosia" ("inattention") in patients with cerebral lesions. *Brain*. 1956;79:68–93.
25. Denny-Brown D, Meyer J, Horenstein S. The significance of perceptual rivalry resulting from parietal lesion. *Brain*. 1952;75(4):433–471.
26. Bender MB. Extinction and other patterns of sensory interaction. *Adv Neurology*. 1977;18:107–110 (0091-3952 (Print)).
27. Ungerstedt U. 6-hydroxydopamine-induced degeneration of the nigrostriatal dopamine pathway: the turning syndrome. *Pharmacol Ther B*. 1976;2(1):37–40.
28. Critchley M, Russell WR, Zangwill OL. Discussion on parietal lobe syndromes. *Proc R Soc Med*. 1951;44(4): 337–346.
29. Heilman KM, Watson RT, Valenstein E. Neglect and related disorders. In: Heilman KM, Valenstein E, eds. *Clinical Neuropsychology*. 5th ed. New York: Oxford University; 2012:296–348.
30. Payne BR, Rushmore RJ. Functional circuitry underlying natural and interventional cancellation of visual neglect. *Exp Brain Res*. 2004;154(2):127–153.
31. Baldassarre A, Ramsey L, Hacker CL, et al. Large-scale changes in network interactions as a physiological signature of spatial neglect. *Brain*. 2014;137(pt 12): 3267–3283.
32. Smith DV, Clithero JA, Rorden C, Karnath HO. Decoding the anatomical network of spatial attention. *Proc Natl Acad Sci U S A*. 2013;110(4):1518–1523.
33. Khurshid S, Trupe LA, Newhart M, et al. Reperfusion of specific cortical areas is associated with improvement in distinct forms of hemispatial neglect. *Cortex*. 2012; 48(5):530–539.
34. Mesulam MM. Spatial attention and neglect: parietal, frontal and cingulate contributions to the mental representation and attentional targeting of salient extrapersonal events. *Philosophical Trans R Soc Lond B Biol Sci*. 1999;354(1387):1325–1346.
35. He BJ, Shulman GL, Snyder AZ, Corbetta M. The role of impaired neuronal communication in neurological disorders. *Curr Opin Neurol*. 2007;20(6):655–660.
36. Catani M, Dell'acqua F, Bizzi A, et al. Beyond cortical localization in clinico-anatomical correlation. *Cortex*. 2012;48(10):1262–1287.
37. Adair JC, Barrett AM. Spatial neglect: clinical and neuroscience review: a wealth of information on the poverty of spatial attention. *Ann N Y Acad Sci*. 2008; 1142:21–43.
38. Eskes GA, Barrett AM. *Neuropsychological Rehabilitation*. *Neurovascular Neuropsychology*. Springer; 2009:281–305.
39. Rapcsak SZ, Watson RT, Heilman KM. Hemispace-visual field interactions in visual extinction. *J Neurol Neurosurg Psychiatry*. 1987;50(9):1117–1124.
40. Heilman KM, Bowers D, Coslett HB, Whelan H, Watson RT. Directional hypokinesia: prolonged reaction times for leftward movements in patients with right hemisphere lesions and neglect. *Neurology*. 1985;35(6): 855–859.
41. Kwon SE, Heilman KM. Ipsilateral neglect in a patient following a unilateral frontal lesion. *Neurology*. 1991; 41(12):2001–2004.
42. Barrett AM, Crosson JB, Crucian GP, Heilman KM. Horizontal line bisections in upper and lower body space. *J Int Neuropsychol Soc*. 2000;6(4):455–459.
43. Triggs WJ, Gold M, Gerstle G, Adair J, Heilman KM. Motor neglect associated with a discrete parietal lesion. *Neurology*. 1994;44(6):1164–1166.
44. Kirshner H, Mark VW. Ischemic stroke syndromes. In: Festa J, Lazar R, eds. *Neurovascular Neuropsychology*. Springer; 2009:36.
45. Barrett AM, Crucian GP, Schwartz RL, Heilman KM. Adverse effect of dopamine agonist therapy in a patient with motor-intentional neglect. *Arch Phys Med Rehabil*. 1999;80(5):600–603.
46. Khurshid S, Longin H, Crucian GP, Barrett AM. Monocular patching affects inattention but not perseveration in spatial neglect. *Neurocase*. 2009;15(4):311–317.
47. Na DL, Adair JC, Williamson DJ, Schwartz RL, Haws B, Heilman KM. Dissociation of sensory-attentional from motor-intentional neglect. *J Neurol Neurosurg Psychiatry*. 1998;64(3):331–338.
48. Bisiach E, Geminiani G, Berti A, Rusconi ML. Perceptual and premotor factors of unilateral neglect. *Neurology*. 1990;40(8):1278–1281.
49. Fortis P, Chen P, Goedert KM, Barrett AM. Effects of prism adaptation on motor-intentional spatial bias in neglect. *Neuroreport*. 2011;22(14):700–705.

50. Goedert KM, Chen P, Boston RC, Foundas AL, Barrett AM. Presence of motor-intentional aiming deficit predicts functional improvement of spatial neglect with prism adaptation. *Neurorehabil Neural Repair.* 2014; 28(5):483–493.

51. Goedert KM, Chen P, Botticello A, Masmela JR, Adler U, Barrett AM. Psychometric evaluation of neglect assessment reveals motor-exploratory predictor of functional disability in acute-stage spatial neglect. *Arch Phys Med Rehabil.* 2012;93(1):137–142.

52. Chen P, Hreha K, Fortis P, Goedert KM, Barrett AM. Functional assessment of spatial neglect: a review of the Catherine Bergego scale and an introduction of the Kessler foundation neglect assessment process. *Top Stroke Rehabil.* 2012;19(5):423–435.

53. Weinstein EA, Kahn RL. *Denial of Illness; Symbolic and Physiological Aspects.* Springfield, Illinois: Thomas; 1955.

54. Gillen G, Nilsen DM, Attridge J, et al. Effectiveness of interventions to improve occupational performance of people with cognitive impairments after stroke: an evidence-based review. *Am J Occup Ther.* 2015;69(1): 6901180040p1–6901180040p9.

55. Barrett AM, Goedert KM, Basso JC. Prism adaptation for spatial neglect after stroke: translational practice gaps. *Nat Rev Neurol.* 2012;8(10):567–577.

56. Champod AS, Frank RC, Taylor K, Eskes GA. The effects of prism adaptation on daily life activities in patients with visuospatial neglect: a systematic review. *Neuropsychol Rehabil.* 2018;28(4):491–514.

57. Yang NY, Zhou D, Chung RC, Li-Tsang CW, Fong KN. Rehabilitation interventions for unilateral neglect after stroke: a systematic review from 1997 through 2012. *Front Hum Neurosci.* 2013;7:187.

58. Robertson IH, North N. Active and passive activation of left limbs: influence on visual and sensory neglect. *Neuropsychologia.* 1993;31(3):293–300.

59. Eskes GA, Butler B, McDonald A, Harrison ER, Phillips SJ. Limb activation effects in hemispatial neglect. *Arch Phys Med Rehabil.* 2003;84(3):323–328.

60. Weinberg J, Diller L, Gordon WA, et al. Visual scanning training effect on reading-related tasks in acquired right brain damage. *Arch Phys Med Rehabil.* 1977;58(11): 479–486.

61. Weinberg J, Diller L, Gordon WA, et al. Training sensory awareness and spatial organization in people with right brain damage. *Arch Phys Med Rehabil.* 1979;60(11): 491–496.

62. Frassinetti F, Angeli V, Meneghello F, Avanzi S, Ladavas E. Long-lasting amelioration of visuospatial neglect by prism adaptation. *Brain.* 2002;125(pt 3):608–623.

63. Cicerone KD, Langenbahn DM, Braden C, et al. Evidence-based cognitive rehabilitation: updated review of the literature from 2003 through 2008. *Arch Phys Med Rehabil.* 2011;92(4):519–530.

64. Antonucci G, Guariglia C, Judica A, et al. Effectiveness of neglect rehabilitation in a randomized group study. *J Clin Exp Neuropsychol.* 1995;17(3):383–389.

65. Pizzamiglio L, Antonucci G, Judica A, Montenero P, Razzano C, Zoccolotti P. Cognitive rehabilitation of the hemineglect disorder in chronic patients with unilateral right brain damage. *J Clin Exp Neuropsychol.* 1992;14(6): 901–923.

66. Wagenaar RC, van Wieringen PC, Netelenbos JB, Meijer OG, Kuik DJ. The transfer of scanning training effects in visual inattention after stroke: five single-case studies. *Disabil Rehabil.* 1992;14(1):51–60.

67. Kelly MP, Ostreicher H. Environmental factors and outcome in hemineglect syndrome. *Rehabil Psychol.* 1985;30(1):35.

68. Adair JC, Barrett AM. Anosognosia. In: Heilman KM, Valenstein E, eds. *Clinical Neuropsychology.* 5th ed. New York: Oxford University Press; 2012:198–213.

69. Babinski J. Contribution a l'etude dies troubles mentaux dans l'hemiplegie organique cerebrale (anosognosie). *Rev Neurol.* 1914;27:845–847.

70. Bisiach E, Vallar G, Perani D, Papagno C, Berti A. Unawareness of disease following lesions of the right hemisphere: anosognosia for hemiplegia and anosognosia for hemianopia. *Neuropsychologia.* 1986;24(4):471–482.

71. Baier B, Karnath HO. Incidence and diagnosis of anosognosia for hemiparesis revisited. *J Neurol Neurosurg Psychiatry.* 2005;76(3):358–361.

72. Hartman-Maeir A, Soroker N, Oman SD, Katz N. Awareness of disabilities in stroke rehabilitation—a clinical trial. *Disabil Rehabil.* 2003;25(1):35–44.

73. Gilmore RL, Heilman KM, Schmidt RP, Fennell EM, Quisling R. Anosognosia during Wada testing. *Neurology.* 1992;42(4):925–927.

74. Durkin MW, Meador KJ, Nichols ME, Lee GP, Loring DW. Anosognosia and the intracarotid amobarbital procedure (Wada test). *Neurology.* 1994;44(5):978–979.

75. Lu LH, Barrett AM, Schwartz RL, et al. Anosognosia and confabulation during the Wada test. *Neurology.* 1997; 49(5):1316–1322.

76. Dywan CA, McGlone J, Fox A. Do intracarotid barbiturate injections offer a way to investigate hemispheric models of anosognosia? *J Clin Exp Neuropsychol.* 1995;17(3):431–438.

77. Healton EB, Navarro C, Bressman S, Brust JC. Subcortical neglect. *Neurology.* 1982;32(7):776–778.

78. Graff-Radford NR, Eslinger PJ, Damasio AR, Yamada T. Nonhemorrhagic infarction of the thalamus: behavioral, anatomic, and physiologic correlates. *Neurology.* 1984; 34(1):14–23.

79. Evyapan D, Kumral E. Pontine anosognosia for hemiplegia. *Neurology.* 1999;53(3):647–649.

80. Levine DN. Unawareness of visual and sensorimotor defects: a hypothesis. *Brain Cogn.* 1990;13(2):233–281.

81. Fotopoulou A, Tsakiris M, Haggard P, Vagopoulou A, Rudd A, Kopelman M. The role of motor intention in motor awareness: an experimental study on anosognosia for hemiplegia. *Brain.* 2008;131(pt 12):3432–3442.

82. Besharati S, Forkel SJ, Kopelman M, Solms M, Jenkinson PM, Fotopoulou A. Mentalizing the body: spatial and social cognition in anosognosia for hemiplegia. *Brain.* 2016;139(pt 3):971–985.

83. Prigatano GP, Matthes J, Hill SW, Wolf TR, Heiserman JE. Anosognosia for hemiplegia with preserved awareness of complete cortical blindness following intracranial hemorrhage. *Cortex*. 2011;47(10):1219–1227.

84. Heilman KM, Barrett AM, Adair JC. Possible mechanisms of anosognosia: a defect in self-awareness. *Philos Trans R Soc Lond B Biol Sci*. 1998;353(1377):1903–1909.

85. Turnbull OH, Solms M. Awareness, desire, and false beliefs: Freud in the light of modern neuropsychology. *Cortex*. 2007;43(8):1083–1090.

86. Nardone IB, Ward R, Fotopoulou A, Turnbull OH. Attention and emotion in anosognosia: evidence of implicit awareness and repression? *Neurocase*. 2007;13(5):438–445.

87. Starkstein SE, Fedoroff JP, Price TR, Leiguarda R, Robinson RG. Anosognosia in patients with cerebrovascular lesions. A study of causative factors. *Stroke*. 1992; 23(10):1446–1453.

88. Orfei MD, Robinson RG, Prigatano GP, et al. Anosognosia for hemiplegia after stroke is a multifaceted phenomenon: a systematic review of the literature. *Brain*. 2007; 130(Pt 12):3075–3090.

89. Prigatano GP. Anosognosia and patterns of impaired self-awareness observed in clinical practice. *Cortex*. 2014;61: 81–92.

90. Toglia J, Kirk U. Understanding awareness deficits following brain injury. *NeuroRehabilitation*. 2000;15(1): 57–70.

91. Prigatano GP. *The Study of Anosognosia*. Vol 17. New York: Oxford University Press; 2010.

92. Barrett AM. Rose-colored answers: neuropsychological deficits and patient-reported outcomes after stroke. *Behav Neurol*. 2010;22(1–2):17–23.

93. Winstein CJ, Stein J, Arena R, et al. Guidelines for adult stroke rehabilitation and recovery: a guideline for healthcare professionals from the American Heart Association/ American Stroke Association. *Stroke*. 2016;47(6): e98–e169.

94. Goverover Y, Johnston MV, Toglia J, Deluca J. Treatment to improve self-awareness in persons with acquired brain injury. *Brain Inj*. 2007;21(9):913–923.

95. Cappa S, Sterzi R, Vallar G, Bisiach E. Remission of hemineglect and anosognosia during vestibular stimulation. *Neuropsychologia*. 1987;25(5):775–782.

96. Besharati S, Kopelman M, Avesani R, Moro V, Fotopoulou AK. Another perspective on anosognosia: self-observation in video replay improves motor awareness. *Neuropsychol Rehabil*. 2015;25(3):319–352.

97. Fotopoulou A, Rudd A, Holmes P, Kopelman M. Self-observation reinstates motor awareness in anosognosia for hemiplegia. *Neuropsychologia*. 2009;47(5):1256–1260.

98. Malec J, Moessner AM. Self-awareness, distress, and post-acute rehabilitation outcome. *Rehabilitation Psychology*. 2000;45(3):227–241. Vol 452000.

99. Ownsworth T, Fleming J, Desbois J, Strong J, Kuipers P. A metacognitive contextual intervention to enhance error awareness and functional outcome following traumatic brain injury: a single-case experimental design. *J Int Neuropsychol Soc*. 2006;12(1):54–63.

100. Ekman P, Sorenson ER, Friesen WV. Pan-cultural elements in facial displays of emotion. *Science*. 1969; 164(3875):86–88.

101. Heilman KM, Blonder LX, Bowers D, Valenstein E. Emotional disorders associated with neurological disorders. In: Heilman KM, Valenstein E, eds. *Clinical Neuropsychology*. 2nd ed. New York, NY: Oxford; 2012: 466–503.

102. Ross ED, Prodan CI, Monnot M. Human facial expressions are organized functionally across the upper-lower facial axis. *Neuroscientist*. 2007;13(5):433–446.

103. Ross ED, Reddy AL, Nair A, Mikawa K, Prodan CI. Facial expressions are more easily produced on the upper-lower compared to the right-left hemiface. *Percept Mot Skills*. 2007;104(1):155–165.

104. Levy J, Heller W, Banich MT, Burton LA. Asymmetry of perception in free viewing of chimeric faces. *Brain Cogn*. 1983;2(4):404–419.

105. Ley RG, Bryden MP. Hemispheric differences in processing emotions and faces. *Brain Lang*. 1979;7(1): 127–138.

106. Suberi M, McKeever WF. Differential right hemispheric memory storage of emotional and non-emotional faces. *Neuropsychologia*. 1977;15(6):757–768.

107. Van Lancker D. Rags to riches: our increasing appreciation of cognitive and communicative abilities of the human right cerebral hemisphere. *Brain Lang*. 1997;57(1): 1–11.

108. Borod JC, Kent J, Koff E, Martin C, Alpert M. Facial asymmetry while posing positive and negative emotions: support for the right hemisphere hypothesis. *Neuropsychologia*. 1988;26(5):759–764.

109. DeKosky ST, Heilman KM, Bowers D, Valenstein E. Recognition and discrimination of emotional faces and pictures. *Brain Lang*. 1980;9(2):206–214.

110. Bowers D, Bauer RM, Coslett HB, Heilman KM. Processing of faces by patients with unilateral hemisphere lesions. I. Dissociation between judgments of facial affect and facial identity. *Brain Cogn*. 1985;4(3):258–272.

111. Heilman KM, Bowers D, Speedie L, Coslett HB. Comprehension of affective and nonaffective prosody. *Neurology*. 1984;34(7):917–921.

112. Bowers D, Heilman KM. Dissociation between the processing of affective and nonaffective faces: a case study. *J Clin Neuropsychol*. 1984;6(4):367–379.

113. Blonder LX, Bowers D, Heilman KM. The role of the right hemisphere in emotional communication. *Brain*. 1991; 114(Pt 3):1115–1127.

114. Bowers D, Blonder LX, Feinberg T, Heilman KM. Differential impact of right and left hemisphere lesions on facial emotion and object imagery. *Brain*. 1991;114(pt 6):2593–2609.

115. Barrett LF, Simmons WK. Interoceptive predictions in the brain. *Nat Rev Neurosci*. 2015;16(7):419–429.

116. Rorden C, Brett M. Stereotaxic display of brain lesions. *Behav Neurol*. 2000;12(4):191–200.

117. Gainotti G. Emotional behavior and hemispheric side of the lesion. *Cortex*. 1972;8(1):41–55.

118. Heilman KM, Schwartz HD, Watson RT. Hypoarousal in patients with the neglect syndrome and emotional indifference. *Neurology.* 1978;28(3):229−232.

119. Buck R, Duffy JR. Nonverbal communication of affect in brain-damaged patients. *Cortex.* 1980;16(3):351−362. Vol 161980.

120. Borod JC, Cicero BA, Obler LK, et al. Right hemisphere emotional perception: evidence across multiple channels. *Neuropsychology.* 1998;12(3):446−458.

121. Kent J, Borod JC, Koff E, Welkowitz J, Alpert M. Posed facial emotional expression in brain-damaged patients. *Int J Neurosci.* 1988;43(1−2):81−87.

122. Ross E, Homan WR, Buck R. Differential hemispheric lateralization of primary and social emotions implications for developing a comprehensive neurology for emotions, repression, and the subconscious. *Neuropsychiatry, Neuropsychology, & Behavioral Neurology.* 1994;7(1): 1−19. Vol 71994.

123. Pichon S, Kell CA. Affective and sensorimotor components of emotional prosody generation. *J Neurosci.* 2013;33(4):1640−1650.

124. Ethofer T, Anders S, Erb M, et al. Impact of voice on emotional judgment of faces: an event-related fMRI study. *Hum Brain Mapp.* 2006;27(9):707−714.

125. Ethofer T, Pourtois G, Wildgruber D. Investigating audio-visual integration of emotional signals in the human brain. *Prog Brain Res.* 2006;156:345−361.

126. Wildgruber D, Ackermann H, Kreifelts B, Ethofer T. Cerebral processing of linguistic and emotional prosody: fMRI studies. *Prog Brain Res.* 2006;156:249−268.

127. Cannon WB. The James-Lange theory of emotion: a critical examination and an alternative theory. *Am J Psychol.* 1927;39:106−124.

128. LeDoux JE, Cicchetti P, Xagoraris A, Romanski LM. The lateral amygdaloid nucleus: sensory interface of the amygdala in fear conditioning. *J Neurosci.* 1990;10(4): 1062−1069.

129. Robinson RG, Starkstein SE. Mood disorders following stroke: new findings and future directions. *J Geriatr Psychiatry.* 1989;22(1):1−15.

130. Zoccolotti P, Caltagirone C, Benedetti N, Gainotti G. Disorders of autonomic responses to emotional stimuli in patients with unilateral hemispherical lesions. *Encephale.* 1986;12(5):263−268.

131. De Raedt S, De Vos A, De Keyser J. Autonomic dysfunction in acute ischemic stroke: an underexplored therapeutic area? *J Neurol Sci.* 2015;348(1−2):24−34.

132. Beissner F, Meissner K, Bar KJ, Napadow V. The autonomic brain: an activation likelihood estimation meta-analysis for central processing of autonomic function. *J Neurosci.* 2013;33(25):10503−10511.

133. Gola KA, Shany-Ur T, Pressman P, et al. A neural network underlying intentional emotional facial expression in neurodegenerative disease. *Neuroimage Clin.* 2017;14: 672−678.

134. Prochnow D, Hoing B, Kleiser R, et al. The neural correlates of affect reading: an fMRI study on faces and gestures. *Behav Brain Res.* 2013;237:270−277.

135. Fruhholz S, Ceravolo L, Grandjean D. Specific brain networks during explicit and implicit decoding of emotional prosody. *Cereb Cortex.* 2012;22(5):1107−1117.

136. Schindler K, Van Gool L, de Gelder B. Recognizing emotions expressed by body pose: a biologically inspired neural model. *Neural Netw.* 2008;21(9):1238−1246.

137. Patel S, Oishi K, Wright A, et al. Right hemisphere regions critical for expression of emotion through prosody. *Front Neurol.* 2018;9:224.

138. Kesler-West ML, Andersen AH, Smith CD, et al. Neural substrates of facial emotion processing using fMRI. *Brain Res Cogn Brain Res.* 2001;11(2):213−226.

139. Tucker DM, Watson RT, Heilman KM. Discrimination and evocation of affectively intoned speech in patients with right parietal disease. *Neurology.* 1977;27(10): 947−950.

140. Yeh ZT, Tsai CF. Impairment on theory of mind and empathy in patients with stroke. *Psychiatry Clin Neurosci.* 2014;68(8):612−620.

141. Heath RL, Blonder LX. Spontaneous humor among right hemisphere stroke survivors. *Brain Lang.* 2005;93(3): 267−276.

142. Radice-Neumann D, Zupan B, Tomita M, Willer B. Training emotional processing in persons with brain injury. *J Head Trauma Rehabil.* 2009;24(5):313−323.

143. Neumann D, Babbage DR, Zupan B, Willer B. A randomized controlled trial of emotion recognition training after traumatic brain injury. *J Head Trauma Rehabil.* 2015;30(3):E12−E23.

144. Leon SA, Rosenbek JC, Crucian GP, et al. Active treatments for aprosodia secondary to right hemisphere stroke. *J Rehabil Res Dev.* 2005;42(1):93−101.

145. Rosenbek JC, Rodriguez AD, Hieber B, et al. Effects of two treatments for aprosodia secondary to acquired brain injury. *J Rehabil Res Dev.* 2006;43(3):379−390.

146. McDonald S, Togher L, Tate R, Randall R, English T, Gowland A. A randomised controlled trial evaluating a brief intervention for deficits in recognising emotional prosody following severe ABI. *Neuropsychol Rehabil.* 2013;23(2):267−286.

147. Goldstein K. Zur lehre von der motorischen apraxie. *J Psychol Neurology.* 1908;11:169−187.

148. Akelaitis AJ. Studies on the corpus callosum IV. Diagnostic dyspraxia in epileptics following partial and complete section of the corpus callosum. *Am J Psychiatry.* 1945;101:494−499.

149. Brion S, Jedynak CP. [Disorders of interhemispheric transfer (callosal disonnection). 3 cases of tumor of the corpus callosum. The strange hand sign]. *Rev Neurol Paris.* 1972;126(4):257−266.

150. Heilman KM, Valenstein E. *Clinical Neuropsychology.* 3rd ed. New York: Oxford University Press; 1993.

151. Schaefer M, Denke C, Apostolova I, Heinze HJ, Galazky I. A case of right alien hand syndrome coexisting with right-sided tactile extinction. *Front Hum Neurosci.* 2016;10:105.

152. Feinberg TE, Schindler RJ, Flanagan NG, Haber LD. Two alien hand syndromes. *Neurology.* 1992;42(1):19−24.

153. Nowak DA, Bosl K, Ludemann-Podubecka J, Gdynia HJ, Ponfick M. Recovery and outcome of frontal alien hand syndrome after anterior cerebral artery stroke. *J Neurol Sci.* 2014;338(1−2):203−206.

154. Chan JL, Chen RS, Ng KK. Leg manifestation in alien hand syndrome. *J Formos Med Assoc.* 1996;95(4):342−346.

155. Hertza J, Davis AS, Barisa M, Lemann ER. Atypical sensory alien hand syndrome: a case study. *Appl Neuropsychol Adult.* 2012;19(1):71−77.

156. Ay H, Buonanno FS, Price BH, Le DA, Koroshetz WJ. Sensory alien hand syndrome: case report and review of the literature. *J Neurol Neurosurg Psychiatry.* 1998;65(3):366−369.

157. Pappalardo A, Ciancio MR, Reggio E, Patti F. Posterior alien hand syndrome: case report and rehabilitative treatment. *Neurorehabil Neural Repair.* 2004;18(3):176−181.

158. Sabrie M, Berhoune N, Nighoghossian N. Alien hand syndrome and paroxystic dystonia after right posterior cerebral artery territory infarction. *Neurol Sci.* 2015;36(9):1709−1710.

159. Rafiei N, Chang GY. Right sensory alien hand phenomenon from a left pontine hemorrhage. *J Clin Neurol.* 2009;5(1):46−48.

160. Marey-Lopez J, Rubio-Nazabal E, Alonso-Magdalena L, Lopez-Facal S. Posterior alien hand syndrome after a right thalamic infarct. *J Neurol Neurosurg Psychiatry.* 2002;73(4):447−449.

161. Olgiati E, Maravita A, Spandri V, et al. Body schema and corporeal self-recognition in the alien hand syndrome. *Neuropsychology.* 2017;31(5):575−584.

162. Assal F, Schwartz S, Vuilleumier P. Moving with or without will: functional neural correlates of alien hand syndrome. *Ann Neurol.* 2007;62(3):301−306.

163. Chang MC, Yeo SS, Jang SH. Callosal disconnection syndrome in a patient with corpus callosum hemorrhage: a diffusion tensor tractography study. *Arch Neurol.* 2012;69(10):1374−1375.

164. Jang SH, Lee J, Yeo SS, Chang MC. Callosal disconnection syndrome after corpus callosum infarct: a diffusion tensor tractography study. *J Stroke Cerebrovasc Dis.* 2013;22(7):e240−e244.

165. Delrieu J, Payoux P, Toulza O, Esquerre JP, Vellas B, Voisin T. Sensory alien hand syndrome in corticobasal degeneration: a cerebral blood flow study. *Mov Disord.* 2010;25(9):1288−1291.

166. Biran I, Chatterjee A. Alien hand syndrome. *Arch Neurol.* 2004;61(2):292−294.

167. Lunardelli A, Sartori A, Mengotti P, Rumiati RI, Pesavento V. Intermittent alien hand syndrome and callosal apraxia in multiple sclerosis: implications for interhemispheric communication. *Behav Neurol.* 2014;2014: 873541.

168. Heilman KM, Valenstein E. *Clinical Neuropsychology.* 4th ed. Oxford, New York: Oxford University Press; 2003.

169. Brainin M, Seiser A, Matz K. The mirror world of motor inhibition: the alien hand syndrome in chronic stroke. *J Neurol Neurosurg Psychiatry.* 2008;79(3):246−252.

170. Hassan A, Josephs KA. Alien hand syndrome. *Curr Neurol Neurosci Rep.* 2016;16(8):73.

171. Pack BC, Stewart KJ, Diamond PT, Gale SD. Posterior-variant alien hand syndrome: clinical features and response to rehabilitation. *Disabil Rehabil.* 2002;24(15):817−818.

172. Romano D, Sedda A, Dell'aquila R, et al. Controlling the alien hand through the mirror box. A single case study of alien hand syndrome. *Neurocase.* 2014;20(3):307−316.

173. Graff-Radford J, Rubin MN, Jones DT, et al. The alien limb phenomenon. *J Neurol.* 2013;260(7):1880−1888.

174. Kikkert MA, Ribbers GM, Koudstaal PJ. Alien hand syndrome in stroke: a report of 2 cases and review of the literature. *Arch Phys Med Rehabil.* 2006;87(5):728−732.

175. Pooyania S, Mohr S, Gray S. Alien hand syndrome: a case report and description to rehabilitation. *Disabil Rehabil.* 2011;33(17−18):1715−1718.

176. Haq IU, Malaty IA, Okun MS, Jacobson CE, Fernandez HH, Rodriguez RR. Clonazepam and botulinum toxin for the treatment of alien limb phenomenon. *Neurologist.* 2010;16(2):106−108.

177. Heilman KM, Rothi LJG. Apraxia. In: Heilman KM, Valenstein E, eds. *Clinical Neuropsychology.* New York, NY: Oxford University Press; 2012:214−237.

178. Smania N, Aglioti SM, Girardi F, et al. Rehabilitation of limb apraxia improves daily life activities in patients with stroke. *Neurology.* 2006;67(11):2050−2052.

179. Smania N, Girardi F, Domenicali C, Lora E, Aglioti S. The rehabilitation of limb apraxia: a study in left-brain-damaged patients. *Arch Phys Med Rehabil.* 2000;81(4):379−388.

180. Mylius V, Ayache SS, Zouari HG, Aoun-Sebaiti M, Farhat WH, Lefaucheur JP. Stroke rehabilitation using noninvasive cortical stimulation: hemispatial neglect. *Expert Rev Neurother.* 2012;12(8):983−991.

181. Lindgren A, Maguire J. Stroke recovery genetics. *Stroke.* 2016;47(9):2427−2434.

182. Barrett AM, Muzaffar T. Spatial cognitive rehabilitation and motor recovery after stroke. *Curr Opinion Neurology.* 2014;27(6):653−658.

CHAPTER 6

Musculoskeletal Pain

RICHARD D. WILSON, MD, MS • JOHN CHAE, MD, MS

Pain is one of the most common complications experienced by stroke survivors. During early recovery, approximately 30% of those who receive care in a rehabilitation facility will have pain.[1] In the 2 years following stroke onset, new pain complaints will be experienced by 39%, an incidence 1.3 times of the non-stroke population.[2] Within the first year of stroke, between 50% and 66% of stroke survivors will have pain, though a majority of the pain precedes or is unrelated to the stroke.[2–6]

The consequences of musculoskeletal complications may affect function, quality of life, and health. Most complaints will be related to pain, yet some complaints are not related to pain but interfere with function. In telephone surveys up to 6 months from stroke, more than 35% describe the effect of stroke-related pain on their daily life as moderate to severe in intensity.[3] Stroke survivors report greater pain interference than the non-stroke population, with worse quality of life, mood, social life, and activities of daily living.[2] Regardless of the onset of pain, the presence of pain increases disability and dependence of stroke survivors.[5]

Stroke survivors experience many different types of pain syndromes, and often more than one. This chapter focuses on musculoskeletal pain in particular, though there is increasing evidence that chronic pain syndromes are associated with alterations of the central nervous system. This chapter will include pain syndromes that tend to occur after stroke and are related to impairments resulting from the stroke. The most common musculoskeletal stroke-related pain complaints are related to the shoulder, other arthralgias, and those related to muscle hypertonicity.[1–3,6–8] The pain syndromes of complex regional pain syndrome and central poststroke pain are covered in Chapter 7.

RISK FACTORS

A few common risk factors appear to be shared for the development of pain after stroke, including younger age, increased severity of stroke impairment, and depression.[2,3,5,6] The association with age changes depending on consideration of incidence or prevalence, with younger stroke survivors being more likely than their older counterparts to develop new pain complaints, though the prevalence of pain is higher in the older stroke survivors.[2] It is possible that comorbid illnesses that are associated with stroke risk also increase the risk for development of pain, such as diabetes mellitus or peripheral vascular disease, or due to medications commonly prescribed to stroke survivors, such as statin medications.[5] There are also unique risk factors that are associated with particular pain syndromes.

There are other factors that may also influence the prevalence of pain in stroke survivors. First, pain is undertreated in stroke survivors and in older adults, which can be due to competing obligations of comorbid illnesses that take precedent or failure to seek treatment.[9–11] Second, pain is not easily recognized in those with impairments in communication or cognition, increasing the potential for undertreatment.[12–14] Third, common stroke comorbidities may affect treatment options, such as long-term use of nonsteroidal antiinflammatory drugs (NSAIDs) or invasive treatments if on medications that affect coagulation. Finally, there are many chronic pain syndromes without adequate treatments that result in prolonged suffering and frustration for patients and providers.[15–17] It is important for providers that care for stroke survivors to inquire about the presence of pain and to treat pain syndromes when able.

Joint Pain

Joint pain is prevalent in the general population and arthritis is the number one comorbidity for stroke survivors.[18,19] Stroke survivors subjectively feel that joint pain interferes with recovery from stroke due to pain, mobility limitations, frustration, and the extra coping required (see Fig. 6.1).[15] There is evidence that the presence of joint pain has many deleterious effects on stroke recovery. Data from a study of national registry that controlled for confounders showed that stroke survivors

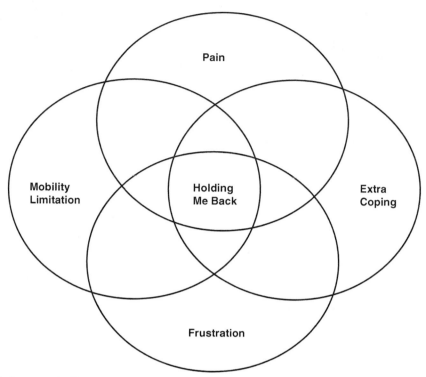

FIG. 6.1 Compound effects of comorbid arthralgia contributing to the experience of feeling like being held back from recovery from stroke. (Adapted from Wood JP, Connelly DM, Maly MR. "Holding me back": living with arthritis while recovering from stroke. *Arch Phys Med Rehabil.* 2009;90(3):494–500; with permission.)

with a comorbid diagnosis of osteoarthritis experience longer lengths of stay in acute rehabilitation settings after stroke, and also realize lower functional gains after discharge than stroke survivors without a diagnosis of osteoarthritis.[20] The effect is stronger than the number of medical comorbidities. In the postacute and chronic phase of recovery, joint pain contributes to difficulty in functional activities, and the effect is greater than the additive effect of having either impairment alone, regardless of whether the joint pain affects the hemiparetic or nonparetic limb.[21] The risk of functional loss of ability in upper limb activities is further increased when the stroke and joint impairment are ipsilateral. The opposite is true for the lower limb, such as standing and walking, where the highest risk is when the stroke and joint impairments are on opposite limbs.[21]

While arthritis is the number one comorbidity in stroke survivors, it is less certain whether stroke-related impairments increase the likelihood of developing joint pain except for shoulder pain. There may be an increased risk for acute arthritis, with crystal arthropathies being more common than other forms, in the weeks following stroke.[22] Such risk may be related

to common medications administered after stroke, such as thiazide diuretics or aspirin. The prevalence of new joint pain increases in the first 6 months following stroke,[3] though a matched population study did not find a difference in development of joint pain over 2 years when compared to a reference cohort, with the exception of shoulder pain.[2] A community-based population study of adults aged 55 years and older found that stroke survivors of all age groups experienced joint pain at a greater prevalence than those without stroke.[21] There was an association with upper limb joint symptoms in the hemiparetic arm, though that association was not present in the lower limb. The study did not find a difference in joint pain in those who reported recovery from their stroke, and those who did not report recovery.

A potential explanation for an association is from population studies which have shown that arthritis increases the risk for stroke, and that the risk is increased with severity of arthritis or arthritis-related disability.[23,24] This risk is independent of the use of NSAIDs, though NSAIDs are also an independent risk factor for stroke. Similarly, those with inflammatory arthropathies are also at an increased risk of stroke.[25,26] The higher prevalence of joint pain in stroke survivors may be due to the elevated risk among those with arthritides. It is also possible that joint pain that develops after stroke is related to undiagnosed, or early onset, arthropathy that was present before the stroke.

It is clear that the comorbid arthralgia has a detrimental effect on stroke survivors, regardless of whether it arises before or after the stroke. The disability related to joint pain further increases the risk of recurrent stroke and heart disease.[24] Treating joint pain is important to improving the recovery and risks after stroke. There are many treatments for osteoarthritis ranging from conservative, nonpharmacologic therapy, to over-the-counter medications, to injections and surgical treatment. A summary of the American College of Rheumatology guidelines[27] can be seen in Table 6.1. Although the full scope of treatment options for joint pain after stroke is not within the scope of this chapter, salient points to the treatment of stroke survivors are included.

Guidelines for the treatment of musculoskeletal pain often include pharmacological treatment with a recommendation of oral NSAIDs for pain reduction. Oral NSAIDs, in particular, should be used with caution, if at all, in stroke survivors. Many stroke survivors will have comorbid hypertension and NSAIDs can raise blood pressure to a level sufficient for clinical concern.[28] The use of any NSAID, even short term, can increase the risk for stroke and myocardial infarction, for which stroke survivors are at higher risk.[29,30] The combined use of NSAIDs with aspirin, even at low doses, increases the risk of gastrointestinal complications more so than either medication alone.[31] Alternative medications include acetaminophen, topical capsaicin, and glucosamine.[32] First line treatment should also include non-pharmacological treatments such as self-management advice, exercise therapy, and psychosocial interventions, whereas corticosteroid interventions can be used for short-term relief of pain.[33]

Shoulder Pain

Hemiplegic shoulder pain (HSP) affects approximately 25% of stroke survivors and has a negative effect on function, functional independence, and quality of life.[34−36] The prevalence in stroke survivors who have moderate to severe impairments are higher. Hemiplegic shoulder pain in rehabilitation settings is estimated to be 37%−55%.[37−40] Vigilance for HSP is important. Early detection followed by appropriate treatment is associated with resolution in 80% of patients.

Unfortunately, many will develop chronic HSP. Approximately 30% of those with moderate to severe impairments will continue to experience HSP many years after their stroke.

The syndrome of HSP is not attributable to a single etiology. Many pathologies contribute to the syndrome of HSP, and more than one pathology may exist within an individual. Shoulder pain after stroke may be associated with impairments from the stroke, soft tissue injury, or altered peripheral and central nervous system activity (see Fig. 6.2).[41] Typically, the syndrome of HSP excludes distinct pathologies of peripheral nerve injury, complex regional pain syndrome, and central post-stroke pain, since they are not specific to the shoulder, even if pain is experienced in the region of the affected shoulder.

Severity of motor impairment is a leading risk factor in the development of HSP, though other risks have been identified.[35,42,43] Additional risk factors include duration of motor impairment,[44] sensory impairment,[43,45] impaired range of motion,[35,46,47] spasticity,[48] central sensitization,[49,50] soft tissue injuries,[51−53] and prior injury.[35]

SOFT TISSUE INJURY

Many soft-tissue injuries have been demonstrated in imaging studies of those with HSP.[52,54−56] Soft-tissue lesions detectable by ultrasound are present in more than 30% of those admitted to rehabilitation settings, are commonly found in the affected shoulder, and are correlated with severity of impairment.[51,53] There is question as to whether abnormalities on imaging studies is relevant in the diagnosis of the etiology of shoulder pain due to the prevalence of such abnormalities in asymptomatic older adults and similarities of findings in those with and without pain.[57,58] The prevalence of shoulder pathology of both the affected and unaffected shoulders increases after stroke.[52,59] Studies have also found that the presence of tears and tendinopathies is not related to the severity of pain.[56,60] Lesions in the unaffected shoulder appear to be correlated with severity of impairment in the affected side, though causation is not known. To avoid misdiagnosis, imaging studies should not be relied upon alone but should be accompanied by a careful evaluation of the upper limb (Table 6.2).

Subacromial Pain Syndrome. Subacromial pain syndrome (SAPS) refers to nontraumatic shoulder problems that cause pain localized around the acromion that is often worse with overhead movement or lifting

TABLE 6.1

American College of Rheumatology Guidelines for Hand, Hip, Knee Osteoarthritis, 2012

	Hand OA	Knee OA	Hip OA
Nonpharmacologic	Conditionally recommend: • Evaluate the ability to perform activities of daily living • Instruct in joint protection techniques • Provide assistive devices, as needed for activities of daily living • Instruct in use of thermal modalities • Provide splints for patients with trapeziometacarpal joint OA	Strongly recommend: • Aerobic and/or resistance land-based exercise • Aquatic exercise • Weight loss (for persons who are overweight) Conditionally recommend: • Self-management programs • Manual therapy with supervised exercise • Psychosocial interventions • Medially directed patellar taping • Medially wedged insoles for lateral compartment OA • Laterally wedged subtalar strapped insoles for medial compartment OA • Be instructed in the use of thermal agents • Receive walking aids, if needed • Tai chi programs • Traditional Chinese acupuncture • Instructed in the use of transcutaneous electrical stimulation[a] No recommendations regarding: • Balance exercises • Laterally wedged insoles • Manual therapy alone • Knee braces • Laterally directed patellar taping	Strongly recommend: • Aerobic and/or resistance land-based exercise • Aquatic exercise • Weight loss (for persons who are overweight) Conditionally recommend: • Self-management programs • Manual therapy with supervised exercise • Psychosocial interventions • Be instructed in the use of thermal agents • Receive walking aids, if needed No recommendations regarding: • Balance exercises • Tai chi • Manual therapy alone
Pharmacologic	Conditionally recommend: • Topical capsaicin • Topical NSAIDs, including trolamine salicylate • Oral NSAIDs • Tramadol Conditionally recommend against: • Intraarticular therapies • Opioid analgesics Conditionally recommend for persons age ≥75 years: • Topical rather than oral NSAIDs.	Conditionally recommend: • Acetaminophen • Oral NSAIDs • Topical NSAIDs • Tramadol • Intraarticular corticosteroid injections Conditionally recommend against: • Chondroitin sulfate • Glucosamine • Topical capsaicin No recommendations regarding: • Intraarticular hyaluronates • Duloxetine • Opioid analgesics	Conditionally recommend: • Acetaminophen • Oral NSAIDs • Tramadol • Intraarticular corticosteroid injections Conditionally recommend against: • Chondroitin sulfate • Glucosamine No recommendations regarding: • Intraarticular hyaluronates • Duloxetine • Opioid analgesics • Topical NSAIDs

No recommendations are provided for initial pharmacologic treatment. *NSAIDs*, nonsteroidal antiinflammatory drugs; *OA*, osteoarthritis.

[a] These modalities are conditionally recommended only when the patient with knee osteoarthritis (OA) has chronic moderate to severe pain and is a candidate for total knee arthroplasty but either is unwilling or unable to undergo the procedure.

Adapted from Hochberg MC, Altman RD, April KT, et al. American College of Rheumatology 2012 recommendations for the use of nonpharmacologic and pharmacologic therapies in osteoarthritis of the hand, hip, and knee. *Arthritis Care Res (Hoboken)*. 2012;64(4):465–474.

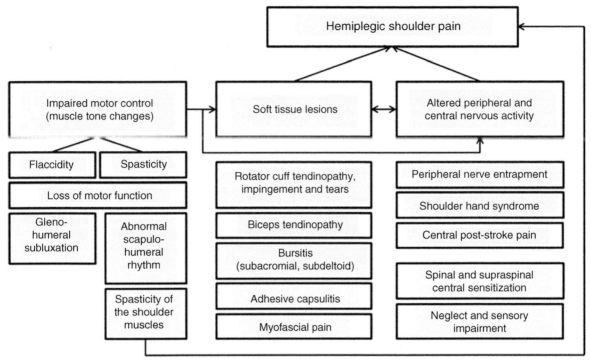

FIG. 6.2 Pathologies contributing to shoulder pain after stroke. (From from Kalichman L, Ratmansky M. Underlying pathology and associated factors of hemiplegic shoulder pain. *Am J Phys Med Rehabil Assoc Acad Physiatr*. 2011;90(9):768–780; with permission.)

TABLE 6.2
Examination for Soft-Tissue Lesions in HSP

	Impingement Syndrome/Rotator Cuff Tendinopathy	Bicipital Tendinopathy	Adhesive Capsulitis	Myofascial Pain
Exam	Positive Abduction Test Positive Drop Arm Test Positive Neer Sign Positive Hawkins Test	Positive Yergason test Positive Speed test	External rotation less than 15 degrees Early scapular motion	Palpation of shoulder and scapular muscles
Diagnostic test	Subacromial lidocaine injection MRI Ultrasound	Tendon sheath injection of lidocaine	MRI Arthrogram	None

MRI, magnetic resonance imaging.
From Wilson RD, Chae J. Hemiplegic shoulder pain. *Phys Med Rehabil Clin N Am*. 2015;26(4):641–655; with permission.

of the arm.[61] The syndrome includes those that have been described as subacromial impingement syndrome, rotator cuff tendinopathy, and subacromial and subdeltoid bursitis. Biomechanical changes due to the stroke such as weakness of muscles that stabilize the joint, flaccidity, hypertonicity, and scapular dyskinesis increase the risk for SAPS. While not rigorously studied, a cross-sectional study utilizing diagnostic anesthetic blocks estimated that approximately 50% of those with HSP are attributable to SAPS.[62]

The weakness and impaired control of the shoulder that accompanies hemiplegia makes prevention an important component of the rehabilitation process. Suggested interventions in practice guidelines include proper positioning, maintenance of shoulder range of motion (ROM), and motor retraining.[63] Range of motion exercises should be overseen by therapists until the patient and caregivers have been trained as injury may occur. The use of overhead pulleys has been implicated as worsening pain and should be avoided.[64]

The diagnosis of SAPS is made clinically through a careful history and physical exam. Imaging studies may support the diagnosis, though, as described above, imaging studies carry the risk of false positive diagnoses due to the high prevalence of asymptomatic anatomical abnormalities at the shoulder. There is not one single physical sign that can differentiate between disorders within SAPS or that will provide the accurate status of rotator cuff muscles.[61] The use of more than one test can increase posttest probability of diagnostic accuracy. Provocative maneuvers include Neer sign, Hawkins–Kennedy test, painful arc test, rotator cuff muscle strength tests, and drop-arm test; however, several of these tests require volitional motor control, which limits their utility among more severely impaired stroke survivors. Neer test, the injection of subacromial anesthetic with monitoring of resultant pain relief, can also provide insight into the diagnosis.

Treatment of SAPS should begin with physical therapeutics overseen by a physical or occupational therapist to improve ROM, strength, motor control, and education. Oral analgesics such as acetaminophen or NSAIDs may provide symptomatic relief, though NSAIDs should be used with caution. If pain is severe or interferes with participation in physical therapeutic treatments, other treatments may be necessary. Subacromial corticosteroid injections have been shown to provide relief of pain for at least 2 months in those with known rotator cuff pathology.[65] Suprascapular nerve block with corticosteroid and anesthetic are efficacious in reducing pain for at least 3 months after treatment.[66] In those in the chronic phase, axillary peripheral nerve stimulation has been shown to reduce pain to a greater extent than physical therapy for at least 3 months after treatment, though the efficacy of combined therapy is not known.[67] When hypertonicity may contribute to abnormal positioning or motor control, it may be necessary to additionally focus treatment on reducing hypertonicity.

BICIPITAL TENDONITIS

Bicipital tendonitis is one of the more common pathologies found on imaging studies among those with HSP,[52,60] though also present, less frequently, in the asymptomatic shoulder.[60] The biceps tendon is more active in those with unstable shoulders,[68] thus bicipital tendonitis may be more common in those with shoulder subluxation,[69] or in those with spasticity or movement synergies that result in overactivation of the biceps as elbow flexors or forearm supinators.

The diagnosis is easily obtained with ultrasound or MRI evaluation; however, physical exam is adequate and the diagnosis is suggested when there is greater tenderness to palpation of the long head of the biceps as it originates from the anterior glenoid on the affected side compared to the unaffected side.[70] Provocative maneuvers, such as Yergason test and Speed test can provide additional diagnostic information for those with sufficient motor control. Injection of an anesthetic agent at the bicipital groove, often combined with a therapeutic corticosteroid, can support the diagnosis and provide treatment.[71] Long-term relief usually requires alleviation of the underlying biomechanical abnormalities through exercise treatment, spasticity reduction, and reduction of subluxation.

SHOULDER SUBLUXATION

Subluxation of the glenohumeral joint is common after stroke for those who have greater upper limb impairment after stroke. There is variability in the prevalence depending on the population studied, though a large cohort study over 12 months reported an incidence of approximately 50%.[48] The prevalence in those with HSP is estimated at 44%.[72] The typical pattern of subluxation is inferior and anterior translation is due to the paralysis of active muscle restraints from the rotator cuff that maintains glenohumeral stability.[73–76] The diagnosis of shoulder subluxation can be made using radiographic studies, though they are not necessary. A commonly used clinical measure of shoulder subluxation is quantification of inferior subluxation by the number of fingerbreadths that can be inserted between the inferior border of the acromion and the superior border of the humeral head while the patient is seated.

Shoulder subluxation is one of the most commonly cited causes of HSP in the literature, though the nature of that relationship is controversial because the evidence is mixed. Multiple studies suggest a correlation between subluxation and HSP,[48,64,77–79] though others have demonstrated no correlation.[38,62,80–83] Both shoulder subluxation and HSP are associated with greater shoulder impairment, which may increase the risk for development of HSP from other injuries. Studies demonstrate a correlation between shoulder subluxation after stroke and the development of other causes of shoulder pain.[64,84–86]

Treatment of subluxation may be beneficial, even if there is not a causal relationship with HSP, due to the association with poor upper limb function.[72,87] Studies of surface neuromuscular electric stimulation (NMES) of shoulder muscles show effectiveness in reduction of subluxation when used early after the stroke, though surface NMES does not reduce pain or improve function.[88,89] It is not clear the reduction in subluxation is due to an increase in muscle tone, improvement in voluntary muscle contraction, or another mechanism. Shoulder slings may be helpful in reducing pain associated with subluxation in select patients, though slings may be detrimental to reduction when used for long periods.[90] Support via slings, or lap trays when sitting in a wheelchair, may be helpful for those with cognitive impairment or neglect.

CAPSULITIS AND RELATED CONDITIONS

Capsulitis, also known as adhesive capsulitis or frozen shoulder, is a common finding after stroke and refers to synovitis and progressive contracture of the joint capsule.[91] The primary clinical presentation includes pain and marked loss of range of motion. The prevalence among all stroke survivors is not known, but studies in select groups of stroke survivors have found a high prevalence of joint capsule thickening and synovial membrane contrast enhancement on magnetic resonance imaging among those with shoulder pain after stroke compared to controls.[60,92] Capsulitis is one of the most common pathological findings among those with HSP.[72] The causative relationship of capsulitis and HSP is not known. Capsulitis may be secondary to the immobility that is a result of the stroke, including shoulder pain itself, rather than a primary pathology.[41,91] There are shared risk factors for capsulitis and stroke, such as diabetes mellitus and cardiac disease which may increase the prevalence among stroke survivors compared to the general population.

The diagnosis of capsulitis can often be supported clinically by physical exam with findings of diffuse shoulder pain and loss of passive and active range of motion (ROM), particularly external ROM. Imaging can confirm the diagnosis if needed. Magnetic resonance imaging is a noninvasive method for diagnosis of capsulitis, with findings of increased thickness and enhancement of the joint capsule and ligaments, as well as evidence for synovitis, whereas arthrography can demonstrate loss of joint volume and scalloped appearance, though it is more invasive.[91]

The natural history of capsulitis is for resolution over 12–24 months with most having a full recovery.[91,93] The syndrome is often described as having 3 phases.[91,93] The initial phase is marked by pain and mild loss of ROM which lasts approximately 3 months. This is followed by a 3–9 period of severe pain and development of contracture that significantly reduces active and passive ROM. As this phase persists, the pain might lessen, though the ROM restriction persists. The resolution phase follows, which may last up to 18 months, in which pain largely abates and ROM gradually improves.

There is limited high-quality evidence to guide treatment of capsulitis, particularly when occurring with stroke. Evidence for treatment relies on nonstroke populations and may not be accurate for stroke survivors. Pain control is often the focus of management because of the self-limiting nature of capsulitis and lack of effective therapies. Conservative treatment with physical therapy and analgesics, such as acetaminophen and NSAIDs, are the mainstays of treatment, though NSAIDs should be used with caution in stroke survivors. The combination of corticosteroid injections and physical therapy appear to be more effective in reducing pain, improving ROM, and improving function than either treatment alone. While not commonly used, short wave diathermy may add short-term pain relief to exercise therapy.[94] There is no evidence that manipulation under anesthesia improves pain, function, or range of motion more than exercise-based therapy, nor evidence for the effectiveness of arthrographic distention.[94] Arthroscopic release and manipulation may not offer better long-term outcomes than a corticosteroid injection, and may contribute to a slower recovery.[95] It is not clear that treatment of any type will alter long-term endpoints compared to no treatment, though treatments may offer sooner relief of pain.[96] If spasticity contributes to pain or predisposes to recurrent capsulitis, additional measures to improve spasticity may be indicated.

SPASTICITY

The principles of assessment and management of spasticity following stroke are presented in Chapter 10. Spasticity is a motor disorder characterized by a velocity dependent increase in tonic stretch reflexes with exaggerated tendon jerks, resulting from augmentation of the stretch reflexes that may be present more commonly in those who experience pain after stroke.[97,98] Other features include spastic dystonia and spastic cocontraction of muscles.[99] The biomechanical forces spasticity places on joints in limbs and trunk can lead to abnormal posture and loss of ROM. There are several mechanisms by which spasticity may contribute to pain.[6] Spasticity may create abnormal loading and strain on muscles and ligaments that can cause pain. Second, pain may enhance spinal reflexes involved in spasticity, thereby worsening spasticity. Finally, the neuronal networks involved in spasticity and pain within the central nervous system may overlap and can be affected by the same stroke-related lesion.

The association between spasticity and HSP is controversial, with studies identifying spasticity as a contributing factor[39,48] and studies failing to find an association.[44,62] There is a great deal of covariance between spasticity and other painful conditions that affect the shoulder, such as capsulitis, subacromial pain syndrome, rotator cuff disease, and bicipital tendonitis. It is possible that there is a shared risk of spasticity and for these pain conditions, though the possibility that biomechanical stresses associated with spasticity increase the risk for injury. Spastic internal rotators and adductors are often seen in those with HSP, with the subscapularis and pectoralis as key muscles in abnormal movements that may contribute to HSP.[100,101]

Potential treatments for pain in the presence of spasticity include stretching and pharmacologic modalities, though no controlled trials have demonstrated efficacy. Thermoplastic splints are often prescribed to prevent contracture associated with spasticity, though splints may not reduce contracture, spasticity, or pain.[102] There is insufficient evidence that botulinum toxin is efficacious in reducing HSP for those with spastic hemiplegia,[103] though there is no consensus about which muscles to target or the appropriate dose.[104]

CENTRAL HYPERSENSITIVITY

There is increasing evidence that chronic musculoskeletal pain may be related to changes within the nervous system rather than a symptom of pathoanatomic changes. The central nervous system changes, termed central hypersensitivity or central sensitization, serve to augment the nociceptive system through adding new inputs to the system, including mechanoreceptors and other nerve types that do not typically provide nociceptive information.[105] This is also accompanied by altered brain processing of sensory inputs, dysfunction of descending inhibition, augmentation of pain facilitatory pathways, and temporal summation and long-term potentiation of neuronal synapses in the anterior cingulate cortex.[106,107] The end result is that patients become more sensitive to pain such that stimuli that were previously nonpainful are perceived as painful, and painful stimuli are perceived as more painful. Central hypersensitivity may be a consequence of ongoing peripheral nociceptive stimuli, or may serve to drive persistent pain in the absence of peripheral injury. Evidence of central hypersensitivity has been identified in those with HSP, SAPS, and osteoarthritis, along with many other chronic pain conditions.[47,49,50,108,109]

Diagnostic tests specific for central hypersensitivity are not available, though some clinical signs can increase the likelihood of central hypersensitivity as playing a role.[110,111] The painful area in question may show evidence of hyperalgesia, or disproportionate pain in response to a stimulus, whether palpation or movement. There may be an expansion of the painful area to include neighboring regions that are innervated by additional spinal segments. There may be diffuse hyperalgesia such that the entire body displays a higher sensitivity to pain. Those that have long-standing pain are more likely to have central hypersensitivity than those who report that pain resolves with rest.

There are no specific treatments for central hypersensitivity. The most efficacious treatments are likely multimodal and will address biopsychosocial contributors to pain and related disability. If pathoanatomical mechanisms that contribute to central hypersensitivity are identified, they should be treated, though many will not have evidence of an ongoing pathology. Exercise therapy, including manual therapy and education to reduce kinesiophobia should be part of treatment, though intensity may need to progress at a slower rate if pain limits participation. Cognitive behavioral therapy and stress management may also be important.[112] There are no approved pharmaceuticals for central hypersensitivity, though trials in pain conditions that have a high likelihood of a neuropathic or central hypersensitivity component may provide insight. Pharmaceuticals such as serotonin-norepinephrine reuptake inhibitors (SNRIs) and calcium-channel alpha(2) delta ligands (such as gabapentin or pregabalin) may be effective in reducing pain, in addition to commonly used medications such as acetaminophen and opioids in exceptional cases.[110,113] It has been suggested that neuromodulatory treatments, such as peripheral nerve stimulation, may alter central hypersensitivity in those with HSP and other chronic shoulder pain, though the mechanism is not yet known.[114–116] Further research is required to determine the best treatments for those with chronic pain and central hypersensitivity.

SUMMARY

Pain is one of the most common complications experienced by stroke survivors, and it may affect function, quality of life, and health. Stroke survivors report greater pain interference than the nonstroke population that can affect many aspects of their lives. Many different pain syndromes can occur as a result of the stroke, and often more than one. The most common musculoskeletal stroke-related pain complaints are related to the shoulder, other arthralgias, and those related to muscle hypertonicity. Careful examination and history can often reveal the diagnosis in most cases, whereas imaging studies increase the risk of false-positive diagnoses due to the high prevalence of asymptomatic anatomical changes. Biomechanical aberrations caused by the stroke should be evaluated and treated with exercise therapy. For some, pharmacological intervention will be necessary. Peripheral nerve stimulation is an example of neuromodulation which may be beneficial for HSP, whereas surface neuromuscular electrical stimulation may improve shoulder subluxation if applied early after the stroke. Early and appropriate treatment of pain is required to ensure that stroke survivors are able to participate in rehabilitation during the postacute phase, and to maintain optimal function during the chronic phase.

DISCLOSURE STATEMENT

R. Wilson is a consultant to SPR Therapeutics. J. Chae is a consultant and chief medical advisor to SPR Therapeutics and owns equity in SPR Therapeutics.

REFERENCES

1. Caglar NS, Akin T, Aytekin E, et al. Pain syndromes in hemiplegic patients and their effects on rehabilitation results. *J Phys Ther Sci.* 2016;28(3):731–737.
2. Klit H, Finnerup NB, Overvad K, Andersen G, Jensen TS. Pain following stroke: a population-based follow-up study. *PLoS One.* 2011;6(11):e27607.
3. Hansen AP, Marcussen NS, Klit H, Andersen G, Finnerup NB, Jensen TS. Pain following stroke: a prospective study. *Eur J Pain.* 2012;16(8):1128–1136.
4. Sackley C, Brittle N, Patel S, et al. The prevalence of joint contractures, pressure sores, painful shoulder, other pain, falls, and depression in the year after a severely disabling stroke. *Stroke.* 2008;39(12):3329–3334.
5. O'Donnell MJ, Diener HC, Sacco RL, et al. Chronic pain syndromes after ischemic stroke: PRoFESS trial. *Stroke.* 2013;44(5):1238–1243.
6. Lundstrom E, Smits A, Terent A, Borg J. Risk factors for stroke-related pain 1 year after first-ever stroke. *Eur J Neurol.* 2009;16(2):188–193.
7. Widar M, Samuelsson L, Karlsson-Tivenius S, Ahlstrom G. Long-term pain conditions after a stroke. *J Rehabil Med.* 2002;34(4):165–170.
8. Zorowitz RD, Smout RJ, Gassaway JA, Horn SD. Usage of pain medications during stroke rehabilitation: the post-stroke rehabilitation outcomes project (PSROP). *Top Stroke Rehabil.* 2005;12(4):37–49.
9. Paolucci S, Iosa M, Toni D, et al. Prevalence and time course of post-stroke pain: a multicenter prospective hospital-based study. *Pain Med.* 2016;17(5):924–930.
10. Denny DL, Guido GW. Undertreatment of pain in older adults: an application of beneficence. *Nurs Ethics.* 2012;19(6):800–809.
11. Makris UE, Higashi RT, Marks EG, et al. Ageism, negative attitudes, and competing co-morbidities—why older adults may not seek care for restricting back pain: a qualitative study. *BMC Geriatr.* 2015;15:39.
12. Kehayia E, Korner-Bitensky N, Singer F, et al. Differences in pain medication use in stroke patients with aphasia and without aphasia. *Stroke.* 1997;28(10):1867–1870.
13. Reynolds KS, Hanson LC, DeVellis RF, Henderson M, Steinhauser KE. Disparities in pain management between cognitively intact and cognitively impaired nursing home residents. *J Pain Symptom Manage.* 2008;35(4):388–396.
14. Closs SJ, Barr B, Briggs M. Cognitive status and analgesic provision in nursing home residents. *Br J Gen Pract.* 2004;54(509):919–921.
15. Wood JP, Connelly DM, Maly MR. "Holding me back": living with arthritis while recovering from stroke. *Arch Phys Med Rehabil.* 2009;90(3):494–500.
16. Dow CM, Roche PA, Ziebland S. Talk of frustration in the narratives of people with chronic pain. *Chronic Illn.* 2012;8(3):176–191.
17. Spitz A, Moore AA, Papaleontiou M, Granieri E, Turner BJ, Reid MC. Primary care providers' perspective on prescribing opioids to older adults with chronic non-cancer pain: a qualitative study. *BMC Geriatr.* 2011;11:35.
18. Helmick CG, Felson DT, Lawrence RC, et al. Estimates of the prevalence of arthritis and other rheumatic conditions in the United States. Part I. *Arthritis Rheum.* 2008;58(1):15–25.
19. Studenski SA, Lai SM, Duncan PW, Rigler SK. The impact of self-reported cumulative comorbidity on stroke recovery. *Age Ageing.* 2004;33(2):195–198.
20. Nguyen-Oghalai TU, Ottenbacher KJ, Granger CV, Goodwin JS. Impact of osteoarthritis on the rehabilitation of patients following a stroke. *Arthritis Rheum.* 2005;53(3):383–387.

21. Hettiarachchi C, Conaghan P, Tennant A, Bhakta B. Prevalence and impact of joint symptoms in people with stroke aged 55 years and over. *J Rehabil Med.* 2011; 43(3):197–203.

22. Chakravarty K, Durkin CJ, al-Hillawi AH, Bodley R, Webley M. The incidence of acute arthritis in stroke patients, and its impact on rehabilitation. *Q J Med.* 1993; 86(12):819–823.

23. Hsu PS, Lin HH, Li CR, Chung WS. Increased risk of stroke in patients with osteoarthritis: a population-based cohort study. *Osteoarthr Cartil.* 2017;25(7): 1026–1031.

24. Hawker GA, Croxford R, Bierman AS, et al. All-cause mortality and serious cardiovascular events in people with hip and knee osteoarthritis: a population based cohort study. *PLoS One.* 2014;9(3):e91286.

25. Dregan A, Chowienczyk P, Molokhia M. Cardiovascular and type 2 diabetes morbidity and all-cause mortality among diverse chronic inflammatory disorders. *Heart.* 2017.

26. Bengtsson K, Forsblad-d'Elia H, Lie E, et al. Are ankylosing spondylitis, psoriatic arthritis and undifferentiated spondyloarthritis associated with an increased risk of cardiovascular events? A prospective nationwide population-based cohort study. *Arthritis Res Ther.* 2017; 19(1):102.

27. Hochberg MC, Altman RD, April KT, et al. American College of Rheumatology 2012 recommendations for the use of nonpharmacologic and pharmacologic therapies in osteoarthritis of the hand, hip, and knee. *Arthritis Care Res Hob.* 2012;64(4):465–474.

28. White WB. Defining the problem of treating the patient with hypertension and arthritis pain. *Am J Med.* 2009; 122(5 Suppl):S3–S9.

29. Bally M, Dendukuri N, Rich B, et al. Risk of acute myocardial infarction with NSAIDs in real world use: bayesian meta-analysis of individual patient data. *BMJ.* 2017; 357:j1909.

30. Park K, Bavry AA. Risk of stroke associated with nonsteroidal anti-inflammatory drugs. *Vasc Health Risk Manag.* 2014;10:25–32.

31. Rafaniello C, Ferrajolo C, Sullo MG, et al. Risk of gastrointestinal complications associated to NSAIDs, low-dose aspirin and their combinations: results of a pharmacovigilance reporting system. *Pharmacol Res.* 2016;104: 108–114.

32. Fogleman CD. Analgesics for osteoarthritis. *Am Fam Physician.* 2013;87(5):354–356.

33. Babatunde OO, Jordan JL, Van der Windt DA, Hill JC, Foster NE, Protheroe J. Effective treatment options for musculoskeletal pain in primary care: a systematic overview of current evidence. *PLoS One.* 2017;12(6): e0178621.

34. Adey-Wakeling Z, Liu E, Crotty M, et al. Hemiplegic shoulder pain reduces quality of life after acute stroke: a prospective population-based study. *Am J Phys Med Rehabil.* 2016;95(10):758–763.

35. Adey-Wakeling Z, Arima H, Crotty M, et al. Incidence and associations of hemiplegic shoulder pain poststroke: prospective population-based study. *Arch Phys Med Rehabil.* 2015;96(2):241 e1–247 e1.

36. Nickel R, Lange M, Stoffel DP, Navarro EJ, Zetola VF. Upper limb function and functional independence in patients with shoulder pain after stroke. *Arq Neuropsiquiatr.* 2017;75(2):103–106.

37. Dromerick AW, Edwards DF, Kumar A. Hemiplegic shoulder pain syndrome: frequency and characteristics during inpatient stroke rehabilitation. *Arch Phys Med Rehabil.* 2008;89(8):1589–1593.

38. Zorowitz RD, Hughes MB, Idank D, Ikai T, Johnston MV. Shoulder pain and subluxation after stroke: correlation or coincidence. *Am J Occ Ther.* 1996;50(3):194–201.

39. Poulin de Courval L, Barsauskas A, Berenbaum B, et al. Painful shoulder in the hemiplegic and unilateral neglect. *Arch Phys Med Rehabil.* 1990;71(9):673–676.

40. Demirci A, Ocek B, Koseoglu F. Shoulder pain in hemiplegic patients. *J PMR Sci.* 2007;1:25–30.

41. Kalichman L, Ratmansky M. Underlying pathology and associated factors of hemiplegic shoulder pain. *Am J Phys Med Rehabil.* 2011;90(9):768–780.

42. Lindgren I, Jonsson AC, Norrving B, Lindgren A. Shoulder pain after stroke: a prospective population-based study. *Stroke.* 2007;38(2):343–348.

43. Roosink M, Renzenbrink GJ, Buitenweg JR, Van Dongen RT, Geurts AC, MJ IJ. Persistent shoulder pain in the first 6 months after stroke: results of a prospective cohort study. *Arch Phys Med Rehabil.* 2011;92(7): 1139–1145.

44. Bohannon RW, Larkin PA, Smith MB, Horton MG. Shoulder pain in hemiplegia: statistical relationship with five variables. *Arch Phys Med Rehabil.* 1986;67:514–516.

45. Lindgren I, Ekstrand E, Lexell J, Westergren H, Brogardh C. Somatosensory impairments are common after stroke but have only a small impact on post-stroke shoulder pain. *J Rehabil Med.* 2014;46(4):307–313.

46. Lindgren I, Lexell J, Jonsson AC, Brogardh C. Left-sided hemiparesis, pain frequency, and decreased passive shoulder range of abduction are predictors of long-lasting poststroke shoulder pain. *PM R.* 2012;4(8):561–568.

47. Roosink M, Renzenbrink GJ, Geurts AC, Ijzerman MJ. Towards a mechanism-based view on post-stroke shoulder pain: theoretical considerations and clinical implications. *NeuroRehabilitation.* 2012;30(2):153–165.

48. VanOuwenaller C, Laplace PM, Chantraine A. Painful shoulder in hemiplegia. *Arch Phys Med Rehabil.* 1986; 67:23–26.

49. Soo Hoo J, Paul T, Chae J, Wilson RD. Central hypersensitivity in chronic hemiplegic shoulder pain. *Am J Phys Med Rehabil.* 2013;92(1):1–13.

50. Roosink M, Renzenbrink GJ, Buitenweg JR, van Dongen RT, Geurts AC, Ijzerman MJ. Somatosensory symptoms and signs and conditioned pain modulation in chronic post-stroke shoulder pain. *J Pain.* 2011; 12(4):476–485.

51. Huang YC, Liang PJ, Pong YP, Leong CP, Tseng CH. Physical findings and sonography of hemiplegic shoulder in patients after acute stroke during rehabilitation. *J Rehabil Med.* 2010;42(1):21–26.

52. Pong YP, Wang LY, Huang YC, Leong CP, Liaw MY, Chen HY. Sonography and physical findings in stroke patients with hemiplegic shoulders: a longitudinal study. *J Rehabil Med.* 2012;44(7):553–557.

53. Pong YP, Wang LY, Wang L, Leong CP, Huang YC, Chen YK. Sonography of the shoulder in hemiplegic patients undergoing rehabilitation after a recent stroke. *J Clin Ultrasound.* 2009;37(4):199–205.

54. Dogun A, Karabay I, Hatipoglu C, Ozgirgin N. Ultrasound and magnetic resonance findings and correlation in hemiplegic patients with shoulder pain. *Top Stroke Rehabil.* 2014;21(Suppl 1):S1–S7.

55. Kim YH, Jung SJ, Yang EJ, Paik NJ. Clinical and sonographic risk factors for hemiplegic shoulder pain: a longitudinal observational study. *J Rehabil Med.* 2014;46(1):81–87.

56. Shah R, Haghpanah S, Elovic E, et al. MRI findings in painful post-stroke shoulder. *Stroke.* 2008;39:1803–1813.

57. Gill TK, Shanahan EM, Allison D, Alcorn D, Hill CL. Prevalence of abnormalities on shoulder MRI in symptomatic and asymptomatic older adults. *Int J Rheum Dis.* 2014;17(8):863–871.

58. Needell SD, Zlatkin MB, Sher JS, Murphy BJ, Uribe JW. MR imaging of the rotator cuff: peritendinous and bone abnormalities in an asymptomatic population. *AJR Am J Roentgenol.* 1996;166(4):863–867.

59. Cho HK, Kim HS, Joo SH. Sonography of affected and unaffected shoulders in hemiplegic patients: analysis of the relationship between sonographic imaging data and clinical variables. *Ann Rehabil Med.* 2012;36(6):828–835.

60. Pompa A, Clemenzi A, Troisi E, et al. Enhanced-MRI and ultrasound evaluation of painful shoulder in patients after stroke: a pilot study. *Eur Neurol.* 2011;66(3):175–181.

61. Diercks R, Bron C, Dorrestijn O, et al. Guideline for diagnosis and treatment of subacromial pain syndrome: a multidisciplinary review by the Dutch Orthopaedic Association. *Acta Orthop.* 2014;85(3):314–322.

62. Joynt RL. The source of shoulder pain in hemiplegia. *Arch Phys Med Rehabil.* 1992;73(5):409–413.

63. Winstein CJ, Stein J, Arena R, et al. Guidelines for adult stroke rehabilitation and recovery: a guideline for healthcare professionals from the American heart association/American stroke association. *Stroke.* 2016;47(6):e98–e169.

64. Najenson T, Yacubovich E, Pikielni SS. Rotator cuff injury in shoulder joints of hemiplegic patients. *Scan J Rehab Med.* 1971;3:131–137.

65. Rah UW, Yoon SH, Moon do J, et al. Subacromial corticosteroid injection on poststroke hemiplegic shoulder pain: a randomized, triple-blind, placebo-controlled trial. *Arch Phys Med Rehabil.* 2012;93(6):949–956.

66. Adey-Wakeling Z, Crotty M, Shanahan EM. Suprascapular nerve block for shoulder pain in the first year after stroke: a randomized controlled trial. *Stroke.* 2013;44(11):3136–3141.

67. Wilson RD, Gunzler DD, Bennett ME, Chae J. Peripheral nerve stimulation compared with usual care for pain relief of hemiplegic shoulder pain: a randomized controlled trial. *Am J Phys Med Rehabil.* 2014;93(1):17–28.

68. Itoi E, Kuechle DK, Newman SR, Morrey BF, An KN. Stabilising function of the biceps in stable and unstable shoulders. *J Bone Joint Surg Br.* 1993;75(4):546–550.

69. Huang SW, Liu SY, Tang HW, Wei TS, Wang WT, Yang CP. Relationship between severity of shoulder subluxation and soft-tissue injury in hemiplegic stroke patients. *J Rehabil Med.* 2012;44(9):733–739.

70. Patton WC, McCluskey 3rd GM. Biceps tendinitis and subluxation. *Clin Sports Med.* 2001;20(3):505–529.

71. Larson HM, O'Connor FG, Nirschl RP. Shoulder pain: the role of diagnostic injections. *Am Fam Physician.* 1996;53(5):1637–1647.

72. Lo SF, Chen SY, Lin HC, Jim YF, Meng NH, Kao MJ. Arthrographic and clinical findings in patients with hemiplegic shoulder pain. *Arch Phys Med Rehabil.* 2003;84(12):1786–1791.

73. Aronen JG, Regan K. Decreasing the incidence of recurrence of first time anterior shoulder dislocations with rehabilitation. *Am J Sports Med.* 1984;12:283.

74. Glousman R, Jobe F, Tibone J, Moynes D, Antonelli D, Perry J. Dynamic electromyographic analysis of the throwing shoulder with glenohumeral instability. *J Bone Joint Surg Am.* 1988;70(2):220–226.

75. Cain PR. Anterior stability of the glenohumeral joint: a dynamic model. *Am J Sports Med.* 1987;15:144.

76. Symeonides PP. The significance of the subscapularis muscle in the pathogenesis of recurrent anterior dislocation of the shoulder. *J Bone Joint Surg.* 1972;54B:476.

77. Griffin JW. Hemiplegic shoulder pain. *Phys Ther.* 1986;66(12):1884–1893.

78. Ring H, Feder M, Berchadsky R, Samuels G. Prevalence of pain and malalignment in the hemiplegic's shoulder at admission for rehabilitation: a preventive approach. *Eur J Phys Med Rehabil.* 1993;3:199–203.

79. Roy CW, Sands MR, Hill LD. Shoulder pain in acutely admitted subjects. *Clin Rehabil.* 1994;8:334–340.

80. Bohannon RW, Andrews AW. Shoulder subluxation and pain in stroke patients. *Am J Occ Ther.* 1990:507–509.

81. VanLangenberghe H, Hogan BM. Degree of pain and grade of subluxation in the painful hemiplegic shoulder. *Scand J Rehab Med.* 1988;20:161–166.

82. Arsenault AB, Bilodeau M, Dutil E, Riley E. Clinical significance of the V-shaped space in the subluxed shoulder of hemiplegics. *Stroke.* 1991;22(7):867–871.

83. Wanklyn P, Forster A, Young J. Hemiplegic shoulder pain (HSP): natural history and investigation of associated features. *Disabil Rehabil.* 1996;18(10):497–501.

84. Chino N. Electrophysiological investigation on shoulder subluxation in hemiplegics. *Scand J Rehab Med.* 1981;13: 17–21.

85. Ring H, Leillen B, Server S, Luz Y, Solzi P. Temporal changes in electrophysiological, clinical and radiological parameters in the hemiplegic's shoulder. *Scand J Rehab Med Suppl.* 1985;12:124–127.

86. Dursun E, Dursun N, Ural CE, Cakci A. Glenohumeral joint subluxation and reflex sympathetic dystrophy in hemiplegic patients. *Arch Phys Med Rehabil.* 2000;81(7): 944–946.

87. Jang SH, Yi JH, Chang CH, et al. Prediction of motor outcome by shoulder subluxation at early stage of stroke. *Med Baltim.* 2016;95(32):e4525.

88. Gu P, Ran JJ. Electrical stimulation for hemiplegic shoulder function: a systematic review and meta-analysis of 15 randomized controlled trials. *Arch Phys Med Rehabil.* 2016.

89. Lee JH, Baker LL, Johnson RE, Tilson JK. Effectiveness of neuromuscular electrical stimulation for management of shoulder subluxation post-stroke: a systematic review with meta-analysis. *Clin Rehabil.* 2017. https://doi.org/10.1177/0269215517700696.

90. van Bladel A, Lambrecht G, Oostra KM, Vanderstraeten G, Cambier D. A randomized controlled trial on the immediate and long-term effects of arm slings on shoulder subluxation in stroke patients. *Eur J Phys Rehabil Med.* 2017; 53(3):400–409.

91. Nagy MT, Macfarlane RJ, Khan Y, Waseem M. The frozen shoulder: myths and realities. *Open Orthop J.* 2013;7: 352–355.

92. Tavora DG, Gama RL, Bomfim RC, Nakayama M, Silva CE. MRI findings in the painful hemiplegic shoulder. *Clin Radiol.* 2010;65(10):789–794.

93. Georgiannos D, Markopoulos G, Devetzi E, Bisbinas I. Adhesive capsulitis of the shoulder. Is there consensus regarding the Treatment? A comprehensive review. *Open Orthop J.* 2017;11:65–76.

94. Maund E, Craig D, Suekarran S, et al. Management of frozen shoulder: a systematic review and cost-effectiveness analysis. *Health Technol Assess.* 2012;16(11):1–264.

95. De Carli A, Vadala A, Perugia D, et al. Shoulder adhesive capsulitis: manipulation and arthroscopic arthrolysis or intra-articular steroid injections? *Int Orthop.* 2012;36(1): 101–106.

96. Vastamaki H, Kettunen J, Vastamaki M. The natural history of idiopathic frozen shoulder: a 2- to 27-year followup study. *Clin Orthop Relat Res.* 2012;470(4): 1133–1143.

97. Lance JW. Symposium synopsis. In: Feldman RG, Young RR, Koella WP, Corporation. C-G, eds. *Spasticity, Disordered Motor Control.* Miami, FL Chicago: Symposia Specialists ; distributed by Year Book Medical Publishers; 1980. xviii, 510 pp.

98. Sommerfeld DK, Welmer AK. Pain following stroke, initially and at 3 and 18 months after stroke, and its association with other disabilities. *Eur J Neurol.* 2012; 19(10):1325–1330.

99. Sheean DG. Is spasticity painful? *Eur J Neurol.* 2009; 16(2):157–158.

100. Yi Y, Lee KJ, Kim W, Oh BM, Chung SG. Biomechanical properties of the glenohumeral joint capsule in hemiplegic shoulder pain. *Clin Biomech (Bristol, Avon).* 2013; 28(8):873–878.

101. Karaahmet OZ, Eksioglu E, Gurcay E, et al. Hemiplegic shoulder pain: associated factors and rehabilitation outcomes of hemiplegic patients with and without shoulder pain. *Top Stroke Rehabil.* 2014;21(3):237–245.

102. Tyson SF, Kent RM. The effect of upper limb orthotics after stroke: a systematic review. *NeuroRehabilitation.* 2011; 28(1):29–36.

103. Singh JA, Fitzgerald PM. Botulinum toxin for shoulder pain: a cochrane systematic review. *J Rheumatol.* 2011; 38(3):409–418.

104. Viana R, Pereira S, Mehta S, Miller T, Teasell R. Evidence for therapeutic interventions for hemiplegic shoulder pain during the chronic stage of stroke: a review. *Top Stroke Rehabil.* 2012;19(6):514–522.

105. Latremoliere A, Woolf CJ. Central sensitization: a generator of pain hypersensitivity by central neural plasticity. *J Pain.* 2009;10(9):895–926.

106. Staud R, Craggs JG, Robinson ME, Perlstein WM, Price DD. Brain activity related to temporal summation of C-fiber evoked pain. *Pain.* 2007;129(1–2):130–142.

107. Nijs J, Van Houdenhove B, Oostendorp RA. Recognition of central sensitization in patients with musculoskeletal pain: application of pain neurophysiology in manual therapy practice. *Man Ther.* 2010;15(2):135–141.

108. Paul TM, Soo Hoo J, Chae J, Wilson RD. Central hypersensitivity in patients with subacromial impingement syndrome. *Arch Phys Med Rehabil.* 2012;93(12): 2206–2209.

109. Roosink M, Buitenweg JR, Renzenbrink GJ, Geurts AC, Ijzerman MJ. Altered cortical somatosensory processing in chronic stroke: a relationship with post-stroke shoulder pain. *NeuroRehabilitation.* 2011;28(4):331–344.

110. Akinci A, Al Shaker M, Chang MH, et al. Predictive factors and clinical biomarkers for treatment in patients with chronic pain caused by osteoarthritis with a central sensitisation component. *Int J Clin Pract.* 2016;70(1):31–44.

111. Woolf CJ. Pain: moving from symptom control toward mechanism-specific pharmacologic management. *Ann Intern Med.* 2004;140(6):441–451.

112. Nijs J, Paul van Wilgen C, Van Oosterwijck J, van Ittersum M, Meeus M. How to explain central sensitization to patients with 'unexplained' chronic musculoskeletal pain: practice guidelines. *Man Ther.* 2011;16(5): 413–418.

113. Nijs J, Meeus M, Van Oosterwijck J, et al. Treatment of central sensitization in patients with 'unexplained' chronic pain: what options do we have? *Expert Opin Pharmacother*. 2011;12(7):1087–1098.

114. Yu DT, Chae J, Walker ME, et al. Intramuscular neuromuscular electric stimulation for poststroke shoulder pain: a multicenter randomized clinical trial. *Arch Phys Med Rehabil*. 2004;85(5):695–704.

115. Wilson RD, Knutson JS, Bennett ME, Chae J. The effect of peripheral nerve stimulation on shoulder biomechanics: a randomized controlled trial in comparison to physical therapy. *Am J Phys Med Rehabil*. 2017;96(3):191–198.

116. Wilson RD, Harris MA, Bennett ME, Chae J. Single-lead percutaneous peripheral nerve stimulation for the treatment of shoulder pain from subacromial impingement syndrome. *PM R*. 2012;4(8):624–628.

CHAPTER 7

Central Pain and Complex Regional Pain Syndromes

ANDREW K. TREISTER, MD • ERIC Y. CHANG, MD

INTRODUCTION

Pain after stroke is a common symptom that is poorly understood by many practitioners. It can be easily overlooked due to its variable characteristics, concurrent medical issues, or impairments in cognition or communication. While pain can create its own disabilities secondary to a decrease in function, its effect on the recovery of post-stroke patients can substantially impact a patient's quality of life. Indeed, as is the case with many other chronic pain syndromes, post-stroke pain (PSP) is often refractory to most medications and thus extremely difficult to control for a wide range of patients.

Estimates of the prevalence of PSP vary widely, with one recent large study estimating that 10.6% of all patients with ischemic stroke experience some type of chronic PSP.[1] Among these patients, central post-stroke pain (CPSP) is the most frequent diagnosis, followed by peripheral neuropathy, pain due to spasticity, and joint subluxation.[1] Additionally, complex regional pain syndrome (CRPS) following stroke has been observed on a similar scale.[2] Pain syndromes after stroke are in some ways unique to each patient and are often insufficiently managed. In this chapter, the most common types of pain encountered by stroke patients are delineated, and a basis for their pathophysiology is provided, though musculoskeletal-related pain is covered in Chapter 6.

CENTRAL POST-STROKE PAIN

Central post-stroke pain (CPSP) is a term used to describe the symptom of pain arising after a stroke that is secondary to a lesion within the central nervous system.[3] As in the case of all strokes, the location of the infarct and the function of the neurologic structures involved dictate the character of the deficit. In the case of CPSP, the lesion includes some portion of central pain pathways, and this damage creates the sensation of pain with minimal or no stimulation of the peripheral pain receptors.

CPSP can be difficult to characterize, as it can be subjectively described by a patient in a variety of ways. Descriptions can range from aching, dull, and throbbing to sharp, stabbing, shooting, or burning pain.[4] The onset of CPSP can be quite variable as well, most commonly beginning 1−3 months after stroke, with the majority of affected patients developing symptoms by 6 months.[5] Additionally, CPSP can be particularly difficult to evaluate since it can be accompanied by other pain syndromes including those resulting from pathology outside of the central nervous system. In a cross-sectional study of 40 CPSP patients, 27 (65.5%) were also diagnosed with myofascial pain syndrome: a non-neuropathic painful disorder characterized by painful, stiffened muscles with taut bands and discernible trigger points.[5,6] Symptoms of CPSP can be induced or spontaneous. Induced pain describes an increase in sensitivity to stimulation (hyperesthesia), which can be further dissected into pain that is evoked by a non-painful stimulus (allodynia), or as an increased sensitivity to a normally painful stimulus (hyperalgesia).[7] Spontaneous pain, however, is independent of stimuli and may be continuous or paroxysmal. Induced pain can be clarified and classified with a careful bedside sensory exam, while spontaneous pain remains subject to the patient's description. Taking these factors into account, CPSP remains a diagnosis of exclusion.

Neuroanatomy of CPSP

CPSP was first described by Dejerine and Roussy in 1906 when they coined the phrase "syndrome thalamique," or thalamic syndrome.[8] The pair described a series of patients with intolerable pain on their hemiplegic sides, who were later found to have suffered strokes to the thalamus. The thalamus was widely accepted for many years as the sole culprit in what became known as "Dejerine—Roussy Syndrome"; however, more recent case reports and studies have shown that the thalamus is only one of many structures that may be implicated in CPSP. It has been found that CPSP can arise in patients whose lesion involves any of the tracts responsible for transmission of pain as they pass throughout the entire central nervous system.[5] Below, some of the relevant tracts and specific brain structures associated with CPSP are listed.

The spinothalamic tract

The most studied tract associated with pain is the spinothalamic tract, which transmits the modalities of pain, temperature, and deep touch from the body. The spinothalamic tract courses from the lateral portion of the spinal cord, through the lateral medulla and pons, to the ventral posterolateral nucleus (VPL) of the thalamus, terminating in the post-central gyrus (Fig. 7.1A). Lesions or injury to any part of this tract can potentially result in CPSP; however, some structures are more highly associated with this syndrome than others.

CPSP was originally described as a thalamic pain syndrome, and the thalamus continues to be the most commonly documented and studied neural structure associated with CPSP.[5,9] Modern studies have shown that specific areas within the thalamus are more correlated to the development of CPSP than others. Studies have shown that CPSP patients have lesions within the VPL and/or the ventral posteromedial (VPM) of the thalamus (Fig. 7.1B).[10–14] A more recent study using MRI and digital radiographic atlases in thalamic stroke patients with and without CPSP found that the CPSP group had lesions largely involving the VPL, with some also involving the VPM nucleus.[15,16] Specifically, lesions in the posterolateral and inferior parts of the VPL were most associated with CPSP. A few of the CPSP patients in this study did have lesions confined to the pulvinar nucleus as well, an area that processes visual input. The development of CPSP in these patients was thought to be due to the shared vascular supply and close proximity to the VPL[15] (Fig. 7.1B); again implying the strong association of the VPL and CPSP. Indeed, another study found that thalamic lesions involving the area where the ventral posterior nuclei and the pulvinar meet were 81 times more likely to lead to CPSP than other thalamic lesions, confirming this area as high risk for CPSP, and opening the door for potential preemptive treatments against CPSP as a future avenue of research.[16]

The medullary tracts

In addition to the spinothalamic pathway, lesions in the trigeminothalamic and the lemniscal pathways can result in CPSP symptoms of both the body and the face. The trigeminothalamic pathway functions for the face in a similar manner as the spinothalamic pathway for the body in that they transmit the same modalities of sensation: pain, temperature, and deep touch. It receives afferent input from cranial nerves (5, 7, 9, and 10), which is relayed to the spinal trigeminal nucleus within the caudal pons and medulla before travelling up to the VPM of the thalamus. Lateral medullary syndrome (Wallenberg Syndrome) is a well-documented constellation of symptoms arising from a stroke to the lateral medulla, which characteristically causes, among other deficits, facial pain and numbness ipsilateral to the lesion with contralateral body and limb numbness. In patients with Wallenberg Syndrome, 25%—44% have been described as suffering from CPSP, most commonly in the face ipsilateral to the lesion, but with a smaller percentage experiencing pain in the contralateral body and limbs.[17,18] These symptoms can arise acutely, within the first few days, but more often, they occur within weeks to the first 6 months after stroke. The most common types of pain described are constant, burning, and lancinating, with frequent allodynia.[17] This association of facial CPSP with bodily sensory deficits can be explained by the proximity of the spinal trigeminal nucleus to the fibers of the spinothalamic tract, both located in the lateral portion of the brainstem.[17]

In contrast to the burning and lancinating pain symptoms associated with infarction of the lateral medulla, a study on medial medullary stroke patients found that 21 out of 59 (35.6%) were diagnosed with CPSP with the pain being described as "numb," "cold," and "painful"; no patients described their pain as burning.[19] It is possible that the qualitative difference in pain in these patients can be attributed to the fact that the pain tracts described above are spared. Instead, the medial medulla contains fibers from the dorsal column-medial lemniscal pathway which governs the transmission of vibratory, positional, and fine touch sensation; as well as the spinoreticulothalamic system which is thought to modify the signal from the spinothalamic tract by projecting to neural structures important for the emotional perceptions of pain.[20] These consistent differences in the characteristics of lesions only millimeters apart illustrate the dependence CPSP has on the affected neural substrate and how infarct location translates into the symptoms patients perceive.

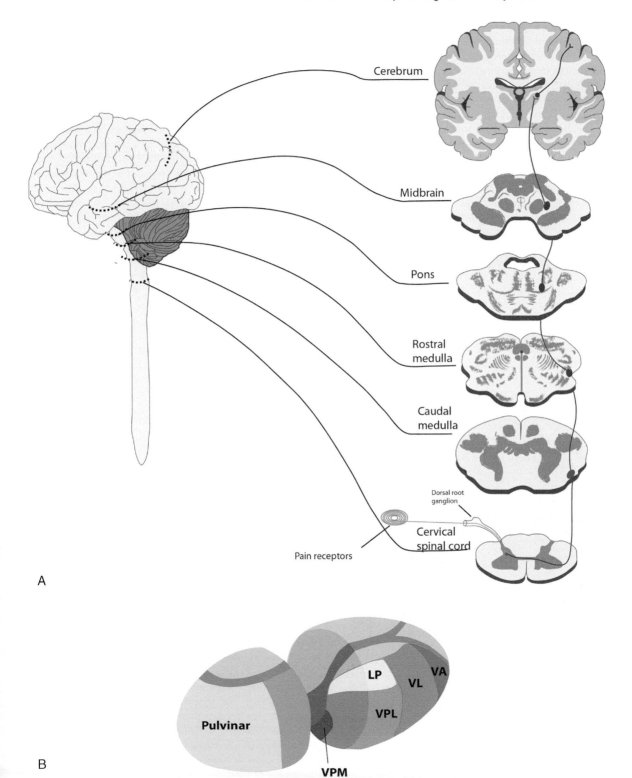

FIG. 7.1 **(A)** The spinothalamic tract. **(B)** The nuclei of the thalamus.

The cerebral cortex

Within the cerebral cortex, some areas have been implicated in CPSP while others have not. The primary sensory cortex, located in the post-central gyrus, is rarely associated with the development of CPSP; however, other cortical structures may be.[5,21] One study of 24 patients found that ischemic injury to the operculum and insular cortex was linked to the development of CPSP, whereas ischemic lesions in the post-central gyrus did not.[21] The posterior insular cortex and medial operculum (Fig. 7.2) have been shown in functional imaging and electrophysiology studies to play a major role in processing pain and temperature signals from the spinothalamic pathway, so much so that these adjacent structures have been argued to make up a "primary area for pain."[22]

What Is Known About the Pathophysiology of CPSP

The pathophysiology by which CPSP arises after stroke remains uncertain. Several factors have been identified as significant predictors for the development of CPSP and may provide some insight into the mechanism of onset. These include previous history of depression, greater stroke severity, younger age, and smoking.[1]

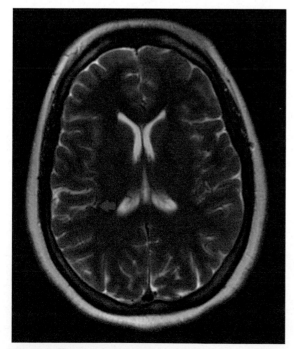

FIG. 7.2 The region including the posterior insular cortex and medial operculum as seen on T2-weighted magnetic resonance imaging.

Shortly after their description of the Thalamic Syndrome, Head and Holmes proposed a theory of disinhibition to explain CPSP: injury to the sensory pathways would lead to a compensatory overactivation within the thalamus, thus causing spontaneous pain or allodynia.[23] This theory continues to be the most widely accepted explanation for CPSP and has been continually reaffirmed using modern technology. For example, a fairly recent study using single photon emission computerized tomography (SPECT) scanning showed that evoking pain on the affected side of CPSP patients leads to hyperactivity in the contralateral thalamus.[24] This theory of disinhibition relies on the fact that some parts of the sensory tract, as described above, must remain intact and some sort of synaptic reorganization or an overall shift in neuronal circuitry occurs for processing pain. Indeed, diffusion tensor tractography studies (a derivation of diffusion weighted MRI that allows for neural tracts to be evaluated) revealed that CPSP is more likely to occur in patients whose lesion only partially involved the spinothalamic tract compared to those whose lesion showed complete involvement.[25] Therefore, some continuity of the spinothalamic tract must be maintained for CPSP to develop.

Opioid receptor (OR) binding has also been linked to clinical pain,[26,27] and it may play a role in the etiology of CPSP. A study by Willoch et al. used a nonselective, radiolabeled OR ligand ([11C]diprenorphine) and PET scanning to assess OR binding in long-term CPSP patients and healthy controls.[28] Their results showed significantly decreased binding in CPSP patients of the OR ligand in the ventroposterior thalamus, periventricular grey matter, the insular cortex, the accessory sensory cortex (S2), the posterior parietal cortex, the lateral prefrontal cortex, and the cingulate cortex; all areas within the pain processing circuitry. This study provides new insights to the neurochemical nature of structures that have already been implicated in CPSP, although it does not provide the entire story of how opioids are involved in the pathophysiology of CPSP. For example, it is interesting that several of these same structures have been shown on other PET scan studies to have *increased* metabolic activity in those with CPSP.[29] With a measured deficit in opioid receptor binding capacity, it may explain the reason that reports on the administration of opioids to CPSP patients have been discouraging,[30] and that opioid use can contribute to heightened pain sensitization in other neuropathic pain syndromes.[31,32] Taken together these studies demonstrate that the role of opioids in the pathophysiology of CPSP is likely complicated and more detailed studies are needed.

More recent studies in mice have implicated the long-chain fatty acid receptor, GPR40. It had previously been shown that GPR40 mediates β-endorphin release,[33] and more recently, shown in an established mouse model of CPSP that providing a GPR40 agonist suppresses pain scoring in experimentally affected mice.[34] While these studies may not be directly translatable to humans, they provide a basis for an additional biochemical pathway, as well as a potential treatment option.

Treatments for CPSP

As with other types of neuropathic pain, a variety of neuromodulating and psychoactive medications have been found to be useful for the treatment of CPSP. While data supporting their use specifically for CPSP may be somewhat limited, a few studies have been performed and have been presented below. We believe that this area will continue to grow as awareness and more studies on CPSP patients are undertaken.

Antidepressants

Amitriptyline, a tricyclic antidepressant, was the first antidepressant to be shown to be significantly effective in CPSP in a small study from 1989.[10] This study showed that the medication was safe and effective in treating CPSP at a dosage of 75 mg daily. Amitriptyline has been considered for use as a prophylactic treatment for CPSP.[35] However, the only trial published had a low sample size, which suggested efficacy but with no clinical significance.[35] The most common side effects of amitriptyline include dry mouth, constipation, urinary retention, and orthostatic hypotension.

Selective serotonin reuptake inhibitors (SSRIs) and serotonin norepinephrine reuptake inhibitors (SNRIs) are also potential candidates for pain patients. In CPSP, the only SSRI that has been tested is fluvoxamine.[36] It has been shown to significantly reduce pain in CPSP patients when started within 1 year of the stroke. However, if started after 1 year, it was found not to be effective.

Venlafaxine, desvenlafaxine, and duloxetine are SNRIs and have been used in a variety of neuropathic pain applications but have yet to be studied specifically in CPSP.[37]

Anticonvulsants

Many antiepileptic drugs have been used in the treatment of neuropathic pain, some of which have been studied in CPSP patients. Calcium channel modulators, such as pregabalin and gabapentin, are a popular choice for neuropathic pain in multiple pain states. Pregabalin

has the most thorough testing in this category, having been used in a placebo-controlled, double-blind study in 219 patients.[38] In this study, the drug did not significantly reduce the mean pain score, but did improve patient reported sleep, anxiety, and other quality of life measures. On the other hand, 70% of patients receiving pregabalin reported adverse effects; dizziness, somnolence, edema, and weight gain were the most commonly reported. A more recent study evaluated the long-term efficacy of pregabalin in central neuropathic pain patients, of which, 60 were diagnosed with CPSP.[39] Among the CPSP patients, 50% reported a 30% reduction in their Short-Form McGill Pain Questionnaire Visual Analog Scale (SF-MPQ VAS), suggesting that there is a significant improvement in subjective pain over a 52-week period. This study is encouraging in its establishment of an effective treatment over a longer period than its predecessors, though limited as an open-label study lacking a placebo control. As such, gabapentin is often the first antiepileptic medication selected in the treatment of neuropathic pain due to its flexibility in dosing and relative affordability. However, data regarding the safety and efficacy of gabapentin in the treatment of CPSP are lacking.

Other anticonvulsants used to treat pain are sodium channel blockers. Carbamazepine is often a secondary treatment in CPSP patients because it has been found to be less efficacious with a higher incidence of adverse effects when compared to other drugs like amitriptyline.[10] It is also known for its side effects, which can include Stevens–Johnson syndrome and aplastic anemia, as well as its interactions with other medications. Lamotrigine has been studied in a placebo-controlled, double-blind study where it significantly reduced global pain scoring in 27 of 30 patients.[40] Clinically significant results were achieved at a dose of 200 mg per day. While lamotrigine may be safer than other antiepileptic drugs, 2 of the 30 patients in this group developed a drug rash, one of which required withdrawal from the study. Phenytoin and zonisamide have both been tested in limited sample sizes, but have shown the potential of offering some relief in CPSP.[41,42] Levetiracetam was recently tested in a placebo-controlled, double-blind study of 42 patients and failed to achieve significant pain relief or any secondary outcome goals.[43]

Corticosteroids

While methylprednisolone has not been studied in any prospective studies of CPSP patients, a retrospective study suggested some potential benefit.[44] In that study, 146 charts of stroke patients admitted to an acute inpatient rehabilitation ward were reviewed, 12 (8.2%) of whom were diagnosed with CPSP. Within this group, it was found that the patients receiving methylprednisolone had significantly reduced pain-scoring 1 day after starting treatment and 1 day prior to discharge. Additionally, these patients required as-needed pain medications less often than those not receiving steroids; however, this result was marginal. Doses of methylprednisolone used in the study were reported as 6-day tapers starting with 24 mg on day one and decreasing by 4 mg daily.

Nonpharmacologic treatments

There are several nonpharmacologic treatments available to treat CPSP in cases refractory to medication or where medications cannot be tolerated. Some of the most promising treatments are listed here. Deep brain stimulation (DBS) is a procedure involving the implantation of a medical device into the brain that sends electrical signals, through stereotactically placed electrodes, to targeted neural structures. It has been effective in managing refractory Parkinson disease, depression, and chronic pain syndromes. Multiple studies and case reports have shown that it can offer various degrees of relief, sometimes even allowing for complete discontinuation of pain medications.[45] A study of 15 patients from 2006 demonstrated effectiveness of DBS implanted in the thalamus and periventricular/periaqueductal grey matter and 12 patients (80%) followed through with permanent implantation after initial trial implantation, 7 of whom were able to discontinue all analgesics and the remaining 5 switched from regular opiates to only as-needed nonopiate analgesics.[46] Among 45 CPSP patients included in a metaanalysis from Bittar (2005), 53% went through with permanent implantation, 58% of whom achieved long-term pain relief.[47] Historically, the most effective target structures are the periventricular grey matter and the VPL of the thalamus[45]; however, one recent case report has also demonstrated a good response to stimulation of the nucleus accumbens in a CPSP patient.[48]

In addition to DBS, other surgical techniques such as cingulotomy, targeted destruction of a small portion of the anterior cingulate cortex, have found success in treating psychiatric illnesses and pain disorders.[49] Few cases have been reported regarding cingulotomy in post-stroke patients; however, a 2012 study of three patients with CPSP showed an improvement in Visual Analog Scoring of 51.9% over the first month following the procedure.[50] These patients also had deep-brain stimulators implanted, which were activated after the 1-month mark making long-term results difficult to predict for cingulotomy alone. Further research is needed

to fully determine whether this is a viable option for medically refractory CPSP.

Repetitive transcranial magnetic stimulation (rTMS) is another treatment that has been used for several neurologic and psychiatric disorders. In rTMS, a coil is placed over the patient's scalp and is used to deliver a magnetic pulse that induces an electrical discharge in a targeted region of cerebral cortex. Multiple studies have been performed on patients with neuropathic pain, including CPSP patients, and have shown it to be associated with minimal side effects.[45] A recent open-label, noncontrolled study from Japan showed that weekly rTMS sessions involving motor cortex stimulation over 12 weeks (18 patients) and 1 year (6 of the original 18 patients) led to significant reductions in Visual Analog Scale scoring.[51] Eight patients with severe dysesthesia were found to have the least relief from pain, suggesting that rTMS may be a therapy better suited for milder CPSP patients. Reported side effects were limited to 2 patients describing transient slight scalp discomfort. While this is a relatively small study that lacks a control group, previous studies have shown significant benefits from rTMS for patients with neuropathic pain syndromes on a wider scale,[52] and given the benign risks of therapy, further studies specifically in CPSP patients are warranted.

COMPLEX REGIONAL PAIN SYNDROME

Complex regional pain syndrome (CRPS), sometimes referred to as reflex sympathetic dystrophy, is a condition characterized by burning pain, increased sensitivity to tactile stimulation, and changes in skin temperature and color.[2] CRPS can be further classified into CRPS Type I, which develops in the absence of evidence of direct injury to a nerve and is generally the subset observed in patients with stroke, and CRPS Type II, which follows discrete peripheral nerve damage. Additionally, the term shoulder-hand syndrome has been used to describe CRPS in hemiplegic patients.[53]

CRPS was first described following stroke in a retrospective study from 1977 in which 68 of 540 (12.5%) inpatient rehabilitation patients were diagnosed with shoulder-hand syndrome.[54] A more recent study among 95 persons with stroke admitted to a Turkish rehabilitation hospital in 2006 showed that 30.5% went on to develop CRPS.[55] Age, gender, side of involvement, and stroke etiology were not shown to predispose one to CRPS; however, flaccidity, glenohumeral subluxation, and poorer functional recovery did significantly increase risk. Aside from acute rehabilitation inpatients, two studies which followed persons with stroke causing hemiplegia longitudinally showed an incidence of CRPS of 23% and 48.8%.[56,57] Both studies implicated spasticity as a risk factor and one also identified shoulder subluxation and loss of range of motion.[56] To fully analyze the burden of CRPS on the stroke community, a large-scale longitudinal study on a broader stroke population is needed.

Pathophysiology of CRPS

The pathophysiology of CRPS in otherwise healthy patients remains a subject of much debate, and can be further obscured by the presence of a stroke. Thus, much of what is known about the onset of CRPS is from studies not involving stroke.

The classic theory holds that CRPS is the result of local hyperactivity of the sympathetic nervous system.[2] This is supported by data showing an alteration in temperature regulation between the affected and nonaffected limbs in CRPS patients,[58] as well as a study showing that stimulation of the sympathetic nervous system with localized cooling and startle stimuli worsened pain in those with CPRS, but less-so after sympathetic blockade.[59] Historically, patients have been treated for CRPS with sympathetic blockade, strengthening the argument for a sympathetic origin of the disorder; however, further analysis of the efficacy of that procedure suggests that this may not always be the case.[60] A comprehensive review of 29 studies, including 1144 patients showed that 29% had a full response to sympatholytic blockade, 41% had a partial response, and 32% had no response,[60] suggesting that other mechanisms may be involved.

Other mechanisms have been proposed including sensitization of the somatic sensory pathway, overactivation of inflammatory responses, and hypoxia;[2] however, there remains limited data attempting to link CRPS to a stroke lesion specifically. One study from 1994 that followed 36 post-stroke CRPS patients was able to examine the shoulder capsules of 7 patients on autopsy and found evidence of previous trauma, suggesting that CRPS may be due in part to preexisting or post-stroke musculoskeletal injury, as much as, or more than the central stroke lesion.[61] Conversely, a case report from 2008 of a patient with a left parietal lobe stroke who also had MRI evidence of an old right thalamic infarct and later developed CRPS, showed an increase in left thalamic regional cerebral blood flow on SPECT imaging, as well as contralateral cerebellar diaschisis, or demonstrated hypoperfusion, and decreased metabolic uptake in the left cerebellum.[62] This report opens a door to further investigation of how central nervous system activity can play a role in CRPS, and with the reported thalamic involvement contralateral to the old injury, raises an important question about a possible relationship between CRPS and CPSP.

Treatment of CRPS in Stroke

As has been mentioned, CRPS and its management are widely studied, though specific studies concerning persons with stroke are limited. With any neurologic deficits following a stroke, physical therapy and early mobility are of vital importance to reducing long-term disability, and seem to help the symptoms associated with CRPS as well. A recent study of 52 patients admitted to an acute rehabilitation facility with a diagnosis of CRPS following stroke participated in a 4-week course of upper extremity aerobic exercise, where 98.9% of patients in the experimental group reported significant pain relief, as well as a reduction in other CRPS-associated symptoms.[63]

Two studies have suggested a benefit from corticosteroids in patients with CRPS following stroke. The first was a placebo-controlled non-blinded clinical trial from 1994 in which 36 patients with hemiplegic stroke who developed CRPS were started on low-dose oral corticosteroids and 31 of the 36 achieved near-total relief from symptoms.[61] More recently, a randomized controlled trial of prednisolone and piroxicam in 60 patients with stroke diagnosed with CRPS showed significant improvement in pain scoring in the prednisolone group, where patients received 40 mg daily of prednisolone for 1 month, with only a modest improvement observed in the piroxicam group.[64]

A longitudinal study comparing post-stroke inpatients to historical controls measured the incidence of CRPS in the setting of prophylactic calcitonin administration, and showed a significant reduction in the onset of CRPS among treated patients.[65] Patients in the experimental group received 20 units of elcalcitonin weekly during admission, and were shown to have the greatest benefit if therapy was started within the first 4 weeks following stroke.

Overall, pharmacologic clinical trials in stroke-related CRPS seem to be greatly lacking and are a potential valuable area for future research; however drugs that have shown benefit or the possibility of being beneficial in patients with CRPS not from stroke include the NMDA receptor agonist memantine, as well as the anticonvulsants gabapentin and carbamazepine.[2]

Mirror therapy is a technique in which a patient watches the unaffected arm perform a motor task in a mirror. With the affected arm hidden behind the mirror, the patient is able to imagine and perceive normal function from the hemiparetic limb. A placebo-controlled randomized trial of 48 post-stroke CRPS patients showed statistical improvements in both pain as measured by Visual Analog Scale scoring, as well as motor function.[66]

Sympathetic blockade, typically by means of targeting the stellate ganglion with anesthetic injection has been used in CRPS in the past. As discussed above, sympathetic block has been shown to offer some degree of relief to CRPS patients, though more recent analyses suggest that it is not effective.[60,67]

In addition to the above therapies, proper management of chronic CRPS should also involve a foundation of routine activity and exercise.

CONCLUSION

Post-stroke pain is a complicated phenomenon encompassing both nociceptive and neuropathic pain etiologies. CPSP and CRPS represent two disorders that commonly disrupt maximal stroke recovery. The management and treatment of these syndromes include pharmacologic, orthotic, biomechanic, electrophysiological and surgical therapies. The optimal treatment for an individual patient will often require a combination of therapy modalities based on the needs of each patient. However, a complete discussion of the basis for development along with current and future treatment options for pain syndromes that impair stroke recovery is the first step in early diagnosis and therapy for patients.

REFERENCES

1. O'Donnell MJ, Diener HC, Sacco RL, et al. Chronic pain syndromes after ischemic stroke: PRoFESS trial. *Stroke*. 2013;44(5):1238–1243.
2. Chae J. Poststroke complex regional pain syndrome. *Top Stroke Rehabil*. 2010;17(3):151–162.
3. Leijon G, Boivie J, Johansson I. Central post-stroke pain—neurological symptoms and pain characteristics. *Pain*. 1989;36(1):13–25.
4. Nicholson BD. Evaluation and treatment of central pain syndromes. *Neurology*. 2004;62(5 suppl 2):S30–S36.
5. Kumar B, Kalita J, Kumar G, Misra UK. Central poststroke pain: a review of pathophysiology and treatment. *Anesth Analg*. 2009;108(5):1645–1657.
6. de Oliveira RA, de Andrade DC, Machado AG, Teixeira MJ. Central poststroke pain: somatosensory abnormalities and the presence of associated myofascial pain syndrome. *BMC Neurol*. 2012;12:89.
7. Pain TFoTotIAftSo. In: Merskey HBN, ed. *Classification of Chronic Pain Descriptions of Chronic Pain Syndromes and Definitions of Pain Terms*. 2nd ed. SEATTLE IASP Press; 1994.
8. Dejerine J, Roussy G. Le syndrome thalamique. *Rev Neurol*. 1906;12:521–532.
9. Kheder A, Nair KP. Spasticity: pathophysiology, evaluation and management. *Pract Neurol*. 2012;12(5):289–298.
10. Leijon G, Boivie J. Central post-stroke pain—a controlled trial of amitriptyline and carbamazepine. *Pain*. 1989; 36(1):27–36.
11. Bogousslavsky J, Regli F, Uske A. Thalamic infarcts: clinical syndromes, etiology, and prognosis. *Neurology*. 1988; 38(6):837–848.
12. Paciaroni M, Bogousslavsky J. Pure sensory syndromes in thalamic stroke. *Eur Neurol*. 1998;39(4):211–217.
13. Bowsher D, Leijon G, Thuomas KA. Central poststroke pain: correlation of MRI with clinical pain characteristics and sensory abnormalities. *Neurology*. 1998;51(5):1352–1358.
14. Kim JS. Pure sensory stroke. Clinical-radiological correlates of 21 cases. *Stroke*. 1992;23(7):983–987.
15. Krause T, Brunecker P, Pittl S, et al. Thalamic sensory strokes with and without pain: differences in lesion patterns in the ventral posterior thalamus. *J Neurol Neurosurg Psychiatry*. 2012;83(8):776–784.
16. Sprenger T, Seifert CL, Valet M, et al. Assessing the risk of central post-stroke pain of thalamic origin by lesion mapping. *Brain*. 2012;135(Pt 8):2536–2545.
17. MacGowan DJ, Janal MN, Clark WC, et al. Central post-stroke pain and Wallenberg's lateral medullary infarction: frequency, character, and determinants in 63 patients. *Neurology*. 1997;49(1):120–125.
18. Nakazato Y, Yoshimaru K, Ohkuma A, Araki N, Tamura N, Shimazu K. Central post-stroke pain in Wallenberg syndrome. *Brain Nerve*. 2004;56(5):385–388.
19. Kim JS, Han YS. Medial medullary infarction: clinical, imaging, and outcome study in 86 consecutive patients. *Stroke*. 2009;40(10):3221–3225.
20. Willis WD, Westlund KN. Neuroanatomy of the pain system and of the pathways that modulate pain. *J Clin Neurophysiol*. 1997;14(1):2–31.
21. Kim JS. Patterns of sensory abnormality in cortical stroke: evidence for a dichotomized sensory system. *Neurology*. 2007;68(3):174–180.
22. Garcia-Larrea L. The posterior insular-opercular region and the search of a primary cortex for pain. *Neurophysiol Clin*. 2012;42(5):299–313.
23. Head H, Holmes G. Sensory disturbances from cerebral lesions. *Brain A J Neurol*. 1911;34:102–254.
24. Cesaro P, Mann MW, Moretti JL, et al. Central pain and thalamic hyperactivity: a single photon emission computerized tomographic study. *Pain*. 1991;47(3):329–336.
25. Hong JH, Choi BY, Chang CH, et al. The prevalence of central poststroke pain according to the integrity of the spino-thalamo-cortical pathway. *Eur Neurol*. 2012;67(1):12–17.
26. Willoch F, Tolle TR, Wester HJ, et al. Central pain after pontine infarction is associated with changes in opioid receptor binding: a PET study with 11C-diprenorphine. *AJNR Am J Neuroradiol*. 1999;20(4):686–690.
27. Zubieta JK, Smith YR, Bueller JA, et al. Regional mu opioid receptor regulation of sensory and affective dimensions of pain. *Science*. 2001;293(5528):311–315.

28. Willoch F, Schindler F, Wester HJ, et al. Central poststroke pain and reduced opioid receptor binding within pain processing circuitries: a [^{11}C]diprenorphine PET study. *Pain.* 2004;108(3):213–220.

29. Peyron R, Garcia-Larrea L, Gregoire MC, et al. Allodynia after lateral-medullary (Wallenberg) infarct. A PET study. *Brain A J Neurol.* 1998;121(Pt 2):345–356.

30. Boivie J. *Central Pain.* Edinburgh: Churchill Livingstone; 1999.

31. Celerier E, Rivat C, Jun Y, et al. Long-lasting hyperalgesia induced by fentanyl in rats: preventive effect of ketamine. *Anesthesiology.* 2000;92(2):465–472.

32. Mayer DJ, Mao J, Holt J, Price DD. Cellular mechanisms of neuropathic pain, morphine tolerance, and their interactions. *Proc Natl Acad Sci USA.* 1999;96(14):7731–7736.

33. Nakamoto K, Nishinaka T, Matsumoto K, et al. Involvement of the long-chain fatty acid receptor GPR40 as a novel pain regulatory system. *Brain Res.* 2012;1432:74–83.

34. Harada S, Haruna Y, Aizawa F, et al. Involvement of GPR40, a long-chain free fatty acid receptor, in the production of central post-stroke pain after global cerebral ischemia. *Eur J Pharmacol.* 2014;744:115–123.

35. Lampl C, Yazdi K, Roper C. Amitriptyline in the prophylaxis of central poststroke pain. Preliminary results of 39 patients in a placebo-controlled, long-term study. *Stroke.* 2002;33(12):3030–3032.

36. Shimodozono M, Kawahira K, Kamishita T, Ogata A, Tohgo S, Tanaka N. Reduction of central poststroke pain with the selective serotonin reuptake inhibitor fluvoxamine. *Int J Neurosci.* 2002;112(10):1173–1181.

37. Miller A, Rabe-Jablonska J. The effectiveness of antidepressants in the treatment of chronic non-cancer pain—a review. *Psychiatr Polska.* 2005;39(1):21–32.

38. Kim JS, Bashford G, Murphy TK, Martin A, Dror V, Cheung R. Safety and efficacy of pregabalin in patients with central post-stroke pain. *Pain.* 2011;152(5):1018–1023.

39. Onouchi K, Koga H, Yokoyama K, Yoshiyama T. An open-label, long-term study examining the safety and tolerability of pregabalin in Japanese patients with central neuropathic pain. *J Pain Res.* 2014;7:439–447.

40. Vestergaard K, Andersen G, Gottrup H, Kristensen BT, Jensen TS. Lamotrigine for central poststroke pain: a randomized controlled trial. *Neurology.* 2001;56(2):184–190.

41. Agnew DC, Goldberg VD. A brief trial of phenytoin therapy for thalamic pain. *Bull Los Angel Neurol Societies.* 1976;41(1):9–12.

42. Takahashi Y, Hashimoto K, Tsuji S. Successful use of zonisamide for central poststroke pain. *J Pain.* 2004;5(3):192–194.

43. Jungehulsing GJ, Israel H, Safar N, et al. Levetiracetam in patients with central neuropathic post-stroke pain—a randomized, double-blind, placebo-controlled trial. *Eur J Neurol.* 2013;20(2):331–337.

44. Pellicane AJ, Millis SR. Efficacy of methylprednisolone versus other pharmacologic interventions for the treatment of central post-stroke pain: a retrospective analysis. *J Pain Res.* 2013;6:557–563.

45. Flaster M, Meresh E, Rao M, Biller J. Central poststroke pain: current diagnosis and treatment. *Top Stroke Rehabil.* 2013;20(2):116–123.

46. Owen SL, Green AL, Stein JF, Aziz TZ. Deep brain stimulation for the alleviation of post-stroke neuropathic pain. *Pain.* 2006;120(1–2):202–206.

47. Bittai RG, Kai-Purkayastha I, Owen SL, et al. Deep brain stimulation for pain relief: a meta-analysis. *J Clin Neurosci.* 2005;12(5):515–519.

48. Mallory GW, Abulseoud O, Hwang SC, et al. The nucleus accumbens as a potential target for central poststroke pain. *Mayo Clin Proc.* 2012;87(10):1025–1031.

49. Brotis AG, Kapsalaki EZ, Paterakis K, Smith JR, Fountas KN. Historic evolution of open cingulectomy and stereotactic cingulotomy in the management of medically intractable psychiatric disorders, pain and drug addiction. *Stereotact Funct Neurosurg.* 2009;87(5):271–291.

50. Kim JP, Chang WS, Park YS, Chang JW. Impact of ventralis caudalis deep brain stimulation combined with stereotactic bilateral cingulotomy for treatment of post-stroke pain. *Stereotact Funct Neurosurg.* 2012;90(1):9–15.

51. Kobayashi M, Fujimaki T, Mihara B, Ohira T. Repetitive transcranial magnetic stimulation once a week induces sustainable long-term relief of central poststroke pain. *Neuromodulation.* 2015;18(4):249–254.

52. Lefaucheur JP, Andre-Obadia N, Antal A, et al. Evidence-based guidelines on the therapeutic use of repetitive transcranial magnetic stimulation (rTMS). *Clin Neurophysiol.* 2014;125(11):2150–2206.

53. Pertoldi S, Di Benedetto P. Shoulder-hand syndrome after stroke. A complex regional pain syndrome. *Eur Medicophys.* 2005;41(4):283–292.

54. Davis SW, Petrillo CR, Eichberg RD, Chu DS. Shoulder-hand syndrome in a hemiplegic population: a 5-year retrospective study. *Arch Phys Med Rehabil.* 1977;58(8):353–356.

55. Gokkaya NK, Aras M, Yesiltepe E, Koseoglu F. Reflex sympathetic dystrophy in hemiplegia. *Int J Rehabil Res.* 2006;29(4):275–279.

56. Kocabas H, Levendoglu F, Ozerbil OM, Yuruten B. Complex regional pain syndrome in stroke patients. *Int J Rehabil Res.* 2007;30(1):33–38.

57. Van Ouwenaller C, Laplace PM, Chantraine A. Painful shoulder in hemiplegia. *Arch Phys Med Rehabil.* 1986;67(1):23–26.

58. Niehof SP, Huygen FJ, van der Weerd RW, Westra M, Zijlstra FJ. Thermography imaging during static and controlled thermoregulation in complex regional pain syndrome type 1: diagnostic value and involvement of the central sympathetic system. *Biomed Eng Online.* 2006;5:30.

59. Drummond PD, Finch PM. Persistence of pain induced by startle and forehead cooling after sympathetic blockade in patients with complex regional pain syndrome. *J Neurol Neurosurg Psychiatry*. 2004;75(1):98−102.

60. Cepeda MS, Lau J, Carr DB. Defining the therapeutic role of local anesthetic sympathetic blockade in complex regional pain syndrome: a narrative and systematic review. *Clin J Pain*. 2002;18(4):216−233.

61. Braus DF, Krauss JK, Strobel J. The shoulder-hand syndrome after stroke: a prospective clinical trial. *Ann Neurol*. 1994;36(5):728−733.

62. Lai MH, Wang TY, Chang CC, Li TY, Chang ST. Cerebellar diaschisis and contralateral thalamus hyperperfusion in a stroke patient with complex regional pain syndrome. *J Clin Neurosci*. 2008;15(10):1166−1168.

63. Topcuoglu A, Gokkaya NK, Ucan H, Karakus D. The effect of upper-extremity aerobic exercise on complex regional pain syndrome type I: a randomized controlled study on subacute stroke. *Top Stroke Rehabil*. 2015;22(4): 253−261.

64. Kalita J, Vajpayee A, Misra UK. Comparison of prednisolone with piroxicam in complex regional pain syndrome following stroke: a randomized controlled trial. *QJM*. 2006;99(2):89−95.

65. Matayoshi S, Shimodozono M, Hirata Y, Ueda T, Horio S, Kawahira K. Use of calcitonin to prevent complex regional pain syndrome type I in severe hemiplegic patients after stroke. *Disabil Rehabil*. 2009;31(21):1773−1779.

66. Cacchio A, De Blasis E, De Blasis V, Santilli V, Spacca G. Mirror therapy in complex regional pain syndrome type 1 of the upper limb in stroke patients. *Neurorehabil Neural Repair*. 2009;23(8):792−799.

67. O'Connell NE, Wand BM, McAuley J, Marston L, Moseley GL. Interventions for treating pain and disability in adults with complex regional pain syndrome. *Cochrane Database Syst Rev*. 2013;4:CD009416.

CHAPTER 8

Upper Limb Impairment

PREETI RAGHAVAN, MD

INTRODUCTION

Stroke is a leading cause of disability worldwide.[1] More than 80% of patients with stroke develop hemiparesis of whom 85% have persistent arm and hand dysfunction.[2] Poor recovery of arm function is a major problem because it limits activities of daily living, participation in society, and the odds of returning to professional activity. Hence, it is imperative to understand the nature of upper limb impairment to develop effective solutions for poststroke arm dysfunction and reduce the burden of disability.[3]

The extent of upper limb motor impairment is proportional to the degree of damage to the corticospinal tract.[4] Patients with mild-to-moderate upper limb impairment within 72 h of their stroke have a good prognosis for functional recovery, and achieve at least some dexterity by 6 months post stroke.[4–7] However, this is not the case for individuals with moderate-to-severe upper limb impairment, who constitute the majority with persistent arm and hand dysfunction after stroke.[5,8] There are few options to train arm function for individuals with moderate-to-severe upper limb impairment, and many of these patients feel abandoned by the healthcare system.

Poor upper extremity recovery may be due to the direct impact of the stroke on the capacity for recovery,[4] as well as due to insufficient, inadequate, or inappropriate therapeutic interventions. Given that recovery is experience-dependent, the lack of appropriate therapeutic interventions may further limit the capacity for recovery in individuals with substantial arm weakness. Studies show that upper limb function can be improved by high-dose, task-specific, repetitive use of the arm in individuals with mild-to-moderate upper limb weakness.[9] However, this is difficult to achieve in individuals with substantial weakness, who depend on a therapist or caregiver to move the arm. Therapy time is increasingly limited due to reduced length of stay in rehabilitation and insurance restrictions, and the focus is on teaching compensatory techniques to maintain overall functional ability rather than on recovery of arm movement. There are at least three main functional consequences of poststroke upper limb impairment: (1) nonuse, (2) bad-use, and (3) lack of dexterity. Nonuse and bad-use are critical barriers to recovery of arm movement in patients with moderate-to-severe upper limb impairment, whereas bad-use and lack of dexterity limit individuals with mild-to-moderate upper limb impairment. Each of these functional consequences and the underlying impairments are elaborated below.

NONUSE

Immediately after a stroke, upper limb impairment is caused by neural disconnection of the lesioned area of the brain,[10] resulting in an inability to use the arm. Initially nonuse may occur because of weakness/paresis or sensory loss. However, as time progresses, nonuse may become habitual and the limb may not be incorporated into functional activities, even though the individual can move it. Now it becomes a learned behavior and is referred to as learned nonuse.

Weakness or paresis is the predominant impairment that contributes to dysfunction after stroke[11,12]; it is a direct consequence of the lack of signal transmission from the motor cortex, which generates the movement impulse, to the spinal cord, which executes the movement via signals to muscles. The lack of signal from the motor cortex results in delayed initiation and termination of muscle contraction,[13] and slowness in developing force,[14] manifested as an inability to move or move quickly with negative functional consequences. Abnormally increased electromyographic (EMG)-force slopes are seen on the affected side compared with the contralateral side, as well as compared with neurologically intact subjects, suggesting that greater EMG activity is necessary to generate a given force in patients with stroke.[15,16] Large interindividual differences exist in the pattern of muscle weakness across muscle groups, but no consistent proximal-to-distal gradient

Stroke Rehabilitation. https://doi.org/10.1016/B978-0-323-55381-0.00008-1

or greater extensor relative to flexor weakness has been found.[17,18]

Sensory loss across tactile, proprioceptive, and/or higher-order sensory modalities such as two-point discrimination, stereognosis, and graphesthesia are common after stroke and may be associated with the degree of weakness and the degree of stroke severity, as well as mobility, independence in activities of daily living, and recovery.[20] Sensory impairments without motor weakness may also occur from specific lesions in the parietal cortex.[21] A study that compared the ability of hemiparetic and healthy subjects to produce symmetric forces with both upper limbs showed that maximum voluntary joint forces and proprioceptive impairments in the affected limb predicted the errors in force matching.[22] These results suggest that sensory impairments can lead to inaccurate motor output, even when motor capacity is adequate to perform the task. The term *learned nonuse* was coined from observations of deafferented monkeys that could move, but did not do so voluntarily.[23] Thus, chronic loss of sensation contributes to upper limb impairment because of an inability to control the motor output appropriately owing to lack of feedback about the consequences of motor actions.

Both weakness and sensory loss contribute to immobility, which can initiate a cascade of problems that further contribute to upper limb impairment (Fig. 8.1). These problems include peripheral soft tissue changes that increase muscle viscosity and stiffness and reduce tissue compliance, potentiate spinal cord hyperreflexia and spasticity, and eventually lead to muscle fibrosis, abnormal limb posturing, pain, and decreased function.[24,25] Immobility also leads to changes in bone mineral density with increased risk of developing osteoporosis on the paralyzed side.[26,27] In fact, fractures are common in the paretic upper limb after stroke.[28] Practitioners need to pay more attention to changes in bone mineral density after stroke and take active measures to prevent problems arising from immobility. Motor and sensory impairments and immobility are also associated with an increased risk for stroke-related pain.[29] Stiffness in the connective tissue of an immobilized limb may stimulate free nerve endings and proprioceptors, such as Pacini and Ruffini corpuscles in the soft tissue producing pain.[30–33] Shoulder pain on the paretic side is common after stroke and is strongly associated with abnormal shoulder joint examination, ipsilateral sensory abnormalities, and arm weakness.[34]

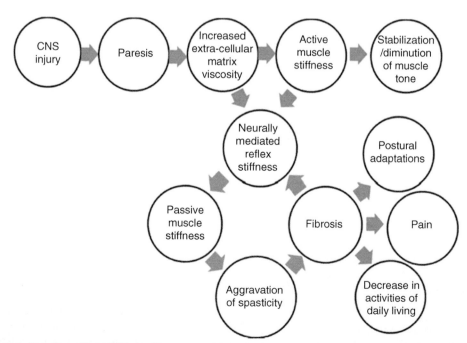

FIG. 8.1 Paresis and immobility lead to nonuse which initiates a cascade of problems that contribute to upper limb impairment. (From Stecco A, Stecco C, Raghavan P. Peripheral mechanisms of spasticity and treatment implications. *Curr Phys Med Rehabil Rep.* 2014;2(2):121–127; with permission.)

Deafferentation and sensory loss may also lead to the development of neuronal hypersensitivity and eventually to chronic central pain.[35,36] Pain can lead to learned nonuse, which may persist even after the pain has resolved. Hence early interventions that reduce immobility and preserve range of motion either passively or actively, despite weakness, are critical to prevent complications such as muscle stiffness, pain, osteoporosis, contractures, deformity, and further dysfunction.

BAD-USE

Weakness, sensory impairments, and pain combined with muscle stiffness, spasticity, and changes resulting from nonuse lead to characteristic abnormal movement patterns on attempted use.[37] These abnormal movement patterns (bad-use) have been well described for animal and human reaching and grasping after stroke.[38,39] For example, reaching requires shoulder flexion and elbow extension; however, attempted reaching post stroke leads instead to involuntary shoulder abduction and extension or shoulder adduction and flexion,[40] often accompanied by elbow, wrist, and finger flexion, making it very difficult to reach normally.[41,42] As a result, patients with stroke use compensatory trunk flexion rather than elbow extension to reach,[43] forearm pronation and wrist flexion rather than neutral forearm position and wrist extension to orient the hand for grasping, and metacarpophalangeal joint flexion rather than proximal interphalangeal joint flexion to grasp objects.[44] Although the use of these abnormal strategies may lead to initial success in completing a task, success is reduced over time because of poor accuracy, which increases the probability of failure with repetition. Reinforcement of the abnormal strategy by occasional successes can lead to bad movement habits,[45] resulting in a decline in performance despite extended training because the abnormal behavior is repeated and reinforced at the cost of the correct pattern of behavior.[46] Thus in the absence of appropriate feedback and correction of the abnormal motor behavior, learned bad-use develops.

The typical abnormal movement or synergy patterns are reliably captured using the Fugl−Meyer scale,[47] which is widely used as a standard measure of the extent of motor impairment.[48] The Fugl−Meyer scale has shown excellent reliability,[49] construct validity and responsiveness,[50] and content validity.[51] The upper limb Fugl−Meyer scale assesses how well a person moves across 33 different tasks by isolating movement at various joints on a three-point rating scale. However,

it does not indicate the range of movement at any particular joint, or the level of function, although it is correlated with measures of function.[52]

Examination of muscle activation patterns in healthy controls and patients with stroke reveals that patients with stroke show increased activation of the pectoral muscles, and the anterior, middle, and posterior deltoids in the chronic phase post stroke compared with controls (Fig. 8.2).[40] Clinically, this is manifested as palpable muscle stiffness in the pectoral and deltoid muscles.[54] This abnormal pattern is responsible for reduced range of motion at multiple upper limb joints, which limits the workspace of paretic arm movements.[55−59] Interestingly, the abnormal movement patterns are gravity-dependent. As the arm is abducted against gravity, the muscle torque required to balance the load on the arm increases. When the muscles in the front of the shoulder, such as the pectoralis major and anterior deltoid, are short and overactivated[40] and the anti-gravity back muscles are underactivated and uncoordinated as has been found after stroke,[60−62] the torque generated to support the load of the arm is inadequate. However, just flexing the elbow can reduce the torque requirement by half, and abducting and laterally rotating the arm increases shoulder joint stability.[63] Thus, patients flex their elbow and abduct their arm when they attempt to reach, leading to abnormal movement patterns and bad-use.

Training strategies that promote movement outside of the abnormal motor patterns are needed to retrain more normal movement patterns. For example, when the trunk is restrained during reach practice, the typical use of a more normal pattern of reaching by extending the elbow is restored along with a reduction in overall impairment.[64,65] Reducing the effect of gravity by passively supporting the arm,[66−69] also leads to instant, albeit temporary, changes in the abnormal movement patterns. Training upper limb movements that potentially activate the antigravity back muscles also lead to improvement in abnormal movement patterns even in severely impaired patients.[70]

LACK OF DEXTERITY

Dexterity requires skill. Skill is learned and necessitates that at least three independent processes occur across multiple timescales.[71] First, precise task-specific sensorimotor mappings occur through trial-and-error adaptation during practice with appropriate error sensing. In other words, one quickly adapts one's movements and forces according to task demands. Adaptation is a fast learning process,[72] which leads to a rapid reduction in

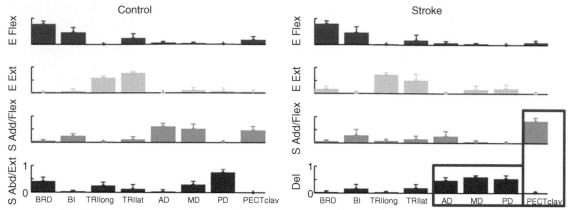

FIG. 8.2 Abnormal activation of the deltoid and pectoral muscles (*red boxes*) poststroke accounts for the shoulder adduction/flexion and shoulder abduction/extension synergies or bad-use during attempted voluntary movement. (From Roh J, Rymer WZ, Perreault EJ, Yoo SB, Beer RF. Alterations in upper limb muscle synergy structure in chronic stroke survivors. *J Neurophysiol*. 2013;109(3):768—781; with permission.)

movement error, and typically takes only a few trials[73]; however it is easily forgotten.[74,75] The second process is repetition, which alters movement biases depending on what is repeated. Repetition leads to a slow tuning of directional biases toward the repeated movement.[76] A task can be repeated with or without adaptation to error and does not require error sensing. The third process is reinforcement, whereby movements are rewarded intrinsically or extrinsically, and reward leads to faster relearning or savings on subsequent attempts.[77] Although these three processes occur independently, it has been shown that learning is most successful when sensorimotor adaptation is combined effectively with repetition (Fig. 8.3).[71] For instance, appropriate sensorimotor mappings learned through adaptation must be repeated over time for sustained and appropriate changes in skill to occur.[78]

Once a motor skill is attained through training, there is an expectation that it will be retained forever, despite intervals of no training (in the same way that one never forgets how to ride a bicycle). However, rats with motor cortex injury show a decline in performance during intervals of no training and additional training is required to get performance back to pretraining levels.[38] Breaks in rehabilitation similarly lead to forgetting of upper extremity motor skills in humans after stroke.[79,80] Impaired sensorimotor adaptation and lack of opportunities for long-term practice can lead to unlearning or forgetting after stroke.[81] Thus sensorimotor adaptation and long-term practice are critically needed to facilitate skill learning and dexterity post stroke.

Studies from several laboratories have shown that adaptation of reach and grasp are impaired after stroke

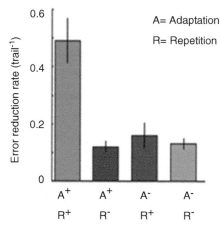

FIG. 8.3 Error reduction reflects motor learning, which is greatest when adaptation and repetition combine. (Adapted from Huang VS, Haith A, Mazzoni P, et al. Rethinking motor learning and savings in adaptation paradigms: Model-free memory for successful actions combines with internal models. *Neuron*. 2011:70(4);793; with permission.)

despite reasonable amounts of repetition with the affected hand.[44,82—84] This suggests that patients may be unable to effectively sense the error with their affected hand and/or subsequently update their motor behavior. Adaptation requires specific sensory inputs: kinesthetic sense from muscle forces used to lift objects is required to produce fingertip load forces appropriate for object weight[85,86]; tactile sensation from touch receptors is required to produce grip forces appropriate for object texture, with higher grip forces needed to hold smoother objects[87,88]; and visual input about object contours determines how the hand is shaped during reach.[89–91] In reaching experiments, both vision and proprioception provide information about arm configuration, but faulty integration of visual and proprioceptive signals may introduce errors in motor planning[92–94]; this might explain why we close our eyes when we want to enhance feeling. Thus, although multiple sensory contexts may collaborate to maintain task performance,[95] they can also compete and interfere with the acquisition of accurate sensorimotor associations.[92,96,97]

In the presence of sensory deficits after a stroke, however, one sensory context may substitute for another to improve the accuracy of sensorimotor maps.[98] Information about how and when sensory substitution should be used is key to the development of effective rehabilitation protocols for the recovery of motor skill. Even mild sensory and/or motor deficits can impair error sensing and affect adaptation of movements and forces with the affected hand after stroke.[44,83] Thus, the first step in improving dexterity is to facilitate the formation of sensorimotor mappings or adaptation, which can then be repeated and reinforced for faster relearning during subsequent encounters.

CONCLUSION

A variety of motor, sensory and learning deficits contribute to poststroke upper limb impairment which leads to nonuse, bad-use, and lack of dexterity. Therapeutic strategies that target the underlying mechanisms of nonuse, bad-use, and lack of dexterity are needed to effectively rehabilitate the upper limb and restore movement and function post stroke.

REFERENCES

1. Feigin VL, Norrving B, Mensah GA. Global burden of stroke. *Circ Res.* 2017;120(3):439–448.
2. Kwakkel G, Kollen BJ, van der Grond J, Prevo AJ. Probability of regaining dexterity in the flaccid upper limb: impact of severity of paresis and time since onset in acute stroke. *Stroke.* 2003;34(9):2181–2186.
3. Kissela BM, Khoury JC, Alwell K, et al. Age at stroke: temporal trends in stroke incidence in a large, biracial population. *Neurology.* 2012;79(17):1781–1787.
4. Feng W, Wang J, Chhatbar PY, et al. Corticospinal tract lesion load: an imaging biomarker for stroke motor outcomes. *Ann Neurol.* 2015;78(6):860–870.
5. Prabhakaran S, Zarahn E, Riley C, et al. Inter-individual variability in the capacity for motor recovery after ischemic stroke. *Neurorehabil Neural Repair.* 2008;22(1):64–71.
6. Winters C, van Wegen EE, Daffertshofer A, Kwakkel G. Generalizability of the proportional recovery model for the upper extremity after an ischemic stroke. *Neurorehabil Neural Repair.* 2015;29(7):614–622.

7. Byblow WD, Stinear CM, Barber PA, Petoe MA, Ackerley SJ. Proportional recovery after stroke depends on corticomotor integrity. *Ann Neurol.* 2015;78(6):848–859.
8. van Kuijk AA, Pasman JW, Hendricks HT, Zwarts MJ, Geurts AC. Predicting hand motor recovery in severe stroke: the role of motor evoked potentials in relation to early clinical assessment. *Neurorehabil Neural Repair.* 2009;23(1):45–51.
9. Pundik S, McCabe JP, Hrovat K, et al. Recovery of post stroke proximal arm function, driven by complex neuroplastic bilateral brain activation patterns and predicted by baseline motor dysfunction severity. *Front Hum Neurosci.* 2015;9:394.
10. Peters DM, Fridriksson J, Stewart JC, et al. Cortical disconnection of the ipsilesional primary motor cortex is associated with gait speed and upper extremity motor impairment in chronic left hemispheric stroke. *Hum Brain Mapp.* 2018;39(1):120–132.
11. Canning CG, Ada L, Adams R, O'Dwyer NJ. Loss of strength contributes more to physical disability after stroke than loss of dexterity. *Clin Rehabil.* 2004;18(3):300–308.
12. Wagner JM, Lang CE, Sahrmann SA, Edwards DF, Dromerick AW. Sensorimotor impairments and reaching performance in subjects with poststroke hemiparesis during the first few months of recovery. *Phys Ther.* 2007;87(6):751–765.
13. Chae J, Yang G, Park BK, Labatia I. Delay in initiation and termination of muscle contraction, motor impairment, and physical disability in upper limb hemiparesis. *Muscle Nerve.* 2002;25(4):568–575.
14. Canning CG, Ada L, O'Dwyer N. Slowness to develop force contributes to weakness after stroke. *Arch Phys Med Rehabil.* 1999;80(1):66–70.
15. Suresh NL, Zhou P, Rymer WZ. Abnormal EMG-force slope estimates in the first dorsal interosseous of hemiparetic stroke survivors. *Conf Proc IEEE Eng Med Biol Soc.* 2008;2008:3562–3565.
16. McCrea PH, Eng JJ, Hodgson AJ. Saturated muscle activation contributes to compensatory reaching strategies after stroke. *J Neurophysiol.* 2005;94(5):2999–3008.
17. Mercier C, Bourbonnais D. Relative shoulder flexor and handgrip strength is related to upper limb function after stroke. *Clin Rehabil.* 2004;18(2):215–221.
18. Tyson SF, Chillala J, Hanley M, Selley AB, Tallis RC. Distribution of weakness in the upper and lower limbs poststroke. *Disabil Rehabil.* 2006;28(11):715–719.
19. Renner CI, Bungert-Kahl P, Hummelsheim H. Change of strength and rate of rise of tension relate to functional arm recovery after stroke. *Arch Phys Med Rehabil.* 2009;90(9):1548–1556.
20. Tyson SF, Hanley M, Chillala J, Selley AB, Tallis RC. Sensory loss in hospital-admitted people with stroke: characteristics, associated factors, and relationship with function. *Neurorehabil Neural Repair.* 2008;22(2):166–172.
21. Bassetti C, Bogousslavsky J, Regli F. Sensory syndromes in parietal stroke. *Neurology.* 1993;43(10):1942–1949.

22. Mercier C, Bertrand AM, Bourbonnais D. Differences in the magnitude and direction of forces during a submaximal matching task in hemiparetic subjects. *Exp Brain Res.* 2004;157(1):32−42.

23. Taub E, Heitmann RD, Barro G. Alertness, level of activity, and purposive movement following somatosensory deafferentation in monkeys. *Ann N Y Acad Sci.* 1977;290: 348−365.

24. Stecco A, Stecco C, Raghavan P. Peripheral mechanisms of spasticity and treatment implications. *Curr Phys Med Rehabil Rep.* 2014;2(2):121−127.

25. Ward AB. A literature review of the pathophysiology and onset of post-stroke spasticity. *Eur J Neurol.* 2012;19(1): 21−27.

26. Hamdy RC, Krishnaswamy G, Cancellaro V, Whalen K, Harvill L. Changes in bone mineral content and density after stroke. *Am J Phys Med Rehabil.* 1993;72(4):188−191.

27. Hamdy RC, Moore SW, Cancellaro VA, Harvill LM. Long-term effects of strokes on bone mass. *Am J Phys Med Rehabil.* 1995;74(5):351−356.

28. Ramnemark A, Nyberg L, Borssen B, Olsson T, Gustafson Y. Fractures after stroke. *Osteoporos Int.* 1998; 8(1):92−95.

29. Lundstrom E, Terent A, Borg J. Prevalence of disabling spasticity 1 year after first-ever stroke. *Eur J Neurol.* 2008; 15(6):533−539.

30. Stecco C, Gagey O, Belloni A, et al. Anatomy of the deep fascia of the upper limb. Second part: study of innervation. *Morphologie.* 2007;91(292):38−43.

31. Tesarz J, Hoheisel U, Wiedenhofer B, Mense S. Sensory innervation of the thoracolumbar fascia in rats and humans. *Neuroscience.* 2011;194:302−308.

32. Yahia L, Rhalmi S, Newman N, Isler M. Sensory innervation of human thoracolumbar fascia. An immunohistochemical study. *Acta Orthop Scand.* 1992;63(2):195−197.

33. Bell J, Holmes M. Model of the dynamics of receptor potential in a mechanoreceptor. *Math Biosci.* 1992;110(2): 139−174.

34. Gamble GE, Barberan E, Laasch HU, Bowsher D, Tyrrell PJ, Jones AK. Poststroke shoulder pain: a prospective study of the association and risk factors in 152 patients from a consecutive cohort of 205 patients presenting with stroke. *Eur J Pain.* 2002;6(6):467−474.

35. Boivie J, Leijon G, Johansson I. Central post-stroke pain−a study of the mechanisms through analyses of the sensory abnormalities. *Pain.* 1989;37(2):173−185.

36. Klit H, Finnerup NB, Jensen TS. Central post-stroke pain: clinical characteristics, pathophysiology, and management. *Lancet Neurol.* 2009;8(9):857−868.

37. Twitchell TE. The restoration of motor function following hemiplegia in man. *Brain.* 1951;74(4):443−480.

38. Whishaw IQ, Alaverdashvili M, Kolb B. The problem of relating plasticity and skilled reaching after motor cortex stroke in the rat. *Behav Brain Res.* 2008;192(1): 124−136.

39. Levin MF, Kleim JA, Wolf SL. What do motor "recovery" and "compensation" mean in patients following stroke? *Neurorehabil Neural Repair.* 2009;23(4):313−319.

40. Roh J, Rymer WZ, Perreault EJ, Yoo SB, Beer RF. Alterations in upper limb muscle synergy structure in chronic stroke survivors. *J Neurophysiol.* 2013;109(3):768−781.

41. Kamper DG, McKenna-Cole AN, Kahn LE, Reinkensmeyer DJ. Alterations in reaching after stroke and their relation to movement direction and impairment severity. *Arch Phys Med Rehabil.* 2002;83(5):702−707.

42. Reinkensmeyer DJ, McKenna Cole A, Kahn LE, Kamper DG. Directional control of reaching is preserved following mild/moderate stroke and stochastically constrained following severe stroke. *Exp Brain Res.* 2002; 143(4):525−530.

43. Cirstea MC, Levin MF. Compensatory strategies for reaching in stroke. *Brain.* 2000;123(Pt 5):940−953.

44. Raghavan P, Santello M, Gordon AM, Krakauer JW. Compensatory motor control after stroke: an alternative joint strategy for object-dependent shaping of hand posture. *J Neurophysiol.* 2010;103(6):3034−3043.

45. Skinner BF, ed. *The Behavior of Organisms: An Experimental Analysis.* New York: Appleton-Century; 1938.

46. Dickinson A. Actions and habits: the development of behavioral anatomy. *Philos Trans R Soc Lond B Biol Sci.* 1985;308:67−78.

47. Fugl-Meyer AR, Jaasko L, Leyman I, Olsson S, Steglind S. The post-stroke hemiplegic patient. 1. A method for evaluation of physical performance. *Scand J Rehabil Med.* 1975; 7(1):13−31.

48. Gladstone DJ, Danells CJ, Black SE. The fugl-meyer assessment of motor recovery after stroke: a critical review of its measurement properties. *Neurorehabil Neural Repair.* 2002; 16(3):232−240.

49. Duncan PW, Propst M, Nelson SG. Reliability of the Fugl-Meyer assessment of sensorimotor recovery following cerebrovascular accident. *Phys Therapy.* 1983;63(10): 1606−1610.

50. Hsieh YW, Wu CY, Lin KC, Chang YF, Chen CL, Liu JS. Responsiveness and validity of three outcome measures of motor function after stroke rehabilitation. *Stroke.* 2009;40(4):1386−1391.

51. Crow JL, Harmeling-van der Wel BC. Hierarchical properties of the motor function sections of the Fugl-Meyer assessment scale for people after stroke: a retrospective study. *Phys Therapy.* 2008;88(12):1554−1567.

52. Ang JH, Man DW. The discriminative power of the Wolf motor function test in assessing upper extremity functions in persons with stroke. *Int J Rehabil Res.* 2006;29(4): 357−361.

53. Canning CG, Ada L, O'Dwyer NJ. Abnormal muscle activation characteristics associated with loss of dexterity after stroke. *J Neurol Sci.* 2000;176(1):45−56.

54. Raghavan P, Lu Y, Mirchandani M, Stecco A. Human recombinant hyaluronidase injections for upper limb muscle stiffness in individuals with cerebral injury: a case series. *EBioMedicine.* 2016;9:306−313.

55. Ellis MD, Sukal-Moulton TM, Dewald JP. Impairment-based 3-D robotic intervention improves upper extremity work area in chronic stroke: targeting abnormal joint torque coupling with progressive shoulder abduction

loading. *IEEE Trans Robotics Publication IEEE Robotics Automation Soc.* 2009;25(3):549−555.

56. Ellis MD, Schut I, Dewald JPA. Flexion synergy overshadows flexor spasticity during reaching in chronic moderate to severe hemiparetic stroke. *Clin Neurophysiol.* 2017; 128(7):1308−1314.

57. Ellis MD, Kottink AI, Prange GB, Rietman JS, Buurke JH, Dewald JP. Quantifying loss of independent joint control in acute stroke with a robotic evaluation of reaching workspace. *Conf Proc IEEE Eng Med Biol Soc.* 2011;2011: 8231−8234.

58. Ellis MD, Lan Y, Yao J, Dewald JP. Robotic quantification of upper extremity loss of independent joint control or flexion synergy in individuals with hemiparetic stroke: a review of paradigms addressing the effects of shoulder abduction loading. *J Neuroeng Rehabil.* 2016; 13(1):95.

59. Cheung VC, Turolla A, Agostini M, et al. Muscle synergy patterns as physiological markers of motor cortical damage. *Proc Natl Acad Sci USA.* 2012;109(36): 14652−14656.

60. De Baets L, Jaspers E, Desloovere K, Van Deun S. A systematic review of 3D scapular kinematics and muscle activity during elevation in stroke subjects and controls. *J Electromyogr Kinesiol.* 2013;23(1):3−13.

61. De Baets L, Jaspers E, Janssens L, Van Deun S. Characteristics of neuromuscular control of the scapula after stroke: a first exploration. *Front Hum Neurosci.* 2014;8:933.

62. De Baets L, Van Deun S, Desloovere K, Jaspers E. Dynamic scapular movement analysis: is it feasible and reliable in stroke patients during arm elevation? *PLoS One.* 2013; 8(11):e79046.

63. Hall SJ, ed. *Basic Biomechanics.* McGraw Hill.

64. Michaelsen SM, Luta A, Roby-Brami A, Levin MF. Effect of trunk restraint on the recovery of reaching movements in hemiparetic patients. *Stroke.* 2001;32(8): 1875−1883.

65. Woodbury ML, Howland DR, McGuirk TE, et al. Effects of trunk restraint combined with intensive task practice on poststroke upper extremity reach and function: a pilot study. *Neurorehabil Neural Repair.* 2009;23(1):78−91.

66. Beer RF, Ellis MD, Holubar BG, Dewald JP. Impact of gravity loading on post-stroke reaching and its relationship to weakness. *Muscle Nerve.* 2007;36(2):242−250.

67. Ellis MD, Carmona C, Drogos J, Dewald JPA. Progressive abduction loading therapy with horizontal-plane viscous resistance targeting weakness and flexion synergy to treat upper limb function in chronic hemiparetic stroke: a randomized clinical trial. *Front Neurol.* 2018;9:71.

68. Ellis MD, Carmona C, Drogos J, Traxel S, Dewald JP. Progressive abduction loading therapy targeting flexion synergy to regain reaching function in chronic stroke: preliminary results from an RCT. *Conf Proc IEEE Eng Med Biol Soc.* 2016;2016:5837−5840.

69. Ellis MD, Holubar BG, Acosta AM, Beer RF, Dewald JP. Modifiability of abnormal isometric elbow and shoulder joint torque coupling after stroke. *Muscle Nerve.* 2005; 32(2):170−178.

70. Raghavan P, Aluru V, Milani S, et al. Coupled bimanual training using a non-powered device for individuals with severe hemiparesis: a pilot study. *Int J Phys Med Rehabil.* 2017;5(3).

71. Huang VS, Haith A, Mazzoni P, Krakauer JW. Rethinking motor learning and savings in adaptation paradigms: model-free memory for successful actions combines with internal models. *Neuron.* 2011;70(4):787−801.

72. Joiner WM, Smith MA. Long-term retention explained by a model of short-term learning in the adaptive control of reaching. *J Neurophysiol.* 2008;100(5):2948−2955.

73. Gordon AM, Westling G, Cole KJ, Johansson RS. Memory representations underlying motor commands used during manipulation of common and novel objects. *J Neurophysiol.* 1993;69(6):1789−1796.

74. Benson BL, Anguera JA, Seidler RD. A spatial explicit strategy reduces error but interferes with sensorimotor adaptation. *J Neurophysiol.* 2011;105(6):2843−2851.

75. Schweighofer N, Lee JY, Goh HT, et al. Mechanisms of the contextual interference effect in individuals poststroke. *J Neurophysiol.* 2011;106(5):2632−2641.

76. Galea JM, Celnik P. Brain polarization enhances the formation and retention of motor memories. *J Neurophysiol.* 2009;102(1):294−301.

77. Haith AM, Huberdeau DM, Krakauer JW. The influence of movement preparation time on the expression of visuomotor learning and savings. *J Neurosci.* 2015;35(13):5109−5117.

78. Bastian AJ. Understanding sensorimotor adaptation and learning for rehabilitation. *Curr Opin Neurol.* 2008;21(6): 628−633.

79. Krakauer JW. Motor learning: its relevance to stroke recovery and neurorehabilitation. *Curr Opin Neurol.* 2006;19(1): 84−90.

80. Takahashi CD, Reinkensmeyer DJ. Hemiparetic stroke impairs anticipatory control of arm movement. *Exp Brain Res.* 2003;149(2):131−140.

81. Kitago T, Ryan SL, Mazzoni P, Krakauer JW, Haith AM. Unlearning versus savings in visuomotor adaptation: comparing effects of washout, passage of time, and removal of errors on motor memory. *Front Hum Neurosci.* 2013;7:307.

82. Hermsdorfer J, Hagl E, Nowak DA, Marquardt C. Grip force control during object manipulation in cerebral stroke. *Clin Neurophysiol.* 2003;114(5):915−929.

83. Raghavan P, Krakauer JW, Gordon AM. Impaired anticipatory control of fingertip forces in patients with a pure motor or sensorimotor lacunar syndrome. *Brain.* 2006; 129(Pt 6):1415−1425.

84. Nowak DA, Hermsdorfer J, Topka H. Deficits of predictive grip force control during object manipulation in acute stroke. *J Neurol.* 2003;250(7):850−860.

85. Johansson RS, Westling G. Coordinated isometric muscle commands adequately and erroneously programmed for the weight during lifting task with precision grip. *Exp Brain Res.* 1988;71(1):59−71.

86. Lu Y, Bilaloglu S, Aluru V, Raghavan P. Quantifying feed-forward control: a linear scaling model for fingertip forces and object weight. *J Neurophysiol.* 2015;114(1):411−418.

87. Johansson RS, Westling G. Roles of glabrous skin receptors and sensorimotor memory in automatic control of precision grip when lifting rougher or more slippery objects. *Exp Brain Res.* 1984;56(3):550–564.

88. Bilaloglu S, Lu Y, Geller D, et al. Effect of blocking tactile information from the fingertips on adaptation and execution of grip forces to friction at the grasping surface. *J Neurophysiol.* 2016;115(3):1122–1131.

89. Marino BF, Stucchi N, Nava E, Haggard P, Maravita A. Distorting the visual size of the hand affects hand preshaping during grasping. *Exp Brain Res.* 2010;202(2):499–505.

90. Sakata H, Taira M, Kusunoki M, Murata A, Tanaka Y. The TINS Lecture. The parietal association cortex in depth perception and visual control of hand action. *Trends Neurosci.* 1997;20(8):350–357.

91. Santello M, Soechting JF. Gradual molding of the hand to object contours. *J Neurophysiol.* 1998;79(3):1307–1320.

92. Gordon AM, Forssberg H, Johansson RS, Westling G. Visual size cues in the programming of manipulative forces during precision grip. *Exp Brain Res.* 1991;83(3):477–482.

93. Sarlegna FR, Przybyla A, Sainburg RL. The influence of target sensory modality on motor planning may reflect errors in sensori-motor transformations. *Neuroscience.* 2009; 164(2):597–610.

94. Scheidt RA, Conditt MA, Secco EL, Mussa-Ivaldi FA. Interaction of visual and proprioceptive feedback during adaptation of human reaching movements. *J Neurophysiol.* 2005;93(6):3200–3213.

95. Holmes NP, Spence C. Visual bias of unseen hand position with a mirror: spatial and temporal factors. *Exp Brain Res.* 2005;166(3–4):489–497.

96. Cole KJ. Lifting a familiar object: visual size analysis, not memory for object weight, scales lift force. *Exp Brain Res.* 2008;188(4):551–557.

97. van Beers RJ, Baraduc P, Wolpert DM. Role of uncertainty in sensorimotor control. *Philos Trans R Soc Lond B Biol Sci.* 2002;357(1424):1137–1145.

98. Quaney BM, He J, Timberlake G, Dodd K, Carr C. Visuomotor training improves stroke-related ipsilesional upper extremity impairments. *Neurorehabil Neural Repair.* 2010; 24(1):52–61.

CHAPTER 9

Lower Limb Impairments After Stroke

JOHN J. LEE, MD

INTRODUCTION

According to the International Classification of Impairments, Disabilities and Handicaps (WHO), an impairment is a problem in muscle function or structure.[1] After stroke, impairments involving the lower limb such as weakness, loss of sensation, spasticity, and impaired motor coordination can lead to activity limitations such as difficulties with transfers, sit-to-stand, balance, gait, and stair ascent and descent. These impairments interact to affect function and can lead to a decreased quality of life.[2]

MOTOR IMPAIRMENT

Motor deficits are the most common impairments after stroke, with decreased strength being the most obvious.[3] Strength is defined as the ability to produce force.[4] Weakness is a cardinal feature of stroke and is the loss of capacity to generate normal muscle force levels, leading to functional impairments.[5] Strength deficits have a greater impact on function and quality of life compared to other common stroke impairments, such as sensation and motor coordination, and thus are an important target for therapy programs post stroke.[6]

Muscle strength is the force produced during a muscle contraction. There are many variables in measuring strength, from the type of contraction (isometric and isotonic) to the choice of the muscle group being tested. Other variables are the speed of contraction (isokinetic), the angle of the joint, and the muscle group to be tested. The most frequently tested muscle groups among chronic stroke patients were the knee extensors, followed by knee flexors, hip flexors, hip extensors, ankle dorsiflexors, and lastly ankle plantarflexors.[7] The knee extensors can be easily and reliably tested and are often viewed as representative of overall lower extremity strength.[8] Greater reliability can be achieved in strength measurements by using consistent test protocols, adhering to variables such as positioning, stabilization, environment, and instruction.[6]

In addition to the impaired supraspinal control caused by stroke, other mechanisms also contribute to motor weakness.[4] These include physiologic changes in paretic muscles such as a decrease in the number of functioning motor units,[9] and decreased recruitment in response to stimulation in the hemiparetic muscle.[10] There is a change in the fiber type proportion from atrophy of fast-twitch, fatigable, high force-producing fiber to hypertrophy of slow-twitch, fatigue-resistance, low-force producing fibers.[11] In addition, there are factors that cause force to be applied in abnormal directions, such as increased tone and the presence of spasticity which can lead to decreased unidirectional force production.[4] Tone is differentiated from spasticity in that tone is due to changes in the intrinsic muscle properties leading to "increased resistance to passive movement and can be attributed to the loss of sarcomeres, remodeling of muscle connective tissue, and altered periarticular connective tissue. Increased tone is also attributed to changes in passive properties of muscle contractile elements, such as alterations in cross-bridge behavior."[4]

Increasing strength in the lower extremities is a major goal of therapies as strength is related to improvement in many functional activities such as sit-to-stand,[12] gait speed,[13] gait distance,[14] and stair ascent.[15] Strength can be measured directly by dynamometers or by manual muscle testing. Strength can also be assessed indirectly through functional tests. Several commonly used functional tests are the 6 Minute Walk Test (6 MWT), 10 Meter Walk Test (10 MWT), the Timed Up-and-Go (TUG), and the Berg Balance Scale (BBS). The 6 MWT is a test to determine the maximum distance a subject can walk in 6 min and is generally used to assess gait endurance. The minimal detectable change is roughly 50 m (in chronic mild to moderate poststroke hemiparesis), and there is excellent concurrent validity with the 10 MWT, TUG, and stair climbing ascend and descend.[16] The 10 MWT measures the time it takes for the subject to walk 10 m at their preferred walking speed or their fastest speed and is used to assess gait speed. A difference of 0.10 m is considered a

Stroke Rehabilitation. https://doi.org/10.1016/B978-0-323-55381-0.00009-3

substantial meaningful change.[17] The TUG assesses the subject's time to change positions from sit to stand, walk 3 m at a comfortable speed, then turn, walk back to the chair, and sit down. It assesses mobility, balance, walking ability, and fall risk. The minimal detectable change for the TUG (in chronic mild to moderate severity stroke patients) is a change of 23%.[16] The BBS has 14 items assessing static and dynamic balance with a maximum score of 56 and classification of subjects into fall risk categories based on score. A difference by a score of 5.8 on the scale indicated a significant change (in stroke patients undergoing inpatient rehabilitation).[18] Gait distance and gait speed are important variables impacting the functionality of gait. To functionally ambulate in the home requires the ability to ambulate a distance of at least 46 m.[19] In comparison, functional community distances can range from 200 to 700 m. Having the ability to achieve speeds of at least 0.9−1.2 m/s is generally recommended for safe community ambulation.[19] Walking speed can be used to classify stroke patients into categories of ambulation ability; <0.4 m/s are household ambulators, 0.4−0.8 m/s are limited community ambulators, and >0.8 m/s are community ambulators.[20]

There are many studies examining the effects of exercise training on strength and lower extremity function; however, the exercise protocols used vary widely. Common themes that emerge are the use of progressive resistance training, power training, eccentric versus concentric training, and task-oriented training. These techniques are used individually or in combination. Due to the wide variety of exercise protocols used, it is difficult to draw comparisons as each has its unique theoretical basis and the ideal exercise program likely will include elements from multiple techniques.

Progressive resistance training (PRT) is used in many exercise programs for the healthy and stroke populations. PRT is resistance strength training using the overload principle which involves progressively increasing resistance as the body adapts to the exercise.[21] The load, or resistance, used generally starts at a certain percentage of the load that can be lifted once (one repetition maximum, 1-RM), with periodic retesting of the 1-RM and readjustment of the load to be used.[22] The 1-RM can be safely determined by using various estimation calculators. There are many options for the exercise mode which can include machines, weights, bands, pulleys, or functional activities. PRT has been shown to be safe and effective in stroke patients to increase measures of strength.[23] It has also been shown that resistance training does not increase spasticity as was once previously thought.[24] The American Heart Association

(AHA) recommends resistance training in stroke survivors but recognizes that there are no research-based guidelines. AHA states that "it may be prudent to prescribe 10 to 15 repetitions for each set of exercises similar to that recommended for patients after myocardial infarction. Such regimens should be performed 2 to 3 days per week and include a minimum of 1 set of 8 to 10 different exercises that involve the major muscle groups of the torso, as well as the upper and lower extremities."[25]

Task-oriented training focuses on improving function through use of exercises that mimic functional tasks. Resistance training principles are often incorporated in task-oriented exercises. A Cochrane review on repetitive task training for improving functional ability after stroke showed improvements in many functional outcomes.[26] The authors conclude that repetitive task-oriented training of the lower limb resulted in significant benefit on lower limb function (walking distance, functional ambulation, standing balance/reach). Many of the interventions in the studies examined were mixed, containing elements of strength training and endurance, in addition to having repetition and functional practice. Thus the mechanism of improvements for lower limb functional gains cannot be elucidated. Examples of some of the types of exercise used can be seen in a study by Yang et al. which showed improvements in strength and functional measures by using a task-oriented resistance training program of the lower extremities in chronic stroke patients.[27] In this study, the exercises used were standing and reaching for objects in different directions; sit-to-stand from various chair heights; stepping forward, backward, and sideways onto blocks of varying heights; and heel raises in standing posture. The exercises were performed in a circuit, with total of 30 min per session, 3 times a week for 4 weeks. Improvements were seen in gait velocity, cadence, stride length, 6 MWT, and TUG. The authors speculate that the functional improvements might be due to motor unit recruitment and motor learning that occurred through the task-oriented training.

Power is a component of muscle function that has been studied in strength training in stroke patients. Power is defined as the product of force and velocity and is the ability to develop force quickly. Power, in addition to strength, has a significant predictive value for functional abilities in activities such as gait, stair climbing, sit-to-stand, and affects balance; more so than muscle strength alone.[28] Power generally requires specialized equipment for measurement, but power has been shown to be associated with more commonly used clinical functional tests involving activities assessing walk speed, sit-to-stand (Five-Times-Sit-to-Stand-Test), or stair climbing ability (Stair Climb Power Test).[29]

In stroke patients, power in the lower extremities is decreased in both the involved and the uninvolved leg.[30] The deficits in power are due to factors starting with decreased voluntary muscle activation from cortical damage, with a subsequent loss of motor units, and with the remaining motor units exhibiting reduced discharge rates and prolonged contraction times.[28] In addition, other muscle changes occurring post stroke such as the reduction in muscle cross-sectional area and in Type II muscle fiber numbers and reduced muscle fiber lengths all contribute to decreased power generation.[27]

Due to the association between power and the ability to perform functional tasks, training programs have been devised targeting power output. Training with the aim to increase power involves exercising with loads that can be moved rapidly and under safe control. Morgan et al. implemented an exercise program aimed at improving muscle power by using several lower extremity exercises (leg press, calf raises, and jump training all performed on a supine exercise device) with the instruction to perform the concentric phase as quickly as possible.[31] There was also a fast walking component to this program (repeated 10 m trials of fast walking, 10 trials per session, at a minimum of 125% of self-selected walking speed). The program consisted of 3 sessions per week for 8 weeks. Using this protocol, stroke patients in the chronic stage had improved power output in the lower extremities (measured with an isokinetic dynamometer at the knee extensors and ankle plantarflexors) and demonstrated an increase in the self-selected and fastest comfortable walking speed. The key to this program and others targeting power is in performing the chosen exercises with sufficient speed to train the velocity component of the power equation. The choice of the appropriate resistance is important as well. For example, power output of the knee extensors at 40% of 1 RM was found to explain more variability in habitual walking speed than 70% of 1 RM.[32] This suggests that different tasks such as walking, sit-to-stand, and stair climbing may have different power requirements, and that there is an optimal training resistance to maximize the power output for each task.

Eccentric muscle actions (motion of the muscle while it is lengthening under load) are an important part of normal muscle function in daily activities. Muscles in the lower extremity utilize concentric and eccentric muscle actions in activities such as ambulation (particularly down a slope) and stairs (particularly in descent). Exercises emphasizing the eccentric component are useful in increasing muscle strength and function. Eccentric muscle actions are able to produce greater force than concentric actions in the healthy[33] and also appear to be more preserved after stroke.[34] Thus a higher load (if emphasizing eccentric actions as compared to concentric) can be used in the post-stroke patient to impart a greater training stimulus to drive recovery. In a study emphasizing eccentric exercise using a unilateral eccentric-overload flywheel leg press machine, there were increases in the quadriceps femoris volume (measured by MRI) and muscle power.[35] In another study by the same group using the same eccentrically focused exercise leg press machine, power improved along with balance (BBS), 30 - s Chair-Stand Test, and TUG scores.[36] Similar results were found in another study training ankle dorsiflexion/plantarflexion, knee extension/flexion, and hip abduction where there was an increase in power output at the quadriceps that was also associated with an increase in gait speed.[37] Despite the lack of intervention on the untrained leg, in both studies, there was improvement in the power of the untrained leg as well. This was thought to be due to cross-education, which is defined as the increase in strength of an untrained limb after training of the contralateral homologous limb.[38]

All the muscles of the lower extremity serve an individual and collective function in gait. When examining higher level outcome measures such as balance, gait speed, and endurance, it is difficult to separate out the individual contributions of each muscle group. The choice of which muscle groups to target in strength training programs invariably will have an impact on gait function. In a literature search on the task specificity of strength training for walking in neurologic conditions, Williams et al. found there to be a predominance of strengthening protocols training the knee flexors and extensors.[19] While the muscles that cross the knee joint serve an important function in gait, the authors comment that these muscles have a relatively minor role in propulsive force generation in gait compared to the three main muscle groups responsible for propulsive strength in gait; (1) ankle plantarflexor power generation at push-off, (2) hip extensor power generation in early stance, and (3) hip flexor power generation terminal stance and early swing phase. Training programs geared toward improving gait propulsive function, that is, gait speed, should target these three muscle groups and should do so in the range of motion and contraction speeds that occur during gait. Thus, the authors proposed that to improve the propulsive function of gait, the ideal training parameters for the three muscle groups should be concentrically focused at high angular velocities and the training range of motion at the ankle plantar flexors should be 5 degrees of dorsiflexion to 20 degrees of plantarflexion, at the hip flexors should be in the range of 10 degrees of hip extension to 10 degrees of hip flexion and at the hip extensors should be in the range from 40 to 20 degrees of hip flexion. This illustrates the concept of training specificity; "the closer the training routine is to the requirements of the desired outcome (i.e., a specific exercise task or performance criteria), the better will be the outcome."[39] There were a wide variety of exercise seen, many functionally based, with some examples being calf raises, seated leg press, sit-to-stand activities, squats, stepping or step-ups. Other exercise variables were use of bodyweight, weights, pneumatic or isokinetic machines, and resistance bands.

In an observational study (of chronic post-stroke independent ambulators) examining the individual and the relative association between the strength of 12 muscle groups in the affected lower extremity and walking speed, when the strength of all the muscle groups were examined individually, nine muscle groups were found to be significantly associated with walking speed, indicating the importance of each muscle group to gait. When the strength of the muscle groups was examined in combination, using multiple regression analysis, only the ankle dorsiflexors were found to have a significant association with walking speed.[40] The authors postulated that this might be because all of the study participants were all able to ambulate without assistive devices, and therefore were able to generate sufficient extensor moment for stability in the stance phase. In this group of subjects, the swing phase of gait might be a greater determinant of overall gait speed where ankle dorsiflexor weakness will have a larger effect. Thus, as can be seen, the choice of which muscle groups to be strengthened and by which method needs to be tailored according to the impairments, functional levels, and desired outcomes.

SOMATOSENSORY IMPAIRMENT

Somatosensory impairments are common post stroke with reported ranges from 11% to 85%.[41] Impaired sensation has been defined as an inability of the nervous system to accurately perceive, process, and interpret cutaneous and proprioceptive feedback. Important sensory modalities are touch, proprioception, pressure, pain, and temperature. Clinically, the most frequently tested sensory modalities post stroke are touch and proprioception. Within each of these

two modalities, two aspects can be tested: detection and discrimination.[42] Detection refers to the ability to sense joint movement and touch. Discrimination is more detailed and refers to the ability to detect the direction of movement and the location of the touch.

Sensory examinations performed in clinical practice are generally not standardized in technique, are subjective in nature, and can be affected by other stroke impairments such as attention, cognition, and language.[43] Standardized assessment tests have been developed, though they are mainly used in research settings to assess sensation. Some of these tests have lower extremity components. The Fugl–Meyer assessment has a sensory scale which assesses light touch (leg, sole of foot) and position sense (great toe, ankle, knee, hip) at various areas on the lower extremity.[44] The Rivermead Assessment of Somatosensory Performance (RASP) tests six sensations: sharp/dull discrimination, surface pressure, tactile localization, temperature discrimination, joint movement, and movement discrimination; in the lower extremities it is tested on the foot,[45] though it requires the use of specialized equipment such as the neurometer (measuring pressure), the neurotemp (measure temperature in temperature discrimination), and the neurodiscriminator (assess two-point discrimination). The Nottingham Sensory Assessment has components assessing light touch, pressure, pinprick, temperature, tactile localization, bilateral simultaneous touch, proprioception, two-point discrimination, and stereognosis.[46]

Sensation has an important role in gait other than motor performance since gait depends on both intact feedforward and intact feedback from afferent inputs.[47] The modalities of touch and proprioception work together to provide the necessary input regarding contact with the ground, the load borne through the limb, and the position and movements of limb segments so that gait can be as symmetrical and as efficient as possible. In particular, the sensory system is vitally important to changing environmental conditions and obstacles.[48]

Sensory impairment has been found to be associated with poor balance[49] and increased incidence of falls.[50] The research on the degree of influence of somatosensory impairments on gait is inconclusive. When compared to other impairments at the ankle, such as motor strength and spasticity, somatosensory impairments have a lesser effect on gait velocity and gait symmetry.[51] In a study examining the relationship of ankle joint position sense to gait velocity and stride length in chronic stroke patients who can ambulate at least 10 m without assistive devices, while the joint position sense at the ankle was found to have contributed significantly to gait velocity and stride length, a direct relationship was not found.[52] The study author theorized that the lack of a direct relationship was due to the redundancy in the afferent control of locomotion, so that if proprioception was impaired other somatosensory pathways, such as the activation of pressure sensation in weight bearing during gait, can be utilized to compensate for the impaired proprioception. Also, in addition to the somatosensory system, locomotion utilizes input from the visual and vestibular systems and that each system can compensate to some degree for impairments elsewhere.[53]

Therapy protocols targeting proprioception have been developed to improve balance and overall gait function. In a review of proprioceptive training for improving motor function, the different types of training methods were classified into five broad categories: (1) active movement/balance training (participants actively move the limb); (2) passive movement training (passive movement of limb); (3) somatosensory stimulation/training (various forms of stimulation such as vibrotactile, thermal, or magnetic stimulation; multisomatosensory stimulation; acupuncture); (4) somatosensory discrimination training (discriminate between two somatosensory stimuli); and, (5) combined/multiple system training.[54] The majority of studies fell into the active movement/balance category. Training activities in this group included single-joint and multijoint active movements, stepping on specific target, walking, stair-stepping, and balance training using single and double limb on surfaces of differing stability. Somatosensory training in stroke studies (most of which involved the upper extremities) yielded the highest levels of improvement compared to studies involving other conditions. From this review, several conclusions were drawn, which may be applicable to the stroke population: (1) Proprioceptive training can be effective in improving proprioceptive function, with the majority of improvement rates greater than 20%; and (2) longer lasting interventions seemed to produce greater benefits, with training regimens lasting longer than 6 weeks resulting in greater improvements in proprioceptive and/or motor function.

The timecourse of recovery of sensory impairments is not as well defined as recovery from motor impairments. In a review by Kessner et al., the general consensus was that somatosensory deficits mainly recover during the first 3−6 months post stroke but not all modalities recover equally.[55] In an observational study of 18 patients 6 months after stroke the proprioception subset of sensation (as assessed by the RASP)

demonstrated the greatest level of recovery.[56] It was theorized that as the proprioceptive sense is closely linked to movement, this might be partly due to the predominant focus on movement during traditional rehabilitation from stroke.

SPASTICITY

Spasticity in the lower extremities is common, affecting approximately 40% of hemiparetic patients 6 months post ischemic stroke.[57] Spasticity is a velocity-dependent increase in tonic stretch reflexes and causes agonist and antagonist muscle coordination issues affecting balance and gait kinematics. In the lower extremities, common areas affected by spasticity are the hip, knee, ankle, and toes.[58] Hip flexor spasticity involving the rectus femoris and the iliopsoas can lead to a crouched gait pattern.[59] Knee extensor spasticity can contribute to a stiff-legged gait pattern with decreased knee flexion during the swing phase of gait, leading to a functional increase in leg length, causing difficulty in clearing the limb during swing phase.[59] Compensatory maneuvers such as circumduction, hip-hiking, or vaulting may be adopted to achieve swing limb advancement.[59] Ankle plantarflexion spasticity may lead to an equinovarus foot with decreased ankle dorsiflexion affecting forward propulsion in stance and limb clearance in swing phase of gait.[59] Due to its negative effects, spasticity has been a frequent target of rehabilitation treatment.

Botulinum neurotoxin injection (BoNT) is a common treatment for spasticity and has been shown to reduce spasticity[60] and increase passive and active joint range of motion.[61] Its effect on measures of gait function has been mixed. In a study of chronic stroke patients who received BoNT for ankle plantarflexor spasticity, all patients had increased ankle joint mobility but no changes in the temporal distance parameters of gait or in kinetic outcomes.[62] Other studies have also found no significant effect of BoNT injection on functional measure[63] while others have found a benefit.[64] These studies have examined the effect of BoNT alone. When BoNT injections have been paired with therapies, improvements in functional outcomes have been demonstrated. BoNT injection combined with therapy interventions have been shown to improve maximal gait speed, ambulation distance, and stair ascent and descent.[65] In this study by Roche et al., patients who underwent BoNT injection were randomized into a therapy or control (no therapy) group. Therapy consisted of a standardized home exercise program (3 parts: task-oriented exercises, stretching, and strengthening exercises; 10 min each). The improvement in the BoNT + therapy group was thought to be due to the gain in strength from the therapy exercises and the task-oriented activities, which had a carryover effect to the functional tests used.

Spasticity can affect the center of pressure excursions in the anteroposterior or mediolateral directions and postural sway,[66] thus leading to balance deficits. Ankle plantarflexor spasticity can cause the foot to be in an equinovarus position leading to a decreased foot surface area contact with the ground and also decreased dorsiflexion in stance phase of gait, both of which can theoretically lead to impaired balance. The unilateral nature of spasticity and limb involvement in stroke can also contribute to impaired balance.[67] Balance, or postural control, is affected by multifactorial causes, with spasticity being only one component; and with stroke patients typically having multiple impairments that may each affect balance, it is difficult to separate the individual contributions. In a review of poststroke spasticity and BoNT injections on standing balance, the overall conclusion was that balance is impaired in subjects with spasticity, but there is insufficient evidence to draw a causal relationship to spasticity.[67] This review also discussed the evidence of the effect of BoNT injections on spastic plantarflexors and found that while there were subjective improvements in balance measures, the evidence is weak due to lack of randomization, control group comparison, objective assessment measures of balance, and standard clinical scales.

Spasticity does have an effect on gait symmetry. In a study assessing the contributions of lower extremity motor strength, somatosensory impairments, and spasticity to gait speed post mild to moderate severity stroke, spasticity was the greatest contributor to gait asymmetry, while motor strength had the greatest impact on gait speed.[68]

MOTOR COORDINATION AND BALANCE

Lower limb motor coordination is impaired post stroke in patients with hemiparesis,[69] and is associated with impaired balance and gait.[70] Improving motor coordination is thus an important target for therapies. However, there is not a clear definition of motor coordination nor is there consistent use of standardized tests. In a general sense, motor coordination or dexterity refers to the ability to perform a motor task in an accurate, rapid, and controlled manner.[71] Krasovsky et al. proposed a more detailed definition, factoring in the spatial and temporal components of locomotion: "the ability to maintain a context-dependent and phase-dependent cyclical relationship between different body segments or joints in both spatial and temporal domains."[72] In their review, the end results of impaired motor coordination were decreased speed, strength, and precision in motor movement, which were caused by decreased supraspinal drive post stroke, and its associated constellation of effects such as increased recurrent inhibition, increased cocontraction, and the remodeling changes of the hemiparetic muscles such as decreased number of fast twitch motor units and increased atrophy of type II fibers.

As seen from its definition, the measurement of motor coordination will assess the speed and quality when performing certain movements. These measures involve spatial and temporal indices of gait symmetry, cross-correlations of lower limb or axial segment displacement, velocity or acceleration trajectories, or measures of relative phase.[73] Two simple clinical examples are the finger-to-nose test in the upper extremity and the heel-to-shin test for the lower extremity. Motor coordination will also be reflected in the more global tests of balance, gait speed, and endurance. To specifically assess lower extremity motor coordination, the Lower Extremity Motor Coordination Test (LEMOCOT) has been developed to more specifically evaluate motor coordination in the lower extremity. It requires subjects to alternatively touch their foot to a proximal and distal target on the floor as fast and accurately as possible in a 20-s span while in a seated position.[74] It has good convergent construct validity with lower extremity motor function (FMA), balance (Berg Balance Scale) and walk speed (5-m walk test), and good discriminant validity for people living in different environments (home, senior residences, or long-term care).[74]

In a review of rehabilitation interventions for coordination of walking following stroke, the various interventions seen were grouped into four categories: (1) task specific practice of walking, (2) ankle-foot orthoses (AFO) or functional electrical stimulation (FES), (3) auditory cueing, and (4) exercise.[73] Exercise and AFO/FES interventions sought to improve coordination by addressing the impairment while task-specific practice and auditory cueing sought to improve coordination by stimulating cortical reorganization through repetition of an activity. Among these categories, auditory cueing and task-specific practice positively influenced gait coordination after stroke; however, many of the studies pooled were of small sample sizes, selected convenience samples, and of nonrandomized design.

Motor coordination is also related to balance. Balance, or postural control, refers to the ability to maintain the center of gravity within the base of support and depends upon effective interactions between sensory input, neural processing, and motor output (strength and motor coordination). Balance control is achieved through the interaction of multiple body systems and depends upon several mechanisms: (1) sensory processes and their integration (sensory afferents), (2) biomechanical constraints, (3) movement strategies, (4) cognitive processing, and (5) perception of verticality.[75] Sensory processes and their integration involves the three main sensory mechanisms—somatosensory, visual, and vestibular. In a healthy individual, the somatosensory afferents account for around 70% of the information needed to maintain postural control; vestibular afferents contribute 20%; and visual input 10%.[76] In poststroke patients who have proprioceptive impairments in the lower extremity, there may be a greater reliance on the visual and vestibular systems to maintain postural control. This is an example of sensory reweighting.[77] Examples of biomechanical constraints are decreased muscle force, range of motion, increased tone, and impaired muscle control. There are three movement strategies used to restore balance: ankle strategy which uses mainly the ankle plantar and dorsiflexors (used when there is mild sway),[78] hip strategy using mainly the hip and trunk muscles (used when there is greater or faster disturbance exceeding what the ankle strategy can handle), and stepping strategy (shifting of the base of support to match a moving center of gravity).[79] Cognitive processing refers to the integration of sensory input and cognitive elements such as attention, experience, and intention. Perception of verticality is the body's perception of vertical position and depends on the CNS integration of the somatosensory, vestibular, and visual information.

Balance can be measured by functional tests such as the BBS, the TUGT, the Tinetti Assessment Tool, the Functional Reach Test, the FMA—Balance subscale, Postural Assessment Scale for Stroke Patients (PASS), the Dynamic Gait Index, the Multidirectional Reach Test, the Activities-Specific Balance Confidence Scale, and the Fullerton Balance Scale.[80] These tests require little equipment and are easy to administer, but are limited in their lack of sensitivity to slight changes, in being susceptible to the ceiling effect, and in their subjective nature. Laboratory measurements of balance, through use of force platforms and accelerometers, are more objective and sensitive in measuring balance than functional tests. Posturography uses force platforms to detect movements in the body and thus can be used to assess forces that affect static and dynamic balance.[81] Accelerometers measure motion velocity and acceleration of body parts in the vertical, horizontal, and transverse axis, and can be used to assess ambulation, posture, and postural changes.[82]

In stroke patients, compared to the general population of elderly people, balance is impaired and falls are very common during the acute inpatient rehabilitation phase (mainly during transfers)[83] as well as the community dwelling chronic phase (mainly during ambulation).[84] Multiple impairments after stroke affect balance; from motor deficits, somatosensory impairments, motor coordination to the cognitive processing needed. Balance is a frequent target of therapies and a wide variety of techniques addressing the different aspects of balance have been devised. Standing on an unstable surface increases the difficulty of maintaining balance, stimulates the somatosensory system, trains posture coordination, and has been found to improve balance in stroke patients.[85] Therapies aimed at trunk control also improve balance as the trunk is involved in postural control by preparing the body for the movement of the extremities against gravity, in smoothing the movement of the center of gravity, and in easing body movement into new postures.[86] Dual task training is another technique with positive results on balance involving simultaneous performance of two tasks, such as gait or balance training while performing a cognitive task or a different motor task (such as involving the upper extremity) to address the effect to balance from dual task-interference.[87] Balance training on force platforms, which can track the patient's center of gravity during weight or posture shifting, with visual feedback given in real time to allow corrective strategies, has been shown to improve balance in chronic stroke patients.[88]

CONCLUSIONS

Lower limb impairments are common after stroke, ranging from motor weakness, somatosensory impairments, and spasticity, to motor coordination affecting static and dynamic balance, gait symmetry, speed, and endurance. These impairments often coexist and need to be addressed and alleviated as best as possible to improve quality of life. Many different therapy options have been devised to address these impairments and functional deficits, with each having its rationale and purported benefit. While there might be general guidelines for various therapy protocols, to increase effectiveness, the therapy regimen should be individualized and multifaceted, addressing multiple impairments and their mechanisms and taking into account the patient's functional status and goals.

REFERENCES

1. World Health Organization. *World Report on Disability.* World Health Organization; 2011.
2. Abubakar SA, Isezuo SA. Health related quality of life of stroke survivors: experience of a stroke unit. *Int Journal Biomedical Science IJBS.* 2012;8(3):183.
3. Bohannon RW. Muscle strength and muscle training after stroke. *J Rehabil Med.* 2007;39(1):14–20.
4. American College of Sports Medicine. *ACSM's Resource Manual for Guidelines for Exercise Testing and Prescription.* Lippincott Williams & Wilkins; 2012.
5. Arene N, Hider J. Understanding motor impairment in the paretic limb after stroke: a review of literature. *Top Stroke Rehabil.* 2009;16(5):346–356.
6. Faria-Fortini I, Basilio ML, Polese JC, et al. Strength deficits of the paretic lower extremity muscles were the impairment variables that best explained restrictions in participation after stroke. *Disability and rehabilitation.* 2016;39. 2016;(21):2158–2163.
7. Rabelo M, Guilherme SN, Amante NM, et al. Reliability of muscle strength assessment in chronic post-stroke hemiparesis: a systematic review and meta-analysis. *Top Stroke Rehabil.* 2016;23(1):26–36.
8. Clark DJ, Condliffe EG, Patten C. Reliability of concentric and eccentric torque during isokinetic knee extension in post-stroke hemiparesis. *Clin Biomech.* 2006;21(4): 395–404.
9. Brooks MH, Engel WK. The histographic analysis of human biopsies with regard to fiber types: 2. Diseases of upper and lower motor neurons. *Neurology.* 1969;19: 378–393.
10. Edstrom L, Grimby L, Hannerz J. Correlation between recruitment order of motor units and muscle atrophy pattern in upper motor neuron lesion: significance of spasticity. *Experimentia.* 1973;29:560–561.
11. Edstrom L. Selective changes in the sizes of red and white muscle fibers in upper motor neuron lesions and Parkinsonism. *J Neurol Sci.* 1970;11:537–550.
12. Bohannon RW. Knee extension strength and body weight determine sit-to-stand independence after stroke. *Physiother Theory Practice.* January 1, 2007;23(5):291–297.
13. Flansbjer U-B, Downham D, Lexell J. Knee muscle strength, gait performance, and perceived participation after stroke. *Arch Phys Med Rehabil.* 2006;87:974–980.
14. Bohannon RW. Selected determinants of ambulatory capacity in patients with hemiplegia. *Clin Rehabil.* 1989; 3:47–53.
15. Bohannon RW, Walsh S. Association of paretic lower extremity muscle strength and standing balance with stair-climbing ability in patients with stroke. *J Stroke Cerebrovasc Dis.* 1991;1(3):129–133.
16. Flansbjer UB, Holmbäck AM, Downham D, Patten C, Lexell J. Reliability of gait performance tests in men and women with hemiparesis after stroke. *J Rehabil Med.* 2005;37(2):75–82.
17. Perera S, Mody S, et al. Meaningful change and responsiveness in common physical performance measures in older adults. *J Am Geriatrics Soc.* 2006;54(5):743–749.
18. Stevenson TJ. Detecting change in patients with stroke using the Berg Balance Scale. *Aust J Physiother.* 2001;47(1): 29–38.
19. Andrews AW, Chinworth SA, Bourassa M, et al. Update on distance and velocity requirements for community ambulation. *J Geriatr Phys Ther.* 2010;33:128–134.
20. Bowden M, Balasubramanian C, et al. Validation of a speed-based classification system using quantitative measures of walking performance poststroke. *Neurorehabil Neural Repair.* 2008;22(6):672.
21. DeLorme TL, Watkins AL. Techniques of progressive resistance exercises. *Arch Phys Med.* 1948;29:263–273.
22. Patten C, Lexell J, Brown HE. Weakness and strength training in persons with poststroke hemiplegia: rationale, method, and efficacy. *J Rehabil Res Dev.* 2004;41(3):293.
23. Lexell J. Muscle structure and function in chronic neurological disorders: the potential of exercise to improve activities of daily living. *Exerc Sport Sci Rev.* 2000;28: 80–84.
24. Ada L, Dorsch S, Canning CG. Strengthening interventions increase strength and improve activity after stroke: a systematic review. *Aust J Physiother.* 2006;52(4):241–248.
25. Billinger SA, Arena R, Bernhardt J, et al. Physical activity and exercise recommendations for stroke survivors. *Stroke.* 2014;45(8):2532–2553.
26. French B, Thomas LH, Coupe J, et al. *Repetitive Task Training for Improving Functional Ability after Stroke.* The Cochrane Library; January 1, 2016.
27. Yang YR, Wang RY, Lin KH, Chu MY, Chan RC. Task-oriented progressive resistance strength training improves muscle strength and functional performance in individuals with stroke. *Clin Rehabil.* October 2006;20(10):860–870.
28. Md JF, Kiely DK, Herman S, et al. The relationship between leg power and physical performance in mobility-limited older people. *J Am Geriatrics Soc.* 2002;50(3):461–467.
29. Bean JF, Kiely DK, LaRose S, et al. Is stair climb power a clinically relevant measure of leg power impairments in at-risk older adults? *Arch Phys Med Rehabil.* 2007;88:604–609.
30. Stavric VA, McNair PJ. Optimizing muscle power after stroke: a cross-sectional study. *J Neuroeng Rehabil.* 2012; 9(67):1–8.
31. Morgan P, Embry A, Perry L, et al. Feasibility of lower-limb muscle power training to enhance locomotor function poststroke. *J Rehabil Res Dev.* 2015;52(1):77–84.
32. Cuoco A, Callahan DM, Sayers S, Frontera WR, Bean J, Fielding RA. Impact of muscle power and force on gait speed in disabled older men and women. *J Gerontol Ser A Biol Sci Med Sci.* 2004;59(11):1200–1206.
33. Tesch PA, Dudley GA, Duvoisin MR, Hather BM, Harris RT. Force and EMG signal patterns during repeated bouts of concentric or eccentric muscle actions. *Acta Physiol.* 1990; 138(3):263–271.

34. Clark DJ, Condliffe EG, Patten C. Activation impairment alters muscle torque-velocity in the knee extensors of persons with post-stroke hemiparesis. *Clin Neurophysiol.* 2006; 17(10):2328–2337.

35. Fernandez-Gonzalo R, Fernandez-Gonzalo S, Turin M, et al. Muscle, functional and cognitive adaptations after flywheel resistance training in stroke patients: a pilot randomized controlled trial. *J Neuroeng Rehabil.* April 6, 2016;13:37.

36. Fernandez-Gonzalo R, Nissemark C, Åslund B, Tesch PA, Sojka P. Chronic stroke patients show early and robust improvements in muscle and functional performance in response to eccentric-overload flywheel resistance training: a pilot study. *J Neuroeng Rehabil.* 2014;11(1):150.

37. Clark DJ, Patten C. Eccentric versus concentric resistance training to enhance neuromuscular activation and walking speed following stroke. *Neurorehabil Neural Repair.* 2013; 27(4):335–344.

38. Zhou S. Chronic neural adaptations to unilateral exercise: mechanisms of cross education. *Exerc Sport Sci Rev.* 2000; 28(4):177–184.

39. Hawley JA. Specificity of training adaptation: time for a rethink? *J Physiol.* 2008;586(1):1–2.

40. Dorsch S, Ada L, Canning CG, et al. The strength of the ankle dorsiflexors has a significant contribution to walking speed in people who can walk independently after stroke: an observational study. *Arch Phys Med Rehabil.* 2012;93(6): 1072–1076.

41. Sullivan JE, Hedman LD. Sensory dysfunction following stroke: incidence, significance, examination, and intervention. *Top Stroke Rehabil.* 2008;15(3):200–217.

42. Tyson SF, Crow JL, Connell L, Winward C, Hillier S. Sensory impairments of the lower limb after stroke: a pooled analysis of individual patient data. *Top Stroke Rehabil.* 2013;20(5):441–449.

43. Pumpa LU, Cahill LS, Carey LM. Somatosensory assessment and treatment after stroke: an evidence-practice gap. *Aust Occup Ther J.* 2015;62(2):93–104.

44. Fugl-Meyer AR, Jääskö L, Leyman I, Olsson S, Steglind S. The post-stroke hemiplegic patient. 1. A method for evaluation of physical performance. *Scand J Rehabil Med.* 1975; 7(1):13–31.

45. Winward CE, Halligan PW, Wade DT. The Rivermead assessment of somatosensory performance (RASP): standardization and reliability data. *Clin Rehabil.* 2002;16(5): 523–533.

46. Lincoln NB, Jackson JM, Adams SA. Reliability and revision of the Nottingham sensory assessment for stroke patients. *Physiotherapy.* 1998;84(8):358–365.

47. O'Sullivan S, Schmitz T. Assessment and treatment. In: O'Sullivan S, Schmitz T, eds. *Physical Rehabilitation.* Philadelphia, PA: FA Davis; 1988.

48. Dietz V, Muller R, Colombo G. Locomotor activity in spinal man: significance of afferent input from joint and load receptors. *Brain.* 2002;125(12):2626–2634.

49. Tyson SF, Hanley M, Chillala J, Selley AB, Tallis RC. Sensory loss in hospital-admitted people with stroke: characteristics, associated factors, and relationship with function. *Neurorehabil Neural Repair.* 2008;22(2):166–172.

50. Yates JS, Lai SM, Duncan PW, et al. Falls in community-dwelling stroke survivors: an accumulated impairments model. *J Rehabil Res Dev.* 2002;39(3):385–394.

51. Lin PY, Yang YR, Cheng SJ, et al. The relationship between ankle impairments and gait velocity and symmetry in people with stroke. *Arch Phys Med Rehabil.* 2006;87(4): 562–568.

52. Lin S. Motor function and joint position sense in relation to gait performance in chronic stroke patients. *Arch Phys Med Rehabil.* 2005;86:197–203.

53. Shumway-Cook A, Woollacott MH. Control of normal mobility. In: *Motor Control: Theory and Practical Applications.* Baltimore: Williams and Wilkens; 2001:p239–p268.

54. Aman JE, Elangovan N, Yeh IL, et al. The effectiveness of proprioceptive training for improving motor function: a systematic review. *Front Hum Neurosci.* January 28, 2015; 8:1075.

55. Kessner SS, Bingel U, Thomalla G. Somatosensory deficits after stroke: a scoping review. *Top Stroke Rehabil.* April 2016;23(2):136–144.

56. Winward CE, Halligan PW, Wade DT. Somatosensory recovery: a longitudinal study of the first 6 months after unilateral stroke. *Disabil Rehabil.* 2007;29(4):293–299.

57. Urban PP, Wolf T, Uebele M, et al. Occurence and clinical predictors of spasticity after ischemic stroke. *Stroke.* 2010; 41(9):2016–2020.

58. Brashear A, Elovic E. *Spasticity: Diagnosis and Management.* Demos Medical Publishing; 2011.

59. Thibaut A, Chatelle C, Ziegler E, Bruno MA, Laureys S, Gosseries O. Spasticity after stroke: physiology, assessment and treatment. *Brain Inj.* 2013;27(10):1093–1105.

60. Burbaud P, Wiart L, Dubos JL, et al. A randomised, double blind, placebo controlled trial of botulinum toxin in the treatment of spastic foot in hemiparetic patients. *J Neurol Neurosurg Psychiatry.* 1996;61(3):265–269.

61. Dengler R, Neyer U, Wohlfarth K, Bettig U, Janzik HH. Local botulinum toxin in the treatment of spastic drop foot. *J Neurology.* 1992;239(7):375–378.

62. Novak AC, Olney SJ, Bagg S, Brouwer B. Gait changes following botulinum toxin A treatment in stroke. *Top Stroke Rehabilitation.* 2009;16(5):367–376.

63. Robertson JV, Pradon D, Bensmail D, Fermanian C, Bussel B, Roche N. Relevance of botulinum toxin injection and nerve block of rectus femoris to kinematic and functional parameters of stiff knee gait in hemiplegic adults. *Gait Posture.* 2009;29(1):108–112.

64. Hutin E, Pradon D, Barbier F, Gracies JM, Bussel B, Roche N. Lower limb coordination in hemiparetic subjects: impact of botulinum toxin injections into rectus femoris. *Neurorehabil Neural Repair.* 2010;24(5): 442–449.

65. Roche N, Zory R, Sauthier A, Bonnyaud C, Pradon D, Bensmail D. Effect of rehabilitation and botulinum toxin injection on gait in chronic stroke patients: a randomized controlled study. *J Rehabil Med.* 2015;47(1):31–37.

66. Sosnoff JJ, Shin S, Motl RW. Multiple sclerosis and postural control: the role of spasticity. *Arch Phys Med Rehabil.* 2010; 91(1):93–99.

67. Phadke CP, Ismail F, Boulias C, Gage W, Mochizuki G. The impact of post-stroke spasticity and botulinum toxin on standing balance: a systematic review. *Exp Rev Neurotherap.* 2014;14(3):319–327.

68. Hsu AL, Tang PF, Jan MH. Analysis of impairments influencing gait velocity and asymmetry of hemiplegic patients after mild to moderate stroke. *Arch Phys Med Rehabil.* 2003; 84(8):1185–1193.

69. Menezes KK, Nascimento LR, Pinheiro MB, et al. Lower-limb motor coordination is significantly impaired in ambulatory people with chronic stroke: a cross-sectional study. *J Rehabil Med.* April 1, 2017;49:322–326.

70. Hyndman D, Ashburn A, Stack E. Fall events among people with stroke living in the community: circumstances of falls and characteristics of fallers. *Arch Phys Med Rehabil.* 2002;83(2):165–170.

71. Bernstein NA. *Dexterity and Its Development.* 1st ed. Mahwah: Lawrence Erlbaum Associates; 1996.

72. Krasovsky T, Levin MF. Toward a better understanding of coordination in healthy and poststroke gait. *Neurorehabil Neural Repair.* 2010;24(3):213–224.

73. Hollands KL, Pelton TA, Tyson SF, Hollands MA, van Vliet PM. Interventions for coordination of walking following stroke: systematic review. *Gait Posture.* 2012; 35(3):349–359.

74. Desrosiers J, Rochette A, Corriveau H. Validation of a new lower-extremity motor coordination test. *Arch Phys Med Rehabil.* 2005;86(5):993–998.

75. Oliveira CB, Medeiros RT, Frota NAF, et al. Balance control in hemiparetic patients: main tools for evaluation. *J Rehabil Res Dev.* 2008;45(8):1215–1226.

76. Peterka JR. Sensorimotor integration in human postural control. *J Neurophysiol.* 2002;88(3):1097–1118.

77. Horak FB. Postural orientation and equilibrium: what do we need to know about neural control and balance to prevent falls? *Age Ageing.* 2006;35(Suppl 2):ii7–ii11.

78. Winter DA. Human balance and posture control during standing and walking. *Gait Posture.* 1995;3(4):193–214.

79. Horak FB, Nashner LM. Central programming of postural movements: adaptation to altered support-surface configurations. *J Neurophysiol.* 1986;55(6):1369–1381.

80. Lendraitienė E, Tamošauskaitė A, Petruševičienė D, Savickas R. Balance evaluation techniques and physical therapy in post-stroke patients: a literature review. *Neurol I Neurochirurgia Polska.* 2017;51(1):92–100.

81. van Nes IJ, Nienhuis B, Latour H, Geurts AC. Posturographic assessment of sitting balance recovery in the sub-acute phase of stroke. *Gait Posture.* 2008;28(3):507–512.

82. Godfrey AC, Conway R, Meagher D, ÓLaighin G. Direct measurement of human movement by accelerometry. *Med Eng Phys.* 2008;30(10):1364–1386.

83. Nyberg L, Gustafson Y. Patient falls in stroke rehabilitation. *Stroke.* 1995;26(5):838–842.

84. Harris JE, Eng JJ, Marigold DS, Tokuno CD, Louis CL. Relationship of balance and mobility to fall incidence in people with chronic stroke. *Phys Therapy.* 2005;85(2): 150–158.

85. Yeun Lee J, Park J, Lee D, Roh H. The effects of exercising on unstable surfaces on the balance ability of stroke patients. *J Phys Ther Sci.* 2011;23(5):789–792.

86. Bae SH, Lee HG, Kim YE, Kim GY, Jung HW, Kim KY. Effects of trunk stabilization exercises on different support surfaces on the cross-sectional area of the trunk muscles and balance ability. *J Phys Ther Sci.* 2013;25(6):741–745.

87. Her JG, Park KD, Yang Y, et al. Effects of balance training with various dual-task conditions on stroke patients. *J Phys Ther Sci.* 2011;23(5):713–717.

88. Srivastava A, Taly AB, Gupta A, Kumar S, Murali T. Post-stroke balance training: role of force platform with visual feedback technique. *J Neurol Sci.* 2009;287(1):89–93.

CHAPTER 10

Current Concepts in Assessment and Management of Spasticity

SHENG LI, MD, PHD • GERARD E. FRANCISCO, MD

INTRODUCTION

According to the U. S. Center for Disease Control (CDC), approximately 800,000 people have a stroke every year in the United States. This results in a total of 7 million stroke survivors. Spasticity and weakness (i.e., spastic paresis) are the primary motor impairments and impose significant challenges for patient care. Spasticity is estimated to be present in about 20%−40% stroke survivors.[1] Clinically, poststroke spasticity is easily recognized as a phenomenon of velocity-dependent increase in tonic stretch reflexes ("muscle tone") with exaggerated tendon jerks, resulting from hyperexcitability of the stretch reflex.[2] Such phenomenon is commonly assessed by passive stretch in clinical practice. It has become common practice to label the finding of increased muscle resistance or muscle tightness as "spasticity." It is important to point out that not all hypertonia (increased muscle resistance) is spasticity.[3] In a study where 24 stroke survivors were recruited nonselectively within 13 months of their stroke, hypertonia was found in 12 subjects, but only 5 of them had spasticity as demonstrated by reflex hyperexcitability.[3]

Spasticity not only causes problems directly, such as pain, distorted joint position, and posture and hygiene difficulties. It also predisposes to other complications, such as joint contractures and permanent deformities. Furthermore, spasticity interacts with and amplifies the effects of other impairments, such as weakness, exaggerated stretch reflexes, clonus, impaired coordination, and motor control/planning, thus contributing to limitations in activity and participation.[4] These numerous abnormalities and interactions produce a dynamic picture of varying clinical presentations after an upper motor neuron (UMN) lesion.[5,6] For example, weakness tends to result in immobilization in a shortened muscle length and predisposes to contracture. This in turn exacerbates the development of spasticity

in the same muscles. Further, spasticity exacerbates contracture and triggers a vicious cycle that worsens the condition.[3,5,6] Overall, spasticity not only has downstream effects on the patient's quality of life, it also lays substantial burdens on the caregivers and society.[1] The continued care of these survivors costs the nation approximately $33 billion annually.[7]

PATHOPHYSIOLOGY

Managing and caring for persons with poststroke spasticity remains a challenge for both clinicians and care providers. This is partly related to the fact that the pathophysiology of poststroke spasticity is still poorly understood. Here we briefly summarize current understandings of poststroke spasticity pathophysiology evolved from decades of research.[5,8−13] As shown in Fig. 10.1, damages to motor cortex and its descending corticospinal tract (CST) occur because of a stroke. These damages cause muscle weakness (usually hemiparesis) immediately after stroke, subsequently resulting in weakness and incoordination, and often leading to joint immobilization. On the other hand, neuroplasticity occurs after stroke as well. Due to lesions of corticobulbar pathways accompanied with lesion of motor cortices and/or descending CST, bulbospinal hyperexcitability develops due to loss of supraspinal inhibition. This is mainly a phenomenon of disinhibition or unmasking effects. There are several potential candidates, including reticulospinal, vestibulospinal, and rubrospinal projections.[12,14,15] Medial reticulospinal (RS) hyperexcitability appears to be the most likely mechanism related to poststroke spasticity. RS hyperexcitability provides unopposed excitatory descending inputs to spinal stretch reflex circuits, resulting in elevated excitability of spinal motor neurons. This adaptive change can account for most clinical findings, for example, exaggerated stretch reflex, velocity-dependent

Stroke Rehabilitation. https://doi.org/10.1016/B978-0-323-55381-0.00010-X

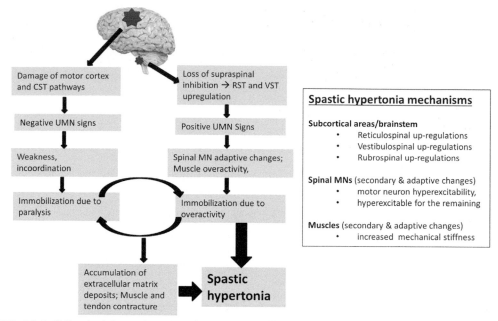

FIG. 10.1 Pathophysiology of post-stroke spasticity. *CST*, corticospinal tract; *MN*, motor neuron; *RST*, reticulospinal tract; *UMN*, upper motor neuron; *VST*, vestibulospinal tract.

resistance to stretch, muscle overactivity, or spontaneous firings of motor units. As mentioned earlier, muscle overactivity also potentiates muscle shortening and weakness in a vicious cycle. Their interactions also facilitate limb immobilization, development of muscle and tendon contractures, and accumulation of extracellular matrix deposits.[13,16] Taken together, three different components have been proposed to account for increased resistance of spastic muscles or spasticity. These components are neither adequately distinguished in clinical examinations[17] nor in laboratory settings.[18]

- **Hyperreflexia and reflex stiffness** Clinically, hyperreflexia and reflex stiffness present as the commonly observed phenomenon of velocity-dependent increase in resistance to passive muscle stretch. It is mediated by hyperexcitability of stretch reflex circuits as a result of unopposed RS hyperexcitability.
- **"Active" muscle stiffness (hyaluronan accumulation)** Hyaluronan is the primary component in the extracellular matrix.[19] Its primary function in the muscle is to smooth the muscle fiber gliding system and to facilitate muscle force transmission, that is, lubrication.[19] Immobilization or paresis decreases the normal turnover of the extracellular matrix, thus increasing its concentration within and between the muscular compartments, subsequently increasing the molecular weight and macromolecular

crowding.[20,21] These changes can increase the fluid viscosity,[22] thus decreasing the gliding and lubrication between the layers of collagen and muscle fibers. This change may be perceived by the stroke survivor as stiffness.[23]

- **Passive muscle stiffness (muscle fiber changes and connective tissue fibrosis)** Due to immobilization, spastic muscles may rest at a shortened length and muscle fibers become more stiff as a result.[24] Furthermore, fibrosis within the muscle tissue could be developed gradually secondary to the deposition of collagen within and between muscle bundles later on in the chronic phase.[25] These changes increase passive, mechanical stiffness of the muscle.

Understanding of different mechanisms for weakness and spasticity, as well as different components of spastic hypertonia, provides a useful theoretical framework to assess spasticity and to guide treatment plans for an effective motor rehabilitation program for motor recovery. For example, difficulty in hand and finger opening could be due to finger extensor weakness and/or masking by overactive spastic finger flexors. Suppression of spasticity and weakening of finger flexors will facilitate hand and finger opening and voluntary use.[12,26] Another example is development of new treatment for spasticity to specifically target the "Active" muscle stiffness component. Hyaluronidase is an enzyme that hydrolyzes hyaluronan. Raghavan et al.,[16] reported that spasticity was significantly reduced in stroke survivors after hyaluronidase injection.

CLINICAL PRESENTATION, ASSESSMENT, AND GOAL-SETTING

Clinical Presentations

Although clinical presentation of spasticity varies widely across individuals within and across patient populations, there are postural patterns that are commonly observed. Table 10.1 lists muscles that, when they are hypertonic, are potentially involved in commonly observed abnormal postures. It has been suggested that knowledge of the abnormal postural patterns help inform dosing, goal-setting, and outcome of interventions, such as chemodenervation.[27] It is important to point out here that treatment plan and goal-setting should not be based on presentations of abnormal joint positions and postures. Clinical problems are more than presentations of muscle hypertonia and abnormal postures.

Abnormal postures are manifestations of imbalance of agonist and antagonist strength and hypertonia. Thus, a flexed elbow posture is not necessarily due to flexor muscle group hypertonia solely, but may be a combination of hypertonic flexors and weak extensors; or it could also be that both flexor and extensor muscle groups are both hypertonic, but the former predominates. Just as it is with abnormal postures, impaired movements usually result from the interaction between spasticity, weakness, and other features of the upper motor neuron syndrome, such as loss of coordination and dexterity, associated reactions and dystonia, or sustained contraction of muscles. Activity limitations are even more complex, as the causes of impaired movements are further aggravated by abnormalities other than the upper motor neuron disorder, but are a direct result of the underlying disease. Tactile and proprioceptive sensory loss, visual field cut and hemi-neglect, and cognitive difficulties, such as learning a novel task and procedural sequencing, can magnify the motor challenges imposed upon by spasticity and weakness. Thus, a rehabilitation effort that will be effective in enhancing activity participation should address not just spasticity and deficits in strength and coordination, but concurrently tackle the related impairments.

Clinical and Quantitative Assessment

When assessing poststroke spasticity, it is important to keep in mind that spasticity is only one component

TABLE 10.1
Common Postural Abnormalities due to Spasticity and Potential Muscle Involvement

Postural Abnormality	Muscles Potentially Involved
Shoulder adduction	Pectoralis major
	Latissimus dorsi
	Coracobrachialis (especially when shoulder is forward flexed)
Shoulder internal rotation	Subscapularis
	Teres major
	Pectoralis major and minor
Elbow flexion	Brachialis
	Biceps
	Brachioradialis
	Pronator teres
Elbow extension	Triceps
	Anconeus
Forearm pronation	Pronator teres
	Pronator quadratus
Wrist extension	Extensor carpi radialis
	Extensor carpi ulnaris
Wrist flexion	Flexor carpi radialis
	Flexor carpi ulnaris
Metacarpophalangeal (knuckle) flexion	Lumbricals
Finger flexion	Flexor digitorum superficialis (proximal phalanx)
	Flexor digitorum profundus (distal phalanx)
Thumb flexion	Flexor pollicis brevis (proximal)
	Flexor pollicis longus (distal phalanx)
Trunk flexion, lateral	Quadratus lumborum
	Latissimus dorsi
Hip Flexion	Psoas
	Iliacus
	Rectus femoris
Hip extension	Gluteus maximus
Hip adduction	Adductor complex
Knee extension	Quadriceps complex

Continued

TABLE 10.1
Common Postural Abnormalities due to Spasticity and Potential Muscle Involvement—cont'd

Postural Abnormality	Muscles Potentially Involved
Knee flexion	Hamstrings
	Gastrocnemius
Ankle plantarflexion	Gastrocnemius
	Soleus
	Tibialis posterior
	Tibialis anterior
	Flexor digitorum longus
Ankle inversion	Tibialis posterior
	Tibialis anterior
	Extensor hallucis longus
Small toe flexion	Flexor digitorum brevis (proximal)
	Flexor digitorum longus (distal)
Great toe hyperextension	Extensor hallucis longus

inability to release a grasped object or difficulty with walking due to an inturned foot. Thus, it is important to obtain a thorough, yet focused, history to guide the examination and formulation of treatment goals and plans. A systematic approach to history-taking and clinical assessment of spasticity that can be modified to suit different clinical scenarios is proposed in Tables 10.2 and 10.3.

Spasticity assessment typically consists of a combination of quantitative and qualitative measures. Clinically, the Ashworth scale, the modified Ashworth scale (MAS), and the Tardieu scale are most commonly used (Tables 10.4 and 10.5). The Tardieu scale has advantages over the MAS because it not only quantifies the muscles' reaction to stretch, but it controls the velocity of the stretch and measures the angle at which the catch, or clonus, occurs. However, neither scale has shown to be more reliable than the other. While it is true that quantitative measures are desirable because of their inherent objectivity and reliability, they may not be practical and may discourage clinicians from assessing and managing spasticity. Ideal measures include biomechanical and electrophysiologic tests, but many of the devices needed to carry these out are not available to a typical clinician, and the time needed to perform them properly may impose excessive demands in a busy practice. Table 10.6 summarizes many of these evaluation tools and techniques. Biomechanical and electrophysiologic assessments are commonly used in the research setting to quantitatively assess spasticity. Biomechanical assessment utilizes the concept of velocity-dependent increase in resistance. The approach has advantages of the ability to

that causes the clinical problem and presentation, as mentioned before. In addition, patients typically complain of the manifestations of spasticity, such as muscle tightness or that a limb could not be moved, or the resultant functional limitations, such as the

TABLE 10.2
Some Important Historical Points in Spasticity Assessment

Is the limb tight all the time or only at certain times?
Does a particular position or movement trigger tightness?
Is the tightness related to spasms?
Does the tightness cause pain?
Have there been episodes of skin compromise due to tightness or spasm?
Does the tightness result in difficulty with cleaning?
Does the tightness result in difficulty donning splints?
Does the tightness limit ability to move limbs, reach for objects, and use the hands?
Does the tightness of the lower limbs result in problems with transferring form one surface to another or with walking?
What treatments for muscle tightness have been tried previously and their outcome?
What are the current medications?
Was there a recent increase in tightness (that may warrant further diagnostic testing to rule out a new neurologic problem)?
Any recent medical problems?

From Francisco GE, Li S. Clinical assessment and management of spasticity and contractures in traumatic brain injury. In: Pandyan AD, Hermens H, Conway B, eds. *Spasticity and Contractures in Neurological Rehabilitation: A Guide to Clinical Practice and Research* (in press).

TABLE 10.3
Practical Clinical Examination Sequence

Examination Phase	What to Look for	What Can Be Gleaned
Observation	Observe limb posture at rest and how they change with position	Abnormal posture at rest—sustained muscle contraction (dystonia), contracture
		Position-dependent postural changes—dynamic tone
Voluntary[a]	How limbs move and how much active range is available	Functional strength, coordination, spastic cocontraction, contractures, presence of other movement disorders, synkinesis, or associated reactions
	Gait characteristics and associated upper limb and trunk postural abnormalities	Pain and discomfort during voluntary movements
Passive	Passive range of motion, strength, muscle tone, velocity-dependent "angle of catch," clonus	Spasticity
		Rigidity
		Contracture
		Clonus
		Pain and discomfort during passive stretch
Functional activities	Performance of specific tests and tasks (both formal tests, such as Frenchay and improvized tasks such as demonstrating ability to pick up a bottle of water and pour its contents to a cup)	Impact of multiple impairments (e.g., spasticity, weakness) on performance

[a] Voluntary movements, such as sit to stand, transfer, and ambulation, could be part of functional tests.

TABLE 10.4
Modified Ashworth Scale

0 No increase in muscle tone

1 Slightly increase in tone, manifested by a catch and release at the end of ROM

1+ Slightly increase in tone, manifested by a catch, followed by minimal resistance throughout the remainder (less than half) of the ROM (catch in the first half of ROM)

2 Marked increase in tone through most of the ROM, still easily moved

3 Considerable increase in tone, passive movement difficult

4 Affected part(s) rigid in flexion or extension by a catch, followed by minimal

TABLE 10.5
Tardieu Scale

QUALITY OF MUSCLE REACTION

0. No resistance

1. Slight resistance

2. Catch followed by a release

3. Fatigable clonus (<10 seconds)

4. Infatigable clonus (>10 seconds)

ANGLE OF MUSCLE REACTION AT DIFFERENT VELOCITIES OF STRETCH

V1. As slow as possible

V2. Speed of limb galling under gravity

V3. As fast as possible

differentiate neural and nonneural component of spastic hypertonia, thus spasticity versus contracture.[28–34] The measurement of electromyographic activity is able to determine the threshold of stretch reflex. The threshold indicates the onset of motoneuronal recruitment in response to external stretch[35] and can be measured with a portable device.[36] This method provides a more physiologically insightful measurement

TABLE 10.6
Measures of Spasticity Categorized Based on WHO International Classification of Function

Domain	Measure	Examples
Body function and Structure	Clinical	Visual Analog Scale
		Goniometric
		Ashworth Scale (and its modified version)[b]
		Tardieu Method
		Tone Assessment Scale
		Spasm Severity Scale
		Spasm Frequency Scale
	Physiologic	Hmax/Mmax Ratio
		Vibratory Inhibitory Index
		Tendon Reflex Gain
		Angular Joint Velocity
		Reflex Threshold Angle
		Torque Measurement
		Pendulum Test
		Myotonometry
Activity	Impairment[a]	Fugl–Meyer
		Jebsen–Taylor Hand Test
		Wolf Motor Test
		Action Research Arm Test
		Berg Balance Scale
	Function[a]	Functional Independence Measure
		Barthel Index
		Disability Assessment Scale[b]
		Frenchay Arm Test
		Timed Walking Test
		Motion Analysis
		Individualized functional tasks
Participation	Quality of Life[a]	SF-36 Health Survey
		Satisfaction With Life Scale
		EuroQol (EQ-5D)

[a]Measure is not specific for spasticity.
[b]Measure was developed specifically for spasticity.
From Francisco GE, Li S. Spasticity. In: *Braddom Physical Medicine & Rehabilitation*. 5th ed.; 2015.

of spasticity, that is, a physiological evidence of the onset of spasticity. The Myotonometer (Neurogenic Technologies, Inc., Missoula, Montana, USA) is a portable device that measures muscle stiffness at rest and during voluntary contraction by recording displacement of a probe that occurs as a result of force applied perpendicularly to the skin over a target muscle. The Myotonometer can provide objective measurement and is found to have good intra- and interrater reliability. The measurement is correlated well with clinical measurement of spasticity by MAS,[37,38] but does not provide insight to the reflex component of the stretch response.

Goal-Setting

Goal-setting is an important component of assessment and management decision-making. The treatment goals should be mutually agreed upon by the patient (or caregiver) and clinician. It is not uncommon for patients to desire goals of regaining normal function, but since this is not always achievable a discussion regarding goal-setting prior to initiating treatment can help manage expectations of treatment outcomes. All factors should be considered, including findings from focused medical history, functional history, patient's realistic expectations, inputs from care provider(s) and therapists, and social support system. For example, a medical cause of a transient increase in the severity of spasticity, such as urinary tract infection or pressure sores, should be considered and treated. Intrathecal baclofen management is not appropriate for a patient without sufficient social support system for follow-up and pump maintenance.

A useful method to set goals for spasticity management is through the use of the SMART acronym, originally developed for use in the business sector (Dornan 1981). Each of the letters in the acronym stands for a criterion that characterizes goals and objectives and that has appeared in various iterations to fit different purposes. For the purpose of goal-setting in spasticity management, SMART or SMARTER[39] can stand for:

S—Specific (well defined and targets a specific problem to be addressed)

M—Measurable (either quantitatively, as for technical goals, or qualitatively as for symptom-directed goals) and meaningful (achievement of the goal should be beneficial to the patient or caregiver)

A—Agreed upon (the patient or caregiver and clinician work toward a common end)

R—Realistic (will the patient's potential for improvement and available resources support achievement of the treatment goal?)

T—Time-bound (achievement of a goal should be within a reasonable amount of time)

E—Evaluated (at predetermined points in time, goal achievement and progress in doing so should be evaluated to determine effectiveness of intervention)

R—Revised (based on evaluation of goal achievement, new treatment goals may be identified or prior ones revised)

MANAGEMENT

There are different ways to approach the management of spasticity. Fig. 10.2 summarizes most commonly used treatment options. Historically, a sequential approach is used, that is, starting with the least invasive treatment and culminating with surgical procedures should nonoperative options fail. More recently, this approach has been abandoned in favor of concurrent use of both "non-invasive" and "invasive" procedures (e.g., injection therapy concurrent with therapeutic exercises, or using injection therapy for residual focal spasticity in persons whose generalized spasticity is simultaneously managed with intrathecal baclofen). Selection of combined treatments is based on severity of spasticity (focal vs. generalized, mild vs. severe) and availability of resources (Table 10.7). This reflects better appreciation of the magnitude of the problem, that is, spasticity alone does not account for presenting problem, and that other features of UMN syndrome contribute significantly, and that concurrent treatments are required to increase the chances of successful outcome.

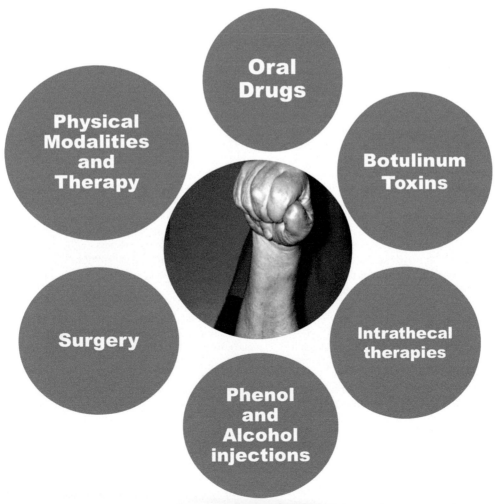

FIG. 10.2 Treatment options.

TABLE 10.7
Treatment Algorithm

	Physical Modalities and Therapy	Oral Drugs	Botulinum Toxin (BoNT)	Neurolysis (Phenol/Alcohol)	Intrathecal Baclofen	Surgery
Focal	+		+	+		
Multifocal	+	+	+	+		
Regional	+	+	+	+	+	+
Generalized	+	+	*BoNT/Phenol should be considered for focal problems that are superimposed on a general presentation		+	+

+, indicating this treatment may be considered.

Physical Modalities

While spasticity is a neurologically based condition, its obvious manifestation is physical. Physical modalities are thus considered to be in the first line of treatment and in combination with other treatment options, since they are widely available and innocuous relative to drugs. Passive stretching has been shown to be effective in reducing tone and increasing Range of motion (ROM) in patients with brain injury.[40] Splinting and casting are often used in the acute setting for sustained stretching to prevent contracture and reduce spasticity.[41–45] Casting alone seems sufficient to prevent contracture and reduce spasticity if the intervention is initiated early after severe brain injury. However, a systematic review on the use of upper extremity casting found high variability in casting protocols which indicates no consensus in technique.[46] Individualized stretching has been shown to be clinically promising to reduce wrist and finger spasticity and increase passive ROM.[47] Electrical stimulation may be utilized to reduce spasticity temporarily,[48] though the efficacy of electrical stimulation on spasticity reduction was not observed in more recent studies.[49,50] A novel technique demonstrated a long-lasting effect on spasticity reduction if electrical stimulation was triggered by voluntary breathing.[51]

Oral Spasmolytics

Various medications have been used to treat spasticity. Oral spasmolytics that have been evaluated for stroke and are currently available in the United States include baclofen, tizanidine, dantrolene, diazepam, and clonazepam (see reviews 52). These oral spasmolytics are generally associated with similar and related adverse events, such as sedation, drowsiness, and weakness. Because of this, and because of the limited evidence of efficacy attributable to inadequate sample size and

lack of quality-of-life measures, it is best to limit the use of these medications. However, oral spasmolytics may be cost-effective for individuals who achieve adequate spasticity reduction without experiencing adverse events. On the other hand, the somnolent effect of oral medications may benefit a stroke survivor who has difficulty sleeping because of muscle spasms. Each of these medications is briefly reviewed here.

Baclofen is an analog of GABA, the most potent inhibitory neurotransmitter. It binds to $GABA_B$ receptors that are widespread in Ia sensory afferent neurons and α motor neurons. It is the most widely studied oral spasmolytic in various patient populations, including spinal cord injury (SCI), multiple sclerosis (MS), cerebral palsy, and acquired brain injuries (traumatic brain injury, stroke, anoxia, or encephalopathy).[52–58] As with many spasticity medication trials, the studies involving baclofen demonstrated reduction in hypertonia and spasms, but did not investigate functional impact. Adverse effects of baclofen include drowsiness and weakness, which are shared by other oral spasmolytics. Abrupt discontinuation of baclofen may result in a withdrawal syndrome, characterized by rebound spasticity, hallucinations, and seizures.

Tizanidine is believed to exert its effects by inhibiting the facilitatory ceruleospinal tracts and the release of excitatory amino acid from spinal interneurons. As a result, presynaptic interneuronal excitation is suppressed, manifesting as reduction in tonic and phasic stretch reflexes and agonist–antagonist cocontraction.[59] Similar to baclofen, its efficacy in reducing muscle hypertonia and clonus, but not in improving function, has been demonstrated by various investigations.[60] In patients with stroke or TBI, tizanidine was deemed inferior to botulinum toxin in efficacy and safety in treating upper limb spasticity.[61] In addition to the typical side effects of oral spasmolytics, hepatotoxicity may also occur. Thus, monitoring liver function test is important, especially in those patients who concomitantly take hepatically cleared drugs. Being a central α2-adrenergic receptor agonist, tizanidine should be used carefully in patients with hypotension or are concomitantly taking other α agonists, such as clonidine. Likewise, caution should be used when coadministering tizanidine with fluoroquinolone antibiotics, which may increase the serum concentration of tizanidine. Tizanidine is a peculiar spasmolytic in that it has a dose-dependent antinociceptive effect, presumably due to a reduction in the release of substance P and activity of excitatory amino acids at the spinal level.[62] This makes tizanidine a suitable choice for those with concurrent spasticity and pain.

Dantrolene is used to manage a myriad of conditions, such as neuroleptic malignant syndrome and 3,4-methylenedioxymethamphetamine (MDMA; "Ecstasy") overdose, but its first reported therapeutic use was for spasticity.[63] Unlike baclofen and tizanidine, which act on the central nervous system, dantrolene acts directly on skeletal muscle. While it is widely regarded to exert its muscle relaxant effect by inhibiting the release of calcium from the sarcoplasmic reticulum during excitation–contraction coupling, its exact mechanism of action has not been elucidated until recently. It appears that a direct or indirect inhibition of the ryanodine receptor, the major calcium release channel of the skeletal muscle sarcoplasmic reticulum, is fundamental in the molecular action of dantrolene in decreasing intracellular calcium concentration.[64] Several investigations have supported dantrolene's beneficial effect on spasticity.[56,63,65,66] Although it is peripherally acting, dantrolene has also been associated with side effects that appear to be centrally mediated, such as drowsiness, dizziness, fatigue, and weakness, perhaps through alteration of neuronal calcium homeostasis.[66,67] Due to its potential for hepatotoxicity, regular monitoring of liver function is recommended.

Similar to baclofen, benzodiazepines (valium and clonazepam) exert their effects through modulation of GABAergic transmission; but unlike baclofen, benzodiazepines bind GABA-A receptors. The use of benzodiazepines as first-line treatment for spasticity has been limited, because of concerns for its side effects, mainly drowsiness, sedation, reduced attention and memory impairment, and the potential for physiological dependence. They appear to be used more often when spasticity is accompanied by other conditions that are also amenable to benzodiazepine therapy, such as seizures, anxiety, insomnia, spasms, and other movement disorders. Similar to baclofen, abrupt discontinuation of benzodiazepines may result in a withdrawal syndrome.

Focal Treatment—Botulinum Toxins

Chemodenervation using botulinum toxins (BoNT) has become a widely used spasticity treatment. It is preferred for the management of focal spasticity, or when the treatment plan targets a particular muscle. Botulinum toxin exerts its effect through inhibition of acetylcholine release at the neuromuscular junction via a complex process.[68] Currently, serotypes A and B of *Clostridium botulinum* are utilized clinically: *abobotulinumtoxinA*, *incobotulinumtoxinA*, *onabotulinumtoxinA*, *rimabotulinumtoxinB*. All these serotypes share common properties in that they are all clostridial neurotoxins with a bichain structure. They all inhibit acetylcholine release and the muscle paralysis they produce is reversible. The clinical effects of BoNT do not manifest until several days following an injection. The clinical effects last about 3 months, and recurrence of spasticity is likely due to functional repair of the neuromuscular junctions previously paralyzed by the toxin.[69] Usually, patients require repeated BoNT injections every 3–4 months.[70,71] However, a major survey of treating physicians and patients found that a majority prefer more frequent injections to achieve better clinical outcome.[72]

Advantages of BoNT treatment over oral medications are target specificity and a more favorable adverse event profile. Drowsiness and sedation are practically nonexistent with BoNT treatment. Consensus and review papers support the use of BoNT for the management of spastic conditions in upper and lower limbs in both pediatric and adult populations.[73–78] While overwhelming evidence demonstrates that BoNT treatment results in significant improvement at the body function and structure level, [73,74,76,77,79–86] it has not been shown unequivocally to be significantly efficacious in improving the activity and participation domains of the International Classification of Functioning.[87–90]

Clinical Issues Related to the Use of BoNT

The use of BoNT as the first-line treatment for focal spasticity after stroke has now been well accepted. The main clinical issue is how to achieve the best outcome with BoNT therapy. The relevant issues are (1) medication related: dosing; dilution; molecular manipulation; and immune-resistance; (2) injection related: injection guidance, motor innervation zone; (3) use of adjunct therapy; (4) relation to motor recovery: therapeutic weakness and central mechanisms.

Dosing. According to the mechanism of action of BoNT, the outcome is determined by the amount of BoNT absorbed at the neuromuscular junctions of spastic muscles. Dosing is an important factor. Clinical experience, regulatory and insurance coverage restrictions, and manufacturers' recommendations based on a few studies largely dictate the choice of doses of the various BoNT. There are a handful of dose-ranging studies that define dose-related therapeutic and adverse effects in spasticity.[91–96] Dosages that are used in current practice, recommended by consensus statements,[74] and described in retrospective studies,[97,98] appear to be higher than doses used in published randomized, controlled, studies. The use of escalating doses of BoNT was a common practice until safety concerns were raised and fueled by mandates from the United States Food and Drug administration (FDA). Responding to reports suggestive of systemic effects of BoNT in 2009 the FDA required new label warnings and a risk mitigation strategy that requires clinicians to discuss the risks and provide written material that details the warnings. The current experience of many clinicians is that using dosages of inco- and onabotulinumtoxinA as high as 600–800 units (U) is effective and safe.[99,100]

Dilution. The volume of BoNT solution is another factor. It is believed that increasing volume magnifies its therapeutic effects by facilitating the toxin's ability to reach more motor endplates. Higher volume of BoNT injections are effective in animal studies,[101,102] but equivocal in human studies.[103,104] In another human study, it was found that high-volume or endplate-targeted BoNT injections result in more profound neuromuscular blockade and spasticity and cocontraction reduction, as compared to low-volume, non-endplate targeted injections.[105] As much as high volume injections appear attractive, it may be a double-edged sword in that it may facilitate distant spread of the toxin. Cases have been reported wherein patients with poststroke spasticity developed transient weakness in the noninjected contralateral upper limb after receiving large dilution volumes in proximal upper limb muscles. Weakness was attributed to spread neuromuscular blockade based on EMG findings.

Molecular weight and subtypes. Recently, a new low-molecular weight subtype BoNT (subtype A2, A2NTX) has been developed for clinical use.[106] In this first human study with patients with poststroke spasticity, A2NTX has a similar time course as compared to onabotulinumtoxin A (subtypeA1), but with greater clinical efficacy (1.5 times more with A2NTX) and less spread to its neighboring muscle. Furthermore, functional independence measure (FIM) was significantly improved with A2NTX, but not with subtypeA1.

Immunoresistance. Immunoresistance accounts for loss of responsiveness to spasmolytic effects from repeated BoNT injections. Based on early reports in the cervical dystonia population, high doses and frequent injections of BoNT were identified as risk factors for immunoresistance.[107,108]This also provided support for the practice of allowing no less than 90 days in between exposures to BoNT. A much higher incidence of antibody formation has been associated with cervical dystonia (1.28%) than in poststroke spasticity (0.32%).[109] Thus, there is growing interest in incobotulinumtoxinA, which is free of excipient proteins and, as such, may have a lower propensity to induce an immunogenic response relative to the other BoNT preparations with complexing proteins.[110,111] Bioassay of neutralizing antibodies to botulinum toxin is considered the gold standard in confirming immunoresistance, but more practical clinical tests, such as the FTAT (frontalis antibody test) or UBI (unilateral brow injection), can be easily performed by injecting a small dose of BoNT in either the frontalis (FTAT) or corrugator (UBI) muscle.[112]

Injection techniques and innervation zone localization. Techniques used to attempt enhancement of BoNT effectiveness include guided injection by listening to EMG activity, identifying motor points through electrical stimulation (ES), or visualizing target sites by sonography. However, there is insufficient evidence to support or refute the superiority of specific techniques for guiding BoNT injection needle placement.[78] It has also been suggested that targeting the muscle innervation zone, not just the motor points, can optimize the effects of BoNT administration.[113,114] Due to advances in EMG technology, high-density surface EMG recordings and analyses allow localization of motor innervation zone (IZ, i.e., neuromuscular injection) on the muscle surface.[115] The effect of IZ-guided BoNT injection has been well examined in healthy subjects.[116] IZs of the right and left extensor digitorum brevis (EDB) muscles in eight healthy volunteers were first localized. On the control side, the same amount of BoNT-A (10 units of abobotulinumtoxinA) was administered into the IZ. The purpose was to examine the duration of BoNT treatment. On the study side BoNT-A (10 units of abobotulinumtoxinA) was injected at different distances randomly between 2 and 12 mm away from the IZ. This was to study how much the BoNT effect reduced when BoNT was injected away from the IZ. The effectiveness of BoNT injection was measurement by compound muscle action potentials (CMAPs). CMAPs reflect the summed activation of the entire muscle if it is fully activated. CMAPs were recorded prior to the injection and 2, 12, and 24 weeks later. On the control side, the mean CMAP reduction 2 weeks after BoNT-A injection was 79.3%. During the follow-up period, the mean CMAP reduction decreased only to 76.4% at 12 weeks (T_2), and to 70.1% at 24 weeks (T_3). This result is of critical clinical importance in that BoNT injection at the IZ could potentially lead to therapeutic effect up to 24 weeks. This long-lasting physiological effect (up to 24 weeks) of IZ-guided BoNT injection is far superior as compared to current clinical practice. The CMAP reduction on the study side, that is, BoNT effect, was linearly and inversely related to the injection distance from the IZ. Reduction of BoNT treatment effect was about estimated to be 46% if BoNT was injected about 1 cm from the IZ. IZ locations have been found to be changed in persons with poststroke spasticity.[117] This could explain variations in BoNT treatment effects in humans studies, including the above mentioned dilution studies.

Adjunct therapies. The beneficial role of adjunctive therapy modalities in enhancing clinical outcomes of BoNT treatment has not been well studied. The few investigations described the potentially beneficial effects of casting[118] and adhesive taping,[119] but in the case of the latter, subsequent studies did not yield consistent results.[120] Casting may also enhance the effect of onabotulinumtoxinA,[121] as prolonged stretching of spastic muscles after BoNT treatment affords long-lasting therapeutic benefit. Another promising technique to magnify the clinical effect of BoNT treatment is pairing it with superficial electrical stimulation, which influences activity of synaptic vesicle 2 receptors[122] that facilitate neuronal binding and subsequent uptake of BoNT.[123-126] More recently, extracorporeal shockwave therapy (ESWT) has been shown to have a greater magnitude of enhancement of BoNT treatment than electrical stimulation, most likely thorough modulation of muscle rheology and neurotransmission.[100,126]

Repeated injections. Most studies involving the use of BoNT for spasticity involve only a few cycles of injection. A rare few have reported safety and sustained efficacy up to 5 injection cycles over a few years.[127-129] In clinical practice many patients receive multiple injections over a period of many years, sometimes decades, and the long-term effects are not systematically documented. The fact that patients continue to receive BoNT over a long period of time implies that the patients continue to benefit from the treatment without experiencing adverse events. Although the few studies claimed that repeated injections were safe, concern remains about the long-term effect of BoNT on muscles. An animal study concluded that the contractile properties of target and nontarget muscles did not fully recover within 6 months of BoNT injections treatment protocol.[130] The same investigators also found that following repeated BoNT injections muscle atrophy sets in and contractile material is replaced by fat.[131] Recognition of BoNTs effects on muscle length and force[132] is also emerging, although how this translates clinically is still unclear. Further research is warranted to study muscle changes after repeat BoNT injections.

Another area that warrants further investigation is the determination of when other treatment interventions should be considered after repeated BoNT injections. For example, how many BoNT injections need to be done to address a spastic-dystonic "clenched fist" before surgical release of the finger and thumb flexor tendons should be entertained? How many times should a person with spastic paraplegia receive BoNT before intrathecal baclofen therapy is considered? The economic impact of these clinical decisions will also need to be weighed to better appreciate the cost-effectiveness of spasticity interventions.

Early treatment. There is no consensus in how early BoNT can be safely and effectively administered. A recent metaanalysis study examined the effect of BoNT treatment as early as 3—6 months after stroke.[133] The authors reported that BoNT injections effectively manage muscle hypertonia and decreases risk of later complications, such as contracture development, and a trend towards reduction in spasticity-related pain as well. However, no improvement in disability or function is reported.

Spasticity reduction and recovery of function. As illustrated in Fig. 10.1 regarding the pathophysiology of poststroke spasticity, spasticity and weakness are mediated by different mechanisms. Recovery of motor function from weakness and development of spasticity are both related to neural plasticity after stroke.[26] Different rehabilitation strategies have been used to promote motor recovery via facilitation and modulation of neural plasticity through early interventions with repetitive goal-oriented intensive therapy, appropriate noninvasive brain stimulation, and pharmacological agents. Though rare, there are unusual cases when the outcome of BoNT injection surpasses its expectation of spasticity reduction and results in increase in functional abilities in chronic stages, particularly when appropriate therapeutic exercise is included in the treatment regimen. Late motor recovery after BoNT injection is likely related to the "therapeutic weakness" effect[12] and the central effect[134] or both.

"Therapeutic weakness." BoNT injection to the spastic muscles concurrently results in both spasticity reduction and muscle weakness. We have observed that in some patients, when this weakness is addressed by

task-specific exercises it could result in improvement of voluntary control of the weakened muscles. For this reason, we coined it "therapeutic weakness." This phenomenon of therapeutic weakening is revealed in a recent case of improved voluntary grip control after BoNT injection.[135] The patient was a 53-year-old female, who sustained a hemorrhagic right middle cerebral artery stroke 3 years earlier. She had finger flexor spasticity and residual weak finger/wrist extension. She received 50 units of onabotulinumtoxin A injection to each of the left flexor digitorum superficialis and flexordigitorum profundus, respectively. As expected, botulinum toxin injection led to weakness and spasticity reduction in the spastic finger flexors. However, she was able to open her hand faster due to improved grip release time. This was accompanied by shortened extensor electromyographic activity. The improved voluntary control of hand opening/grip release was likely realized by decreased cocontraction of spastic finger flexors during voluntary finger extension. This case demonstrated that reduction in finger flexor spasticity can improve voluntary control of residual finger extension. Improvement in voluntary control of extensor muscles likely results from reduced reciprocal inhibition from the spastic flexors after injection. Previous results have shown that injections can paralyze afferent fibers,[136] in addition to blocking acetylcholine release presynaptically at neuromuscular junctions, as such, resulting in reduced inhibition from paralyzed flexors after injection. Consequently, weak finger extensors became functional and motor function of the hand improved.

This concept is further supported by another study,[86] where 15 patients with spastic hemiparesis from stroke or traumatic brain injury were instructed to perform reaching movements within the available range of motion before and 1 month after BoNT injections. BoNT was administered to the elbow, wrist, and finger flexors based on assessment of hypertonia of individual muscles. All patients were able to subsequently perform reaching movements better. Additionally, reaching velocity and smoothness improved. However, the other clinical outcomes, such as the Action Research Arm Test and the Box and Block Test remained unchanged. These findings cannot be explained by spasticity reduction alone. Though EMGs from flexors and extensors were not recorded, the authors postulated that improved reaching performance after injections to the flexors was likely related to better control of antagonist extensor muscles. In other words, voluntary control of extensor muscles during reaching movements is improved from decreased flexors spasticity and weakening of flexors after injections.

"Central effects." In addition to the concept of "therapeutic weakness" after BoNT injection, central mechanisms of BoNT treatment have been considered to play an important role. In our recent review article,[134] a number of plausible explanations for a centrally mediated late motor recovery after BoNT injection are listed: (1) direct action of botulinum neurotoxin at distant sites in the central nervous system, mediated by retrograde transport of the neurotoxin into the spinal cord, and (2) cortical reorganization due to botulinum neurotoxin–induced decrease in peripheral sensory input at the local injection site. Consequently, the central effect of BoNT treatment converts the neuromotor system into a transient labile state.[137] This allows regrowth or strengthening of appropriate synapses and suppression of inappropriate ones, that is, neural plasticity and motor relearning, if coupled with sustained activity-based, goal-oriented training programs.[138] This is particularly important for motor recovery in chronic stroke when motor recovery is usually plateaued or arrested, as demonstrated in the above case. However, in order to better understand and utilize "therapeutic weakness" and "central effects" of BoNT to promote late motor recovery, more research is needed to elucidate dosing specifications, patient selection criteria, and the interplay with other therapeutic modalities.

Focal Treatment—Nerve Block (Neurolysis)

Prior to the introduction of BoNT, nerve block using either alcohol or phenol was the only option for focal spasticity management. It was used in the 1950s to chemically ablate nerve to manage cancer-related pain, and subsequently applied for spasticity management. Over time, neurolysis with phenol or alcohol are proved to be effective in controlling focal spasticity across different populations, including cerebral palsy, traumatic brain injuries, and stroke.[139,140] Phenol (5%–7%) and alcohol (35%–60%) denature proteins in the nerves, leading to blockade of nerve transmission. In addition, phenol appears to result in degeneration of muscle spindles (Wolf 2000) and damage to both afferent and efferent nerve fibers.[141] This chemical denervation is thought to be irreversible and leads to permanent control of spasticity; however, this is not commonly observed clinically, as spasticity tends to return several months after the percutaneous block. This may be explained by partial nerve regrowth and sprouting.

Percutaneous injections can either be at the nerve or motor branch level, guided by electrical stimulation or ultrasound. Since phenol is also an anesthetic, especially at concentrations less than 3%, muscle relaxation commonly observed immediately after injection is due to the anesthetic effect. The neurolytic effect may not set in until a few hours later as it takes some time for the effects on neural tissues to develop. Commonly injected upper limb nerves are pectoral and musculocutaneous nerves. In the lower limb, the obturator, sciatic, and tibial nerves and their branches are commonly treated. Care must be exercised in injecting nerves with significant sensory component to mitigate risk of developing postinjection dysesthesia. Other side effects include localized swelling and excessive weakness. Inadvertent intravascular injection or systemic absorption may result in cardiovascular or central nervous system effects, including hypotension and tremor or convulsions, respectively. In a recent article, we summarized 293 procedures of phenol neurolysis over 3 years in our institution.[142] Overall, phenol neurolysis has a relatively favorable safety profile, including pain (4.0%), swelling and inflammation (2.7%), dysesthesia (0.7%), and hypotension (0.7%).

Neurolysis with phenol and alcohol has taken a backseat to BoNT injections, which appear to have a better safety profile and are easier to administer. While both treatments are effective when applied to the appropriate clinical indication and performed well, there is no evidence demonstrating superiority of one over the other in managing spasticity. To date there is only one peer-reviewed publication comparing onabotulinumtoxinA and phenol 5%.[143] In this study, both onabotulinumtoxinA and phenol were effective in reducing spasticity as measured by the Ashworth scores of ankle plantarflexors and invertors, but the former was better in decreasing muscle tone and ankle clonus at 2 and 4 weeks, but not at 8 and 12 weeks, following injection. Table 10.8 presents a comparison of the clinical characteristics of BoNT and phenol.

Intrathecal Baclofen (ITB) Therapy

When delivered directly to the intrathecal space, baclofen has the advantage of more direct access to $GABA_B$ receptors in the spinal cord, since the blood–brain barrier does not have to be traversed. At the cellular level, ITB's mechanism of action is similar to that of the oral form; however, intrathecal administration allows greater hypertonia reduction and reflex inhibition at doses lower than the oral form, thus decreasing its risk of adverse events. Continuous ITB therapy was introduced in the 1980s to treat spasticity in SCI. Since then, several trials

demonstrated similar beneficial effects in other patient populations, such as cerebral palsy,[144] brain injuries,[145] stroke,[146] and multiple sclerosis.[147]

The intrathecal system consists of a programmable pump that has an accessible drug reservoir that is implanted subcutaneously in the abdominal area. A catheter that is connected to the implanted pump's

TABLE 10.8
Comparison of Clinical Characteristics of Botulinum Toxins and Phenol

	Phenol	Botulinum Toxin (BoNT)
Mechanism of action	Neurolysis via protein denaturation	Blockade of acetylcholine release into neuromuscular junction
Onset	Immediate (anesthetic effect); within 24–48 h (neurolytic effect)	5–10 days
Duration	Variable–dose-dependent	~3 months
Dose titration to desired effect	Yes	Yes
Injection technique	Nerves, preferably motor branches using electrical stimulation or sonographic guidance	Muscle (motor endplates), using intramuscular EMG, electrical stimulation, or sonographic guidance
Ease of administration	Requires more training and expertise	Relatively easy
Evidence of efficacy	No RCT	RCTs published
Pain during injection	More	Some
Pain days after injection	Higher risk	Rare
Adverse events	Higher incidence of dysesthetic pain and swelling as compared to BoNT	Less common
Cost	Very affordable	Expensive

RCT, randomized control trial.

side port is tunneled under the skin and enters the spine at the lumbar level. The catheter tip is advanced cephalad and usually left at the thoracic level, although it is not uncommon for it to be placed at the cervical area,[148] or sometimes intraventricularly.[149] Common side effects of ITB are similar to the oral form but occur less frequently, largely because much lower intrathecal doses are needed to exert therapeutic effects. Additional potential adverse effects are procedure-related or device-related, such as surgical infection, pump malfunction, or catheter interruption.

ITB therapy requires interdisciplinary collaboration, including physiatrist, neurosurgeon, nurses and therapists, and patient and care provider's support and commitment. Prior to surgical implantation of the catheter and pump, a "trial" is performed to confirm ITB's effectiveness in decreasing spasticity, spasms, or pain. Management does not end with implantation of the pump; frequent dose adjustments will be needed subsequently to reach appropriate ITB dose. Therefore, when planning ITB therapy, nonmedical conditions need to be considered, such as the patient's ability to comply with dose titration and pump management, which requires regular visits with the clinician. Recommendations from an expert panel on best practices for ITB therapy have been recently published.[150–153] These recommendations address issues related to different aspects of ITB therapy individually, including patient selection, screening test ("trial"), dosing and long-term management, and troubleshooting.

ITB has been increasingly used to treat generalized or regional spasticity that is unsatisfactory with oral medications or injection therapy in the past decade. ITB therapy has been shown to be effective in managing poststroke spasticity; furthermore, ITB is also potentially effective to improve gait[154] and upper limb use,[155] and to improve quality of life.[156] Previous concerns that an intrathecally administered medication is not selective and, thus, will result in weakness of the noninvolved side were unfounded.[154,156] A consensus statement by a panel of experts recommended that ITB therapy be considered as early as 3–6 months post stroke, whenever it causes significant functional impact or hinders progress in rehabilitation.[157] ITB therapy should be considered as a safe and effective treatment for poststroke spasticity when less invasive treatments fail to provide optimum reduction in problematic spasticity. Despite the potential benefits and safety profiles of ITB, there are only a very small portion of stroke patients (<1%) with severe disabling spasticity treated with ITB.[158] Possible reasons for ITB underutilization include surgical risks, excessive weakness, less

effect on upper limbs, and limited functional improvement. These concerns are alleviated by above mentioned studies and the benefits of ITB therapy outweigh the risks.

Surgical Intervention

Surgical management of spasticity is a well-accepted treatment option for contractures, as it primarily addresses joint deformities rather than spasticity itself. Surgical interventions include neuroablative procedures, such as peripheral neurotomies and dorsal rhizotomies, and orthopedic reconstructive procedures, such as tendon lengthening and tendon transfer. Surgical intervention is a permanent treatment. Optimal management of spasticity by nonsurgical means should be attempted before surgical treatment is employed. Therefore, it is often viewed as a treatment of "last resort." However, surgical intervention could be pursued earlier in cases where other options are unavailable due to lack of availability or resources. When excessive spasticity and contracture are not sufficiently controlled by therapy and focal interventions, tendon lengthening is often considered. This involves correction of abnormal joint posture alignment, allowing for improved ability to move joints and in many cases facilitate activity and exercise.[159] Common tendon procedures include split anterior tibial tendon transfer (SPLATT) and Achilles tendon lengthening to manage spastic equinovarus.[160] Tendon lengthening and release can also help with upper limb management.[161] Surgical interventions primarily manage joint deformities rather than spasticity itself. Tendon lengthening elongates the tendon, and subsequently corrects the abnormal joint position. But it does not change the contractile and mechanical properties of muscle and its innervation. In other words, the unchanged spastic muscle has a new resting position at a corrected joint position via the elongated tendon. The reflex responses are both velocity and muscle (not tendon) length dependent[33] and related to muscle fiber length and sarcomere numbers.[24,162,163] The exaggerated reflex responses are still expected to remain unchanged, if the same stretch is applied with reference to the new resting position. Therefore, tendon lengthening can improve posture, but is not likely to correct altered stretch reflex in spastic muscles. Other procedures, such as neurotomy, have also been shown to benefit spastic conditions.[164,165]

Emerging Therapy—Hyaluronidase Injections

Advances in understanding pathogenesis of poststroke spasticity (as illustrated in Fig. 10.1) not only allow a better understanding of the relation between spasticity and motor recovery, but lead to the development of new treatments as well. One example is the use of human recombinant hyaluronidase to address the active muscle stiffness component of spastic hypertonia.[16] The accumulation of hyaluronan within spastic muscles is considered as the primary extracellular mechanism promoting development of muscle stiffness. It was then hypothesized that hyaluronidase, the enzyme of hyaluronan, is expected to reduce muscle stiffness if it is injected into the muscles.[10] In their pioneering study, Raghavan and colleagues injected human recombinant hyaluronidase with saline in 20 patients with unilateral upper limb spasticity at a single visit. The outcome measures included safety, passive and active movement, and muscle stiffness at eight upper limb joints. There were assessed at four time points: pre-injection (T0), within 2 weeks (T1), within 4–6 weeks (T2), and within 3–5 months post injection (T3). No clinically significant adverse effects were observed from the injections. Passive movement at all joints, and active movement at most joints increased at T1, and persisted at T2 and T3 for most joints. The modified Ashworth scores also declined significantly over time post injection. This study provides preliminary evidence that hyaluronidase injections are safe and potentially efficacious for muscle stiffness reduction. This treatment is very promising in that it reduces muscle stiffness without producing weakness, and increases voluntary movement of the treated limb. However, further research is warranted, such as a large-scale clinical study, dosing, duration of effects, the effect on neural component, etc.

Other Emerging Therapies

In addition to the various treatment options described above other modalities are emerging as potential primary or adjunctive spasticity management options. These include acupuncture,[166,167] vibration [168,169] and noninvasive brain,[170–173] spinal [174] and transcutaneous [175,176] nerve stimulation. The effect of peripheral nerve stimulation appears inconsistent.[177] Extracorporeal shock wave therapy is also being investigated.[100,178,179] Currently there is very little research evidence or clinical experience to support the use of these interventions and, as such, they are not widely used in clinical practice.

REFERENCES

1. Zorowitz RD, Gillard PJ, Brainin M. Poststroke spasticity: sequelae and burden on stroke survivors and caregivers. *Neurology.* 2013;80(3 Supplement 2):S45–S52.
2. Lance JW. Symposium synopsis. In: Feldman RG, Young RR, Koella WP, eds. *Spasticity: Disordered Motor Control.* Chicago: Year Book Medical Publishers; 1980: 485–494.
3. O'Dwyer N, Ada L, Neilson P. Spasticity and muscle contracture following stroke. *Brain.* 1996;119(5): 1737–1749.
4. Mayer NH, Esquenazi A. Muscle overactivity and movement dysfunction in the upper motoneuron syndrome. *Phys Med Rehabil Clin N Am.* 2003;14(4):855–883. vii–viii.
5. Gracies JM. Pathophysiology of spastic paresis. II: Emergence of muscle overactivity. *Muscle Nerve.* 2005;31(5): 552–571.
6. Gracies JM. Pathophysiology of spastic paresis. I: paresis and soft tissue changes. *Muscle Nerve.* 2005;31(5):535–551.
7. Mozaffarian D, Benjamin EJ, Go AS, et al. Heart disease and stroke statistics-2016 update a report from the American Heart Association. *Circulation.* 2016;133(4): e38–e48.
8. Burke D, Wissel J, Donnan GA. Pathophysiology of spasticity in stroke. *Neurology.* 2013;80(3 suppl. 2):S20–S26.
9. Mukherjee A, Chakravarty A. Spasticity mechanisms – for the clinician. *Front Neurol.* 2010;1:149.
10. Nielsen JB, Crone C, Hultborn H. The spinal pathophysiology of spasticity – from a basic science point of view. *Acta Physiol.* 2007;189(2):171–180.
11. Brown P. Pathophysiology of spasticity. *J Neurol Neurosurg Psychiatry.* 1994;57(7):773–777.
12. Li S, Francisco G. New insights into the pathophysiology of post-stroke spasticity. *Front Hum Neurosci.* 2015;9:192. https://doi.org/10.3389/fnhum.2015.00192.
13. Stecco A, Stecco C, Raghavan P. Peripheral mechanisms contributing to spasticity and implications for treatment. *Curr Phys Med Rehabil Rep.* 2014;2:121–127.
14. Owen M, Ingo C, Dewald JPA. Upper extremity motor impairments and microstructural changes in bulbospinal pathways in chronic hemiparetic stroke. *Front Neurol.* 2017;8(257).
15. Miller DM, Klein CS, Suresh NL, Rymer WZ. Asymmetries in vestibular evoked myogenic potentials in chronic stroke survivors with spastic hypertonia: evidence for a vestibulospinal role. *Clin Neurophysiol.* 2014;125(10): 2070–2078.
16. Raghavan P, Lu Y, Mirchandani M, Stecco A. Human recombinant hyaluronidase injections for upper limb muscle stiffness in individuals with cerebral injury: a case series. *eBioMedicine.* 2016;9:306–313.
17. Vattanasilp W, Ada L, Crosbie J. Contribution of thixotropy, spasticity, and contracture to ankle stiffness after stroke. *J Neurol Neurosurg Psychiatry.* 2000;69:34–39.
18. Malhotra S, Pandyan AD, Day CR, Jones PW, Hermens H. Spasticity, an impairment that is poorly defined and poorly measured. *Clin Rehabil.* 2009;23(7):651–658.
19. Fraser JR, Laurent TC, Laurent UB. Hyaluronan: its nature, distribution, functions and turnover. *J Intern Med.* 1997; 242(1):27–33.
20. Nishimura M, Yan W, Mukudai Y, et al. Role of chondroitin sulfate-hyaluronan interactions in the viscoelastic properties of extracellular matrices and fluids. *Biochim Biophys Acta.* 1998;1380(1):1–9.

21. Cowman MK, Schmidt TA, Raghavan P, Stecco A. Viscoelastic properties of hyaluronan in physiological conditions. *F1000Research*. 2015;4:622.

22. Knepper PA, Covici S, Fadel JR, Mayanil CS, Ritch R. Surface-tension properties of hyaluronic Acid. *J Glaucoma*. 1995;4(3):194–199.

23. Stecco A, Gesi M, Stecco C, Stern R. Fascial components of the myofascial pain syndrome. *Curr Pain Headache Rep*. 2013;17(8):352.

24. Friden J, Lieber RL. Spastic muscle cells are shorter and stiffer than normal cells. *Muscle Nerve*. 2003;27(2):157–164.

25. Booth CM, Cortina-Borja MJ, Theologis TN. Collagen accumulation in muscles of children with cerebral palsy and correlation with severity of spasticity. *Dev Med Child Neurol*. 2001;43(5):314–320.

26. Li S. Spasticity, motor recovery, and neural plasticity after stroke. *Front Neurol*. 2017;8(120).

27. Hefter H, Jost WH, Reissig A, Zakine B, Bakheit AM, Wissel J. Classification of posture in poststroke upper limb spasticity: a potential decision tool for botulinum toxin A treatment? *Int J Rehabil Res*. 2012;35(3):227–233.

28. Chung SG, van Rey E, Bai Z, Rymer WZ, Roth EJ, Zhang LQ. Separate quantification of reflex and nonreflex components of spastic hypertonia in chronic hemiparesis. *Arch Phys Med Rehabil*. 2008;89(4):700–710.

29. Zhang LQ, Chung SG, Bai Z, et al. Intelligent stretching of ankle joints with contracture/spasticity. *IEEE Trans Neural Syst Rehabil Eng*. 2002;10(3):149–157.

30. Zhang L-Q, Wang G, Nishida T, Xu D, Sliwa JA, Rymer WZ. Hyperactive tendon reflexes in spastic multiple sclerosis: measures and mechanisms of action. *Arch Phys Med Rehabil*. 2000;81(7):901–909.

31. Kamper DG, Harvey RL, Suresh S, Rymer WZ. Relative contributions of neural mechanisms versus muscle mechanics in promoting finger extension deficits following stroke. *Muscle Nerve*. 2003;28(3):309–318.

32. Kamper DG, Rymer WZ. Quantitative features of the stretch response of extrinsic finger muscles in hemiparetic stroke. *Muscle Nerve*. 2000;23(6):954–961.

33. Li S, Kamper DG, Rymer WZ. Effects of changing wrist positions on finger flexor hypertonia in stroke survivors. *Muscle Nerve*. 2006;33(2):183–190.

34. Sinkjaer T, Magnussen I. Passive, intrinsic and reflex-mediated stiffness in the ankle extensors of hemiparetic patients. *Brain*. 1994;117(Pt 2):355–363.

35. Levin MF, Feldman AG. The role of stretch reflex threshold regulation in normal and impaired motor control. *Brain Res*. 1994;657(1–2):23–30.

36. Calota A, Feldman AG, Levin MF. Spasticity measurement based on tonic stretch reflex threshold in stroke using a portable device. *Clin Neurophysiol*. 2008;119(10):2329–2337.

37. Leonard CT, Deshner WP, Romo JW, Suoja ES, Fehrer SC, Mikhailenok EL. Myotonometer intra- and interrater reliabilities. *Arch Phys Med Rehabil*. 2003;84(6):928–932.

38. Leonard CT, Stephens JU, Stroppel SL. Assessing the spastic condition of individuals with upper motoneuron involvement: validity of the myotonometer. *Arch Phys Med Rehabil*. 2001;82(10):1416–1420.

39. Francisco GE, Li S. *Spasticity. Physical Medicine and Rehabilitation*. 5th ed. 2015.

40. Starring DT, Gossman MR, Nicholson Jr GG, Lemons J. Comparison of cyclic and sustained passive stretching using a mechanical device to increase resting length of hamstring muscles. *Phys Ther*. 1988;68(3):314–320.

41. Preissner KS. The effects of serial casting on spasticity: a literature review. *Occup Therapy Health Care*. 2002;14(2):99–106.

42. Booth BJ, Doyle M, Montgomery J. Serial casting for the management of spasticity in the head-injured adult. *Phys Ther*. 1983;63(12):1960–1966.

43. Mortenson PA, Eng JJ. The use of casts in the management of joint mobility and hypertonia following brain injury in adults: a systematic review. *Phys Ther*. 2003;83(7):648–658.

44. Pohl M, Mehrholz J, Ruckriem S. The influence of illness duration and level of consciousness on the treatment effect and complication rate of serial casting in patients with severe cerebral spasticity. *Clin Rehabil*. 2003;17(4):373–379.

45. Bovend'Eerdt TJ, Newman M, Barker K, Dawes H, Minelli C, Wade DT. The effects of stretching in spasticity: a systematic review. *Arch Phys Med Rehabil*. 2008;89(7):1395–1406.

46. Lannin NA, Novak I, Cusick A. A systematic review of upper extremity casting for children and adults with central nervous system motor disorders. *Clin Rehabil*. 2007;21(11):963–976.

47. Copley J, Kuipers K, Fleming J, Rassafiani M. Individualised resting hand splints for adults with acquired brain injury: a randomized, single blinded, single case design. *NeuroRehabilitation*. 2013;32(4):885–898.

48. Seib TP, Price R, Reyes MR, Lehmann JF. The quantitative measurement of spasticity: effect of cutaneous electrical stimulation. *Arch Phys Med Rehabil*. 1994;75(7):746–750.

49. Leung J, Harvey LA, Moseley AM, et al. Electrical stimulation and splinting were not clearly more effective than splinting alone for contracture management after acquired brain injury: a randomised trial. *J Physiotherapy*. 2012;58(4):231–240.

50. Malhotra S, Rosewilliam S, Hermens H, Roffe C, Jones P, Pandyan AD. A randomized controlled trial of surface neuromuscular electrical stimulation applied early after acute stroke: effects on wrist pain, spasticity and contractures. *Clin Rehabil*. 2013;27(7):579–590.

51. Li S, Rymer WZ. Voluntary breathing influences corticospinal excitability of nonrespiratory finger muscles. *J Neurophysiol*. 2011;105(2):512–521.

52. Francisco GE, McGuire J. Physiology and management of spasticity after stroke. In: Stein J, Harvey RL, Macko RF, Winstein CJ, Zorowitz RD, eds. *Stroke Recovery and Rehabilitation*. DemosMedical; 2009.

53. Pinto OD, Polikar M, Debono G. Results of international clinical trials with Lioresal. *Postgrad Med J.* 1972;48(5): 18–23.
54. Duncan GW, Shahani BT, Young RR. An evaluation of baclofen treatment for certain symptoms in patients with spinal cord lesions: a double blind cross over study. *Neurology.* 1976;26(5):441–446.
55. Milla PJ, Jackson ADM. A controlled trial of baclofen in children with cerebral palsy. *J Int Med Res.* 1997;5: 398–404.
56. Beard S, Hunn A, Wight J. Treatments for spasticity and pain in multiple sclerosis: a systematic review. *Health Technol Assess.* 2003;7(40):1–111.
57. Meythaler JM, Clayton W, Davis LK, Guin-Renfroe S, Brunner RC. Orally delivered baclofen to control spastic hypertonia in acquired brain injury. *J Head Trauma Rehabil.* 2004;19(2):101–108.
58. Medaer R, Hellebuyk H, Van Den Brande E, et al. Treatment of spasticity due to stroke: a double-blind, cross-over trial comparing baclofen with placebo. *Acta Therapeutica.* 1991;17(4):323–331.
59. Stevenson VL, Jarrett L. *Spasticity Management: A Practical Multidisciplinary Guide.* London: Informa Healthcare; 2006.
60. Medici M, Pebet M, Ciblis D. A double-blind, longterm study of tizanidine ('Sirdalud') in spasticity due to cerebrovascular lesions. *Curr Med Res Opin.* 1989;11(6): 398–407.
61. Simpson DM, Gracies JM, Yablon SA, Barbano R, Brashear A. Botulinum neurotoxin versus tizanidine in upper limb spasticity: a placebo-controlled study. *J Neurol.* 2009;80(4):380–385.
62. Royal M, Wienecke G, Movva V, et al. Retrospective study of efficacy of tizanidine in the treatment of chronic pain. *Pain Med.* 2001;2(3):249.
63. Ketel WB, Kolb ME. Long-term treatment with dantrolene sodium of stroke patients with spasticity limiting the return of function. *Curr Med Res Opin.* 1984;9:161–169.
64. Krause T, Gerbershagen MU, Fiege M, Weisshorn R, Wappler F. Dantrolene — a review of its pharmacology, therapeutic use and new developments. *Anaesthesia.* 2004;59(4):364–373.
65. Weiser R, Terenty T, Hudgson P, Weightman D. Dantrolene sodium in the treatment of spasticity in chronic spinal cord disease. *Practitioner.* 1978;221:123–127.
66. Katrak PH, Cole AMD, Poulos CJ, McCauley JCK. Objective assessment of spasticity, strength, and function with early exhibition of dantrolene sodium after cerebrovascular accident: a randomised double-blind controlled study. *Arch Phys Med Rehabil.* 1992;73:4–9.
67. Flewellen EH, Nelson PE, Jones WP, Arens JF, Wagner DL. Dantrolene dose–response in awake man: implications for management of malignant hyperthermia. *Anesthesiology.* 1983;59:275–280.
68. Neuroscience JR. A neuronal receptor for botulinum toxin. *Science.* 2006;312(5773):540–541.
69. de Paiva A, Meunier FA, Molgó J, Aoki KR, Dolly JO. Functional repair of motor endplates after botulinum neurotoxin type A poisoning: biphasic switch of synaptic activity between nerve sprouts and their parent terminals. *Proc Natl Acad Sci.* 1999;96(6):3200–3205.
70. Jankovic J, Brin MF. Therapeutic uses of botulinum toxin. *N Engl J Med.* 1991;324(17):1186–1194.
71. Jankovic J, Orman J. Botulinum a toxin for cranial-cervicaldystonia: a double-blind, placebo-controlled study. *Neurology.* 1987;37(4):616–623.
72. Bensmail D, Hanschmann A, Wissel J. Satisfaction with botulinum toxin treatment in post-stroke spasticity: results from two cross-sectional surveys (patients and physicians). *J Med Econ.* 2014;17(9):618–625.
73. Rosales RL, Chua-Yap AS. Evidence-based systematic review on the efficacy and safety of botulinum toxin-A therapy in post-stroke spasticity. *J Neural Transmission.* 2008; 115(4):617–623.
74. Wissel J, Ward AB, Erztgaard P, et al. European consensus table on the use of botulinum toxin type A in adult spasticity. *J Rehabil Med.* 2009;41(1):13–25.
75. Davis TL, Brodsky MA, Carter VA, et al. Consensus statement on the use of botulinum neurotoxin to treat spasticity in adults. *P and T.* 2006;31(11):666–682.
76. Simpson DM, Gracies JM, Graham HK, et al. Assessment: botulinum neurotoxin for the treatment of spasticity (an evidence-based review) report of the therapeutics and technology assessment subcommittee of the American Academy of Neurology. *Neurology.* 2008;70(19):1691–1698.
77. Sheean G, Lannin NA, Turner-Stokes L, Rawicki B, Snow BJ. Botulinum toxin assessment, intervention and after-care for upper limb hypertonicity in adults: international consensus statement. *Eur J Neurol.* 2010; 17(suppl 2):74–93.
78. Simpson DM, Hallett M, Ashman EJ, et al. Practice guideline update summary: botulinum neurotoxin for the treatment of blepharospasm, cervical dystonia, adult spasticity, and headache report of the guideline development subcommittee of the American Academy of Neurology. *Neurology.* 2016;86(19):1818–1826.
79. Rosales RL, Kong KH, Goh KJ, et al. Botulinum toxin injection for hypertonicity of the upper extremity within 12 weeks after stroke a randomized controlled trial. *Neurorehabil Neural Repair.* 2012;26(7):812–821.
80. Bakheit AMO, Thilmann AF, Ward AB, et al. A randomized, double-blind, placebo-controlled, dose-ranging study to compare the efficacy and safety of three doses of botulinum toxin type A (Dysport) with placebo in upper limb spasticity after stroke. *Stroke.* 2000;31(10):2402–2406.
81. Burridge JH, Wood DE, Hermens HJ, et al. Theoretical and methodological considerations in the measurement of spasticity. *Disabil Rehabil.* 2005;27(1–2):69–80.
82. Shaw LC, Price CI, van Wijck FM, et al. Botulinum toxin for the upper limb after stroke (BoTULS) trial: effect on impairment, activity limitation, and pain. *Stroke.* 2011; 42(5):1371–1379.
83. Lampire N, Roche N, Carne P, Cheze L, Pradon D. Effect of botulinum toxin injection on length and lengthening velocity of rectus femoris during gait in hemiparetic patients. *Clin Biomech.* 2013;28(2):164–170.

84. Tenniglo MJ, Nederhand MJ, Prinsen EC, Nene AV, Rietman JS, Buurke JH. Effect of chemodenervation of the rectus femoris muscle in adults with a stiff knee gait due to spastic paresis: a systematic review with a meta-analysis in patients with stroke. *Arch Phys Med Rehabil.* 2014;95(3):576–587.

85. Holman Barden HL, Baguley IJ, Nott MT, Chapparo C. Measuring spasticity and fine motor control (pinch) change in the hand following botulinum toxin-A injection using dynamic computerised hand dynamometry. *Arch Phys Med Rehabil.* 2014;95(12):2402–2409.

86. Bensmail D, Robertson JV, Fermanian C, Roby-Brami A. Botulinum toxin to treat upper-limb spasticity in hemiparetic patients: analysis of function and kinematics of reaching movements. *Neurorehabil Neural Repair.* 2010; 24(3):273–281.

87. Brashear A, Gordon MF, Elovic E. Intramuscular injection of botulinum toxin for the treatment of wrist and finger spasticity after a stroke. *N Engl J Med.* 2002;347:395–400.

88. Francis HP, Wade DT, Turner-Stokes L, Kingswell RS, Dott CS, Coxon EA. Does reducing spasticity translate into functional benefit? An exploratory meta-analysis. *J Neurol Neurosurg Psychiatry.* 2004;75(11): 1547–1551.

89. Caty GD, Detrembleur C, Bleyenheuft C, Deltombe T, Lejeune TM. Effect of upper limb botulinum toxin injections on impairment, activity, participation, and quality of life among stroke patients. *Stroke.* 2009;40(7): 2589–2591.

90. Foley N, Pereira S, Salter K, et al. Treatment with botulinum toxin improves upper-extremity function post stroke: a systematic review and meta-analysis. *Arch Phys Med Rehabil.* 2013;94(5):977–989.

91. Simpson DM, Alexander DN, O'Brien CF, et al. Botulinum toxin type A in the treatment of upper extremity spasticity: a randomized, double-blind, placebo-controlled trial. *Neurology.* 1996;46(5):1306–1310.

92. Hyman N, Barnes M, Bhakta B, et al. Botulinum toxin (Dysport) treatment of hip adductor spasticity in multiple sclerosis: a prospective, randomised, double blind, placebo controlled, dose ranging study. *J Neurol Neurosurg Psychiatry.* 2000;68(6):707–712.

93. Baker R, Jasinski M, Maciag-Tymecka I, et al. Botulinum toxin treatment of spasticity in diplegic cerebral palsy: a randomized, double-blind, placebo-controlled, dose-ranging study. *Dev Med Child Neurol.* 2002;44(10): 666–675.

94. Childers MK, Brashear A, Jozefczyk P, et al. Dose-dependent response to intramuscular botulinum toxin type A for upper-limb spasticity in patients after a stroke. *Arch Phys Med Rehabil.* 2004;85(7):1063–1069.

95. Bhakta BB, Cozens JA, Bamford JM, Chamberlain MA. Use of botulinum toxin in stroke patients with severe upper limb spasticity. *J Neurol Neurosurg Psychiatry.* 1996; 61(1):30–35.

96. Gracies JM, Bayle N, Goldberg S, Simpson DM. Botulinum toxin type B in the spastic arm: a randomized, double-blind, placebo-controlled, preliminary study. *Arch Phys Med Rehabil.* 2014;95(7):1303–1311.

97. Goldstein EM. Safety of high-dose botulinum toxin type A therapy for the treatment of pediatric spasticity. *J Child Neurol.* 2006;21(3):189–192.

98. Dressler D, Benecke R. Pharmacology of therapeutic botulinum toxin preparations. *Disabil Rehabil.* 2007;29(23): 1761–1768.

99. Wissel J, Manack A, Brainin M. Toward an epidemiology of poststroke spasticity. *Neurology.* 2013;(3 suppl. 2):80.

100. Santamato A, Notarnicola A, Panza F, et al. SBOTE study: extracorporeal shock wave therapy versus electrical stimulation after botulinum toxin type a injection for post-stroke spasticity-a prospective randomized trial. *Ultrasound Med Biol.* 2013;39(2):283–291.

101. Shaari CM, Sanders I. Quantifying how location and dose of botulinum toxin injections affect muscle paralysis. *Muscle Nerve.* 1993;16(9):964–969.

102. Kim HS, Hwang JH, Jeong ST, et al. Effect of muscle activity and botulinum toxin dilution volume on muscle paralysis. *Dev Med Child Neurol.* 2003;45(3):200–206.

103. Francisco GE. Botulinum toxin: dosing and dilution. *Am J Phys Med Rehabil.* 2004;83(10 suppl.):S30–S37.

104. Lee LR, Chuang YC, Yang BJ, Hsu MJ, Liu YH. Botulinum toxin for lower limb spasticity in children with cerebral palsy: a single-blinded trial comparing dilution techniques. *Am J Phys Med Rehabil.* 2004;83(10): 766–773.

105. Gracies JM, Lugassy M, Weisz DJ, Vecchio M, Flanagan S, Simpson DM. Botulinum toxin dilution and endplate targeting in spasticity: a double-blind controlled study. *Arch Phys Med Rehabil.* 2009;90(1):9–16.e12.

106. Kaji R. Clinical differences between A1 and A2 botulinum toxin subtypes. *Toxicon.* 2015;107:85–88.

107. Zuber M, Sebald M, Bathien N, De Recondo J, Rondot P. Botulinum antibodies in dystonic patients treated with type A botulinum toxin: frequency and significance. *Neurology.* 1993;43(9):1715–1718.

108. Greene P, Fahn S, Diamond B. Development of resistance to botulinum toxin type A in patients with torticollis. *Mov Disord.* 1994;9(2):213–217.

109. Naumann M, Carruthers A, Carruthers J, et al. Meta-analysis of neutralizing antibody conversion with onabotulinumtoxinA (BOTOX(R)) across multiple indications. *Mov Disord.* 2010;25(13):2211–2218.

110. Benecke R, Jost WH, Kanovsky P, Ruzicka E, Comes G, Grafe S. A new botulinum toxin type A free of complexing proteins for treatment of cervical dystonia. *Neurology.* 2005;64(11):1949–1951.

111. Jost WH, Blumel J, Grafe S. Botulinum neurotoxin type A free of complexing proteins (XEOMIN) in focal dystonia. *Drugs.* 2007;67(5):669–683.

112. Brin MF, Comella CL, Jankovic J, Lai F, Naumann M. Long-term treatment with botulinum toxin type A in cervical dystonia has low immunogenicity by mouse protection assay. *Mov Disord.* 2008;23(10): 1353–1360.

113. Guzman-Venegas RA, Araneda OF, Silvestre RA. Differences between motor point and innervation zone locations in the biceps brachii. An exploratory consideration for the treatment of spasticity with botulinum toxin. *J Electromyogr Kinesiol.* 2014;2(14): 00153−00159.

114. Im S, Park JH, Son SK, Shin JE, Cho SH, Park GY. Does botulinum toxin injection site determine outcome in post-stroke plantarflexion spasticity? Comparison study of two injection sites in the gastrocnemius muscle: a randomized double-blind controlled trial. *Clin Rehabil.* 2014;28(6):604−613.

115. Barbero M, Merletti R, Rainoldi A. *Atlas of Muscle Innervation Zones: Understanding Surface Electromyography and Its Applications.* Springer; 2012.

116. Lapatki B, Van Dijk J, Van de Warrenburg B, Zwarts M. Botulinum toxin has an increased effect when targeted toward the muscle's endplate zone: a high-density surface EMG guided study. *Clin Neurophysiol.* 2011;122(8): 1611−1616.

117. Bhadane M, Liu J, Rymer WZ, Zhou P, Li S. Re-evaluation of EMG-torque relation in chronic stroke using linear electrode array EMG recordings. *Sci Rep.* 2016; 6:28957.

118. Park ES, Rha DW, Yoo JK, Kim SM, Chang WH, Song SH. Short-term effects of combined serial casting and botulinum toxin injection for spastic equinus in ambulatory children with cerebral palsy. *Yonsei Med J.* 2010;51(4): 579−584.

119. Santamato A, Micello MF, Panza F, et al. Adhesive taping vs. daily manual muscle stretching and splinting after botulinum toxin type A injection for wrist and fingers spastic overactivity in stroke patients: a randomized controlled trial. *Clin Rehabil.* 2014;29(1):50−58. https://doi.org/10.1177/0269215514537915.

120. Karadag-Saygi E, Cubukcu-Aydoseli K, Kablan N, Ofluoglu D. The role of kinesiotaping combined with botulinum toxin to reduce plantar flexors spasticity after stroke. *Top Stroke Rehabil.* 2010;17(4):318−322.

121. Farina S, Migliorini C, Gandolfi M, et al. Combined effects of botulinum toxin and casting treatments on lower limb spasticity after stroke. *Funct Neurol.* 2008;23(2): 87−91.

122. Rummel A, Häfner K, Mahrhold S, et al. Botulinum neurotoxins C, e and F bind gangliosides via a conserved binding site prior to stimulation-dependent uptake with botulinum neurotoxin F utilising the three isoforms of SV2 as second receptor. *J Neurochem.* 2009;110(6): 1942−1954.

123. Bayram S, Sivrioglu K, Karli N, Ozcan O. Low-dose botulinum toxin with short-term electrical stimulation in poststroke spastic drop foot: a preliminary study. *Am J Phys Med Rehabil.* 2006;85(1):75−81.

124. Hesse S, Reiter F, Konrad M, Jahnke MT. Botulinum toxin type A and short-term electrical stimulation in the treatment of upper limb flexor spasticity after stroke: a randomized, double-blind, placebo-controlled trial. *Clin Rehabil.* 1998;12(5):381−388.

125. Mayer NH, Whyte J, Wannstedt G, Ellis CA. Comparative impact of 2 botulinum toxin injection techniques for elbow flexor hypertonia. *Arch Phys Med Rehab.* 2008; 89(5):982−987.

126. Wilkenfeld AJ. Review of electrical stimulation, botulinum toxin, and their combination for spastic drop foot. *J Rehabil Res Dev.* 2013;50(3):315−326.

127. Lagalla G, Danni M, Reiter F, Ceravolo MG, Provinciali L. Post-stroke spasticity management with repeated botulinum toxin injections in the upper limb. *Am J Phys Med Rehabil.* 2000;79(4):377−384.

128. Gordon MF, Brashear A, Elovic E, et al. Repeated dosing of botulinum toxin type A for upper limb spasticity following stroke. *Neurology.* 2004;63(10):1971−1973.

129. Elovic EP, Brashear A, Kaelin D, et al. Repeated treatments with botulinum toxin type a produce sustained decreases in the limitations associated with focal upper-limb poststroke spasticity for caregivers and patients. *Arch Phys Med Rehabil.* 2008;89(5):799−806.

130. Fortuna R, Horisberger M, Vaz MA, Herzog W. Do skeletal muscle properties recover following repeat onabotulinum toxin A injections? *J Biomech.* 2013;46(14):2426−2433.

131. Fortuna R, Vaz MA, Youssef AR, Longino D, Herzog W. Changes in contractile properties of muscles receiving repeat injections of botulinum toxin (Botox). *J Biomech.* 2011;44(1):39−44.

132. Turkoglu AN, Huijing PA, Yucesoy CA. Mechanical principles of effects of botulinum toxin on muscle length-force characteristics: an assessment by finite element modeling. *J Biomech.* 2014;47(7):1565−1571.

133. Rosales RL, Efendy F, Teleg ES, et al. Botulinum toxin as early intervention for spasticity after stroke or non-progressive brain lesion: a meta-analysis. *J Neurol Sci.* 2016;371:6−14.

134. Mas MF, Li S, Francisco GE. Centrally mediated late motor recovery after Botulinum toxin injection: case reports and a review of current evidence. *J Rehabil Med.* 2017;49(8): 609−619.

135. Chang SH, Francisco GE, Li S. Botulinum toxin (BT) injection improves voluntary motor control in selected patients with post-stroke spasticity. *Neural Regener Res.* 2012;7(18):1436−1439.

136. Filippi GM, Errico P, Santarelli R, Bagolini B, Manni E. Botulinum A toxin effects on rat jaw muscle spindles. *Acta Otolaryngol.* 1993;113(3):400−404.

137. Krishnan RV. Botulinum toxin: from spasticity reliever to a neuromotor re-learning tool. *Int J Neurosci.* 2005; 115(10):1451−1467.

138. Kaji R. Direct central action of intramuscularly injected botulinum toxin: is it harmful or beneficial? *J Physiol.* 2013;591(4):749.

139. Khalili AA, Betts HB. Peripheral nerve block with phenol in the management of spasticity. Indications and complications. *JAMA.* 1967;200(13):1155−1157.

140. Chua KS, Kong KH. Alcohol neurolysis of the sciatic nerve in the treatment of hemiplegic knee flexor spasticity: clinical outcomes. *Arch Phys Med Rehabil.* 2000; 81(10):1432−1435.

141. Bodine-Fowler SC, Allsing S, Botte MJ. Time course of muscle atrophy and recovery following a phenol-induced nerve block. *Muscle Nerve.* 1996;19(4):497–504.

142. Karri J, Mas MF, Francisco GE, Li S. Practice patterns for spasticity management with phenol neurolysis. *J Rehabil Med.* 2017;49(6):482–488.

143. Kirazli Y, On AY, Kismali B, Aksit R. Comparison of phenol block and botulinus toxin type A in the treatment of spastic foot after stroke: a randomized, double-blind trial. *Am J Phys Med Rehabil.* 1998;77(6):510–515.

144. Albright AL. Baclofen in the treatment of cerebral palsy. *J Child Neurol.* 1996;11(2):77–83.

145. Meythaler JM, Guin-Renfroe S, Grabb P, Hadley MN. Long-term continuously infused intrathecal baclofen for spastic-dystonic hypertonia in traumatic brain injury: 1-year experience. *Arch Phys Med Rehabil.* 1999;80(1):13–19.

146. Meythaler JM, Guin-Renfroe S, Brunner RC, Hadley MN. Intrathecal baclofen for spastic hypertonia from stroke. *Stroke.* 2001;32(9):2099–2109.

147. Peskine A, Roche N, Mailhan L, Thiébaut JB, Bussel B. Intrathecal baclofen for treatment of spasticity of multiple sclerosis patients. *Mult Sclerosis.* 2006;12(1):101–103.

148. Albright AL, Turner M, Pattisapu JV. Best-practice surgical techniques for intrathecal baclofen therapy. *J Neurosurg Pediatr.* 2006;104(4):233–239.

149. Turner M, Nguyen HS, Cohen-Gadol AA. Intraventricular baclofen as an alternative to intrathecal baclofen for intractable spasticity or dystonia: outcomes and technical considerations. *J Neurosurgery Pediatr.* 2012;10(4):315–319.

150. Boster AL, Adair RL, Gooch JL, et al. Best practices for intrathecal baclofen therapy: dosing and long-term management. *Neuromodulation.* 2016;19(6):623–631.

151. Boster AL, Bennett SE, Bilsky GS, et al. Best practices for intrathecal baclofen therapy: screening test. *Neuromodulation.* 2016;19(6):616–622.

152. Saulino M, Anderson DJ, Doble J, et al. Best practices for intrathecal baclofen therapy: troubleshooting. *Neuromodulation.* 2016;19(6):632–641.

153. Saulino M, Ivanhoe CB, McGuire JR, Ridley B, Shilt JS, Boster AL. Best practices for intrathecal baclofen therapy: patient selection. *Neuromodulation.* 2016;19(6):607–615.

154. Francisco GE, Boake C. Improvement in walking speed in poststroke spastic hemiplegia after intrathecal baclofen therapy: a preliminary study. *Arch Phys Med Rehabil.* 2003;84(8):1194–1199.

155. Schiess MC, Oh IJ, Stimming EF, et al. Prospective 12-month study of intrathecal baclofen therapy for post-stroke spastic upper and lower extremity motor control and functional improvement. *Neuromodulation.* 2011;14(1):38–45 (discussion 45).

156. Ivanhoe CB, Francisco GE, McGuire JR, Subramanian T, Grissom SP. Intrathecal baclofen management of poststroke spastic hypertonia: implications for function and quality of life. *Arch Phys Med Rehabil.* 2006;87(11):1509–1515.

157. Francisco GE, Yablon SA, Schiess MC, Wiggs L, Cavalier S, Grissom S. Consensus panel guidelines for the use of intrathecal baclofen therapy in poststroke spastic hypertonia. *Top Stroke Rehabil.* 2006;13(4):74–85.

158. Dvorak EM, Ketchum NC, McGuire JR. The underutilization of intrathecal baclofen in poststroke spasticity. *Top Stroke Rehabil.* 2011;18(3):195–202.

159. Keenan MA. Management of the spastic upper extremity in the neurologically impaired adult. *Clin Orthop Relat Res.* 1988;233:116–125.

160. Deltombe T, Decloedt P, Jamart J, Costa D, Split Anterior Tibialis Tendon Transfer (Splatt) PL, Tendon A. Lengthening for the correction of the varus foot after stroke a prospective longitudinal study. *Int J Phys Med Rehabil.* 2014:S5, 006.

161. Anakwenze OA, Namdari SEHJ, Benham J, Keenan MA. Myotendinous lengthening of the elbow flexor muscles to improve active motion in patients with elbow spasticity following brain injury. *J Shoulder Elbow Surg.* 2013;22(3):318–322.

162. Lieber RL, Friden J. Spasticity causes a fundamental rearrangement of muscle-joint interaction. *Muscle Nerve.* 2002;25(2):265–270.

163. Foran JR, Steinman S, Barash I, Chambers HG, Lieber RL. Structural and mechanical alterations in spastic skeletal muscle. *Dev Med Child Neurol.* 2005;47(10):713–717.

164. Buffenoir K, Decq P, Hamel O, Lambertz D, Perot C. Long-term neuromechanical results of selective tibial neurotomy in patients with spastic equinus foot. *Acta Neurochir.* 2013;155(9):1731–1743.

165. Dudley RW, Parolin M, Gagnon B, et al. Long-term functional benefits of selective dorsal rhizotomy for spastic cerebral palsy: clinical article. *J Neurosurg Pediatr.* 2013;12(2):142–150.

166. Hou LJ, Han SK, Gao WN, Xu YN, Yang XW, Yang WH. Aligned acupuncture at muscle regions plus cutaneous needle for upper limb spasticity after stroke: a multicenter randomized controlled trial. *J Acupunct Tuina Sci.* 2014;12(3):141–145.

167. Cai Y, Zhang CS, Liu S, et al. Electroacupuncture for post-stroke spasticity: a systematic review and meta-analysis. *Arch Phys Med Rehabil.* 2016;98(12):2578–2589.e4.

168. Caliandro P, Celletti C, Padua L, et al. Focal muscle vibration in the treatment of upper limb spasticity: a pilot randomized controlled trial in patients with chronic stroke. *Arch Phys Med Rehabil.* 2012;93(9):1656–1661.

169. Sadeghi M, Sawatzky B. Effects of vibration on spasticity in individuals with spinal cord injury: a scoping systematic review. *Am J Phys Med Rehabil.* 2014;16:16.

170. Kumru H, Murillo N, Samso JV, et al. Reduction of spasticity with repetitive transcranial magnetic stimulation in patients with spinal cord injury. *Neurorehabil Neural Repair.* 2010;24(5):435–441.

171. Wu D, Qian L, Zorowitz RD, Zhang L, Qu Y, Yuan Y. Effects on decreasing upper-limb poststroke muscle tone using transcranial direct current stimulation: a randomized sham-controlled study. *Arch Phys Med Rehabil.* 2013;94(1):1–8.

172. Barros Galvao SC, Borba Costa dos Santos R, Borba dos Santos P, Cabral ME, Monte-Silva K. Efficacy of coupling repetitive transcranial magnetic stimulation and physical therapy to reduce upper-limb spasticity in patients with stroke: a randomized controlled trial. *Arch Phys Med Rehabil.* 2014;95(2):222−229.

173. Gunduz A, Kumru H, Pascual-Leone A. Outcomes in spasticity after repetitive transcranial magnetic and transcranial direct current stimulations. *Neural Regen Res.* 2014;9(7):712−718.

174. Pinter MM, Gerstenbrand F, Dimitrijevic MR. Epidural electrical stimulation of posterior structures of the human lumbosacral cord: 3. Control of spasticity. *Spinal Cord.* 2000;38(9):524−531.

175. Oo WM. Efficacy of addition of transcutaneous electrical nerve stimulation to standardized physical therapy in subacute spinal spasticity: a randomized controlled trial. *Arch Phys Med Rehabil.* 2014;19(14):00432−00438.

176. Hofstoetter US, McKay WB, Tansey KE, Mayr W, Kern H, Minassian K. Modification of spasticity by transcutaneous spinal cord stimulation in individuals with incomplete spinal cord injury. *J Spinal Cord Med.* 2014;37(2):202−211.

177. Krewer C, Hartl S, Muller F, Koenig E. Effects of repetitive peripheral magnetic stimulation on upper-limb spasticity and impairment in patients with spastic hemiparesis: a randomized, double-blind, sham-controlled study. *Arch Phys Med Rehabil.* 2014;95(6):1039−1047.

178. Moon SW, Kim JH, Jung MJ, et al. The effect of extracorporeal shock wave therapy on lower limb spasticity in subacute stroke patients. *Ann Rehabil Med.* 2013;37(4):461−470.

179. Dymarek R, Ptaszkowski K, Slupska L, et al. Extracorporeal shock waves (ESW) as an alternative treatment method for improving the limb muscles' spasticity after cerebral stroke − a systematic review of the literature. *Wiadomosci Lekarskie. (Warsaw, Poland: 1960).* 2017; 70(3 pt. 2):667−676.

CHAPTER 11

Depression and Other Neuropsychiatric Issues Following Stroke

MELISSA JONES, MD • RICARDO E. JORGE, MD

DISCLOSURE STATEMENT

Dr. Jorge received lecture honoraria from Xiang-Jansen Pharmaceuticals. Dr. Jones has no financial disclosures to report.

INTRODUCTION

A stroke occurs on average every 40 seconds in the United States and is the second leading cause of death worldwide.[1] By 2030, 4% of the United States population is projected to have suffered a stroke.[2] Improvements in acute stroke management have contributed to the increasing number of stroke survivors.[2] However, the suffering caused by the emotional and cognitive sequelae of stroke remains underrecognized and underaddressed by clinicians.[3]

Poststroke depression (PSD) is a frequent neuropsychiatric complication of stroke and contributes to stroke-related disability, mortality, and poor quality of life.[4] The identification of PSD is especially important in the rehabilitation setting, where depression can interfere with participation, weaken the efficacy of interventions, and diminish medication adherence.[5] Furthermore, treatment of PSD may improve motor, functional, cognitive, and possibly, mortality outcomes.[6]

The focus of this chapter is to increase the clinician's awareness of the management of PSD. The prevalence, risk factors, negative impact, possible mechanisms, and diagnosis of PSD will be discussed. We will provide a brief overview of the differential diagnosis and treatment of potentially comorbid neuropsychiatric conditions. We will then consider the evidence supporting the use of pharmacotherapy and other treatment modalities for depression.

PREVALENCE

Meta-analysis of prevalence studies have confirmed that PSD will affect nearly a third of stroke patients throughout their course of recovery. A metaanalysis by Hackett and colleagues of 61 studies comprising 25,488 subjects found depression to occur in 31% (95% CI 28%–35%) of stroke patients at any time up to 5 years post stroke.[7] The frequency estimates for patients with a history of depression, aphasia, and first-ever stroke were not significantly different from the overall pooled estimate.[7] Another metaanalysis by Ayerbe and colleagues of 43 cohorts comprising 20,293 subjects found a pooled prevalence of depression at any time point to be 22% (95% CI 17–28) in population studies, 30% (95% CI 24–36) in hospital studies, and 30% (95% CI 25–36) in rehabilitation studies.[8] The overall course of depression appears to be dynamic post stroke, with new cases and recovery of depression occurring over time.[8]

Of note, many of the studies included in these metaanalyses diagnosed depression with severity measures alone. An earlier metaanalysis of studies utilizing diagnostic criteria and structured interviews to diagnose depression found the prevalence to vary according to the study setting, with a higher prevalence reported in acute hospital or rehabilitation settings (19% major depression, 30% minor depression) than in community populations (14% for major depression and 9% for minor depression).[9] In any case, clinicians should expect that at least one in three post-stroke patients undergoing inpatient or outpatient rehabilitation will have depression at any given time.

RISK FACTORS

Predictive factors for PSD have varied across studies. Disability and a prior history of depression are factors most consistently reported in the literature.[8,10] The severity of neurological deficit also appears to be predictive.[10] As discussed later, there is a complex relationship between the effects of depression, disability, and stroke severity on each other and on long-term outcomes.[11]

Stroke Rehabilitation. https://doi.org/10.1016/B978-0-323-55381-0.00011-1

Other factors identified in the literature include a personal history of anxiety and lack of social support.[8,10,12] Sex, age, and family history of depression have been less consistently identified as predictors.[6,12] Genetic and epigenetic risk factors also likely contribute to PSD risk. Polymorphisms and the methylation statuses of the serotonin transporter and brain-derived neurotrophic factor (BDNF) genes have been linked to PSD in prospective samples.[13–15] However, assessment of these risk factors is restricted to the research setting.

Despite the well-known association between cerebrovascular disease burden and depression in older individuals,[16–18] the only vascular risk factor associated with PSD appears to be diabetes.[12] Importantly, stroke type (ischemic vs. hemorrhagic), laterality, and lesion size do not appear to be risk factors for PSD.[8,12]

IMPACT

The prompt recognition and treatment of depression is critical to deter the detrimental effects of depression on stroke recovery. Overall, PSD has been linked to greater disability, cognitive impairment, and even mortality, as discussed below.

Disability

Depression has been associated with reduced participation and efficiency of rehabilitation interventions, leading to poorer mobility outcomes and less recovery of independence.[19,20] Several researchers have found PSD to be independently associated with greater disability, dependency, and poorer quality of life.[4,10,21,22] A prospective study by Pohjasvaara and colleagues of 390 stroke patients found depression at 3 months post-stroke correlated with poor functional outcome (Rankin Scale > II) at 15 months (OR 2.5, 95% CI 1.6–3.8).[22] There was no correlation of poor functional outcome at 3 months with depression at 15 months in this sample, providing some evidence that depression was not just a reaction to disability.[22] In contrast, other authors have proposed that depressive symptoms occur in response to the new deficits associated with acute stroke.[23] A more inclusive view is that depression and functional recovery have a bidirectional relationship, with depression worsening recovery, and greater disability worsening depression.[6] Finally, PSD and disability may be linked by another shared mechanism, such as impaired neuroplasticity, as discussed later.

Nevertheless, interventions targeting depression could help improve functional outcomes post stroke. In one prospective sample of 55 depressed stroke patients with similar rates of neurological deficits, physical therapy, and antidepressant use, patients with remitted depression showed better recovery of activities of daily living at 6 months compared to nonremitters (even if their depression remitted spontaneously).[24]

Cognition

Depression is also associated with deterred cognitive recovery. Patients with PSD underperform on tests of multiple neuropsychological domains and on general cognitive screening measures beyond what is expected from lesion size or location.[25] Executive dysfunction is common in PSD.[26] However, as with physical disability, it is difficult to fully disentangle a cause-and-effect relationship between depression and cognitive impairment. Although cognitive impairment has been reported to be a predictor of PSD,[10,27] Tene and colleagues recently concluded that depressive symptoms in the early to subacute poststroke period are independently predictive of cognitive and functional decline 2 years following admission for a stroke or transient ischemic attack.[28]

The complex relationship between late-life depression and neurodegenerative disorders further complicates matters, with late-onset depression potentially heralding a neurodegenerative process, and PSD being a possible risk factor for post-stroke dementia.[29,30] From a clinical standpoint, serial cognitive assessments before and after treatment of depression are required to determine whether cognitive impairment can be solely attributed to a mood disturbance.

Mortality

The most serious consequence of PSD is its association with increased mortality. In one cohort study, the odds of dying at 10 years post-stroke was 3.7 times (95% CI 1.1–12.2) greater for inpatients with major or minor PSD compared to nondepressed stroke patients after adjusting for stroke characteristics and sociodemographic and disability measures.[21] A more recent metaanalysis of 13 studies comprising 59,598 subjects reported a pooled odds ratio for mortality in patients with PSD of 1.22 (95% confidence interval 1.02–1.47).[31] Currently, the specific causes of this increased mortality are unclear. The associations between PSD and greater stroke severity and disability may be confounding, or depression may hinder adherence to treatment regimens. Another possible mechanism may be that depression is associated with an increased risk of cardiovascular events. In support of this hypothesis, Robinson and colleagues found heart rate variability (HRV) to be reduced in patients with major and minor PSD in comparison to nondepressed stroke patients.[32] HRV represents the balance between parasympathetic and sympathetic influences on the sinoatrial node, and reduced HRV has been associated with depression and increased mortality following myocardial infarction.[32] Nevertheless, the specific factors linking PSD with increased mortality is a topic requiring further research.

Another potential contributor to the increased mortality risk in patients with PSD is suicide. Approximately 12% of stroke survivors experience suicidal ideation according to a recent metaanalysis of 10,400 subjects.[33] Factors associated with suicidal ideation included recurrent stroke, poorer general cognition, and greater stroke severity.[33] Current or previous depression increased the odds of suicidal ideation by approximately 12- and 7-fold, respectively.[33] Thus, screening for PSD should also always include screening for suicidal ideation.

MECHANISM

Several etiologies of PSD have been proposed, and there is evidence supporting the roles of both psychosocial and biological factors. As previously discussed, there is some indication that depressive symptoms may be "reactive" to new onset physical and cognitive symptoms associated with acute stroke.[23,27] On the other hand, depressive symptoms have also been reported in patients with anosognosia who are unaware of their deficits.[4,34] Furthermore, depressive symptoms are common in patients with small vessel cerebrovascular disease who do not have an acute stroke.[16–18]

Other neurobiological explanations have included dysregulation of the hypothalamic-pituitary-adrenal axis, as demonstrated by abnormal dexamethasone suppression tests in some samples of patients with PSD.[35] Stroke may injure ascending monoaminergic axonal projections and disrupt serotonin and norepinephrine production, as supported by lower concentrations of the serotonin metabolite, 5-hydroxy-indoleacetic acid (5-HIAA), in the cerebrospinal fluid of depressed stroke patients.[36] There may also be an excess of proinflammatory cytokines in depressed patients, as evidenced by the higher levels of these cytokines in the serum of patients with PSD.[36] However, a single unifying mechanism has yet to be elucidated.

As previously mentioned, poorer physical and cognitive recovery have been associated with PSD, and impaired neuroplasticity may be a shared pathophysiological mechanism. In support of this hypothesis, antidepressants used to treat depression have been shown to increase expression of brain-derived neurotrophic actor (BDNF) in the prefrontal cortex and hippocampus.[37] In animal models, social isolation of mice following experimentally induced stroke led to depressive behaviors, reduced BDNF production, and greater histological injury.[38] Thus, even psychosocial stressors associated with PSD may exert their negative influence by disrupting mechanisms of neuroplasticity. Recently, mice knocked out of the myelocyte-specific P2X4 receptor, an immune-cell receptor mediating cytokine and BDNF release, led to depressive behaviors in the poststroke period.[39] This finding suggests a possible link between poststroke depressive behaviors, altered inflammatory responses, and reduced BDNF-signaling in the stroke recovery phase, but more work is needed to elucidate these relationships.

Another interesting line of research has taken advantage of functional and diffusion-weighted magnetic resonance imaging (MRI) techniques to investigate the integrity of neuronal networks in PSD. For instance, altered connectivity of the default network in the early poststroke period correlated with depressive symptoms at 3 months in one cohort,[40] and increased fractional anisotropy of the internal capsule correlated with improved depression severity in another.[41] Further advances in our understanding of the anatomy of the brain connectome and the dynamic functional configuration of neural networks may illuminate how lesions of different sizes and locations could alter networks governing mood and cognition in susceptible individuals. However, a coherent "neural signature" binding changes in affective processing and antidepressant response has yet to be confirmed.

DIAGNOSIS

The symptoms of PSD are similar to depressive episodes in patients without a history of acquired brain injury. Thus, the criteria for a depressive episode set forth by the *Diagnostic Statistical Manual (DSM)* are the gold standard for PSD.[42] Per the Fifth Edition of the *DSM (DSM-5)*, the diagnosis of PSD would fall under Depressive Disorder Due to Another Medical Condition (see Box 11.1). If full criteria for a major depressive episode are met (see Box 11.2), then the specifier "with major depressive-like episode" is appropriate. Even patients with "depressive features," or so called "minor depression," who do not meet full criteria for a major depressive episode may benefit from pharmacologic or psychologic interventions, especially if depressive symptoms are interfering with rehabilitation, impairing quality of life, or are associated with suicidal ideation.

Screening measures for depression that have been validated in the stroke population can be utilized in the rehabilitation setting. A systematic review of screens

---

BOX 11.1
Criteria for Major Depressive Disorder Due to Another Medical Condition

A. Prominent or persistent period of depressed mood or markedly diminished interest or pleasure in all, or almost all, activities
B. Evidence that the disturbance is the direct pathophysiological consequence of another medical condition.
C. The disturbance is not better explained by another mental disorder (for example, adjustment disorder).
D. The disturbance does not occur exclusively during the course of a delirium.
E. The disturbance causes clinically significant distress or impairment in social, occupational, or other important areas of functioning.

Specify if:
1. With depressive features: Full criteria are not met for a major depressive episode.
2. With major depressive episode: Full criteria are met for a major depressive episode.
3. With mixed features: Symptoms of mania or hypomania are also present but do not predominate the clinical picture.

BOX 11.2
Criteria for a Major Depressive Episode

At least five of the following symptoms are present for the same 2-week period and represent a change from previous functioning; criteria (1) or (2) must be present.
1. Depressed mood for most of the day, nearly every day. This can be determined with subjective report or observations made by others.
2. Markedly diminished interest or pleasure in all, or almost all, activities most of the day, nearly every day; this can also be determined with subjective or observer account.
3. Significant weight loss when not dieting or weight gain (more than 5% change in body weight in a month) or decrease or increase in appetite nearly every day.
4. Insomnia or hypersomnia nearly every day.
5. Psychomotor agitation or retardation nearly every day (must be observable by others, not merely subjective restlessness or feeling slowed down).
6. Fatigue or loss of energy nearly everyday.
7. Feelings of worthlessness or excessive or inappropriate guilt nearly every day (not merely self-reproach or guilt about being sick).
8. Diminished ability to think or concentrate or indecisiveness nearly every day (by subjective account or observation).
9. Recurrent thoughts of death (not just fear of dying), recurrent suicidal ideation without a specific plan, or a suicide attempt or a specific plan for committing suicide.

---

for PSD identified the 20-item Center of Epidemiological Studies-Depression Scale (CES-D) (sensitivity 75%, specificity 88%), 21-item Hamilton Depression Rating Scale (HDRS) (sensitivity 84%, specificity 83%), and 9-item Patient Health Questionnaire (PHQ-9) (sensitivity 86%, specificity 79%) to be the three most optimal measures.[43] The American Heart Association recommends the use of the PHQ-9 in clinical practice due to its rapid administration.[4] However, these measures do not obviate the need for clinical interview to confirm the diagnosis of PSD.[43] In the research setting, the most rigorous method of diagnosing PSD is with a semistructured interview, such as the Structured Clinical Interview for the *DSM* or the M.I.N.I neuropsychiatric interview.

Inquiring about depressive symptoms can be especially difficult in patients with communication deficits. The 10-item Stroke Aphasic Depression Questionnaire (SADQ) and its 10-item hospital version assess clinician-observed behaviors consistent with depressed mood, such as episodes of tearfulness, avoidance of social activities, restless sleep, anger, and poor eye contact. These screens are available to clinicians and do not require training to administer.[44] Importantly, self-assessments in patients with aphasia should be used with caution due to problems with understanding the instructions and completing the scales correctly.

Overall, more high-quality studies of depression screening measures for patients with aphasia are needed.[44]

DIFFERENTIAL DIAGNOSIS

Sadness, worry, and frustration can all be normal reactions to a recent stroke. Depressive symptoms are considered pathologic when they are interfering with rehabilitation interventions, pace of recovery, social or occupational functioning, and quality of life. Prior to starting treatment for depression, the differential diagnosis must be considered.

Adjustment Disorder

Adjustment disorder occurs when distress reaches an intensity excessive to the severity of the inciting stressor. The distress must begin within 3 months of the onset of the stressor and must be causing some degree of impairment in functioning. However, the patient cannot meet criteria for Major Depressive Disorder Due to Another Medical condition as discussed above.

Again, we would still recommend treating depressive symptoms that are interfering with rehabilitation or quality of life.

Apathy

Apathy is a disorder of motivation characterized by a lack of goal-directed behavior and cognition. Patients lack initiative and can appear to be indifferent. Apathetic symptoms, such as a loss of interest in usual activities and social withdrawal, can be prominent in major depression. However, apathy can occur independently from mood disturbances. Two separate meta-analysis of prevalence studies both concluded that over a third of stroke patients are affected by apathy, and in 24%–40% of cases, apathy occurs independently of depression.[45,46] On the other hand, Caeiro and colleagues concluded that cooccurring depression increases the odds of apathy by more than twofold, as did cognitive impairment.[45]

Rating scales that may be helpful for differentiating apathy from depression or for monitoring the response of apathy symptoms to treatment include The Apathy Evaluation Scale and the Neuropsychiatric Inventory.[47] Apathy occurring independently from depression is usually treated with stimulants, such as methylphenidate; other prodopaminergic agents, such as levodopa or amantadine; or anticholinesterase inhibitors, such as donepezil.[46]

Aprosodia

Affective aprosodia is defined as the impaired ability to express, repeat, or comprehend the variations in pitch, loudness, rate, or rhythm that convey emotional intent and meaning to language. Patients with expressive aprosodia may sound blunted and monotonous, but they do not necessarily have concomitant mood disturbances. This condition must be considered in patients with right-hemispheric lesions.[48] We screen for this condition by assessing the patient's ability to correctly comprehend, repeat, and express three variants of a single sentence: "*He's* going to sing?" (surprise); "He's *going* to sing?!" (anger); "He's going to *sing*!" (happiness).[49] When aprosodias are suspected, a consultation with a speech therapist is recommended.

Delirium

Delirium is defined as a disturbance of attention and impaired orientation that develops within hours to days and tends to fluctuate throughout the course of the day. Mood symptoms, sleep alterations, and/or psychosis can be prominent. Delirium in the acute phase post stroke is not uncommon, with an incidence ranging from 10% to 48%.[50] Furthermore, delirium is associated with an increased risk of poststroke dementia and mortality.[50] The Delirium Rating Scale and Confusion Assessment Method are commonly used screening measures in the hospital setting[50,51] and might also be helpful in the rehabilitation setting.

Stroke lesions may incite an acute confusional state, such as the one observed with certain thalamic infarctions.[52] However, in the rehabilitation setting, other causes of altered mental status must actively be sought, including secondary hemorrhagic transformation or hemorrhage expansion, anticholinergic or sedating drug effects, infections, poststroke seizures, vitamin deficiencies, and endocrinologic and other metabolic abnormalities. We would recommend addressing any potentially reversible causes and waiting until the delirium improves prior to initiating pharmacotherapy for depression to ensure that mood symptoms are persistent. Avoidance of any potential exacerbating medication and simplification of the medication regimen are important aspects of delirium management.

Psychosis

Psychosis secondary to stroke is rare, and there is limited data examining its prevalence. Rabins and colleagues identified only five participants (0.4%) as having psychosis (hallucinations and delusions) attributable to an acute stroke in a hospital-based registry of acute stroke patients.[47,53] Older age, family psychiatric history, right-hemispheric infarcts (especially in the region of the parietal-temporal-occipital junction), seizure disorders, and subcortical atrophy were possible predictors in their limited sample. However, more than one predisposing factor is likely needed.[54]

Peduncular hallucinosis is another infrequent manifestation of acute infarction of the posterior circulation usually involving pontine, midbrain, or thalamic regions. Hallucinations are well-formed, complex visual hallucinations that may or may not be combined with acoustic or tactile aspects.[55] However, given the rarity of new onset psychosis in stroke patients, we recommend a thorough evaluation for delirium and other contributing conditions.

Pathological Laughing and Crying

Pathological laughing and crying (PLC) is characterized by sudden, stereotyped (i.e., of similar intensity or duration) displays of emotion that do not need to be triggered by a stimulus of appropriate valence.[56] Also, these episodes need not be accompanied by a congruent emotional feeling (i.e., an episode of crying may be preceded by a humorous joke). If episodes are not stereotyped and are always preceded by an affectively congruent stimulus, emotional lability is a more appropriate term.[56]

The prevalence of the disorders of involuntary emotional expression is not entirely clear due to heterogeneity in definitions. Estimates of the prevalence of PLC range from 6% to 34% in the acute to subacute poststroke period.[57] Anger proneness may also be considered a form of impaired affective modulation post stroke. In one cohort, excessive episodes of anger and irritability were more closely tied to "emotional incontinence" than PSD.[58]

The Pathological Laughing and Crying Scale has been validated in the stroke population and may be useful for dissociating PLC from underlying mood disturbances or for monitoring treatment response.[59] Fortunately, SSRIs are considered first-line treatment for both depressed mood and disorders of involuntary emotional expression. Other options for PLC include venlafaxine, mirtazapine, tricyclic antidepressants, lamotrigine, levodopa, or amantadine.[57,60]

Fatigue

The prevalence of poststroke fatigue has been difficult to ascertain due to a lack of consensus on its definition. It is usually conceptualized as a general feeling of exhaustion or aversion to exerting effort.[47] Fatigue is common post stroke, affecting up to 85% of stroke survivors.[61,62] Not all patients with fatigue have depression. Furthermore, SSRI antidepressants do not appear to be efficacious for fatigue. Scales that may be useful for the assessment of fatigue or monitoring for its response to treatment include the Fatigue Severity Scale or the Multidimensional Fatigue Inventory.[61]

Potential interventions for fatigue occurring independently of PSD or for fatigue nonresponsive to treatment for PSD include increasing the patient's physical activity or the use of stimulants, such as modafinil.[47,62] In a recent double-blind, cross-over randomized controlled trial (RCT) of 36 subacute to chronic poststroke patients, modafinil 200 mg was found to decrease fatigue compared to placebo, but there were no significant differences in depression or anxiety measures.[63] Finally, other medical issues (e.g., anemia, hypothyroidism, B12 deficiency) should be considered.

Untreated sleep apnea may cause fatigue and depressive symptoms. Sleep apnea affects up to 75% of poststroke patients[64] and has been associated with delirium and poorer functional outcomes.[65] Patients should be referred for a sleep medicine evaluation where appropriate.

Anxiety

Anxiety is frequently comorbid with depression, but anxiety disorders can also occur independently post stroke. Anxiety disorders are generally characterized by excessive worries or anxious foreboding causing some degree of functional, social, and/or occupational impairment.

Concern about having another stroke, future falls, and the impact of the stroke on other family members are examples of normal reactions to an acute stroke. When it is excessive, interfering with rehabilitation efforts, or impacting quality of life, treatment should be considered.

A metaanalysis of 44 publications comprising 5760 stroke patients found a pooled prevalence of poststroke anxiety to be 18%–25%, depending on whether anxiety was diagnosed with clinical interview or rating scales, respectively.[66] Generalized anxiety is most common, but phobic and panic disorders are other possible manifestations.[67]

According to the *DSM-5*, poststroke anxiety would be classified as "anxiety disorder due to another medical condition." As is the case with depression, anxiety disorders post stroke are best diagnosed with semistructured, standardized, clinical interviews. However, the Hamilton Anxiety and Depression Scale, Hospital Anxiety and Depression Scale, and Beck Anxiety Index are commonly used as measures of anxiety symptom severity.[57,67]

Although not as extensively studied as PSD, predictors for anxiety include current or previous depression, stroke severity, anxiety occurring in the acute phases of stroke, and cognitive impairment or dementia.[68] Furthermore, anxiety comorbid with depression appears to worsen recovery in activities of daily living and social function in comparison to depression alone.[69]

Generally, treatment is similar to depression, with SSRI antidepressants as first-line agents. However, a recent systematic review of placebo-controlled RCTs of interventions for poststroke anxiety found little high-quality evidence to support any particular intervention.[70]

While there is limited evidence of the efficacy of paroxetine for poststroke anxiety,[67,70] we caution against the use of this SSRI due to its undesirable side-effect profile, as discussed later. Buspirone,[67,70] serotonin, and norepinephrine reuptake inhibitors (SNRIs), and less preferably, tricyclic antidepressants (TCAs), are secondary options. Benzodiazepines are not recommended due to their potential to cause cognitive impairment, falls, and dependence.

Bipolar Depression

Bipolar disorder is characterized by current or past episodes of hypomania or mania in addition to episodes of major depression. Little is known regarding the rates of poststroke depressive episodes occurring in the context of an underlying bipolar mood disorder. Despite the uncertainty of the frequency of poststroke bipolar depression, we would still recommend screening for current and previous hypomanic or manic symptoms (see below). The rationale is that in patients with bipolar mood disorders, antidepressants alone may be ineffective or cause a switch to hypomania or mania.

In terms of patients with a premorbid history of bipolar disorder presenting with poststroke depression, there is a lack of evidence guiding treatment. Atypical antipsychotics with evidence for idiopathic bipolar depression (i.e., lurasidone, aripiprazole, quetiapine, or olanzapine) can be considered.[71] However, elderly patients are more at risk of developing orthostatic hypotension, extrapyramidal side effects, and/or anticholinergic toxicity from these medications,[72] and cardiovascular side effects may hinder secondary prevention efforts. Antipsychotics should be avoided for unipolar depression, unless it is refractory to conventional treatment.

Poststroke Mania

Poststroke mania is a rare neuropsychiatric consequence of stroke. For instance, Robinson and colleagues prospectively identified only two cases of mania out of 379 patients hospitalized for acute stroke.[73] A systematic review by Santos and colleagues identified only 74 cases of mania spanning over 50 years of literature.[74]

Hypomanic and manic episodes are characterized by elevated, expansive, or irritable mood and increased activity or energy that last for at least 1 week (or 4 days in the case of hypomania). Three or more additional symptoms must be present (four if the mood is only irritable), including grandiosity or elevated self-esteem; decreased need for sleep (e.g., feeling rested after 3 hours per night); excessive talkativeness or pressured speech; flight of ideas or racing thoughts; distractibility; increased goal-directed activity or psychomotor agitation; and engagement in disinhibited, pleasure-seeking behaviors despite their negative consequences (e.g., hypersexuality or shopping sprees). If psychotic features are present or acute hospitalization is required, then the episode is deemed to be a manic episode. In the *DSM-5*, poststroke mania or bipolar disorder would be categorized as "Bipolar and Related Disorder Due to Another Medical Condition." The specifiers "with hypomanic or manic-like episode" and "with manic or hypomanic features" are used when full criteria are met or only partially met, respectively. If depressive symptoms are also present but do not predominate the clinical picture, then "with mixed features" is appropriate.

Early studies investigating predictors of poststroke mood disorders found right-hemispheric infarctions to occur more frequently in mania, whereas left-hemispheric infarctions occurred more frequently in depression.[73] However, more recent reviews have not found support for a relationship between stroke laterality and mood disorders.[10,74,76]

The evidence for the treatment of poststroke mania and hypomania is based on case reports. Mood stabilizers (i.e., lithium, valproic acid, carbamazepine) and antipsychotics (i.e., haloperidol, olanzapine, risperidone) have been utilized in some reports.[74] Elderly, brain-injured patients may be especially vulnerable to side effects of these medications, and again, we would recommend consultation with a psychiatrist. Electroconvulsive therapy may also be considered.

TREATMENT

Pharmacologic interventions are currently first-line treatment for PSD. However, there is no conclusive evidence supporting the efficacy of one antidepressant over another, or that treatment response is influenced by such factors such as stroke mechanism, infarct location, or history of depression. The choice of antidepressant ultimately depends on concurrent medical or psychiatric comorbidities, previous treatment response, and patient preference.

We generally recommend reviewing the prescribing information and routinely using an interaction checker prior to initiating pharmacotherapy. As previously discussed, we also recommend screening for cognitive impairment and prior episodes of mania or hypomania prior to initiating pharmacotherapy.

Patients may not achieve response for at least four to 6 weeks, and after that time, dose increases can be considered. The standardized measures of depressive symptoms mentioned previously may be useful for monitoring treatment efficacy. The ideal length of treatment for new onset PSD is not known, but it is currently recommended that treatment be continued for at least 6 months.[47] If the patient has a history of recurrent episodes, treatment can be continued indefinitely at the lowest, effective dose possible.

As previously mentioned, suicidal ideation should be screened for in every patient, especially since treatment of coexistent depression is an important part of safety risk management.[77] If a patient is actively suicidal or the patient's safety is a concern, one-to-one monitoring and/or urgent involvement of a psychiatrist is advised, depending on the clinical setting.

Selective Serotonin Reuptake Inhibitors

SSRIs are the most-studied and widely used pharmacotherapies for PSD. Fluoxetine has been increasing in popularity since the publication of the Fluoxetine for Motor Recovery after Acute Ischemic Stroke (FLAME) trial.[78] However, double-blind RCTs of fluoxetine for the treatment of PSD have been conflicting.[79–82] RCTs examining the efficacies of other SSRIs, such as paroxetine, sertraline, citalopram, and escitalopram, have also reported conflicting findings.[57,83–85] Despite this, SSRIs are preferred due to their favorable tolerability profiles and efficacy in treating other comorbid neuropsychiatric disorders, such as anxiety, PLC, and emotional lability.

The most common side effects reported in RCTs of SSRIs are gastrointestinal.[79–83,85–87] It can be helpful to inform patients that gastrointestinal side effects tend to improve in the first few weeks of treatment. Sexual side effects are also common among the SSRIs as a class, but they do not tend to improve with treatment duration. If this is a concern, mirtazapine, duloxetine, and the sustained or extended release versions of bupropion can be considered,[88] but there is less evidence supporting their safety and efficacy in PSD. Of note, we usually recommend against the use of paroxetine in brain-injured patients due to its undesirable side-effect profile, including anticholinergic side effects (sedation, urinary retention, constipation, dry mouth, etc.), weight gain, the potential for withdrawal symptoms due to its short half-life, and its propensity for drug-drug interactions.

Less common side effects that have been associated with SSRIs include gastrointestinal, intracerebral, and postsurgical hemorrhage[89–91]; cerebral vasoconstriction[92,93]; increased risk of falls and/or fractures[94,95]; hyponatremia and seizures.[96] However, to our knowledge, no RCT of SSRI therapy for PSD has ever been discontinued because of these severe adverse reactions.

In terms of bleeding risk, medications with serotonin reuptake inhibitor activity deplete platelet serotonin and are thought to increase the risk of gastrointestinal hemorrhage.[89] Gastric acid suppressing drugs may lower the risk,[91] but caution should be used in patients with previous gastrointestinal hemorrhage, concurrent antiplatelet or anticoagulant use, and other conditions that increase bleeding risk, such as liver disease. Other antidepressants, such as duloxetine or the

sustained or extended release versions of bupropion, can be considered as alternatives. Mirtazapine may also be an option, but this antidepressant has also been implicated in increasing the risk of gastrointestinal hemorrhages.[89]

The risk of intracranial hemorrhage is more controversial, especially in patients who have had a stroke.[97,98] However, there is currently insufficient evidence to support withholding SSRIs or pharmacotherapy for depression due to concern for recurrent ischemic or hemorrhagic stroke when mood disturbances are interfering with recovery and quality of life.[99] One exception is in the case of reversible cerebral vasoconstriction syndrome (Call–Fleming Syndrome), which is thought to be precipitated by serotonergic and sympathomimetic medications.[92]

In addition to treating depression, there are other potential benefits of SSRIs that may outweigh the potential risks. A metaanalysis of 52 trials (n = 4060) comparing poststroke SSRI administration to placebo/standard care concluded SSRIs were associated with reduced dependency, disability, and anxiety.[100]

As previously mentioned, fluoxetine has been increasingly used in the post-stroke period to improve motor outcomes following the publication of the FLAME trial. In this study, 118 patients were randomly assigned to receive fluoxetine 20 mg or placebo for 12 weeks along with standardized rehabilitation. The fluoxetine group showed significantly greater improvement in motor deficit, stroke severity, and functional independence measures compared to the placebo group. The positive effects of fluoxetine on motor recovery remained significant after adjusting for rates of depression onset and thrombolysis administration.[78] There are additional ongoing RCTs of fluoxetine for motor recovery following ischemic[101] and hemorrhagic[102] strokes.

There is some evidence suggesting that SSRIs may improve cognitive recovery, even in patients who are not depressed. In an RCT of escitalopram 5–10 mg, problem-solving therapy, or placebo, subjects in the escitalopram group showed greater improvements in memory and general cognitive measures independently of depression severity, stroke-subtype, and time post stroke.[103] Overall, other than paroxetine, SSRIs appear to have little, if any, negative cognitive side effects in stroke patients.

Other Antidepressants

The SNRIs are additional treatment options for PSD, including for patients with cooccurring chronic pain, headache, and comorbid anxiety disorders. However, there is limited evidence supporting the use of duloxetine[104,105] or venlafaxine[106,107] in the treatment of PSD. It is also important to note that venlafaxine has been associated with mild increases in blood pressure, and we would recommend avoiding its use in patients with difficult to control hypertension.

There is also limited evidence supporting the use of mirtazapine, an alpha-2 adrenergic receptor antagonist.[108] Due to its sedating properties at lower dosages ($\leq$15 mg) and propensity to cause weight gain, this medication can be useful for patients with insomnia and poor appetite.

Trazodone, a serotonin receptor antagonist, has been studied in two small RCTs for PSD.[109,110] However, it is rarely used as monotherapy due to sedating and orthostatic properties.

There is a paucity of literature on the use of bupropion, a norepinephrine and dopamine reuptake inhibitor. Perhaps this is due to its potential to lower the seizure threshold.[111] The immediate release formulation should especially be avoided for this reason.[112] However, bupropion sustained or extended release can be considered in the context of smoking cessation, bleeding risk, sexual side effects from SSRIs, or apathy that is comorbid with depression.

Older antidepressants, such as TCAs and monoamine oxidase inhibitors (MAOIs), are less preferred due to their poor side-effect profiles. MAOIs are not recommended because of the risk of hypertensive reactions with coadministration of sympathomimetic medications and foods containing tyramine. Of the TCAs, nortriptyline appears to be efficacious for PSD based on double-blind RCTs.[81,113] Generally, secondary amine TCAs (nortriptyline, desipramine) have less anticholinergic, antihistaminergic, and anti-alpha-1 receptor blocking activity compared to the tertiary amine TCAs (amitriptyline, doxepin, imipramine). If needed for refractory depression, migraine, or chronic pain, we recommend using the lowest effective dose possible, monitoring serum levels, and assessing for delirium, orthostatic hypotension, falls, reflex tachycardia, and electrocardiographic abnormalities, especially in patients with cardiac disease.

Stimulants, such as methylphenidate or amphetamine formulations, have limited evidence for the treatment of PSD.[114,115] An RCT of methylphenidate (maximum dose 15 mg twice daily) combined with physiotherapy for one to 3 weeks found significantly lower depressive symptoms, better motor recovery, and greater improvement in activities of daily living in the methylphenidate group.[115] To our knowledge,

amphetamine formulations have not been studied for PSD, but they have been studied in the context of post-stroke motor recovery (with inconsistent results).[116] If used for comorbid fatigue, apathy, or to enhance processing speed, clinicians should monitor for irritability, emotional lability, psychosis, anxiety, appetite suppression, insomnia, or tic exacerbations. Patients should also be monitored for emergent tachycardia and hypertension. Also, stimulants should be used cautiously in patients with cardiac disease.[117] Modafinil has not, to our knowledge, been specifically studied for PSD. However, it could be an adjunctive medication for hypersomnolence and fatigue.[63] This stimulant also has the capacity to cause anxiety, insomnia, and hypertension.

Additional Interventions

We encourage a multidisciplinary approach to treating patients with PSD that includes secondary stroke prophylaxis. Intuitively, the best method to limit the effects of cerebrovascular disease on mood and cognition would be with adequate control of vascular risk factors. Although evidence is lacking, acetylcholinesterase inhibitors or memantine can be considered in the context of depression cooccurring with vascular cognitive impairment. Neurostimulation techniques are generally reserved for refractory cases. Electroconvulsive therapy has been used for many years to treat depression, but there are no RCTs supporting its use for PSD.

Repetitive transcranial magnetic stimulation (rTMS) may be an option for treatment of refractory depression.[118] For instance, Jorge and colleagues previously demonstrated the efficacy of left dorsolateral prefrontal cortex rTMS in patients with vascular depression who failed at least one trial of antidepressant therapy.[119] However, there is concern for inducing seizures, and more work is needed to optimize stimulation protocols. A recent trial of transcranial direct current stimulation (tDCS) concurrently with occupational therapy found benefit for depressive symptoms and quality of life,[120] but this evidence is too preliminary to recommend the use of tDCS for PSD.

Psychotherapy is another potential intervention that can be considered for the treatment of depression in conjunction with pharmacotherapy. Unfortunately, there is a lack of RCTs supporting its efficacy in PSD.[121] Problem-solving therapy may be effective to prevent or treat depression in stroke patients.[122] According to the American Heart Association, brief psychosocial interventions may be useful, but further research is required.[4] More high-quality studies of psychotherapeutic interventions are greatly needed.

Prevention of Poststroke Depression

The development of interventions for the prevention of depression in stroke patients is an important step forward in combating the potential morbidity and mortality associated with this prevalent neuropsychiatric complication. Psychosocial interventions, such as motivational interviewing, problem-solving therapy, and home-based therapy, may be useful for the prevention of PSD.[4]

Antidepressants administered to nondepressed stroke patients also appear to be efficacious in reducing the onset of depression.[4,123] For instance, Robinson and colleagues found that administering escitalopram to nondepressed stroke patients successfully prevented PSD, with the placebo group being four times more likely to develop depression (adjusted hazard ratio [HR], 4.5; 95% CI, 2.4–8.2; $P < .001$), even after controlling for age, gender, severity of stroke, and severity of disability.[122]

A more recent metaanalysis of pharmacological interventions by Salter and colleagues in 776 nondepressed stroke patients also found a reduced likelihood of developing depression for active compared to placebo groups (OR 0.34, 95% CI 0.22–0.53).[123] Despite potential concerns related to patient acceptability and tolerability of pharmacologic preventive strategies, this metaanalysis did not find a significant difference in the rates of side effects between groups.[123] At this time, more research is needed to support the widespread implementation of preventive strategies in the clinical setting.

CONCLUSION

PSD is a common and disabling condition in stroke survivors. Patients with PSD are more likely to have poorer rates of functional and cognitive recovery. Recognition and treatment of this condition is necessary to combat the negative impact of depression on rehabilitation outcomes. The defining feature of PSD is the persistence of low mood or lack of pleasure for most of the day, nearly every day. Other neuropsychiatric conditions that may be comorbid or occur independently from depression include anxiety, apathy, delirium, affective aprosodia, pathological laughing and crying, and rarely, poststroke bipolar or psychotic disorders. SSRIs are the treatment of choice for depression due to their relatively benign side-effect profile. Newer generation antidepressants and/or stimulants may also be considered depending on coexistent neuropsychiatric or medical conditions and prior treatment responsiveness. Neurostimulation, psychotherapy, and preventive techniques are significant areas of future research.

FINANCIAL DISCLOSURE AND ACKNOWLEDGMENTS

This work was supported by the use of resources and facilities at the Houston VA HSR&D Center for Innovations in Quality, Effectiveness and Safety (CIN13-413). The opinions expressed reflect those of the authors and not necessarily those of the Department of Veterans Affairs, the US government, or Baylor College of Medicine. Dr. Jorge received lecture honoraria from Xiang-Jansen Pharmaceuticals. Dr. Jones has no financial disclosures to report.

REFERENCES

1. Benjamin EJ, Blaha MJ, Chiuve SE, et al. Heart disease and stroke Statistics-2017 update: a report from the American heart association. *Circulation*. 2017;135(10): e146–e603.
2. Ovbiagele B, Goldstein LB, Higashida RT, et al. Forecasting the future of stroke in the United States: a policy statement from the American Heart Association and American Stroke Association. *Stroke*. 2013;44(8): 2361–2375.
3. Walsh ME, Galvin R, Loughnane C, Macey C, Horgan NF. Community re-integration and long-term need in the first five years after stroke: results from a national survey. *Disabil Rehabil*. 2015;37(20):1834–1838.
4. Towfighi A, Ovbiagele B, El Husseini N, et al. Poststroke depression: a scientific statement for healthcare professionals from the American Heart Association/American Stroke Association. *Stroke*. 2017;48(2):e30–e43.
5. Belagaje SR. Stroke rehabilitation. *Contin (Minneap Minn)*. 2017;23(1, Cerebrovascular Disease):238–253.
6. Robinson RG, Jorge RE. Post-stroke depression: a review. *Am J Psychiatry*. 2016;173(3):221–231.
7. Hackett ML, Pickles K. Part I: frequency of depression after stroke: an updated systematic review and meta-analysis of observational studies. *Int J Stroke*. 2014;9(8): 1017–1025.
8. Ayerbe L, Ayis S, Wolfe CD, Rudd AG. Natural history, predictors and outcomes of depression after stroke: systematic review and meta-analysis. *Br J Psychiatry*. 2013; 202(1):14–21.
9. Robinson RG. Prevalence of depressive disorders. In: *The Clinical Neuropsychiatry of Stroke: Cognitive, Behavioral and Emotional Disorders Following Vascular Brain Injury*. 2nd ed. New York: Cambridge University Press; 2006: 52–59.
10. Kutlubaev MA, Hackett ML. Part II: predictors of depression after stroke and impact of depression on stroke outcome: an updated systematic review of observational studies. *Int J Stroke*. 2014;9(8):1026–1036.
11. Ayerbe L, Ayis SA, Crichton S, Rudd AG, Wolfe CD. Explanatory factors for the association between depression and long-term physical disability after stroke. *Age Ageing*. 2015;44(6):1054–1058.

12. De Ryck A, Brouns R, Fransen E, et al. A prospective study on the prevalence and risk factors of poststroke depression. *Cerebrovasc Dis Extra*. 2013;3(1):1−13.

13. Kim JM, Stewart R, Bae KY, et al. Serotonergic and BDNF genes and risk of depression after stroke. *J Affect Disord*. 2012;136(3):833−840.

14. Kim JM, Stewart R, Kang HJ, et al. A longitudinal study of SLC6A4 DNA promoter methylation and poststroke depression. *J Psychiatr Res*. 2013;47(9):1222−1227.

15. Kohen R, Cain KC, Mitchell PH, et al. Association of serotonin transporter gene polymorphisms with post-stroke depression. *Arch Gen Psychiatry*. 2008;65(11): 1296−1302.

16. Aizenstein HJ, Baskys A, Boldrini M, et al. Vascular depression consensus report − a critical update. *BMC Med*. 2016;14(1):161.

17. Alexopoulos GS, Meyers BS, Young RC, Kakuma T, Silbersweig D, Charlson M. Clinically defined vascular depression. *Am J Psychiatry*. 1997;154(4):562−565.

18. van Uden IW, Tuladhar AM, de Laat KF, et al. White matter integrity and depressive symptoms in cerebral small vessel disease: the RUN DMC study. *Am J Geriatr Psychiatry*. 2015;23(5):525−535.

19. Gillen R, Tennen H, McKee TE, Gernert-Dott P, Affleck G. Depressive symptoms and history of depression predict rehabilitation efficiency in stroke patients. *Arch Phys Med Rehabil*. 2001;82(12):1645−1649.

20. Paolucci S, Di Vita A, Massicci R, et al. Impact of participation on rehabilitation results: a multivariate study. *Eur J Phys Rehabil Med*. 2012;48(3):455−466.

21. Morris PL, Robinson RG, Andrzejewski P, Samuels J, Price TR. Association of depression with 10-year post-stroke mortality. *Am J Psychiatry*. 1993;150(1):124−129.

22. Pohjasvaara T, Vataja R, Leppavuori A, Kaste M, Erkinjuntti T. Depression is an independent predictor of poor long-term functional outcome post-stroke. *Eur J Neurol*. 2001;8(4):315−319.

23. Nys GM, van Zandvoort MJ, van der Worp HB, de Haan EH, de Kort PL, Kappelle LJ. Early depressive symptoms after stroke: neuropsychological correlates and lesion characteristics. *J Neurol Sci*. 2005;228(1):27−33.

24. Chemerinski E, Robinson RG, Kosier JT. Improved recovery in activities of daily living associated with remission of poststroke depression. *Stroke*. 2001;32(1):113−117.

25. Robinson RG. Relationship to cognitive impairment and treatment. In: *The Clinical Neuropsychiatry of Stroke: Cognitive, Behavioral and Emotional Disorders Following Vascular Brain Injury*. 2nd ed. New York: Cambridge University Press; 2006:148−170.

26. Sibolt G, Curtze S, Melkas S, et al. Post-stroke depression and depression-executive dysfunction syndrome are associated with recurrence of ischaemic stroke. *Cerebrovasc Dis*. 2013;36(5−6):336−343.

27. Nys GM, van Zandvoort MJ, van der Worp HB, et al. Early cognitive impairment predicts long-term depressive symptoms and quality of life after stroke. *J Neurol Sci*. 2006;247(2):149−156.

28. Tene O, Shenhar-Tsarfaty S, Korczyn AD, et al. Depressive symptoms following stroke and transient ischemic attack: is it time for a more intensive treatment approach? Results from the TABASCO cohort study. *J Clin Psychiatry*. 2016;77(5):673−680.

29. Dichgans M, Leys D. Vascular cognitive impairment. *Circ Res*. 2017;120(3):573−591.

30. Panza F, Frisardi V, Capurso C, et al. Late-life depression, mild cognitive impairment, and dementia: possible continuum? *Am J Geriatr Psychiatry*. 2010;18(2):98−116.

31. Bartoli F, Lillia N, Lax A, et al. Depression after stroke and risk of mortality: a systematic review and meta-analysis. *Stroke Res Treat*. 2013;2013:862978.

32. Robinson RG, Spalletta G, Jorge RE, et al. Decreased heart rate variability is associated with poststroke depression. *Am J Geriatr Psychiatry*. 2008;16(11):867−873.

33. Bartoli F, Pompili M, Lillia N, et al. Rates and correlates of suicidal ideation among stroke survivors: a meta-analysis. *J Neurol Neurosurg Psychiatry*. 2017;88(6): 498−504.

34. Starkstein SE, Fedoroff JP, Price TR, Leiguarda R, Robinson RG. Anosognosia in patients with cerebrovascular lesions. A study of causative factors. *Stroke*. 1992; 23(10):1446−1453.

35. Noonan K, Carey LM, Crewther SG. Meta-analyses indicate associations between neuroendocrine activation, deactivation in neurotrophic and neuroimaging markers in depression after stroke. *J Stroke Cerebrovasc Dis*. 2013; 22(7):e124−e135.

36. Spalletta G, Bossu P, Ciaramella A, Bria P, Caltagirone C, Robinson RG. The etiology of poststroke depression: a review of the literature and a new hypothesis involving inflammatory cytokines. *Mol Psychiatry*. 2006;11(11): 984−991.

37. Harmer CJ, Duman RS, Cowen PJ. How do antidepressants work? New perspectives for refining future treatment approaches. *Lancet Psychiatry*. 2017;4(5):409−418.

38. O'Keefe LM, Doran SJ, Mwilambwe-Tshilobo L, Conti LH, Venna VR, McCullough LD. Social isolation after stroke leads to depressive-like behavior and decreased BDNF levels in mice. *Behav Brain Res*. 2014;260:162−170.

39. Verma R, Cronin CG, Hudobenko J, Venna VR, McCullough LD, Liang BT. Deletion of the P2X4 receptor is neuroprotective acutely, but induces a depressive phenotype during recovery from ischemic stroke. *Brain Behav Immun*. 2017;66:302−312.

40. Lassalle-Lagadec S, Sibon I, Dilharreguy B, Renou P, Fleury O, Allard M. Subacute default mode network dysfunction in the prediction of post-stroke depression severity. *Radiology*. 2012;264(1):218−224.

41. Yasuno F, Taguchi A, Yamamoto A, et al. Microstructural abnormalities in white matter and their effect on depressive symptoms after stroke. *Psychiatry Res*. 2014;223(1): 9−14.

42. Spalletta G, Robinson RG. How should depression be diagnosed in patients with stroke? *Acta Psychiatr Scand*. 2010;121(6):401−403.

43. Meader N, Moe-Byrne T, Llewellyn A, Mitchell AJ. Screening for poststroke major depression: a meta-analysis of diagnostic validity studies. *J Neurol Neurosurg Psychiatry.* 2014;85(2):198–206.

44. van Dijk MJ, de Man-van Ginkel JM, Hafsteinsdottir TB, Schuurmans MJ. Identifying depression post-stroke in patients with aphasia: a systematic review of the reliability, validity and feasibility of available instruments. *Clin Rehabil.* 2016;30(8):795–810.

45. Caeiro L, Ferro JM, Costa J. Apathy secondary to stroke: a systematic review and meta-analysis. *Cerebrovasc Dis.* 2013;35(1):23–39.

46. van Dalen JW, Moll van Charante EP, Nederkoorn PJ, van Gool WA, Richard E. Poststroke apathy. *Stroke.* 2013; 44(3):851–860.

47. Hackett ML, Kohler S, O'Brien JT, Mead GE. Neuropsychiatric outcomes of stroke. *Lancet Neurol.* 2014;13(5): 525–534.

48. Ross ED, Monnot M. Neurology of affective prosody and its functional-anatomic organization in right hemisphere. *Brain Lang.* 2008;104(1):51–74.

49. Arciniegas DB. Mental status examination. In: Arciniegas DBA, Alan C, Filley CM, eds. *Behavioral Neurology & Neuropsychiatry.* New York: Cambridge University Press; 2013:344–393.

50. Klimiec E, Dziedzic T, Kowalska K, Slowik A, Klimkowicz-Mrowiec A. Knowns and unknowns about delirium in stroke: a review. *Cogn Behav Neurol.* 2016; 29(4):174–189.

51. Shi Q, Presutti R, Selchen D, Saposnik G. Delirium in acute stroke: a systematic review and meta-analysis. *Stroke.* 2012;43(3):645–649.

52. Schmahmann JD. Vascular syndromes of the thalamus. *Stroke.* 2003;34(9):2264–2278.

53. Rabins PV, Starkstein SE, Robinson RG. Risk factors for developing atypical (schizophreniform) psychosis following stroke. *J Neuropsychiatry Clin Neurosci.* 1991; 3(1):6–9.

54. Robinson RG. Psychosis. In: *The Clinical Neuropsychiatry of Stroke: Cognitive, Behavioral and Emotional Disorders Following Vascular Brain Injury.* 2nd ed. New York: Cambridge University Press; 2006:357–365.

55. Benke T. Peduncular hallucinosis: a syndrome of impaired reality monitoring. *J Neurol.* 2006;253(12): 1561–1571.

56. Lauterbach EC, Cummings JL, Kuppuswamy PS. Toward a more precise, clinically–informed pathophysiology of pathological laughing and crying. *Neurosci Biobehav Rev.* 2013;37(8):1893–1916.

57. Kim JS. Post-stroke mood and emotional disturbances: pharmacological therapy based on mechanisms. *J Stroke.* 2016;18(3):244–255.

58. Kim JS, Choi S, Kwon SU, Seo YS. Inability to control anger or aggression after stroke. *Neurology.* 2002;58(7): 1106–1108.

59. Robinson RG, Parikh RM, Lipsey JR, Starkstein SE, Price TR. Pathological laughing and crying following stroke: validation of a measurement scale and a double-blind treatment study. *Am J Psychiatry.* 1993;150(2): 286–293.

60. Hackett ML, Yang M, Anderson CS, Horrocks JA, House A. Pharmaceutical interventions for emotionalism after stroke. *Cochrane Database Syst Rev.* 2010;(2): CD003690.

61. Cumming TB, Packer M, Kramer SF, English C. The prevalence of fatigue after stroke: a systematic review and meta-analysis. *Int J Stroke.* 2016;11(9):968–977.

62. Hinkle JL, Becker KJ, Kim JS, et al. Poststroke fatigue: emerging evidence and approaches to management: a scientific statement for healthcare professionals from the American Heart Association. *Stroke.* 2017;48(7): e159–e170.

63. Bivard A, Lillicrap T, Krishnamurthy V, et al. MIDAS (modafinil in debilitating fatigue after stroke): a randomized, double-blind, placebo-controlled, cross-over trial. *Stroke.* 2017;48(5):1293–1298.

64. Culebras A. Sleep apnea and stroke. *Curr Neurol Neurosci Rep.* 2015;15(1):503.

65. Sandberg O, Franklin KA, Bucht G, Gustafson Y. Sleep apnea, delirium, depressed mood, cognition, and ADL ability after stroke. *J Am Geriatr Soc.* 2001;49(4):391–397.

66. Campbell Burton CA, Murray J, Holmes J, Astin F, Greenwood D, Knapp P. Frequency of anxiety after stroke: a systematic review and meta-analysis of observational studies. *Int J Stroke.* 2013;8(7):545–559.

67. Ferro JM, Caeiro L, Figueira ML. Neuropsychiatric sequelae of stroke. *Nat Rev Neurol.* 2016;12(5):269–280.

68. Menlove L, Crayton E, Kneebone I, Allen-Crooks R, Otto E, Harder H. Predictors of anxiety after stroke: a systematic review of observational studies. *J Stroke Cerebrovasc Dis.* 2015;24(6):1107–1117.

69. Shimoda K, Robinson RG. Effects of anxiety disorder on impairment and recovery from stroke. *J Neuropsychiatry Clin Neurosci.* 1998;10(1):34–40.

70. Knapp P, Campbell Burton CA, Holmes J, et al. Interventions for treating anxiety after stroke. *Cochrane Database Syst Rev.* 2017;5:CD008860.

71. Vieta E, Valenti M. Pharmacological management of bipolar depression: acute treatment, maintenance, and prophylaxis. *CNS Drugs.* 2013;27(7):515–529.

72. Aziz R, Lorberg B, Tampi RR. Treatments for late-life bipolar disorder. *Am J Geriatr Pharmacother.* 2006;4(4): 347–364.

73. Robinson RG. Prevalence and clinical symptoms. In: *The Clinical Neuropsychiatry of Stroke: Cognitive, Behavioral and Emotional Disorders Following Vascular Brain Injury.* 2nd ed. New York: Cambridge University Press; 2006:283–287.

74. Santos CO, Caeiro L, Ferro JM, Figueira ML. Mania and stroke: a systematic review. *Cerebrovasc Dis.* 2011;32(1): 11–21.

75. Robinson RG, Boston JD, Starkstein SE, Price TR. Comparison of mania and depression after brain injury: causal factors. *Am J Psychiatry.* 1988;145(2):172–178.

76. Carson AJ, MacHale S, Allen K, et al. Depression after stroke and lesion location: a systematic review. *Lancet.* 2000;356(9224):122–126.

77. Pompili M, Venturini P, Lamis DA, et al. Suicide in stroke survivors: epidemiology and prevention. *Drugs Aging.* 2015;32(1):21–29.

78. Chollet F, Tardy J, Albucher JF, et al. Fluoxetine for motor recovery after acute ischaemic stroke (FLAME): a randomised placebo-controlled trial. *Lancet Neurol.* 2011; 10(2):123–130.

79. Choi-Kwon S, Han SW, Kwon SU, Kang DW, Choi JM, Kim JS. Fluoxetine treatment in poststroke depression, emotional incontinence, and anger proneness: a double-blind, placebo-controlled study. *Stroke.* 2006; 37(1):156–161.

80. Fruehwald S, Gatterbauer E, Rehak P, Baumhackl U. Early fluoxetine treatment of post-stroke depression—a three-month double-blind placebo-controlled study with an open-label long-term follow up. *J Neurol.* 2003;250(3): 347–351.

81. Robinson RG, Schultz SK, Castillo C, et al. Nortriptyline versus fluoxetine in the treatment of depression and in short-term recovery after stroke: a placebo-controlled, double-blind study. *Am J Psychiatry.* 2000;157(3): 351–359.

82. Wiart L, Petit H, Joseph PA, Mazaux JM, Barat M. Fluoxetine in early poststroke depression: a double-blind placebo-controlled study. *Stroke.* 2000;31(8):1829–1832.

83. Andersen G, Vestergaard K, Lauritzen L. Effective treatment of poststroke depression with the selective serotonin reuptake inhibitor citalopram. *Stroke.* 1994;25(6): 1099–1104.

84. Kim JS, Lee EJ, Chang DI, et al. Efficacy of early administration of escitalopram on depressive and emotional symptoms and neurological dysfunction after stroke: a multicentre, double-blind, randomised, placebo-controlled study. *Lancet Psychiatry.* 2017;4(1):33–41.

85. Murray V, von Arbin M, Bartfai A, et al. Double-blind comparison of sertraline and placebo in stroke patients with minor depression and less severe major depression. *J Clin Psychiatry.* 2005;66(6):708–716.

86. De Ryck A, Brouns R, Geurden M, Elseviers M, De Deyn PP, Engelborghs S. Risk factors for poststroke depression: identification of inconsistencies based on a systematic review. *J Geriatr Psychiatry Neurol.* 2014; 27(3):147–158.

87. Ponzio F. An 8-week, double-blind, placebo controlled, parallel group study to assess the efficacy and tolerability of paroxetine in patients suffering from depression following stroke. *PAR.* 2005;625.

88. Clayton AH, Alkis AR, Parikh NB, Votta JG. Sexual dysfunction due to psychotropic medications. *Psychiatr Clin North Am.* 2016;39(3):427–463.

89. Andrade C, Sharma E. Serotonin reuptake inhibitors and risk of abnormal bleeding. *Psychiatr Clin North Am.* 2016; 39(3):413–426.

90. Hackam DG, Mrkobrada M. Selective serotonin reuptake inhibitors and brain hemorrhage: a meta-analysis. *Neurology.* 2012;79(18):1862–1865.

91. Jiang HY, Chen HZ, Hu XJ, et al. Use of selective serotonin reuptake inhibitors and risk of upper gastrointestinal bleeding: a systematic review and meta-analysis. *Clin Gastroenterol Hepatol.* 2015;13(1):42–50.e43.

92. Cappelen-Smith C, Calic Z, Cordato D. Reversible cerebral vasoconstriction syndrome: recognition and treatment. *Curr Treat Options Neurol.* 2017;19(6):21.

93. Ramasubbu R. Cerebrovascular effects of selective serotonin reuptake inhibitors: a systematic review. *J Clin Psychiatry.* 2004;65(12):1642–1653.

94. Marcum ZA, Perera G, Thorpe JM, et al. Antidepressant use and recurrent falls in community-dwelling older adults: findings from the Health ABC study. *Ann Pharmacother.* 2016;50(7):525–533.

95. Warden SJ, Fuchs RK. Do selective serotonin reuptake inhibitors (SSRIs) cause fractures? *Curr Osteoporos Rep.* 2016;14(5):211–218.

96. Carvalho AF, Sharma MS, Brunoni AR, Vieta E, Fava GA. The safety, tolerability and risks associated with the use of newer generation antidepressant drugs: a critical review of the literature. *Psychother Psychosom.* 2016;85(5): 270–288.

97. Mortensen JK, Larsson H, Johnsen SP, Andersen G. Post stroke use of selective serotonin reuptake inhibitors and clinical outcome among patients with ischemic stroke: a nationwide propensity score-matched follow-up study. *Stroke.* 2013;44(2):420–426.

98. Young JB, Singh TD, Rabinstein AA, Fugate JE. SSRI/SNRI use is not associated with increased risk of delayed cerebral ischemia after aSAH. *Neurocrit Care.* 2016;24(2): 197–201.

99. Mortensen JK, Andersen G. Safety of selective serotonin reuptake inhibitor treatment in recovering stroke patients. *Expert Opin Drug Saf.* 2015;14(6):911–919.

100. Mead GE, Hsieh CF, Lee R, et al. Selective serotonin reuptake inhibitors (SSRIs) for stroke recovery. *Cochrane Database Syst Rev.* 2012;11:CD009286.

101. Mead G, Hackett ML, Lundstrom E, Murray V, Hankey GJ, Dennis M. The FOCUS, AFFINITY and EFFECTS trials studying the effect(s) of fluoxetine in patients with a recent stroke: a study protocol for three multicentre randomised controlled trials. *Trials.* 2015;16:369.

102. Marquez-Romero JM, Arauz A, Ruiz-Sandoval JL, et al. Fluoxetine for motor recovery after acute intracerebral hemorrhage (FMRICH): study protocol for a randomized, double-blind, placebo-controlled, multicenter trial. *Trials.* 2013;14:77.

103. Jorge RE, Acion L, Moser D, Adams Jr HP, Robinson RG. Escitalopram and enhancement of cognitive recovery following stroke. *Arch Gen Psychiatry.* 2010;67(2): 187–196.

104. Karaiskos D, Tzavellas E, Spengos K, Vassilopoulou S, Paparrigopoulos T. Duloxetine versus citalopram and sertraline in the treatment of poststroke depression, anxiety, and fatigue. *J Neuropsychiatry Clin Neurosci.* 2012; 24(3):349–353.

105. Zhang LS, Hu XY, Yao LY, et al. Prophylactic effects of duloxetine on post-stroke depression symptoms: an open single-blind trial. *Eur Neurol*. 2013;69(6):336–343.

106. Kucukalic A, Bravo-Mehmedbasic A, Kulenovic AD, Suljic-Mehmedika E. Venlafaxine efficacy and tolerability in the treatment of post-stroke depression. *Psychiatr Danub*. 2007;19(1–2):56–60.

107. Spalletta G, Ripa A, Bria P, Caltagirone C, Robinson RG. Response of emotional unawareness after stroke to antidepressant treatment. *Am J Geriatr Psychiatry*. 2006; 14(3):220–227.

108. Niedermaier N, Bohrer E, Schulte K, Schlattmann P, Heuser I. Prevention and treatment of poststroke depression with mirtazapine in patients with acute stroke. *J Clin Psychiatry*. 2004;65(12):1619–1623.

109. Raffaele R, Rampello L, Vecchio I, Tornali C, Malaguarnera M. Trazodone therapy of the post-stroke depression. *Arch Gerontol Geriatr*. 1996;22(suppl 1): 217–220.

110. Reding MJ, Orto LA, Winter SW, Fortuna IM, Di Ponte P, McDowell FH. Antidepressant therapy after stroke. A double-blind trial. *Arch Neurol*. 1986;43(8):763–765.

111. Kanner AM. Most antidepressant drugs are safe for patients with epilepsy at therapeutic doses: a review of the evidence. *Epilepsy Behav*. 2016;61:282–286.

112. Tripp AC. Bupropion, a brief history of seizure risk. *Gen Hosp Psychiatry*. 2010;32(2):216–217.

113. Lipsey JR, Robinson RG, Pearlson GD, Rao K, Price TR. Nortriptyline treatment of post-stroke depression: a double-blind study. *Lancet*. 1984;1(8372):297–300.

114. Delbari A, Salman-Roghani R, Lokk J. Effect of methylphenidate and/or levodopa combined with physiotherapy on mood and cognition after stroke: a randomized, double-blind, placebo-controlled trial. *Eur Neurol*. 2011;66(1):7–13.

115. Grade C, Redford B, Chrostowski J, Toussaint L, Blackwell B. Methylphenidate in early poststroke recovery: a double-blind, placebo-controlled study. *Arch Phys Med Rehabil*. 1998;79(9):1047–1050.

116. Cramer SC. Drugs to enhance motor recovery after stroke. *Stroke*. 2015;46(10):2998–3005.

117. Prince J, Wilens T, Spencer TJ, Biederman J. Pharmacotherapy of attention-deficit/hyperactivity disorder across the life span. In: Stern TA, Fava M, Wilens TE, Rosenbaum JF, eds. *Massachusetts General Hospital Comprehensive Clinical Psychiatry*. 2nd ed. China: Elsevier Inc.; 2016:538–550.

118. McIntyre A, Thompson S, Burhan A, Mehta S, Teasell R. Repetitive transcranial magnetic stimulation for depression due to cerebrovascular disease: a systematic review. *J Stroke Cerebrovasc Dis*. 2016;25(12):2792–2800.

119. Jorge RE, Moser DJ, Acion L, Robinson RG. Treatment of vascular depression using repetitive transcranial magnetic stimulation. *Arch Gen Psychiatry*. 2008;65(3): 268–276.

120. An TG, Kim SH, Kim KU. Effect of transcranial direct current stimulation of stroke patients on depression and quality of life. *J Phys Ther Sci*. 2017;29(3):505–507.

121. Hackett ML, Anderson CS, House A, Xia J. Interventions for treating depression after stroke. *Cochrane Database Syst Rev*. 2008;(4):CD003437.

122. Robinson RG, Jorge RE, Moser DJ, et al. Escitalopram and problem-solving therapy for prevention of poststroke depression: a randomized controlled trial. *JAMA*. 2008; 299(20):2391–2400.

123. Salter KL, Foley NC, Zhu L, Jutai JW, Teasell RW. Prevention of poststroke depression: does prophylactic pharmacotherapy work? *J Stroke Cerebrovasc Dis*. 2013;22(8): 1243–1251.

CHAPTER 12

Visuospatial Impairment

JOHN-ROSS RIZZO, MD, MSCI • MAHYA BEHESHTI, MD •
NEERA KAPOOR, OD, MS, FAAO, FCOVD-A

OVERVIEW OF VISION-RELATED PRESENTATIONS FOLLOWING STROKE

Following stroke, a constellation of vision symptoms and signs may manifest, typically falling into three major categories: afferent (sensory), efferent (motor), and higher-level visual perceptual. This chapter provides the rehabilitation clinician with high-yield symptoms, a vision screening protocol, criteria for when to refer for detailed vision assessment, as well as generalized treatment options for vision dysfunctions that are amenable to intervention. Subsequently, key neurologic findings with related diagnostics and therapeutic approaches are described following this categorical structure for more common vision problems post-stroke.

VISION SCREENING FOR THE REHABILITATION PROFESSIONAL

The more common vision symptoms following stroke include blurred vision, missing objects in one's peripheral vision, and double vision.[1] These symptoms, among others (see Table 12.1, for the common vision symptoms and possible differential diagnostic conditions), may impact a patient's quality of life by impairing the ability to independently, safely, and efficiently ambulate, drive, perform household-related activities, read hard copy and computer screens, and perform work-related activities.[1] Therefore, identifying and addressing symptoms and signs related to vision impairment following stroke become increasingly important.

Blurred vision at one or all viewing distances falls into two principal categories: (1) constant and (2) intermittent. Constant blur may be due to uncorrected refractive error (i.e., needing an update of spectacle correction for all, or one, viewing distances); media opacity (i.e., opacity of the cornea, lens, or vitreous); optic nerve damage (due to neuritis or neuropathy); or cortical vision loss. Intermittent blur that changes as a patient blinks is probably related to impaired tear film integrity and is not age-dependent. Another cause of intermittent blur is a deficit of accommodation, which is autonomically mediated. While accommodation function is age-dependent and physiologically declines for those in their 40's, it can be impacted prematurely for those under 40 years of age due to neurological insult such as stroke. The remaining symptoms, especially missing or bumping into objects in one's peripheral vision, as well as double vision, reading difficulty, and feeling off-balance, will be discussed in greater detail under the respective afferent and efferent sections of this chapter.

After obtaining the patient's symptoms, a recommended approach (see Table 12.2) to screen for the nature of vision deficits following stroke involves assessing clarity of vision, peripheral vision, eye movements, and pupillary function.

Often following stroke, there are cognitive, language-based, and visual perceptual deficits that may impede the examiner's ability to assess visual acuity accurately. Therefore, for those with alexia or expressive aphasia who can understand what is being asked of them, using a near visual acuity chart with numbers and asking the patient to nod if (s)he is able to accurately see and identify, yet not verbally name, the numbers in a specified row may aid in assessing visual acuity. For those with agnosia, or those who are unable to understand what is being asked of them, a referral is indicated for a more detailed vision evaluation, including a dilated eye examination to assess retinal integrity and possibly visual evoked potential testing to determine the extent of cortical visual processing. Regarding peripheral vision, eye movements, and pupils, criteria indicating the need to refer for a detailed vision evaluation are noted in Table 12.3.

Once a preliminary category of vision deficit has been determined, patients and caregivers may inquire about treatment options. While, for changes in refractive error, updating their spectacle correction is a known treatment, Table 12.4 outlines the generalized compensatory, habituative, and restorative approaches for the sensorimotor vision deficits. For all seven of these vision deficits, there are compensatory approaches

Stroke Rehabilitation. https://doi.org/10.1016/B978-0-323-55381-0.00012-3

TABLE 12.1
Symptoms Secondary to Vision Dysfunction

Symptom	Qualifiers for Differential Diagnosis	Diagnostic Category
Blurred vision/Trouble seeing	Constant blur at one or all viewing distances for one (monocular) or both eyes (binocular)	Improved visual acuity with pinhole → residual uncorrected refractive error (glasses: missing/outdated)
		Improved visual acuity with pinhole → eye media opacity → problems with the cornea, lens [e.g., cataract], or vitreous
		No change with pinhole visual acuity, optic nerve swelling or pallor (monocular or binocular), and anomalous pupillary response (with probable afferent pupillary defect) → unilateral or bilateral optic neuropathy or neuritis
		No change with pinhole visual acuity, intact optic nerve and retina, with pupillary response → cortical vision loss
	Intermittent blur/distorted clarity of vision that varies as the patient blinks	Cranial nerve dysfunction → impaired tear film integrity → dry eye
	Intermittent at all viewing distances, or when changing focus between distances, or at near	Accommodative dysfunction (changes may also be due to cranial nerve III palsy, autonomic dysfunction, or senescence)
Bumping/Missing things (field cuts)	Overall (tunnel) or partial (hemi- or quad-) field restriction [peripheral vision]	Optic pathway dysfunction (from optic nerve to visual cortex)
Double vision (diplopia)	Double vision eliminated w/one eye covered	Cranial nerve dysfunction → impaired range of motion → paralytic strabismus
		Eye movement deficits (vergence dysfunction, nonstrabismic)
	Double vision evident w/both eyes open, as well as w/one eye covered	Polyopia, attributable to: refractive error, eye media opacity, retinal detachment or macular injury, cortical injury or may be psychogenic
Reading difficulty	Slower reading speed with skipping lines; use of finger-guide to improve accuracy/speed	Eye movement deficits (saccades and fixation) and/or cranial nerve dysfunction
	Slower reading with rereading to improve comprehension. Use of finger-guide futile	Possible cognitive deficits, which may or may not be compounded by age

Off-balance/Dizzy	Balance problems exacerbated by: • visually stimulating environments • compound movements (eye—head—body)	Impaired visual-vestibular interaction
	Balance problems regardless of visual stimuli and compound movements	Possible impaired vestibular function, particular attention to posterior circulation strokes
Light sensitive (photosensitivity)	Sensitivity or phobia to light	Poor tolerance to changes in light, possibly related to hyperactive sympathetic innervation.
Headache	Visual problem-induced headache	All previous categories may precipitate a headache; headache should be considered a potential "gateway" symptom for visual dysfunction
Eye fatigue (asthenopia)	Generalized tired sensation from overworked eyes	All previous categories may precipitate generalized eye fatigue

TABLE 12.2
Screening Vision Protocol for Rehabilitation Physicians

Clinical Encounter	Areas of Assessment	Components
History	General questions	Trouble seeing? Blurry vision?
		Bumping into things frequently or missing things often when looking for them?
		Seeing double or triple when viewing objects or things?
		Reading difficulty due to skipping lines, missing words, or rereading words/lines?
		Losing balance? Feeling dizzy or spinning sensation in visually crowded environments?
		Feeling more sensitive to light? To all lights? More so to fluorescent and computer lights?
		Headaches?
		Feeling strain in the eyes or tired sensation regarding vision?
Physical Examination	Visual acuity	Assess with patient's current spectacle or contact lens correction
	Peripheral field	Confrontation visual field testing
	Ocular motor	**Fixation**: patient should be able to maintain fixation for at least 10 s without any loss of fixation or nystagmus.
		Pursuit: evaluate the patient's ability to follow a smoothly and slowly moving target with their eyes in all positions of gaze (up, down, left, right, and obliquely, e.g., H-pattern). Assess for gaze-evoked nystagmus and any restrictions in range.
		Saccades: evaluate the patient's ability to rapidly move the eyes from one target to the next: horizontally, obliquely, and vertically.
	Pupil	Assess pupillary responses

TABLE 12.3
Referral Criteria for a Comprehensive Vision Evaluation

Areas of Assessment	Referral Criteria → Vision Specialist
General questions	Trouble seeing/blurry vision
	Bump or missing things
	Diplopia/polyopia
	Reading difficulty
	Loss of balance/dizziness
	Light sensitivity
	Headaches
	Eye strain
Visual acuity	Poorer than 20/40 with correction or different between eyes at near or far distances
Peripheral field	Deficits in portions or aspects of field (overall, hemi-, or quad-)
Ocular motor	Fixation: nystagmus on fixation assessment
	Pursuit: restriction of eye movements on testing
	Saccades: dysmetria/restriction in any specific direction or speed on testing (slow = loss of darting nature, or ability to witness trajectory of eye movement, as opposed to the "jump")
Pupil	Unequal, irregular, fixed or minimally responsive

that the patient can be taught to increase visual comfort and improve function to a degree. However, the restorative treatment option of vision therapy, which involves neuromotor relearning, is effective for deficits of accommodation (i.e., the ability to change focus or clarity of vision from far to near and back), versional ocular motility (i.e., fixation, saccades, and pursuit), vergence (i.e., eye movements in depth), and vestibular (exacerbated with visual stimulation) function. For example, regarding accommodation and vergence, patients work on increasing and relaxing the accommodative response monocularly (i.e., one eye at a time) and vergence response binocularly (i.e., with both eyes open at the same time) repeatedly and on-command, respectively, to restore some degree of accommodative and vergence function.

COMMON AFFERENT VISION DEFICITS

Following stroke, the more common afferent visual consequences include visual field defects, with or without inattention, and blurred vision due to changes in refractive error or optic nerve damage. If blurred vision is intermittent, it may be related to pre-mature accommodative dysfunction (i.e., for those under 40 years of age), and potentially impaired tear film integrity, which is addressed under the "Efferent Section's Cranial nerve palsies."

Visual Field Impairment

Assessing visual field deficits and hemi-spatial inattention, also known as visual neglect or visual hemi-neglect, requires understanding the categories across the spectrum of visual field integrity[2,3]: (1) a full field with perimetric testing, accompanied by complete awareness of both hemifields; (2) a hemi-/quadrant-visual field defect with perimetric testing, without unilateral hemi-/quadrant-spatial inattention; (3) a hemi-/quadrant-visual field defect with perimetric testing, with unilateral hemi-/quadrant-spatial inattention; (4) an incomplete hemi-/quadrant-visual field defect with perimetric testing, with unilateral hemi-/quadrant-spatial inattention; and (5) a full field with perimetric testing, with unilateral hemi-spatial inattention. Category one is intuitive in that there are no visual field defects with confrontation and perimetric testing, and the person is fully aware of the entire visual field. Category two is intuitive as, for this category, the patient presents with a hemi-field defect, with confrontation and standard perimetric testing, of which he or she is aware. Given rehabilitation clinicians' understanding of visual neglect, even categories three and four are reasonably intuitive, since the patient is still manifesting some degree of a visual field defect with confrontation and perimetric testing, despite the patient's lack of awareness of this defect. Category five is the least intuitive because there is no frank visual field defect with confrontation or perimetric testing, yet the patient seems consistently unaware of one side of his/her peripheral vision.[2,3]

The neurology for impairment of visual field integrity is related to the location along the primary visual pathway that an infarct or hemorrhage occurs. Therefore, understanding the path that optic fibers travel as they leave the optic nerve chiasm is beneficial. At the optic nerve chiasm, there is a partial decussation of the optic nerve fibers occurring prior to travelling as the optic tract onward to the lateral geniculate body. Once at the lateral geniculate body, additional nonvisual input is processed prior to the optic fibers leaving

TABLE 12.4
Treatment Options for Vision Dysfunction

Vision Dysfunction	Treatment Options
Accommodation	*Compensatory approach*: prescription of spectacles for prolonged near vision tasks: instead of, before, in conjunction with, or following restorative vision therapy
	Restorative approach: vision therapy
Tear film integrity	*Compensatory approach*: prescribing synthetic tears, lid hygiene, and/or punctal plugs
Visual field integrity	*Compensatory approach*: prescription of optical aids, including yoked prism, field-expanding lenses, half prisms, and sector or spotting prisms
	Compensatory/adaptive approach: vision therapy for scanning strategies and awareness of the affected visual field
Vergence (ocular motor in depth)	*Compensatory approach*: fusional prism when possible and occlusion as indicated
	Restorative approach: vision therapy
Ocular motor	*Compensatory approach*: using large print books (for those with best-corrected visual acuity poorer than 20/50) and a typoscopic approach highlighting the text of regard and obscuring irrelevant text on the page
	Adaptive approach: using audio books for those with low vision (i.e., best-corrected visual acuity with no letters perceived on the 20/100 line or less than 20-degree diameter of peripheral vision in either eye)
	Restorative approach: vision therapy
Balance (visual-vestibular)	*Compensatory/adaptive approach*: habituate tolerance to eye/head movement
	Restorative approach: vision therapy
Sensitivity to light	*Compensatory approach*: prescription of tinted spectacle lenses and donning brimmed hats (block light superiorly); consider environmental modifications to lighting

for one of three possible locations: superior colliculus for integrated sensory function, pretectum and tectum for pupillary function, and occipital cortex for early processing of visual information. It should be noted the bulk of the optic fibers traverse to the occipital cortex and constitute the optic radiations of the primary visual pathway.[4]

Infarction or hemorrhage occurring more anteriorly along the primary visual pathway results in a visual field defect that is less dense and less congruous (i.e., may present as restricted hemi-field or quadrant-field, rather than a complete field cut respecting the midline) compared to those occurring more posteriorly along the pathway, in particular, more proximal to the occipital lobe. In terms of visual spatial hemi-inattention or visual hemi-neglect, vascular compromise to the posterior parietal cortex, in particular for the right hemisphere, with reasonable predictability results in some degree of visual inattention or neglect.[2,3,5] Middle cerebral artery (MCA) strokes

impacting the angular gyrus of the parietal lobe, right basal ganglia, or the thalamus are reported more commonly to manifest with neglect.[2,5] Right posterior cerebral artery infarction may impact white matter fibers of the occipital lobe that connect the parahippocampal gyrus with the angular gyrus of the right parietal lobe, thereby resulting in some degree of visual inattention or neglect.[5]

For all patients with symptoms related to possible impaired visual field integrity, assessing confrontation visual fields with single, as well as double (i.e., simultaneous extinction), presentation along with performance tests is beneficial. Confrontation visual field testing should first be assessed with single presentation in all eight quadrants of peripheral vision: superior, superior right, right, inferior right, inferior, inferior left, left, and superior left. If confrontation testing with the single presentation is full, then confrontation visual field testing with simultaneous presentation, also referred to as the test for extinction, should be performed. For confrontation testing with simultaneous presentation, one or two fingers from each hand in two different portions of the visual field simultaneously (i.e., simultaneous double stimulus presentation) are used. For this task, if a patient has a left-sided inattention, the patient will consistently report the number of fingers corresponding to the hand presented to the patient's right visual field only.[3] Performance tests include the "draw a clock" test, cancellation test, and line-bisection task, to name a few, and the details on administering these tests are described in Parton et al.[2]

Potential Causes of Blurred Vision: Changes in Refractive Error, Optic Nerve Damage, or Cortical Vision Loss

For constant blurred vision at one or all viewing distances, if the visual acuity improves with pinhole assessment, then the rehabilitation provider knows that there is either an issue of uncorrected (or a change in) refractive error or some media opacity. If the visual acuity is unchanged or slightly poorer than the standard visual acuity measurement, then the reduced acuity is either due to optic nerve changes (where pupil responses are evident but anomalous) or cortical vision loss (where pupil responses are present). The symptom of blurred vision warrants a referral to an eye care provider to verify its underlying cause.

MANAGEMENT OF AFFERENT DEFICITS
Post-Stroke Impaired Visual Field Integrity

Scanning strategies and compensatory/adaptive approaches benefit impaired postchiasmal visual field integrity with or without inattention. While saccadic scanning and searching rehabilitative approaches do subjectively improve the patient's ability to scan into the affected visual field more efficiently, current evidence does not support the ability of these approaches to restore visual field integrity.[6-14] Future research that objectively assesses eye movements to record the speed and accuracy of a patient's ability to scan into the affected field pre- and postrehabilitation is needed to better understand the efficacy of this approach in improving visual field integrity.

When managing postchiasmal hemianopic or quadrantanopic visual inattention, with or without a visual field defect, vision rehabilitation eye care providers may prescribe full-field yoked prisms, mirrors, or field expanding lenses, in conjunction with saccadic scanning strategies as well as compensatory and adaptive approaches. Conversely, when managing postchiasmal

hemianopic or quadrantanopic visual field defects without inattention, vision rehabilitation eye care providers may prescribe sector prisms and spotting prisms, along with saccadic scanning and compensatory and adaptive approaches. However, there has been little evidence at present in the literature supporting this management.[15,16] In fact, Rowe et al. reported adverse responses in approximately 69% of study participants with homonymous hemianopia who were treated with prisms.[15] The adverse responses to the prism may have been related to the optical degradation evident when affixing temporary, or Fresnel, prisms to a person's spectacles. Alternatively, the issue may have been that optical compensation, such as Fresnel prism, is not appropriate for homonymous hemianopia, but, rather, it may be more appropriate for visual inattention or neglect.[17,18] For example, Vaes et al. in 2016 reported a guarded favorable response with experimental prism compared to placebo training over a 7- to 12-day period for most of the 43 stroke participants with right-hemisphere neglect. The majority of the study participants demonstrated an improvement for navigational, drawing, and memory functions up to 3 months after the intervention. However, there was no effect at any time regarding visual search or visual cancellation performance ability with the experimental prism intervention relative to the placebo.[18] Therefore, while optical compensatory rehabilitation may likely continue to be utilized clinically, further studies regarding its efficacy are required to determine if it is predictably effective, when it should be used, what magnitude should be used, and for how long it should be used.

Poststroke Blurred Vision

As was mentioned, blurred vision requires a referral to an eye care provider to confirm its etiology, including uncorrected refractive error, media opacity, optic neuropathy, cortical vision loss, impaired tear film integrity, or accommodative dysfunction. Once the etiology is confirmed, then management can be initiated.

There are four principal causes of *constant* blur: uncorrected refractive error, media opacity, optic neuropathy, and cortical vision loss. When uncorrected refractive error is the cause of the blur, updated spectacle correction can be determined and prescribed, depending upon the patient's systemic and neurologic stability poststroke. Typically, it is advised to wait 4–6 weeks postarousal from stroke prior to prescribing any change in spectacle correction. This delay is advised due to potential initial side effects of medications and fluctuations in systemic health, which may impact refractive error. Regarding the impact of media opacity on clarity of vision, a referral to an ophthalmologist specializing in cornea and cataracts is indicated pending the stabilization of the patient's systemic and neurologic health. If optic neuropathy is the cause of the blurred vision, the patient will be monitored for change by an eye care provider regularly with dilation and automated visual field testing. Lastly, if cortical vision loss is the presumed cause of the blurred vision, the patient will be monitored for any change in presentation by an eye care provider and either neurology or physiatry.

Two principal causes for *intermittent* blur include: (1) impaired accommodation or (2) impaired tear film integrity. There is a predictable, physiologic age-related progressive decline in accommodation, referred to as presbyopia that typically commences when individuals reach their mid-40s. This type of blur is relatively constant (usually), rather than intermittent, and is classified as a change in the person's refractive, or spectacle prescription, status. However, if persons are under 40 years of age and their accommodation is impacted prematurely, then they may report intermittent far vision blur, intermittent near vision blur, or intermittent blur when looking from far to near or near to far: such symptoms relate to the sensorimotor vision category of impaired accommodation. Unlike accommodation, there is no predictable, age-related, physiologic decline in tear film integrity, per se. Therefore, if a patient reports intermittent blur where the clarity of vision changes as the patient blinks, that may be impaired tear film integrity, which is also referred to as dry eye(s) or ocular surface disease.

Regardless of the patient's age, blurred vision of any kind requires assessment. For those over 40 years of age reporting blurred vision, this symptom is typically constant, rather than intermittent, and often involves updating the spectacle prescription. For those under 40 years of age reporting intermittent blur at any viewing distance, a more extensive evaluation is required, which may result in an eye care provider either prescribing accommodative restorative therapy or near vision glasses in lieu of, in conjunction with or subsequent to, accommodative restorative therapy.[19]

When tear film integrity is impaired, an eye care provider will often incorporate over-the-counter artificial tears three to four times daily for each eye into the patient's medication regimen, which is frequently sufficient to ensure a stable tear film and improved clarity of vision. For more moderate to severe bilateral dry eye, using prescription ophthalmic solutions to address the possible underlying immune modulation deficit, inflammation, tear film mucin deficit, and/or infection may be required.[20]

COMMON EFFERENT VISION DEFICITS

Following stroke, the more common efferent visual consequences, that is to say eye movement or eye lid movement consequences, include cranial nerve III, IV, and/or VI palsies, internuclear ophthalmoplegia, one-and-a-half syndrome, Weber syndrome, ptosis, and lagophthalmos.

Cranial Nerve Palsies

A palsy of cranial nerve III (the oculomotor nerve, or CN III) may present as partial or complete with possible lid and pupillary involvement.[21] The oculomotor nerve's superior division innervates the superior rectus and levator palpebrae superioris muscles, while its inferior division innervates the inferior rectus muscle, medial rectus muscle, inferior oblique muscle, and lower part of the ciliary ganglion to impact accommodative and pupillary function.[21]

An incomplete palsy of the superior division of CN III may result in ipsilateral ptosis and restriction of ipsilateral supraversion. An incomplete palsy of the inferior division may restrict ipsilateral accommodation, ipsilateral pupillary function, ipsilateral adduction, and ipsilateral supraversion. A complete third nerve palsy presents with impairment of both divisions, resulting in the ipsilateral eye being positioned down and out with partial or complete ptosis and potential pupillary involvement.[21]

For those under the age of 40 years with intermittent blurred vision, which does not change as the patient blinks, the etiology is probably an underlying accommodative dysfunction due to impairment either along CN III or with the underlying balance of autonomic nervous system. The autonomic innervation for accommodation is transmitted with the inferior division of CN III, commencing with the parasympathetic fibers joining CN III at the level of the Edinger–Westphal nucleus in the pretectum. The combined autonomic-motor fibers then traverse anteriorly within the third cranial nerve toward the ciliary ganglion where the sympathetic fibers join without synapsing. The third cranial nerve's combined fibers continue via the short ciliary nerve to innervate the ciliary muscle effecting a change in the contraction of the muscle, shape of the crystalline lens, and the state of accommodation. There is a normal, age-related physiologic decline in accommodation, referred to as presbyopia, which manifests as individuals reach their early to mid-40s.[19]

There are two additional potential cranial nerve inputs which could contribute to intermittent blurred vision, but are related to blurred or distorted vision that changes as a patient blinks. This category of blurred or distorted vision may occur due to facial nerve palsy, as the seventh cranial nerve (CN VII) innervates the lacrimal gland. Alternatively, damage along the trigeminal nerve (CN V) may impair tear film integrity since the superior division of CN V is responsible for corneal nerve sensitivity, and reduced corneal nerve sensitivity may concurrently slow down a patient's blink rate.

Pupillary involvement with a third nerve palsy is typically related to an aneurysm, specifically of the posterior communicating artery, which is a medical emergency given that a patient may die if that particular aneurysm remains undetected and ruptures. Therefore, upon initial presentation of signs of a third nerve palsy with pupillary involvement, a patient should immediately be sent to the emergency department for surgical management of a presumed posterior communicating artery aneurysm.[21]

A palsy of cranial nerve IV (the trochlear nerve or CN IV) presents with an ipsilateral hypertropia.[21] Since the trochlear nerve innervates the ipsilateral superior oblique muscle, which depresses the eye most prominently upon ipsilateral adduction, the associated hypertropia evident with a CN IV palsy tends to be of larger magnitude at closer viewing distances. In addition, the ipsilateral hypertropia is greater in contralateral gaze and with an ipsilateral head tilt for CN IV palsies.[21]

A palsy of cranial VI (the abducens nerve, or CN VI) presents with an ipsilateral esotropia since the abducens nerve innervates the ipsilateral lateral rectus muscle, which abducts the eye.[21] Since adduction is not impaired and minimal abduction is required in primary gaze at closer viewing distances, the associated ipsilateral esotropia with a CN VI palsy is of larger magnitude at farther viewing distances and ipsilateral horizontal gaze.[21]

Internuclear Ophthalmoplegia

An internuclear ophthalmoplegia (INO) typically presents as a complete adduction deficit of the ipsilateral eye when trying to look contralaterally, with associated abduction nystagmus of the contralateral eye.[21] For example, with a right INO, initially, the right frontal eye fields (FEF) would transmit a signal via the superior colliculus to the left paramedian pontine reticular formation (PPRF) to stimulate leftward eye movements. The left PPRF would stimulate the left CN VI to innervate its associated lateral rectus muscle to abduct. Concurrently, the left CN VI attempts to communicate via the right medial longitudinal fasciculus (MLF) with the right CN III to innervate its associated medial rectus muscle to adduct. However, since the right MLF is impaired, the right eye's ability to adduct becomes

restricted or absent, and this is often accompanied by abduction nystagmus of the left eye with attempted conjugate left gaze.[21]

Gaze Palsies

The initiation of eye movements rests to a significant degree with the frontal eye fields (FEF).

For horizontal gaze, it is the paramedian pontine reticular formation (PPRF) in the mid-pons region that represents the horizontal gaze center generating conjugate horizontal movements for each eye.[21] For example, a horizontal right conjugate gaze palsy would involve the left FEF sending a signal via the superior colliculus to the right PPRF. For a horizontal right conjugate gaze palsy, the right PPRF would be affected preventing transmission of the neural signal to the right CN VI for innervation of the right lateral rectus muscle and the left CN III for innervation of the left medial rectus muscle. Therefore, the patient would present with complete abduction deficit of the right eye and complete adduction deficit of the left eye upon attempted conjugate rightward movement of both eyes. This results in a horizontal right conjugate gaze palsy, or an inability to move both eyes rightward under binocular viewing conditions.[21]

For vertical gaze, the rostral interstitial MLF and, to a lesser extent, the interstitial nucleus of Cajal (INC), are involved and both are supranuclear structures located in the rostral midbrain reticular formation. These two supranuclear neurological substrates comprise the vertical gaze center generating vertical eye movements,[21,22] such that an infarction involving these substrates commonly results in a vertical gaze palsy. Damage, especially bilaterally, to the rostral interstitial MLF may result in slowness, restricted range, or absence of vertical saccades. The rostral interstitial MLF areas project bilaterally to the motor neurons for supraversion and unilaterally to those for infraversion. Therefore, a lesion to the right rostral interstitial MLF may impact all vertical saccades, but it may more likely result in a bilateral upgaze palsy with diplopia, due to a variable-magnitude left hypotropia, on attempted downgaze.[21,23,24]

Special notable exceptions, for which bilateral upgaze is impacted while downgaze remains intact, include thalamic brainstem lesions and dorsal midbrain syndrome (also referred to as Parinaud syndrome). Thalamic lesions in the brainstem may extend into the midbrain, which provides the potential for partial impact from the rostral interstitial MLF.[25] This potential contribution of the supranuclear rostral interstitial MLF may result in increased convergence tone and bilateral adduction in downgaze, which has been referred to as thalamic esotropia.[26] Parinaud syndrome presents with multiple signs, including: supranuclear upgaze palsy, convergence-retraction nystagmus typically evident on attempted upgaze, Collier sign (lid retraction), and pupillary light-near dissociation.[21] The more common causes of this syndrome include hydrocephalus, pineal gland tumors, and midbrain hemorrhage or infarction, with the upgaze palsy likely being due to impairment of INC fibers.

One-and-a-Half Syndrome

A "one and a half" syndrome involves lesions of ipsilateral PPRF, or abducens, along with ipsilateral MLF.[27,28] The ipsilateral abducens nucleus or PPRF lesion results in an ipsilateral horizontal gaze palsy, while the ipsilateral MLF lesion produces an ipsilateral INO with impaired ipsilateral adduction. This manifests as "one and a half" of the horizontal eye movements being impaired, with abduction of the contralateral eye being the remaining intact horizontal eye movement. An intermittent contralateral exotropia is often present, which would be more pronounced on contralateral gaze. If the ipsilateral abducens, rather than the PPRF, is involved, the contralateral adduction deficit may be less pronounced, but an ipsilateral facial palsy may now manifest.[29,30] For example, a right one-and-a-half syndrome would involve the right PPRF or abducens restricting rightward gaze and the right MLF restricting adduction of the right eye. Therefore, the remaining horizontal eye movement would be abduction of the left eye, with an associated right facial palsy if the right abducens, rather than PPRF, were involved.

Weber Syndrome

Weber syndrome results from a compromise to the paramedian branches of either the basilar artery, or else the posterior cerebral artery, causing an infarct in the ventromedial crural region of the mesencephalon.[31,32] This type of infarction manifests as the patient perceiving diplopia due to an ipsilateral third nerve palsy and hemiparesis or hemiplegia of contralateral extremities due to the crural region of the infarct as that impacts the corticospinal tracts. For example, an infarct in the right ventromedial crural region would result in a right CN III palsy and a left hemiparesis.[31,32]

Ptosis

Ptosis is typically accompanied by associated neurological signs related to eye movements, pupils, and/or facial muscles, as with partial or complete third nerve palsy, Horner syndrome, orbital myositis, and myasthenia gravis. However, unilateral isolated ptosis may also occur due to isolated myositis of the levator palpebrae superioris.[33] During the acute few days following stroke, a patient's systemic and neurologic health may be more volatile and isolated areas of neurological inflammation may occur. Therefore, awareness of possible isolated unilateral ptosis as a consequence is beneficial.

Lagophthalmos

An infarct of the seventh cranial nerve (i.e., CN VII, also known as the facial nerve) may result an ipsilateral facial droop and lagophthalmos (i.e., incomplete lid closure) of the ipsilateral eyelids.[34,35] The ipsilateral lagophthalmos results in increased exposure of the ocular surface of the cornea which concurrently increases risk in the affected eye for keratitis, corneal ulcers, and possible long-standing reduction of vision. In the acute phase, the priority is to ensure adequate corneal protection, while in the long term, the ability to sustain corneal integrity and maintain clarity of vision with an increased ability to blink completely becomes more important.[34,35]

MANAGEMENT OF EFFERENT DEFICITS

Poststroke Eye Movement Disorders

Monocular patching of the contralateral eye to increase range of motion of the affected eye may benefit the patient during the first 3 months post stroke. Despite the absence of randomized clinical trials to support or negate the efficacy of such treatment, Rowe et al.[36] performed a prospective observational cohort study of 915 patients, in which they reported that the more common management options for double vision related to stroke-related cranial nerve palsies III, IV, and VI included fusional prism prescription, occlusion with range of motion techniques, and advice about compensatory strategies.

Poststroke Eyelid Disorders

The more traditional treatment options for the affected eye include the use of frequent artificial tears and ophthalmic ointments, protective taping, and occlusive moisture chambers. In addition, for acute lagophthalmos, ophthalmology may incorporate systemic steroids as part of medical management.[34,35]

For more long-standing and chronic lagophthalmos, ophthalmology and optometry also may utilize punctal plugs, soft contact lenses, and scleral shells for the affected eye to ensure protection of its ocular surface. In addition, for chronic lagophthalmos, ophthalmology may employ procedural or surgical techniques to protect the corneal integrity such as botulinum toxin injection, tarsorrhaphy, and eyelid weight implants.[34,35]

Alternative therapy, such as facial physical, "mime," therapy[37] was found to be effective in improving the functional outcomes, and it includes exercises of self-massage, relaxation, and breathing, combined with the performance of movements of the face (trying to open eyes very widely and trying hard to close both eyes very tightly) and the pronunciation of letters and words.[37]

VISUAL PERCEPTUAL DISORDERS

As we review vision-related presentations following stroke, high-order visual perceptual disorders is the last of the three categories. Perception is an extraordinary feat during which light is continually transforming into meaningful signals that are deciphered by the brain. Visual perception, more formally defined, is the day-to-day experience of "seeing" or the conscious representations that occur when the eyes are open.[38] Visual perceptual disorders often follow acquired brain injury or stroke, and are frequently presented as a wide-ranging set of neurological disorders, including apraxias, agnosias, neglects, body scheme disorders, etc., with little attention given to contextualizing signs and/or symptoms. Here we provide a tabular review that highlights the visual end of the spectrum in many perceptual deficits, while providing a more comprehensive framework to better comprehend the sight-relevant and/or sight-irrelevant nature to the condition and related conditions.

A comprehensive overview of management and treatment options is not within the scope of this chapter, however basic screening tests and assessments that may be implemented bedside and in the clinic, to aid in diagnosis, are provided in the rightmost column of the following two tables (Tables 12.5 and 12.6).

TABLE 12.5
Apraxia

Type	Definition	Test(s)
Constructional apraxia	An impairment of performing tasks that require the manipulation of objects in space whether upon command or spontaneously (Ref. 39)	Drawing performance, Copy geometric design test (Refs. 40, 41), Butters and Barton "Stick Test" (Ref. 39)
Coordinate	Right hemisphere lesions cause errors of the coordinate type, i.e., metric distance and angular distortions (Ref. 39)	
Categorical	Left hemisphere lesions cause errors of the categorical type, i.e., reversals of patterns or elements, and/or exchanges of position between elements	
Ocular motor apraxia (Ref. 42)	The absence of, or a defect in, the control of voluntary purposeful eye movement	
Cogan syndrome (saccadic initiation failure)	Congenital disorder characterized by a defect in side-to-side (horizontal) eye movements	Genetic testing
Balint syndrome (Ref. 43)	A disorder of spatial perception comprising three aspects: ocular motor apraxia (inability to direct gaze to a visual target), optic ataxia (inability to reach by hand for targets presented visually), and simultanagnosia (in brief: the inability to comprehend a complex scene in its entirety, see below)	Physical examination, Clinical findings

Visual-imitative apraxia	Deficits in the imitation of novel, meaningless gestures (with meaningful actions spared) (Ref. 44) (nondominant parietal lobe lesions)	Imitation of meaningless gestures
Ideomotor apraxia	Impaired performance of skilled motor acts despite intact sensory, motor, and language function. Patients reveal temporal and spatial errors affecting timing, sequencing, amplitude, configuration, and limb position in space. There is a "voluntary-automatic dissociation"[a] (Ref. 45) (frontal and parietal area lesions, basal ganglia lesions) (Refs. 46, 47)	Movement imitation test, Demonstration-of-use test[46,47]
Ideational apraxia	An impairment of carrying out a sequence of actions requiring the use of various objects in the correct way and order necessary to achieve an intended goal and/or performance of a complex, multistep task (e.g., making a cup of tea) (Refs. 46, 47) (left hemisphere damage, dementia, or delirium) (Ref. 48)	Praxis subtest of the LOTCA[b] (Ref. 47)
Conceptual apraxia (Ref. 47)	A defect of action semantics and mechanical knowledge (Ref. 49). An inability to understand the function of tools. Patients misuse objects and have difficulty matching objects and actions (posterior regions of the left hemisphere lesions)[49]	
Associative	An impairment of object or action knowledge	FLART[c] (Ref. 50)
Tool–action associations	The knowledge of the type of actions associated with tools is impaired or lost	
Tool–object associations	Unable to associate specific tools with the objects that these tools are designed to act upon	
Mechanical	Unable to understand the mechanical nature of problems and the advantages that tools may afford	FLART[c] (Ref. 47)
Apraxia of eyelid opening	Nonparalytic motor abnormality characterized by difficulty in opening the eyes at will in the absence of visible contraction of the orbicularis oculi muscle (Ref. 47) (supranuclear control impairment)	Periocular electromyography

[a] Voluntary-automatic dissociation, means that the patient does not complain about the deficit because the execution of the movement in the natural context is relatively well preserved, and the deficit appears mainly in the clinical setting when the patient is required to represent explicitly the content of the action outside situational props (Ref. 50).

[b] LOTCA, Lowenstein Occupational Therapy Cognitive assessment.

[c] FLART, Florida Action Recall Test.

TABLE 12.6
Agnosias, Neglects, Body Scheme Dysfunction

Type	Definition	Test(s)
Visual agnosia	A modality-specific perceptual disorder, characterized by impaired shape recognition, and should not be explainable by primary sensory deficits such as poor visual acuity, visual field defects, or problems in color, movement, or depth perception[50]	VO-LOTCA,[c] VOSP[d]
Apperceptive agnosia	A person cannot reliably name, match, or discriminate visually presented objects, despite adequate elementary visual function (visual fields, acuity, and color vision)[51] (lateral occipital lobes damage)	Shape-copying tests
Associative agnosia	A person cannot use the derived perceptual representation to access stored knowledge of the object's functions and associations but is able to copy and match the drawing even though unable to identify it[52] (ventral temporal cortex damage)[52]	BORB[g,53]
Ventral simultanagnosia	A reduction in the ability to rapidly recognize multiple visual stimuli, such that recognition proceeds in a part-by-part fashion[54] (posterior temporal or temporal-occipital cortical lesions)	H-R-R Color test[b,55]
Dorsal simultanagnosia	An inability to detect more than one object at a time, with difficulty shifting attention from one object to another,[1] frequently occurs in the context of Balint syndrome (posterior parietal cortex and occipital region lesion)[56]	H-R-R Color test[b,52]
Asomatognosia	Right—left disorientation: difficulty reliably identifying the right and left sides of his or her own body or those of the examiner (temporal-parietal lesions)[52,57]	Body visualization by command/imitation[58]
Prosopagnosia (facial agnosia)	Inability to recognize faces (occipital-temporal region impairment)[52,57]	CFMT[a,59]
Achromatopsia (color agnosia)	Selective loss of color vision (ventral occipital cortex lesions)	The Ishihara plates, The Farnsworth—Munsell 15- or 100-hue test[60,61]
Metamorphopsia	Size and object distortion (temporal lobe lesions or macular disease)	Amsler grid[62]
Stereopsis (depth perception disorder)	An impairment of depth perception that affects activities that require the judgment of spatial relationships (visual cortex lesions, V1, V2)[63]	Stereotests[64]

Palinopsia	Images persist or recur after the visual stimulus has been removed (occipital-temporal region lesions, ocular abnormalities, psychiatric conditions)	Negative afterimages test[65]
Akinetopsia	Selective loss of fast motion perception (lateral occipital motion—specialized cortex impairment)	Computer-animated displays[66]
Visual–spatial neglect	A deficiency of orienting attention to one hemi-field (usually left) and (may) fail to perceive stimuli in this region (usually right hemisphere damage)[67]	BIT[f,68]
Representational (imagery) neglect	Inability to process the contralesional side of visual mental images	O'clock test, Familiar square description test[69]
Form discrimination	An inability of distinguishing different types of forms (right hemisphere).	VFD[e,58]
Alexia	Loss of the ability to comprehend the meaning of written or printed words and sentences[70]	
Cortical alexia (isolated pure alexia)	An impairment in reading, in which reasonable vision, intelligence, and most language functions other than reading remain intact (occipital-temporal cortex lesions)	Number/letter reading[71]
Disconnection alexia	An impairment in reading, after posterior and dorsal lesions involving the splenium of the callosal corpus or the paraventricular white matter, often associated with visual deficits	Number/letter reading[72]
Charles Bonnet syndrome (visual release hallucinations)	Hallucinations in patients who have no neurological and no psychological abnormalities but with significant visual impairment secondary to ocular disease (spontaneous activity of the ventral occipital lobe)	fMRI[73]
Cortical blindness	Total or partial loss of vision in a normal eye (normal pupillary responses, normal fundus, and no nystagmus) caused by damage to the brain's occipital cortex	MRI
Riddoch syndrome	Ability to perceive and discriminate visual motion in otherwise blind visual field, when stimulated with fast motion (primary visual cortex [area VI])	fMRI[74]

[a] CFMT—Cambridge Face Memory Test, CFPT—Cambridge Face Perception Test.

[b] H-R-R test—Hardy Rand and Rittler test.

[c] VO (Visual Object recognition) subtests of the LOTCA (Lowenstein Occupational Therapy Cognitive Assessment).

[d] VOSP—Visual Object and Space Perception Battery.

[e] VFD—Visual Form Discrimination test.

[f] BIT: Behavioral Inattention Test.

[g] Birmingham Object Recognition Battery—BORB.

ACKNOWLEDGMENTS

We would like to thank Dr. Janet Rucker, and the NYULMC Rusk & Neuro Research Teams for their thoughts, suggestions, and contributions.

REFERENCES

1. Hanna KL, Hepworth LR, Rowe F. Screening methods for post-stroke visual impairment: a systematic review. *Disabil Rehabil*. 2017;39(25):2531–2543.
2. Parton A, Malhotra P, Husain M. Hemispatial neglect. *J Neurol Neurosurg Psychiatry*. 2004;75(1):13–21.
3. Suchoff IB, Ciuffreda KJ. A primer for the optometric management of unilateral spatial inattention. *Optometry J Am Optometric Assoc*. 2004;75(5):305–318.
4. Miller NR, Walsh FB, Hoyt WF. *Walsh and Hoyt's Clinical Neuro-ophthalmology*. Vol. 2. Lippincott Williams & Wilkins; 2005.
5. Bird CM, Malhotra P, Parton A, Coulthard E, Rushworth MFS, Husain M. Visual neglect after right posterior cerebral artery infarction. *J Neurol Neurosurg Psychiatry*. 2006;77(9):1008.
6. Aimola L, Lane AR, Smith DT, Kerkhoff G, Ford GA, Schenk T. Efficacy and feasibility of home-based training for individuals with homonymous visual field defects. *Neurorehabil Neural Repair*. 2014;28(3):207–218.
7. de Haan GA, Melis-Dankers BJ, Brouwer WH, Tucha O, Heutink J. The effects of compensatory scanning training on mobility in patients with homonymous visual field defects: further support, predictive variables and follow-up. *PLoS One*. 2016;11(12):e0166310.
8. Elshout JA, van Asten F, Hoyng CB, Bergsma DP, van den Berg AV. Visual rehabilitation in chronic cerebral blindness: a randomized controlled crossover study. *Front Neurol*. 2016;7:92.
9. Jacquin-Courtois S, Bays PM, Salemme R, Leff AP, Husain M. Rapid compensation of visual search strategy in patients with chronic visual field defects. *Cortex J Devoted Study Nervous Syst Behav*. 2013;49(4):994–1000.
10. Levy-Bencheton D, Pelisson D, Prost M, et al. The effects of short-lasting anti-saccade training in homonymous hemianopia with and without saccadic adaptation. *Front Behav Neurosci*. 2015;9:332.
11. Mannan SK, Pambakian ALM, Kennard C. Compensatory strategies following visual search training in patients with homonymous hemianopia: an eye movement study. *J Neurol*. 2010;257(11):1812–1821.
12. Modden C, Behrens M, Damke I, Eilers N, Kastrup A, Hildebrandt H. A randomized controlled trial comparing 2 interventions for visual field loss with standard occupational therapy during inpatient stroke rehabilitation. *Neurorehabil Neural Repair*. 2012;26(5):463–469.
13. Spitzyna GA, Wise RJ, McDonald SA, et al. Optokinetic therapy improves text reading in patients with hemianopic alexia: a controlled trial. *Neurology*. 2007;68(22):1922–1930.
14. Roth T, Sokolov AN, Messias A, Roth P, Weller M, Trauzettel-Klosinski S. Comparing explorative saccade and flicker training in hemianopia: a randomized controlled study. *Neurology*. 2009;72(4):324–331.
15. Rowe FJ, Conroy EJ, Bedson E, et al. A pilot randomized controlled trial comparing effectiveness of prism glasses, visual search training and standard care in hemianopia. *Acta Neurol Scand*. 2017;136(4):310–321.
16. Pouget MC, Levy-Bencheton D, Prost M, Tilikete C, Husain M, Jacquin-Courtois S. Acquired visual field defects rehabilitation: critical review and perspectives. *Ann Phys Rehabil Med*. 2012;55(1):53–74.
17. Rossetti Y, Rode G, Pisella L, et al. Prism adaptation to a rightward optical deviation rehabilitates left hemispatial neglect. *Nature*. 1998;395(6698):166–169.
18. Vaes N, Nys G, Lafosse C, et al. Rehabilitation of visuospatial neglect by prism adaptation: effects of a mild treatment regime. A randomised controlled trial. *Neuropsychol Rehabil*. 2016:1–20.
19. Scheiman M, Wick B. *Clinical Management of Binocular Vision: Heterophoric, Accommodative, and Eye Movement Disorders*. 4th ed. Philadelphia, PA: Lippincott Williams and Wilkins; 2014.
20. Fahmy AM, Hardten DR. Treating ocular surface disease: new agents in development. *Clin Ophthalmol*. 2011;5:465–472.
21. Leigh RJ, Zee DS. *The Neurology of Eye Movements*. 4th ed. New York Oxford University Press; 2006.
22. Horn AK, Helmchen C, Wahle P. GABAergic neurons in the rostral mesencephalon of the macaque monkey that control vertical eye movements. *Ann NY Acad Sci*. 2003;1004:19–28.
23. Moschovakis AK, Scudder CA, Highstein SM. Structure of the primate oculomotor burst generator. I. Medium-lead burst neurons with upward on-directions. *J Neurophysiol*. 1991;65(2):203–217.
24. Moschovakis AK, Scudder CA, Highstein SM, Warren JD. Structure of the primate oculomotor burst generator. II. Medium-lead burst neurons with downward on-directions. *J Neurophysiol*. 1991;65(2):218–229.
25. Choi KD, Jung DS, Kim JS. Specificity of "peering at the tip of the nose" for a diagnosis of thalamic hemorrhage. *Arch Neurol*. 2004;61(3):417–422.
26. Gomez CR, Gomez SM, Selhorst JB. Acute thalamic esotropia. *Neurology*. 1988;38(11):1759–1762.
27. Bronstein AM, Rudge P, Gresty MA, Du Boulay G, Morris J. Abnormalities of horizontal gaze. Clinical, oculographic and magnetic resonance imaging findings. II. Gaze palsy and internuclear ophthalmoplegia. *J Neurol Neurosurg Psychiatry*. 1990;53(3):200–207.

28. de Seze J, Lucas C, Leclerc X, Sahli A, Vermersch P, Leys D. One-and-a-half syndrome in pontine infarcts: MRI correlates. *Neuroradiology.* 1999;41(9):666−669.

29. Eggenberger E. Eight-and-a-half syndrome: one-and-a-half syndrome plus cranial nerve VII palsy. *J Neuroophthalmol.* 1998;18(2):114−116.

30. Oommen KJ, Smith MS, Labadie EL. Pontine hemorrhage causing Fisher one-and-a-half syndrome with facial paralysis. *J Clin Neuroophthalmol.* 1982;2(2): 129−132.

31. Algin DI, Taser F, Aydin Ş, Aksakallı E. Midbrain infarction presenting with Weber's syndrome and central facial palsy: a case report/Orta beyin infarktina bagli gelisen Weber sendromu ve santral fasyal parezi: olgu sunumu. *Arch Neuropsychiat.* 2009;46(4):197−200.

32. Ruchalski K, Hathout GM. A medley of midbrain maladies: a brief review of midbrain anatomy and syndromology for radiologists. *Radiol Res Pract.* 2012;2012:258524.

33. Court JH, Janicek D. Acute unilateral isolated ptosis. *BMJ Case Rep.* 2015:2015.

34. Portelinha J, Passarinho MP, Costa JM. Neuro-ophthalmological approach to facial nerve palsy. *Saudi J Ophthalmol.* 2015;29(1):39−47.

35. Vasquez LM, Medel R. Lagophthalmos after facial palsy: current therapeutic options. *Ophthal Res.* 2014;52(4):165−169.

36. Rowe F. Prevalence of ocular motor cranial nerve palsy and associations following stroke. *Eye (Lond).* 2011;25(7): 881−887.

37. Baricich A, Cabrio C, Paggio R, Cisari C, Aluffi P. Peripheral facial nerve palsy: how effective is rehabilitation? *Otol Neurotol.* 2012;33(7):1118−1126.

38. Ffytche DH, Blom JD, Catani M. Disorders of visual perception. *J Neurol Neurosurg Psychiatry.* 2010;81(11): 1280−1287.

39. Laeng B. Constructional apraxia after left or right unilateral stroke. *Neuropsychologia.* 2006;44(9):1595−1606.

40. Mayer-Gross W. *The Question of Visual Impairment in Constructional Apraxia.* SAGE Publications; 1936.

41. Lorenze E, Cancro R. Dysfunction in visual perception with hemiplegia: its relation to activities of daily living. *Arch Phys Med Rehabil.* 1962;43:514−517.

42. DG C. *Congenit Ocular Motor Apraxia.* 1966;1(4).

43. Greene JDW. Apraxia, agnosias, and higher visual function abnormalities. *J Neurol Neurosurg Psychiatry.* 2005; 76(suppl 5):v25.

44. Canzano L, Scandola M, Gobbetto V, Moretto G, D'Imperio D, Moro V. The representation of objects in apraxia: from action execution to error awareness. *Front Hum Neurosci.* 2016;10:39.

45. Poeck K. The clinical examination for motor apraxia. *Neuropsychologia.* 1986;24(1):129−134.

46. Leiguarda R. Limb apraxia: cortical or subcortical. (1053-8119 (Print)).

47. Goldmann Gross R, Grossman M. Update on apraxia. *Curr Neurol Neurosci Rep.* 2008;8(6):490−496.

48. De Renzi E, Motti F, Nichelli P. Imitating gestures: a quantitative approach to ideomotor apraxia. *Arch Neurol.* 1980; 37(1):6−10.

49. Jongbloed L, Stacey S, Brighton C. Stroke rehabilitation: sensorimotor integrative treatment versus functional treatment. *Am J Occup Therapy.* 1989;43(6):391−397.

50. Schwartz RL, Adair JC, Raymer AM, et al. Conceptual apraxia in probable Alzheimer's disease as demonstrated by the Florida Action Recall Test. *J Int Neuropsychol Soc.* 2000;6(3):265−270.

51. Yoon WT, Chung EJ, Lee SH, Kim BJ, Lee WY. Clinical analysis of blepharospasm and apraxia of eyelid opening in patients with parkinsonism. *J Clin Neurol.* 2005;1(2): 159−165.

52. Baugh LA, Desanghere L, Marotta J. Agnosia. 2010.

53. *Chapter 6-The Art of Seeing. Fundamentals of Cognitive Neuroscience.* San Diego: Academic Press; 2013:141−173.

54. McCarthy RA, Warrington EK. Visual associative agnosia: a clinico-anatomical study of a single case. *J Neurol Neurosurg Psychiatry.* 1986;49(11):1233.

55. Baars BJ, Gage NM. *Cognition, Brain, and Consciousness: Introduction to Cognitive Neuroscience.* Academic Press; 2010.

56. Devinsky O, J Farah M, Barr W. *Chapter 21 Vis Agnosia.* Vol. 882008.

57. Lee AG, Brazis PW, Kline LB, eds. *Curbside Consultation in Neuro-Ophthalmology-49 Clinical Questions.* Thorofare, NJ SLACK Incorporated. 2009.

58. Li K, Malhotra PA. Spatial neglect. *Pract Neurol.* 2015; 15(5):333−339.

59. Feinberg TE, Venneri A, Simone AM, Fan Y, Northoff G. The neuroanatomy of asomatognosia and somatoparaphrenia. *J Neurol Neurosurg Psychiatry.* 2010;81(3): 276.

60. Boone Dr Fau − Landes BA, Landes BA. Left-right discrimination in hemiplegic patients. (0003-9993 (Print)).

61. Cumming WJ. The neurobiology of the body schema. *Br J Psychiatry Suppl.* 1988;(2):7−11.

62. Barton JJS, Press DZ, Keenan JP, O'connor M. Lesions of the fusiform face area impair perception of facial configuration in prosopagnosia. *Neurology.* 2002;58(1): 71−78.

63. Bowles DC, McKone E, Dawel A, et al. Diagnosing prosopagnosia: effects of ageing, sex, and participant−stimulus ethnic match on the Cambridge face memory test and Cambridge face perception test. *Cogn Neuropsychol.* 2009; 26(5):423−455.

64. Bouvier SE, Engel SA. Behavioral deficits and cortical damage loci in cerebral achromatopsia. *Cereb Cortex.* 2005; 16(2):183−191.

65. Simunovic MP. Metamorphopsia and its quantification. (1539-2864 (Electronic)).

66. H Ffytche D, Blom JD, Catani M. *Disorders of Visual Perception.* Vol. 812010.

67. Fricke TR, Siderov J. Stereopsis, stereotests, and their relation to vision screening and clinical practice. *Clin Exp Optometry.* 1997;80(5):165−172.

68. Van der Stigchel S, Nijboer TCW, Bergsma DP, Barton JJS, Paffen CLE. Measuring palinopsia: characteristics of a persevering visual sensation from cerebral pathology. *J Neurol Sci.* 2012;316(1):184−188.

69. Barton JJS. Chapter 9-Disorders of higher visual processing. In: Kennard C, Leigh RJ, eds. *Handbook of Clinical Neurology*. Vol. 102.

70. Stone SP, Wilson B, Wroot A, et al. The assessment of visuo-spatial neglect after acute stroke. *J Neurol Neurosurg Psychiatry*. 1991;54(4):345.

71. Guariglia C, Palermo L, Piccardi L, Iaria G, Incoccia C. Neglecting the left side of a city square but not the left side of its clock: prevalence and characteristics of representational neglect. *PLoS One*. 2013;8(7):e67390.

72. Kasai M, Ishizaki JF-IH, Ishii HF-YS, Yamaguchi SF-YA, Yamadori AF-MK, Meguro K. Normative data on Benton visual form discrimination test for older adults and impaired scores in clinical Dementia rating 0.5 participants: community-based study. Osaki-Tajiri Proj. (1440-1819 (Electronic)).

73. Rodriguez-Lopez CA-O, Guerrero Molina MP, Martinez Salio A. Pure alexia: two cases and a new neuroanatomical classification. Lid — https://doi.org/10.1007/s00415-017-8691-9. (1432-1459 (Electronic)).

74. Starrfelt R, Behrmann M. Number reading in pure alexia—a review. (1873-3514 (Electronic)).

CHAPTER 13

Pharmacological Interventions to Enhance Stroke Recovery

STEVEN R. FLANAGAN, MD • HEIDI FUSCO, MD

INTRODUCTION

795,000 people sustain a new stroke each year in the United States[1] which is a leading cause of death and adult disability. The estimated yearly costs of stroke in the United States is estimated to $33 billion, which includes the cost of Text care, medicines to treat stroke and missed days of work,[2] with the economic burden of ischemic stroke expected to expand to enormous proportions over the next several decades.[3] Significant strides have been made in both primary and secondary prevention of stroke, predominantly through identifying and controlling modifiable risk factors. Reperfusion therapies have become common practice and reduced morbidity and mortality by limiting the degree of cerebral injury. However, they are effective only for a minority of patients when provided during a short therapeutic window after stroke onset. Restoration of functional and cognitive skills lost from stroke occurs over a much longer period and rely on several mechanisms to achieve desirable outcomes. These mechanisms include neuronal genesis and plasticity; the natural ability of the brain to adapt to environmental stimulation, disease, or injury by forming new neurons and synapses and altering surviving neuronal connections that accounts for new learning and behaviors. Rehabilitation plays a vital role in recovery from cerebral injury that enhances plasticity as well as by teaching compensatory techniques that result in patients performing tasks in alternative ways or by using tools that compensate for lost skills. The goal of rehabilitation following stroke or brain injury is to maximize a person's mobility, daily living, and communication and cognitive skills to live as independently as possible. Rehabilitation occurs over a variable period, although it is likely most effective when provided early post stroke when the majority of recovery ensues. The most intense rehabilitation following stroke typically occurs during the acute and immediate postacute stages, often in Inpatient Rehabilitation Facilities (IRFs). However, health care trends over the past several decades have curtailed the amount of time patients with stroke receive IRF level care, thus placing increasing pressure to find means to facilitate and hasten the recovery process. This has led to research examining means to facilitate recovery and the rehabilitation process by using technology and medications.

Although definitive pharmacological means to enhance recovery during the postacute period are not nearly as standardized as reperfusion therapies, notable strides are being made to examine various agents that appear to have promise. Several neurotransmitter systems are believed to play a role in recovery following stroke and brain injury, including the noradrenergic, dopaminergic, acetylcholinergic, serotonergic, and glutamatergic systems. Other medications, including growth factors, monoclonal antibodies, stem cells, and medications that modify inflammation have also been theorized to play a role in recovery. Despite a growing literature on this topic with some promising results, a considerable amount of information remains unknown, and several caveats need to be considered when either investigating or using medications for this purpose.

Physiologic changes in response to stroke occur and change over time; thus, there is likely an ideal window to provide specific drugs to enhance recovery but also a period where they may be either ineffective or detrimental.[4–8] It has also been long known that drugs alone are unlikely to promote recovery noting that some form of training, typically in the form of rehabilitation, is required to induce a positive effect on recovery. Following experimental stroke, rodents provided with amphetamines only resulted in improved outcomes when paired with training,[9] which was confirmed in several follow-up studies.[10–13] Rehabilitation therapies are felt to be necessary as behavioral recovery depends on experience to direct new neuronal connections.[14]

A drug's effectiveness in enhancing recovery may be dependent on numerous factors, including but not

Stroke Rehabilitation. https://doi.org/10.1016/B978-0-323-55381-0.00013-5

limited to the specific impairments being targeted, severity of impairment, time post stroke, genetics, and location and extent of injury. A robust area of investigation is currently examining means to identify phenotypic characteristics that predict response to specific interventions. Failure of some past translational research resulted in part from insufficient patient selection, including prescreening for potential markers of responsiveness. A trial investigating epidural stimulation to improve motor recovery post stroke failed, in part because subjects were included who did not have a preserved motor evoked response prior to stimulator implantation.[15] A posthoc analysis revealed subjects with preserved evoked responses were much more likely to respond to treatment,[16] indicating that specific patient characteristics play an important role in which interventions will be beneficial. Identifying biomarkers, such as responsiveness to electrical stimulation in the previous example, will be useful in future studies of stroke recovery that permit selection of subjects most likely to respond to a specific intervention. It would also potentially assist with identifying the most effective timing, dose, and duration of treatment.

GENERAL PRINCIPLES

When considering the use of pharmacological agents to enhance recovery after stroke, it is important to consider what specific function or skill is being targeted; agree to a treatment goal with the patient, their family, and the other members of the treating team; and choose the appropriate means to assess its effectiveness. This may be through formalized objective assessments of motor, language, or cognitive abilities, or more globally by assessment of how an individual's functional abilities change in response to treatment. Additional and vital information will often come from family members or others on the rehabilitation team. Involving families and other rehabilitation team members is a critical component to the rehabilitation process, particularly as medication enhancement is typically effective only when paired with a behavioral intervention. When initiating medications, it is best to start at low doses and slowly titrate upward until the desired outcome is achieved or a ceiling effect has been reached. Limiting polypharmacy, particularly in elderly patients, is another important consideration, as drug-drug interactions become more difficult to disentangle the more medications a person takes at any given time. In many situations, decreasing or eliminating unneeded medications provides a successful pathway to recovery. Only one medication should be added or dose changed at any given time, with enough time

provided to assess for changes in functional skills, to most meaningfully assess its impact on recovery. The adage of "start low, go slow" is particularly important as patients are typically on multiple medications, and those with brain injuries can respond more aggressively to pharmacological interventions. Physical abilities and stroke-related impairments naturally change over time, making it important to provide periodic medication holidays to ascertain the continued need for pharmacological agents. This can assess whether medications successfully used to enhance recovery are still required at the same dose previously prescribed. While many of the effects desired from medication enhancement of functional skills post stroke are considered "side-effects," other undesirable effects need to be monitored closely. These include but are not limited to tachycardia, nausea, hypotension, lethargy, insomnia, and worsening function. These side effects may be manageable by either lowering doses or by timing the medications in a manner that limits their adverse effect (e.g., prescribing sedating medications closer to time of sleep).

NEUROTRANSMITTER ANATOMY AND PHYSIOLOGY

In order to gain an appreciation of the rationale underlying the use of medications to enhance stroke recovery, it is useful to understand the neural anatomy and basic physiology of the major neurotransmitter systems in the central nervous system (CNS). This will help to envision theories underlying recovery following brain injury and the role medications that affect these systems play in neurological and functional outcomes.

Norepinephrine (NE) containing cell bodies in the brain are predominantly located in the locus coeruleus in the pons. Although occupying a small region of the brain, NE fibers widely project throughout the CNS, including the prefrontal cortex, cerebellum, limbic system, brain stem, and spinal cord, thus having widespread effect on multiple motor and cognitive skills. Synaptic NE is inactivated by several means, including presynaptic reuptake and enzymatic degradation by either monoamine oxidase (MAO) or catechol-O-methyltransferase. Presynaptic receptors also foster a negative feedback mechanism to inhibit NE release. NE modulates several cognitive functions, including but not limited to memory and various aspects of attention.

There are multiple dopaminergic pathways in the brain arising from various locations, including but not limited to the mesolimbic, mesocortical, and nigrostriatal systems. Dopaminergic activity is widespread throughout the brain affecting multiple functions including movement, reward, and learning and neural plasticity. Both the mesolimbic and mesocortical pathways originate from the ventral tegmentum, with fibers from the former projecting to the nucleus accumbens, amygdala, and anterior cingulate cortex and the latter to the cortex and limbic structures with a predominate role in modulating cognitive functions. The nigrostriatal dopaminergic system projects from the substantia nigra to the basal ganglia. Synaptic dopaminergic activity is enzymatically reduced in a similar manner as NE, as well as inhibition of presynaptic release by activation of specific serotonin receptors.

Serotonin containing neurons are in the brainstem, predominantly in the raphe nuclei. Serotonergic fibers project widely throughout the CNS including the frontal cortex, basal ganglia, limbic area, hypothalamus, brain stem, and spinal cord. It mediates a variety of physiological activities including cognition, mood, motor control, appetite, sleep, and sexual responses. Synaptic concentration is decreased enzymatically by MOA or by presynaptic reuptake.

The nucleus basalis of Meynert in the basal forebrain houses the predominant acetylcholine (ACh) containing neurons in the brain with widespread cerebral projections to the hippocampus, amygdala, and neocortex. In the CNS, ACh modulates several cognitive functions, including memory, learning, problem solving, attention, and judgment. Cerebral ACh is enzymatically degraded by either acetylcholinesterase or butyrylcholinesterase, the latter being more concentrated in glial cells.

Glutamate is among the most ubiquitous excitatory neurotransmitters in the CNS, affecting a wide range of cognitive and physiological processes, either by direct postsynaptic receptor activation or by affecting the activity of other neurotransmitters. Exaggerated release of glutamate after brain injury from trauma and ischemia activates N-methyl-D-aspartate (NMDA) receptors, causing neuronal influx of calcium which has been implicated in postinjury neurotoxicity and the development of several neurodegenerative diseases.

MEDICATIONS TO PROMOTE MOTOR RECOVERY
Selective Serotonin Reuptake Inhibitors
Rationale
Several potential mechanisms provide a reasonable rationale to consider selective serotonin reuptake inhibitors (SSRIs) as a pharmacological modulator of recovery post stroke. Neurogenesis refers to the ability to form new neurons, which may take place in certain cerebral regions, including the subventricular zone (SVZ) and the dentate gyrus of the hippocampus. Evidence

suggests that after experimental stroke, nascent cells from SVZ and the hippocampus migrate to areas of ischemic injury and take on the phenotypic characteristics of the injured neurons.[17,18] Several animal studies provide evidence that SSRIs support stimulation of neurogenesis and synaptogenesis that contribute to structural and functional recovery from ischemic lesions and that the newly formed cells can migrate to the injured regions.[19-24] Fluoxetine has been shown to increase hippocampal cell proliferation,[25,26] and pharmacological treatment of major depression has been shown to increase adult hippocampal neurogenesis and expression of neurotropic factors in the hippocampus.[27,28] Fluoxetine has also been demonstrated to enhance plasticity in the adult visual cortex of animals[29,30] by stimulating gene expression known to be important in plasticity.[31,32] Brain-derived neurotrophic factor (BDNF) is associated with neuronal plasticity, and is increased in response to chronic infusion of antidepressants in animals[33-35] and humans.[36]

It is also well-known that inflammation plays a role in ischemic injury and contributes to deterioration of neurological function and poor outcome.[31,37] SSRIs have demonstrated antiinflammatory and neuroprotective effects. They have been shown to decrease postischemia infarct volume associated with less severe neurological deficits in rats by suppressing microglia activation and neutrophil infiltration[38] and protect neurons post ischemia by decreasing inflammation via inhibition of microglia and neutrophil granulocytes[37] Fluoxetine has also been shown to inhibit interleukin 1-β—induced apoptosis and upregulating an antiapoptosis protein.[39]

SSRI Evidence Supporting Recovery
Animal and human evidence support the beneficial effect of SSRIs on motor recovery post stroke. A metaanalysis of 21 experiments reporting the efficacy of fluoxetine in 252 animals revealed that neurobehavioral scores improved by 41% although there was insufficient evidence to determine the likely underlying mechanisms.[40] The strongest clinical evidence of the beneficial effect of SSRIs on recovery comes from the Fluoxetine for Motor Recovery After Acute Ischemic Stroke (FLAME) trial.[41] This study enrolled 118 nondepressed patients within 10 days of an ischemic stroke and randomized them to either 3 months of fluoxetine 20 mg daily or placebo. The fluoxetine group achieved significantly better gains on the arm and leg Fugl—Meyer compared to the placebo group. Subjects receiving fluoxetine were also more likely to be deemed independent based on modified Rankin scores. Metaanalyses of trials examined multiple outcomes of

SSRI post stroke.[42,43] Of the studies examining disability post treatment, there was a large beneficial effect of SSRIs which was greatest for patients with depression at the time of recruitment. However, the effect size was smallest in studies with the lowest risk of bias. In general, secondary measures including neurological impairments, depression, and anxiety were also better in the SSRI groups, although there was a nonsignificant trend for more gastrointestinal and seizure-related complications. In addition to the numerous mechanisms that have been postulated to account for the beneficial effect of SSRIs on motor recovery post stroke, it is possible that an antidepressant effect played a role as well. The antidepressant effects of SSRIs are achieved through inhibiting serotonin removal from the synapse and the downregulation and desensitization of serotonin receptors after longterm use. Although the FLAME trial controlled for depression, increasing depressive symptomology in the absence of a definitive diagnosis of depression affects brain function along a continuum. When present, depression is associated with larger effect sizes when examining the effectiveness of SSRI following stroke.[44,45] Functional recovery following stroke is associated with lower depressive symptoms which decrease over time.[8,46] Thus, decreasing depressive symptoms in the absence of a definitive diagnosis of depression may contribute to recovery. Timing of SSRI administration post stroke may affect recovery, as noted by a small study indicating earlier administration post stroke was more beneficial than delaying intervention.[46]

Catecholaminergic Agents
Rationale
Catecholamines are a class of neurotransmitters that include epinephrine, norepinephrine and dopamine. Several theories have been proposed as a rationale to use catecholaminergic drugs to enhance recovery after brain injury. Reversal in diaschisis, when an intact or uninjured neural structure does not function properly due to loss of afferent input from an injured distal region, is one potential mechanism. Administration of amphetamines, which promote the release of NE and DA, may provide some degree of afferent input that was lost from injury or disease.[47–49] Amphetamine-induced neuronal plasticity, manifested by increased neural sprouting, has also been demonstrated in animals, potentially accounting for restoration of lost function following stroke.[49] Amphetamines have also been shown to increase metabolic activity in regions adjacent to damaged neural areas,[50] potentially enhancing functional activity in structurally related cortex.[51]

Several neurotransmitters, including noradrenaline,[52] serotonin,[53] dopamine,[54] and acetylcholine[55] are known to impart an effect on longterm potentiation; a neuronal process involved in learning and memory.[56] Longterm potentiation is thought to be involved with training-induced plasticity of the primary motor cortex, thus providing a rationale for their use to enhance motor recovery after stroke.[57] While longterm potentiation is physiologically defined by strengthening of synaptic connections via glutamate receptors, longterm depression is defined as decreasing synaptic strength, but also plays a role in the development of motor behaviors and is affected by DA activity.[58] DA activity has also been shown to promote the coordination of vision with action-related information, which plays an important role in motor activity.[59,60] It is well established that DA terminals in the motor cortex play an important role in cortical plasticity and are needed for motor learning.[61,62] The role of DA on motor recovery may be related to its functions on nonmotor functions such as motivation and reward, and not directly on its effect on motor systems.[8]

Amphetamines
Amphetamines increase the synaptic concentration of several neurotransmitters believed to be beneficial in recovery following brain injury, including norepinephrine, dopamine, and serotonin. Multiple studies have examined the potential utility of amphetamines, typically D-amphetamine, in enhancing motor and/or functional recovery after stroke. Nearly all trials provided rehabilitation therapies well within the half-life of the study medication, indicating a consensus among researchers of the importance of rehabilitation interventions in securing positive changes when using drugs to modulate outcomes. Assessing these studies reveals a considerable degree of heterogeneity regarding methodologies and subject selection, including stroke chronicity, type, and severity; outcome measures; and dosing schedules. Not surprisingly, study conclusions have been variable, with outcomes either favoring amphetamine use,[61–67] indicating no beneficial effect,[68–70] or mixed results suggesting acute but no longterm benefit.[71] A Cochrane review of studies examining amphetamine use post stroke, including 287 subjects, found that they did not reduce death or dependence.[72] Similarly, in a review of randomized controlled trials examining amphetamines, only three studies that included 34 patients demonstrated an improvement, while six studies including 227 subjects failed to demonstrate a benefit on motor skills.[73] Given the mixed results of multiple trials, no recommendation can be made with confidence regarding the use of amphetamines to promote motor recovery post stroke at this time.

Other medications that enhance norepinephrine may be beneficial in stroke recovery, although evidence is scarce. Two trials evaluating reboxetine, a medication that blocks reuptake of norepinephrine from the synapse, in subjects with subacute to chronic stroke revealed improvements in finger tapping velocity and grip strength.[74,75] Functional MRI data revealed that the improved motor activity after reboxetine ingestion was associated with a reduction in cortical hyperactivity toward physiologic levels and an improvement in connectivity between motor areas in the injured hemisphere.[75] The study investigators suggested that reboxetine may help to modulate stroke induced abnormal motor network architecture thus improving motor function.[75] However, to date only 21 subjects have been studied; thus, recommendations cannot be made regarding its use to enhance motor recovery after stroke.

Dopamine

Most studies examining the role of DA agonists in enhancing stroke recovery have used levodopa. Results of studies during the subacute phase following stroke are mixed. Some studies revealed improvements in arm function, mobility, and motor skills,[76,77] while others did not.[78,79] One of the studies did reveal a benefit of levodopa when combined with methylphenidate and physiotherapy.[78] Studies on chronic stroke subjects are equally mixed, with some indicating a beneficial response of levodopa[80–82] and others not.[83] Ropinirole, another DA agonist, was also not found to be beneficial in subjects with chronic stroke with regards to gait speed or Fugyl–Meyer scores.[84]

Similar to other trials examining the effect of medications on recovery, a definitive conclusion regarding DA agonism's effectiveness is elusive due to the heterogeneity of the studies and subsequently their variable results. Studies are heterogeneous with regards to time post stroke, lesion size and location, stroke type (ischemic and/or hemorrhagic), variable severity of impairments, outcome measures, and sample size. In addition to the heterogeneity, genotype may play a role in who responds to DA agents, as certain genotypes may predispose response to injury and pharmacologic interventions.[85–87]

Medications to Promote Language Recovery

Aphasia is a common stroke-related impairment, affecting approximately one-third of first-time hospitalized stroke patients.[88–93] Approximately one-third of those experience severe language impairment[88,94] that is associated with poor shortterm and longterm prognosis regarding mortality and dependence.[90,95,96] Speech language therapy is the mainstay of rehabilitation treatments to improve language skills in patients with poststroke aphasia. Despite a growing consensus that speech therapies are effective,[97–101] people are often left with significant language impairments that adversely affect their daily lives and reintegration into their prestroke roles. Efforts to enhance language skills post stroke include various forms of magnetic or electrical stimulation, as well as medications felt to potentially enhance recovery. Similar to motor recovery, the rationale to use drugs to promote language skills include reversal of diaschisis and enhancement of plasticity.[102–104] Several classes of drugs have been trialed over the span of more than half a century, but consensus on their use has not been reached due to multiple reasons. Results from trials vary considerably, with some indicating a beneficial response while others not. Many studies were implemented without a clear theoretical rationale.[104,105] Many studies failed to account for different size, location, and number of cerebral lesions; type of aphasia; subject age; and level of education, handedness, chronicity, concomitant rehabilitation, and many other comorbid factors that affect outcomes. A majority of studies were small, had various methodological limitations, and were not validated in large, well-controlled, multicentered trials. Despite that, the potential promise of pharmacologically improving language function remains an active area of research and interest.

Catecholaminergic Agents

Of all the catecholaminergic drugs, bromocriptine has been studied the most with regards to aphasia recovery. Bromocriptine is a D2 dopaminergic receptor agonist that has been used in several trials with varying results. Studies demonstrating a beneficial response were generally small, often in open-labeled trials, and were tested in subjects with transcortical motor and Broca aphasia of moderate severity with predominantly subcortical lesions.[106–109] Other trials demonstrated a potential beneficial effect on various language characteristics, including length of utterances[110] and word retrieval.[111] Its use in more severe Broca or global aphasia was not successful, nor were randomized trials that attempted to confirm findings in prior open label studies.[112–115] Additional research is needed to more definitely confirm or repute the effectiveness of bromocriptine that addresses important methodological issues. Dosing in these studies varied widely, with lower doses tending to be more beneficial than higher doses. It is conceivable that there is a narrow range of DA agonism corresponding to optimal function. Subject selection varied widely with regards to type and severity of aphasia, as well as with concomitant speech therapy.

The effect of other catecholaminergic drugs has been examined, including levodopa, amantadine, and dextroamphetamine. Levodopa combined with speech therapy was found to improve fluency and repetition ability in chronic aphasic patients with the greatest improvement noted in those with frontal lesions.[116] Other studies have not shown an added benefit of levodopa paired with speech therapy in either subacute[117] or chronic subjects.[118] Several small trials of amantadine have demonstrated promising results in improving various aspects of language in subjects with aphasia of different etiologies, which all need to be replicated in larger controlled trials.[119,120] Studies examining amphetamine, predominantly dextroamphetamine, with one examining methylphenidate, revealed mixed results. Dextroamphetamine paired with speech therapy revealed better language performance at the end of treatment in subjects in the subacute phase of recovery but was no longer significant at 6-month follow-up.[102] Amphetamine use in chronic aphasia patients has resulted in mixed results[121,122] and is not currently recommended for use for that purpose.[123,124] However, a recent proof-of-concept trial pairing dextroamphetamine, melodic intonation speech therapy, and transcranial direct current stimulation in a crossover, placebo-controlled, double-blind study in 10 chronic nonfluent aphasia patients resulted in improvement in some aspects of language function without adverse effect,[125] indicating the potential of combining different modalities to improve language function.

Piracetam

Piracetam belongs to a class of drugs known as nootropics. It is a derivative of gamma aminobutyric acid that has been used for decades in Europe as an enhancer of various cognitive stills. The precise actions of piracetam are not well delineated, although it is thought to enhance acetylcholine and glutamate transmission with evidence suggesting it facilitates memory and learning in humans.[126] Other reported physiological actions include increasing cerebral blood flow and glucose metabolism in infarcted cerebral tissue and its penumbra and neuroprotective effects in an animal stroke model.[127] Thus, it is a seemingly attractive agent to potentially ameliorate or limit functional loss from stroke. However, a Cochrane review of its use in acute ischemic stroke failed to reveal a significant difference between active drug and control groups on functional outcome and dependence, but did detect a nonsignificant trend for early death in the piracetam group, possibly related to an imbalance in one study with more severe stroke receiving the drug.[128] An earlier

Cochrane review examining the effectiveness of several pharmacologic agents in poststroke aphasia found weak evidence supporting piracetam, noting the strength of the findings were hindered by a large number of drop outs from the trials included in the analysis. However, similar to the latter Cochrane review, there was a nonsignificant trend of increased mortality associated with piracetam use.[129] The most recent trial examining its effectiveness in poststroke aphasia failed to demonstrate a benefit in subjects with large left hemisphere strokes.[130]

Aceytlcholine

Acetylcholine-enhancing medications have been considered as potential pharmacological agents to ameliorate aphasia impairments post stroke, based on data suggesting their effectiveness in improving communication skills in patients with dementia.[131–134] Cholinergic drugs have also been associated with improved cognitive and language skills[135,136] making them attractive agents to consider as facilitating improvement in poststroke aphasia. Cholinergic pathways linking the basal forebrain and peri-Sylvian language are known to be disrupted in vascular lesions,[137,138] suggesting that drugs that enhance cholinergic activity could potentially ameliorate language impairments post stroke. Cholinergic-related improvement in various cognitive skills related to language function, including attention, learning, and memory, may also contribute to improvement in poststroke aphasia.[139] Cholinergic blockade has been shown to impair verbal fluency, and naming, reading, and written language skills in healthy adults.[140] Several small studies and reports support the use of cholinergic agonists, most typically acetylcholinesterase inhibitors or direct acting cholinergic agonists, paired with speech language therapy[141–144] which was confirmed in larger trials.[145–147] A review of several studies examined the percentage of patients responding to donepezil, an acetylcholinesterase inhibitor, revealing that 82% of subjects showed significant improvement, and 73% of those completing a 6-month extension continued to show a response.[148] Responders tended to have conduction and Broca aphasia of mild to moderate severity with nonresponders more likely to have moderate to severe Broca or Wernicke aphasia.

Memantine

Acute brain injury caused by trauma or ischemia leads to neuronal injury through many mechanisms, including massive release of glutamate leading to overstimulation of NDMA receptors. In the chronic phase post injury, there can be loss of glutamatergic activity potentially impairing functional skills. Glutamate, which is the most abundant excitatory neurotransmitter in the CNS, acts on multiple receptors. Memantine is a noncompetitive antagonist of NMDA receptors that may offer neuroprotective effects acutely post brain injury, but may also modulate glutamatergic activity in the chronic phase, thereby enhancing plasticity.[149] Studies have shown that the dosing of memantine can have variable results on outcomes post stroke, with short-term low-dose administration limiting experimentally induced lesion volume and improving behavioral outcomes in stroke, while higher doses increased lesion volume.[150] Longterm memantine administration in mice may improve stroke outcomes, as it has been associated with increased levels of brain-derived neurotrophic factor and improved vascularization.[151] Memantine has been shown to improve language skills in patients with Alzheimer disease,[152] which combined with other evidence makes it a potentially attractive agent to enhance language recovery post stroke.

Clinical evidence supporting its use post stroke is limited. Two studies indicated that it facilitated language recovery, particularly when paired with intensive speech-language therapy.[153,154] However, more evidence will be needed prior to establishing it has a definitive means to enhance language recovery post stroke.

MEDICATIONS FOR COGNITIVE IMPAIRMENT AFTER STROKE

In addition to motor and language impairments, cognitive difficulties post stroke and brain injury are common and adversely affect reintegration into desired societal roles. Although most literature pertaining to pharmacologic enhancement of cognitive skills after brain injury have examined traumatic brain injury, some have specifically assessed subjects with stroke. A recent metaanalysis identified 44 randomized controlled trials between drug treatment and placebo to determine the effects of medications on recovery after stroke.[155] Studies were evaluated for method quality using a 5-point Jadad scale. The authors concluded that while SSRIs improved gross motor functions after stroke, as discussed earlier, there was insufficient evidence of any benefit on cognitive recovery. Although the authors found insufficient evidence to recommend any medications to mitigate cognitive deficits after stroke, some medications may offer cognitive enhancing benefits with relatively low risk of undesired side effects, particularly as several of them have been shown to have potential benefit on motor and language impairments. In a study of 129 poststroke patients

without depression, escitalopram was found to increase the total score on the Repeatable Battery for the Assessment of Neuropsychological Status (RBANS), particularly on measures of verbal and visual memory compared to placebo or problem-solving therapy.[156]

Donepezil has also been identified as a possible beneficial drug to improve cognition after stroke. In a small trial in subjects with right hemispheric stroke examining the potential cognitive effects of donepezil, scores on the Mini Mental Status Examination were enhanced as compared to placebo. Function MRI revealed increased activation in the prefrontal areas, inferior frontal lobes, and the left inferior parietal lobe associated with donepezil use. The investigators proposed that donepezil benefits the cognitive pathway in patients with right hemispheric stroke via the same mechanism of action as in both vascular and Alzheimer dementia.[157] However, an open-label trial examining the effectiveness of donepezil and galantamine, both acetylcholinesterase inhibitors titrated to subject tolerance, in poststroke subjects revealed that participants receiving donepezil had better functional recovery than participants receiving galantamine or historical comparators. The investigators suggested that the improvement may have reflected efficacy at the starting dose for donepezil but not galantamine.[158]

CONCLUSION

Stroke is an epidemic in the United States and throughout the world resulting in considerable morbidity and mortality. While survival and morbidity have improved secondary to advances in acute management, many treatments are not available for a large percentage of those with acute stroke, leaving many with longterm disabilities. Research in rehabilitation is focused on improving cerebral plasticity, learning, and functional recovery, which includes the potential use of medications. However, much of the literature on this topic is limited by diverse methodologies and designs that prevent making definitive recommendations regarding the use of medications post stroke. Not surprisingly, multiple pharmacological agents have been studied with mixed results regarding their effectiveness. The most robust response favoring drug enhancement is for SSRI and motor recovery. Evidence supporting the use of medications to enhance other aspects of recovery in decidedly mixed and large, well-designed, placebo-controlled, randomized trials are scarce. Thus, there exist no structured guidelines on timing and dosing of medications after stroke. However, given the worldwide burden of stroke, the importance of enhancing the recovery process and diminishing its related disabilities is of paramount importance. Additional research is warranted that addresses the limitations of past studies that lead to evidence-based recommendations and improved outcomes.

REFERENCES

1. CDC, NCHS. Underlying Cause of Death 1999–2014 on CDC WONDER Online Database, released 2015. Data are from the Multiple Cause of Death Files, 1999–2013, as compiled from data provided by the 57 vital statistic jurisdiction through the Vital Statistics Cooperative Program. OR https:www.cdc.gov/stroke/facts.htm. CDC Centers for Disease Control and Prevention. CDC/24/7: Saving Lives, Protecting People.
2. Mozzafarian D, Benjamin EJ, Go AS, et al. Heart disease and strike statistics-2016 update: a report from the American Heart Association. *Circulation.* 2016;133(4): e38–e360.
3. Brown DL, Boden-Albala B, Langa KM, et al. Projected costs of ischemic stroke in the United States. *Neurology.* 2006;67:1390–1395.
4. Green AR, Hainsworth AH, Jackson DM. GABA potentiation: a logical pharmacological approach for the treatment of acute ischaemic stroke. *Neuropharmacology.* 2000;39:1483–1494.
5. Kozlowski DA, Jones TA, Schallert T. Pruning of dendrites and restoration of function after brain damage: role of the NMDA receptor. *Restor Neurol Neurosci.* 1994;7: 119–126.
6. Narasimhan P, Liu J, Song YS, Massengale JL, Chan PH. VEGF stimulates the ERK ½ signaling pathway and apoptosis in cerebral endothelial cells after ischemic conditions. *Stroke.* 2009;40:1467–1473.
7. Zhao BQ, Tejima E, Lo EH. Neurovascular proteases in brain injury, hemorrhage and remodeling after stroke. *Stroke.* 2007;38(suppl 2):748–752.
8. Cramer SC. Drugs to enhance motor recovery after stroke. *Stroke.* 2015;46(10):2998–3005, 591–608.
9. Feeney DM, Gonzalez A, Law WA. Amphetamine, haloperidol, and experience interact to affect recovery after motor cortex injury. *Science.* 1982;217:855–857.
10. Fang PC, Barbay S, Plautz EJ, Hoover E, Strittmatter SM, Nudo RJ. Combination of NEP 1-40 treatment and motor training enhances behavioral recovery after a focal cortical infarct in rats. *Stroke.* 2010;41:5544–5549.
11. Starkey ML, Schwab ME. Anti-Nogo-A and training: can one plus one equal three? *Exp Neurol.* 2012;235:53–61.
12. Hovda DA, Fenney DM. Amphetamine with experience promotes recovery of locomotor function after unilateral frontal cortex injury in the cat. *Brain Res.* 1984;298: 3358–3361.
13. Adkins-Muir DL, Jones TA. Cortical electrical stimulation combines with rehabilitative training: enhanced functional recovery an dendritic plasticity following focal cortical ischemia in rats. *Neurol Res.* 2003;25: 78–788.
14. Garcia-Alias G, Barkhuysen S, Buckle M, Fawcett JW. Chondroitinase ABC treatment opens a window of opportunity for task-specific rehabilitation. *Nat Neurosci.* 2009;12:1145–1151.
15. Levy RM, Harvey RL, Kissela BM, et al. Epidural electrical stimulation for stroke rehabilitation: results of the prospective, multicenter, randomized, single-blinded Everest trial. *Neurorehabil Neural Repair.* 2016;30(2):107–119.
16. Nouri S, Cramer SC. Anatomy and physiology predict response to motor cortex stimulation after stroke. *Neurology.* 2011;77:1076–1083.
17. Santareilli L, Saxe M, Gross C, et al. Requirement of hippocampal neurogenesis antidepressant treatments and animal model of depressive-like behaviour. *Science.* 2003;301:805–809.
18. Hicks AU, Hewlett K, Windle V, et al. Enriched environment enhances transplanted subventricular zone stem cell migration and functional recovery after stroke. *Neuroscience.* 2007;146:31–40.
19. Liu J, Solway K, Messing RO, Sharp FR. Increased neurogenesis in the dentate gyrus after transient global ischemia in gerbils. *J Neurosci.* 1998;18:7768–7778.
20. Gu W, Brannstrom T, Wester P. Cortical neurogenesis in adult rats after eversible photothrombic stroke. *J Cereb Blood Metab.* 2000;20:1166–1173.
21. Jiang W, Gu W, Brannstrom T, Rosqvist R, Wester P. Cortical neurogenesis in adult rats after transient middle cerebral artery occlusion. *Stroke.* 2001;32:1201–1207.
22. Dempsey RJ, Sailor KA, Bowen KK, Tureyen K, Vemuganti R. Stroke-induced progenitor cell proliferation in adult spontaneously hypertensive rat brain: effect of exogenous IGF-1 and GDNF. *J Neurochem.* 2003;87:586–597.
23. Wiltrout C, Lang B, Yan Y, Dempsey RJ, Vemuganti R. Repairing brain after stroke: a review on post-ischaemic neurogenesis. *Neurochem Int.* 2007;50:1028–1041.
24. Hajszan T, MacLusky NJ, Leranth C. Short-term treatment with the antidepressant fluoxetine triggers pyramidal dendritic spine synapse formation in rat hippocampus. *J Neurosci.* 2005;21:1299–1303.
25. Malberg JE, Eisch AJ, Neslter EJ, Duman RS. Chronic antidepressant treatment increases neurogenesis in adult rat hippocampus. *J Neurosci.* 2000;20:9104–9110.
26. Malberg JE, Duman RS. Cell proliferation in adult hippocampus is decreased by inescapable stress: reversal by fluoexetine treatment. *Neuropharmacol.* 2003;28:1562–1571.
27. Duman RS, Monteggia LM. A neurotropic model for stress-related mood disorders. *Biol Psychiatry.* 2006;59: 1116–1127.
28. Dranovsky A, Hen R. Hippocampal neurogenesis: regulation by stress and antidepressants. *Biol Pychiatry.* 2006;59: 1136–1143.
29. Maya Vetencourt JF, Sale A, Viegi, et al. The antidepressant fluoxetine restores plasticity in the adult visual cortex. *Science.* 2008;320:385–388.
30. Bachatene L, Bharmauria V, Cattan S, Molotchnikoff S. Fluoxetine and serotonin facilitate attractive-adaptation-induced orientation plasticity in adult cat visual cortex. *Eur J Neurosci.* 2013;38:2065–2077.

31. Kirino T. Delayed neuronal death. *Neuropathology*. 2000; 20(suppl):S95–S97.
32. Walker FR. A critical review of the mechanism of action for the selective serotonin reuptake inhibitors: do these drugs possess anti-inflammatory properties and how relevant is this in the treatment of depression? *Neuropharmacol*. 2013;67:304–317.
33. Nibuya M, Morinobu S, Duman RS. Regulation of BDNF and trkB mRNA in rat brain by chronic electroconvulsive seizure and antidepressant drug treatment. *J Neurosci*. 1995;15(11):7539–7547.
34. Dias BG, Banerjee RS, Vaidya. Differential regulation of brain derived neurotropic factor transcripts by antidepressant treatments in the adult rat. *Neuropharmacol*. 2003;45:553–563.
35. Altar CA, Whitehead RE, Chen R, Wortwein G, Madsen TM. Effects of electroconvulsive seizures and antidepressant drugs on brain-derived neurotrophic factor protein in rat brain. *Biol Psychiatry*. 2003;54:703–709.
36. Chen B, Dowlatshahi D, MacQueen GM, Wang JF, Young LT. Increased hippocampal BDNF immunoreactivity in subjects treated with antidepressant medication. *Biol Psychiatry*. 2001;50:260–265.
37. Dirnagl U, Iadecla C, Moskowitz MA. Pathobiology of ischaemic stroke: an integrated view. *Trends Neurosci*. 1999;22:391–397.
38. Lim CM, Kim SW, Park YJ, Kim C, Yoon SH, Lee JK. Fluoxetine affords robust neuroprotection in the postischemic brain via its anti-inflammatory effect. *Neurosci Res*. 2009;87:1037–1045.
39. Mead GE, Hsieh CF, Lee R, et al. Selective serotonin reuptake inhibitors (SSRIs) for stroke recovery. *Cochrane Database Syst Rev*. 2012;11:CD009286.
40. Shan H, Bian Y, Shu Z, et al. Fluoxetine protects against IL-1β-induced neuronal apoptosis via downregulation of p53. *Neuropharmacology*. 2016;107:68–78.
41. McCann SK, Irvine C, Mead GE, et al. Efficacy of antidepressants in animal models of ischemic stroke: a systematic review and meta-analysis. *Stroke*. 2014;45:3055–3063.
42. Chollet F, Tardy J, Albucher JF, et al. Fluoxetine for motor recovery after acute ischemic stroke (FLAME): a randomized placebo-controlled trial. *Lancet Neurol*. 2011;10:123–130.
43. Mead GE, Hankey GJ, Kutlubaev MA, Lee R, Bailey M, Hackett ML. Selective serotonin reuptake inhibitors (SSRIs) for stroke. *Cochrane Database Syst Rev*. 2011;(Issue 11): CD009286. https://doi.org/10.1002/14651858.CD009286.
44. da Rocha e Silva CE, Alves Brasil MA, Matos do Nascimento E, de Braganca Pereira B, Andre C. Is poststoke depression a major depression? *Cerebrovasc Dis*. 2013;35:385–391.
45. Spalletta G, Ripa A, Caltagirone C. Symptom profile of DSM-IV major and minor depressive disorders in first-ever stroke patients. *Am J Geriatr Psychiatry*. 2005;13:108–115.
46. Guo Y, He Y, Tang B, et al. Effect of using fluoxetine at different time windows on neurological functional prognosis after ischemic stroke. *Neurol Neurosci*. 2016;34: 177–187.
47. Feeney DM. From laboratory to clinic: noradrenergic enhancement of physical therapy for stroke or trauma patients. *Adv Neurol*. 1997;73:383–394.
48. Hovda DA, Sutton RL, Feeney DM. Recovery of tactile placing after visual cortex ablation in cat: a behavioral and metabolic study of diaschisis. *Exp Neurol*. 1987;97: 391–402.
49. Stroemer RP, Kent TA, Hulsebosch CE. Enhanced neocortical neural sprouting, synaptogenesis, and behavioral recovery with D-Apmphetamine therapy after neocortical infarction In rats. *Stroke*. 1998;29:2381–2395.
50. Dietrich WD, Alonso O, Busto R, Watson BD, Loor Y, Ginsberg MD. Influence of amphetamine treatment on somatosensory function of the normal and infarcted rat brain. *Stroke*. 1990;21(suppl 11):III147–I150.
51. Goldstein LB. Pharmacology of recovery after stroke. *Stroke*. 1990;21(suppl 11):III139–I142.
52. Tully K, Li Y, Tsvetkov E, Bolshakov VY. Norepinephrine enables the induction of associative long-term potentiation at thalamo-amygdala synapses. *Proc Natl Acad Sci USA*. 2007;104:14146–14150.
53. Kojic L, Gu Q, Douglas RM, Cynader MS. Serotonin facilitates synaptic plasticity in kitten visual cortex. An in vitro study. *Brain Res Dev Brain Res*. 1997;101:299–304.
54. Suzuki T, Miura M, Nishimura K, Aosaki T. Dopamine-dependent synaptic plasticity in the striatal cholinergic interneurons. *J Neurosci*. 2001;21:6492–6501.
55. Leung LS, Shen B, Rajakumar N, Ma J. Cholinergic activity enhances hippocampal long-term potentiation in CA1 during walking in rats. *J Neurosci*. 2003;23:9297–9304.
56. Dunwiddie TV, Roberson NL, Worth T. Modulation of long term potentiation. Effects of adrenergic and neuroleptic drugs. *Pharmacol Biochem Behav*. 1982;17:1257–1264.
57. Butefisch CM, Davis BC, Wise SP, et al. Mechanism of use-dependent plasticity in the human cortex. *Proc Natl Acad Sci USA*. 2000;97:3661–3665.
58. Tran DA, Pajaro-Blazquez M, Daneault JF, et al. Combining dopaminergic facilitation with robot-assisted upper limb therapy in stroke survivors: a focused review. *Am J Phys Med Rehabil*. 2016;95:459–474.
59. Colzato LS, van Wouwe NC, Hommel B. Feature binding and affect: emotional modulation of visuomotor integration. *Neuropsychologia*. 2007;45:440–466.
60. Colzato LS, van Wouwe NC, Hommel B. Spontaneous eyeblink rate predicts the strength of visuomotor binding. *Neuropsychologia*. 2007;45:2387–2392.
61. Molina-Luna K, Pekanovic A, Rohrich S, et al. Dopamine in motor cortex is necessary for skill learning and synaptic plasticity. *PLoS One*. 2009;4:e7082.
62. Hosp JA, Pekanovic A, Rioult-Pedotti MS, Luft AR. Dopaminergic projections from midbrain to primary motor cortex mediates motor skill learning. *J Neurosci*. 2011; 31:2481–2487.
63. Schuster C, Maunz G, Lutz K, Kischka U, Sturzenegger R, Ettlin T. Dextroampehtamine improves upper extremity outcome during rehabilitation after stroke: a pilot randomized controlled trial. *Neurorehabil Beural Repair*. 2011;25:749–755.

64. Crisostomo EA, Duncan PW, Propst M, Dawson DV, Davis JN. Evidence that amphetamine with physical therapy promotes recovery of motor function in stroke patients. *Ann Neurol.* 1988;23:94–97.

65. Walker-Batson D, Smith P, Curtis S, Unwin H, Greenlee R. Amphetamine paired with physical therapy accelerates motor recovery after stroke: further evidence. *Stroke.* 1995;26:2254–2259.

66. Grade C, Redford B, Chrostowski J, Toussaint L, Blackwell B. Methylphenidate in early poststroke recovery: a double-blind, placebo-controlled study. *Arch Phys Med Rehabil.* 1998;79:1047–1050.

67. Tardy J, Pariente J, Leger A, et al. Methylphenidate modulates cerebral post-stroke reorganization. *Neuroimage.* 2006;33:913–922.

68. Sonde L, Nordstrom M, Nilsson CG, Nilsson CG, Lokk J, Viitanen M. A double-blind placebo-controlled study of the effects of amphetamine and physiotherapy after stroke. *Cerebrovasc Dis.* 2001;12:253–257.

69. Treig T, Werner C, Sachse M, Hesse S. No benefit from D-amphetamine when added to physiotherapy after stroke: a randomized, placebo-controlled study. *Clin Rehabil.* 2003;17:590–599.

70. Gladstone DJ, Danells CJ, Armesto A, et al. Physiotherapy coupled with dextroamphetamine for rehabilitation after hemiparetic stroke: a randomized, double-blind, placebo-controlled trial. *Stroke.* 2006;37:179–185.

71. Martinsson L, Wahlgren NG. Safety of dexamphetamine in acute ischemic stroke: a randomized, double-blind, controlled dose-escalation trial. *Stroke.* 2003;34:475–481.

72. Martinsson L, Hardemark HG, Eksborg S. Amphetamines for improving recovery after stroke. *Cochrane Database Syst Rev.* 2007;1:CD002090.

73. Lieprt J. Update on pharmacotherapy for stroke and traumatic brain injury in recovery during rehabilitation. *Curr Opin Neurol.* 2016;29:700–705.

74. Zittel S, Weiller C, Liepert J. Reboxetine improves motor function in chronic stroke. A pilot study. *J Neurol.* 2007;254:197–201.

75. Wang LE, Fink GR, Diekhoff S, Rehme AK, Eickhoff SB, Grefkes C. Noradrenergic enhancement improves motor network connectivity in stroke patients. *Ann Neurol.* 2011;69:375–388.

76. Masihuzzaman AM, Uddin MJ, Majumder S, Barman KK, Ullah MA. Effect of low dose levodopa on motor outcomes of different types of stroke. *Mymensingh Med J.* 2011;20:689–693.

77. Scheidtmann K, Fries W, Muller F, Koenig E. Effect of levodopa in combination with physiotherapy on functional motor recovery after stroke: a prospective, randomised, double-blind study. *Lancet.* 2001;358:787–790.

78. Lokk J, Salman Roghani R, Delbari A. Effect of methylphenidate and/or levodopa coupled with physiotherapy on functional and motor recovery after stroke – a randomized, double-blind, placebo-controlled trial. *Acta Neurol Scand.* 2011;123:255–273.

79. Sonde L, Lokk J. Effects of amphetamine and/or l-dopa on physiotherapy after stroke – a blinded randomized study. *Acta Neurol Scand.* 2007;115:55–59.

80. Floel A, Hummel F, Breitenstein C, Knecht S, Cohen LG. Dopaminergic effects on encoding of a motor memory in stroke. *Neurology.* 2005;65:472–474.

81. Acler M, Fiaschi A, Manganotti P. Long-term levodopa administration in chronic stroke patients. A clinical and neurophysiologic single-blind, placebo controlled, cross-over pilot study. *Restor Neurol Neurosci.* 2009;27:277–283.

82. Rosser N, Heuschmann P, Wersching H, Breitenstein C, Knetch S, Floel A. Levodopa improves procedural motor learning in chronic stroke patients. *Arch Phys Med Rehabil.* 2008;89:1633–1641.

83. Restemeyer C, Weiller C, Liepert J. No effect of a levodopa single dose on motor performance and motor excitability in chronic stroke. A double-blind placebo controlled cross-over pilot study. *Resotr Neurol Neurosci.* 2007;25:143–150.

84. Cramer SC, Dobkin BH, Noser EA, Rodriguez RW, Enney LA. Randomized, placebo-controlled, double-blind study of ropinirol in chronic stroke. *Stroke.* 2009;40:3034–3038.

85. Pearson-Fuhrhop KM, Minton B, Acevedo D, Shahbaba B, Cramer SC. Genetic variation in the human brain dopamine system influences motor learning and its modulation by L-Dopa. *PLoS One.* 2013;8:e61197.

86. Pearson-Fuhrhop KM, Dunn EC, Mortero S, et al. Dopamine genetic risk score predicts depressive symptoms in health adults and adults with depression. *PLoS One.* 2014;9:e93772.

87. Pearson-Fuhrhop KM, Cramer SC. Pharmacogenetics of neural injury recovery. *Pharmacogenomics.* 2013;14:1635–1643.

88. Pedersen PM, Jorgensen HS, Nakayama H, Raaschou HO, Olsen TS. Aphasia in acute stroke: incidence, determinant, and recovery. *Ann Neurol.* 1995;38:659–666.

89. Laska AC, Hellblom A, Murray V, Kahan T, Von Arbin M. Aphasia in acute stroke and relation to outcome. *J Int Med.* 2001;249:413–422.

90. Engelter ST, Gostynski M, Papa S, et al. Epidemiology of aphasia attributable to first ischemic stroke: incidence, severity, fluency, etiology, and thrombolysis. *Stroke.* 2006;37:1379–1384.

91. Bersano A, Burgio F, Gattinoni M, Candelisem L, PROSIT Study Group. Aphasia burden to hospitalized acute stroke patients: need for an early rehabilitation programme. *Int J Stroke.* 2009;4:443–447.

92. Tsouli S, Kyritsis AP, Tsagalis G, Virvidaki E, Vemmos KN. Significance of aphasia after first-ever acute stroke: impact on early and late outcomes. *Neuroepidemiol.* 2009;33:96–102.

93. Dickey L, Kagan A, Lindsay MP, Fang J, Rowland A, Black S. Incidence and profile of inpatient stroke-induced aphasia in Ontario, Canada. *Arch Phys Med Rehabil.* 2010;91:196–202.

94. Law J, Rush R, Pringle AM, et al. The incidence of cases of aphasia following first stroke referred to speech and language therapy services in Scotland. *Aphasiology*. 2009;23:1266−1275.

95. Lazar RM, Antoniello D. Variability in recovery from aphasia. *Curr Neurol Neurosci Rep*. 2008;8:497−502.

96. Lazar RM, Minzer B, Antoniello D, Festa JR, Krakauer JW, Marshall RS. Improvement in aphasia score after stroke is will predicted by initial severity. *Stroke*. 2010;41:1185−1488

97. Cappa SF, Benke T, Clarke S, Rossi B, Stemmer B, van Heugten CM. European Federation of neurological societies. EFNS guidelines on cognitive rehabilitation: report of an EFNS task force. *Eur J Neurol*. 2003;10:11−23.

98. Cicerone KD, Langenbahn DM, Braden C, et al. Evidence-based cognitive rehabilitation: updated review of the literature form 2003−2008. *Arch Phys Med Rehabil*. 2011;92:519−530.

99. Kelly H, Brady MC. Enderby. Speech and language therapy for aphasia following stroke. *Cochrane Database Syst Rev*. 2010;12(5):CD000425.

100. Olesen J, Baker MG, Freund T, et al. Consensus documents on European brain research. *J Neurol Neurosurg Psychiatry*. 2006;77(suppl I):i1−49.

101. Brady MC, Kelly H, Godwin J, Enderby P, Campbell P. Speech and language therapy for aphasia following stroke. *Cochrane Database Rev*. 2016;6:CD000425.

102. Walker-Batson D, Curtis S, Natarajan R, et al. Double-blind, placebo-controlled-controlled study of the use of amphetamine in the treatment of aphasia. *Stroke*. 2001;32:2093−2098.

103. Hilis AE. Pharmacological, surgical, and neurovascular interventions to augment acute aphasia recovery. *Am J Phys Med Rehabil*. 2007;86:426−434.

104. Small SL, Llano DA. Biological approaches to aphasia treatment. *Curr Neurol Neurosci Rep*. 2009;9:443−450.

105. Albert ML, Bachman D, Morgan A, Helm-Eastbrook N. Pharmacotherapy of aphasia. *Neurol*. 1988;38:877−879.

106. Bertheir ML. Poststroke aphasia: epidemiology, pathophysiology and treatment. *Drugs Aging*. 2005;22:163−182.

107. Raymer AM. Treatment of adynamia in aphasia. *Bioscience*. 2003;8:s845−s851.

108. Raymer A, Bandy D, Adair JC. Effects of bromocriptine in a patient with crossed nonfluent aphasia: a case report. *Arch Phys Med Rehabil*. 2001;82:1390144.

109. Gupta SR, Mlcoch AG. Bromocriptine treatment of non-fluent aphasia. *Arch Phys Med Rehabil*. 1992;73:373−376.

110. Reed DA, Johnson NA, Thompson C, Weinraub S, Mesulam MM. A clinical trial of bromocriptine for treatment of primary progressive aphasia. *Ann Neurol*. 2004;56:750.

111. Gold M, VanDam D, Silliman ER. An open-label trial of bromocriptine in nonfluent aphasia: a qualitative analysis of word storage and retrieval. *Brain Lang*. 2000;74:141−156.

112. Gupta SR, Mlcoch AG, Scolaro C, Moritz T. Bromocriptine treatment of nonfluent aphasia. *Neurology*. 1995;45:2170−2173.

113. Ozeren A, Sarica Y, Mavi H, Demirkiran M. Bromocriptine is ineffective in the treatment of chronic nonfluent aphasia. *Acta Neurol Belg*. 1995;95:235−238.

114. Sabe L, Leiguarda R, Starkstein SE. An open-label trial of bromocriptine in nonfluent aphasia. *Neurology*. 1992;42:1637−1638.

115. Ashtary F, Janghorbani M, Chitsaz A, Reisi M, Bahrami A. A randomized, double-blind trial of bromocriptine efficacy in nonfluent aphasia after stroke. *Neurology*. 2006;66:914−916.

116. Seniow J, Litwin M, Litwin T, Lesniak M, Czionkowska A. New approach to the rehabilitation of post-stroke focal cognitive syndrome: effect of levodopa combined with speech and language therapy on functional recovery from aphasia. *J Neurol Neurosci*. 2009;283:214−218.

117. Leeman B, Laganaro M, Chetelat-Mabillard D, Schnider A. Crossover trial of subacute computerized aphasia therapy for anomia with the addition of either levodopa or placebo. *Neurorehabil Neural Repair*. 2011;25:43−47.

118. Breitenstein C, Korsukewitz C, Baumqartner A, et al. L-dopa does not add to the success of high-intensity language training in aphasia. *Restor Neurol Neurosci*. 2015;33:115−120.

119. Arciniegas DB, Frey KL, Anderson CA, Brousseau KM, Harris SN. Amantadine for neurobehavioral deficits following delayed post-hypoxic encephalopathy. *Brain Inj*. 2004;18:1309−1318.

120. Barrett M, Eslinger PJ. Amantadine for adynamic speech: possible benefit for aphasia. *Am J Phys Med Rehabil*. 2007;86:605−612.

121. McNeil MR, Doyle PJ, Spencer KA, Goda AJ, Flores D, Small SL. A double-blind, placebo-controlled study of pharmacological and behavioural treatment of lexical-semantic deficits in aphasia. *Aphasiology*. 1997;11:385−400.

122. Whiting E, Chenery HJ, Chalk J, Darnell R, Copland DA. The explicit learning of new names for known objects is improved by dexamphetamine. *Brain Lang*. 2008;104:254−261.

123. Martinsson L, Eksborg S. Drugs for stroke recovery: the example of amphetamines. *Drugs Aging*. 2004;21:67−79.

124. Floel A, Cohen LG. Recovery of function in humans: cortical stimulation and pharmacological treatment after stroke. *Neurobiol Dis*. 2010;37:243−251.

125. Keser Z, Dehgan MW, Shadravan S, Yozbatiran N, Maher LM, Franscisco GE. Combined dextroamphetamine and transcranial direct current stimulation in poststroke aphasia. *Am J Phys Med Rehabil*. June 2, 2017. https://doi.org/10.1097/PHM.0000000000000780 [Epub ahead of print].

126. Vernon MW, Sorkin EM. Piracetam. An overview of its pharmacological properties and a review of its therapeutic use in senile cognitive disorders. *Drugs Aging*. 1991;1:17−35.

127. Wheble PC, Sena ES, Macleod MR. A systematic review and meta-analysis of the efficacy of piracetm and piracetam-like compounds in experimental stroke. *Cerebrovasc Dis*. 2008;25:5−11.

128. Ricci S, Celani MG, Cantisani TA, Righetti E. Piracetam for acute stroke. *Cochrane Database Syst Rev.* 2012;9: CD000419.

129. Greener J, Enderby P, Whurr R. Pharmacological treatment for aphasia following stroke. *Cochrane Database Rev.* 2001;4:CD000424.

130. Gungor J, Terzi M, Onar MK. Does long term use of piracetam improve speech disturbance due to ischemic cerebrovascular diseases? *Bain Lang.* 2011; 117:23—27.

131. Roman GC, Wilkinson DG, Doody RS, Black SE, Salloway SP, Schindler RJ. Donepezil in vascular dementia: combined analysis of two large-scale clinical trials. *Dement Geriatr Cogn Disord.* 2005;20:338—344.

132. Ferris S, Ihl R, Robert P, et al. Treatment effects of memantine on language in moderate to severe Lasheimer's disease patients. *Alzheimers Dement.* 2009;5:369—374.

133. Wilkinson D, Roman G, Salloway S, et al. The long-term efficacy and tolerability of donepezil in patients with vascular dementia. *Int J Geriatr Psychiatry.* 2010;25: 305—313.

134. Kertesz A, Morlog D, Light M, et al. Galantamine in frontotemporal dementia and primary progressive aphasia. *Dement Geriatr Cogn Disord.* 2008;25: 178—185.

135. FitzGerald DB, Crucian GP, Miekle JB, et al. Effects of donepezil on verbal memory after semantic processing in healthy older adults. *Cogn Behav Neurol.* 2008;21: 57—64.

136. Yesavage JA, Mumenthaler MS, Taylor JL, et al. Donepezil and flight simulator performance: effects on retention of complex skills. *Neurology.* 2002;59: 123—125.

137. Selden NR, Gitelman DR, Salamon-Murayama N, Parrish TB, Mesulam MM. Trajectories of cholinergic pathways within the cerebral hemispheres of the human brain. *Brain.* 1998;121:2249—2257.

138. Simic G, Mrzljak L, Fucic A, Winblad B, Lovric H, Kostovic I. Nucleus subputaminalis (Ayala): the still disregarded magnocellular component of the basal forebrain may be human specific and connected with the cortical speech area. *Neuroscience.* 1999;89: 73—89.

139. Sarter M, Hasselmo ME, Bruno JP, Givens B. Unraveling the attentional functions of cortical cholinergic inputs: interactions between signal-driven and cognitive modulation of signal detection. *Brain Res Rev.* 2005;48: 98—111.

140. Aarsland D, Larsen JP, Reinvang I, Aasland AM. Effects of cholinergic blockade on language in healthy young women. Implications for the cholinergic hypothesis in dementia of the Alzheimer type. *Brain.* 1994;117: 1377—1384.

141. Tanaka Y, Muyazak M, Albert ML. Effects of increased cholinergic activity on naming in aphasia. *Lancet.* 1997; 350:116—117.

142. Yoon SY, Kim JK, An YS, Kim YW. Effect of donepezil on Wernicke aphasia after bilateral middle cerebral artery infarction; Subtraction analysis of brain F-18 fluorodeoxyglucose positron emission tomography images. *Clin Neuropharmacol.* 2015;38:147—150.

143. Bertheir ML, De Torres I, Paredes-Pacheco J, et al. Cholinergic potentiation and audiovisual repetition-imitation therapy improve speech production and communication deficits in a person with crossed aphasia by indwelling structural plasticity in white matter tracts. *Front Hum Neurosci.* 2017;11:304.

144. Berthier ML, Hinojosa J, Martin MC, Fernandez I. Open-label study of donepezil in chronic poststroke aphasia. *Neurology.* 2003;60:1218—1219.

145. Paschek GV, Bachman DL. Cognitive, linguistic, and motor speech of donepezil hydrochloride in a patient with stroke-related aphasia and apraxia of speech. *Brain Lang.* 2003;87:179—180.

146. Woodhead ZV, Crinion J, Teki S, Penny W, Price CJ, Leff AP. Auditory training changes temporal lobe connectivity in "Wernicke's aphasia": a randomized trial. *J Neurol Neurosurg Psychiatry.* 2017. https://doi.org/10.1136/jnnp-2016-314621 [Epub ahead of print].

147. Netheir ML, Green C, Higueras C, Fernandez I, Hinojosa J, Martic MC. A randomized, placebo-controlled study of donepezil in poststroke aphasia. *Neurology.* 2006;67:1687—1689.

148. Hong JM, Shin DH, Lim TS, Huh K. Galantamine administration in chronic post-stroke aphasia. *J Neurol Neurosurg Psychiatry.* 2012;83:675—680.

149. Berthier ML, Pilvermuller DG, Casares NG, Gutierrez A. Drug therapy of post-stroke aphasia: a review of current evidence. *Neuropsychol Rev.* 2011;21:302—317.

150. Parsons CG, Stöffler A, Danysz W. Memantine: a NMDA receptor antagonist that improves memory by restoration of homeostasis in the glutamatergic system — too little activation is bad, too much is even worse. *Neuropharmacology.* 2007;53:699—723.

151. Trotman M, Vermehren P, Gibson CL, Fern R. The dichotomy of memantine treatment for ischemic stroke: dose-dependent protective and detrimental effects. *J Cereb Blood Flow Metab.* 2015;35:230—239.

152. López-Valdés H, Clarkson AN, Ao Y, et al. Memantine enhances recovery from stroke. *Stroke.* 2014;45:2093—2100.

153. Nakamura Y, Kitamura S, Homma A, Shiosakai K, Matsui D. Efficacy and safety of memantine in patients with moderate-to-severe Alzheimer's disease: results of a pooled analysis of two randomized, double-blind, placebo-controlled trials in Japan. *Expert Opin Pharmacother.* 2014;15:913—925.

154. Barbancho MA, Berthier L, Navas-Sánchez P, et al. Bilateral brain reorganization with memantine and constraint-induced aphasia therapy in chronic poststroke aphasia: an ERP study. *Brain Lang.* 2015:145—146.

155. Berthier ML, Green C, Lara JP, et al. Memantine and constraint-induced aphasia therapy in chronic poststroke aphasia. *Ann Neurol.* 2009;65:577—585.

156. Yeo SH, Lim ZI, Mao J, Yau WP. Effects of central nervous system drugs on recovery after stroke: a systematic review and meta-analyses of randomized controlled trials. *Clin Drug Investig.* July 29, 2017. https://doi.org/10.1007/s40261-017-0558-4 [Epub ahead of print].
157. Jorge RE, Acion L, Moser D, Adams HO, Robinson RG. Escitalopram and enhancement of cognitive recovery following stroke. *Arch Gen Psychiatry.* 2010;67:187−196.
158. Chang WH, Park YH, Ohn SH, Park CH, Lee PK, Kim YH. Neural correlates of donepezil-induced cognitive improvement in patients with right hemisphere stroke: a pilot study. *Neuropsychol Rehabil.* 2011;21:502−514.

FURTHER READING

1. Saxena SK, Ng TP, Koh G, Fong NP. Is improvement in impaired cognition and depressive symptoms in post-stroke patients associated with recovery in activities of daily living? *Acta Neurol Scand.* 2007;115:339−346.
2. Whyte EM, Lenze EJ, Butters M, et al. An open-label pilot study of acetylcholinesterase inhibitors to promote functional recovery in elderly cognitively impaired stroke patients. *Cerebrovasc Dis.* 2008;26(3):317−321.

CHAPTER 14

Neuromuscular Electrical Stimulation and Stroke Recovery

MICHAEL J. FU, PHD • JAYME S. KNUTSON, PHD

INTRODUCTION

Motor impairment is common after cerebral vascular injury and can negatively affect an individual's ability to walk or use their hands in everyday life. More than 50% of individuals survive 5 years beyond their stroke,[1] but over 75% of survivors are challenged by upper or lower extremity disability due to motor impairment.[2] Although around 15% of individuals experience nearly complete spontaneous recovery of lost motor abilities within 6 months of cortical injury,[3] the majority of survivors require rehabilitation interventions or orthotic devices to regain lost volitional movement. There is increasing evidence that neuromuscular electrical stimulation (NMES) may benefit survivors of stroke by enhancing the recovery of lost volitional movement (referred to as a therapeutic effect) or replacing lost volitional movement (referred to as a neuroprosthetic effect).

This chapter first presents the poststroke motor impairments that can be addressed by NMES rehabilitation therapy or neuroprostheses. Next, the fundamentals of NMES and relevant NMES device configurations are introduced. Then, clinical applications of NMES for stroke rehabilitation and their efficacy will be discussed. Finally, a strengths, weaknesses, opportunities, and threats (SWOT) analysis of NMES for stroke rehabilitation will be presented. The focus of this chapter is upon NMES interventions applied to intact lower motor neurons to produce functional contractions of paralyzed or paretic muscles. A separate chapter in this book discusses brain stimulation for stroke rehabilitation (Chapter 18).

MOTOR DYSFUNCTION AFTER STROKE

Cerebrovascular accidents leave 80% of survivors with arm and/or hand motor impairment and 75% with lower limb impairment.[2] The majority of these impairments include paresis, loss of fractionated movements, abnormal tone, and somatosensory changes. These impairments are typically uniform across the length of the upper limb and present on the side of the body contralateral to the injured cortical hemisphere (though ipsilateral presentations can occur in brainstem lesions).[4]

Paresis presents clinically as muscle weakness, reduced muscle activation speed, and inability to generate functionally useful movement of the affected limb.[4] This is caused by reduced volitional ability to activate motor units. For the upper limb, paresis of muscles for reaching and hand opening is the most common impairment and the strongest contributor to the loss of ability to use the hand after stroke.[5] Paresis of the shoulder can also lead to shoulder subluxation and pain. For the lower extremities, the most common impairment is the inability to fully dorsiflex the ankle. This causes the foot to drag during the swing phase of gait, which impairs walking ability.

Fractionated movement is the ability to independently move different joints of the limb and coordinate them to perform tasks. However, individuals with stroke may lose this ability and instead exhibit synergy patterns, in which multiple joints flex or extend together—even if the individual intended to move only one of the joints.[6] A typical presentation of this is flexion of the fingers and elbow during shoulder abduction, which makes reaching forward and opening the hand difficult.

Muscle tone is the resistance of muscle fibers to passive stretch, which is often decreased in the early stages after stroke, but typically increases to abnormal levels afterward.[7] Clinically, hypertonia or spasticity presents as increased velocity-dependent resistance to passive stretch, which can lead to range of movement loss and painful joint contractures.

Somatosensory changes that can be caused by stroke are multimodal and can affect perception of pain,

Stroke Rehabilitation. https://doi.org/10.1016/B978-0-323-55381-0.00014-7

temperature, vibration, and proprioception.[8] Hypersensitivity to pain or reduced proprioception can lead to deficits in function and recovery.

Reduction of limb impairment is a primary focus of rehabilitation medicine because limb impairment (the ability to move or position joints) is highly correlated to limb function (the ability to use the limb to walk or perform actions useful in daily life).[9–11] Hemiplegia, or paresis of the limbs on one side of the body, is highly prevalent after stroke, which causes the individual to rely more on the unaffected limb.[12] Eventually, bimanual tasks become extremely challenging, the affected limb becomes unused, and can suffer pain and contractures.

PURPOSES OF NMES IN STROKE MOTOR REHABILITATION

Given these common motor impairments, NMES-based interventions that aim to improve motor function and quality of life will ideally be able to contract weak muscles along the affected limb to address the problem of paresis, facilitate individual joint control and coordination to restore fractionated movement, and reduce abnormal synergy patterns and hypertonia. Also, because there will typically be residual volitional movement and ability, another ideal for NMES interventions is to be able to work in "closed loop" fashion by providing movement assistance that compensates for the difference between the individual's movement intent and residual movement ability.

Furthermore, NMES interventions may achieve these purposes while serving either as a motor training tool or as a neuroprosthesis. As a training tool, NMES interventions can enhance the affected limb's ability to participate in novel, repetitive, goal-oriented movement practice. This type of activity has been shown to result in motor relearning, which is demonstrated by changes in brain activity that are associated with reacquisition of lost motor skills.[13] If the skills are maintained after use of NMES is discontinued, then a therapeutic effect has been achieved. In other words, the desired therapeutic effect is to apply the NMES intervention for a limited period of time to facilitate a permanent recovery of the individual's volitional movement.

Alternatively, for individuals who do not benefit from motor training or do not regain sufficient use of an affected limb, NMES may serve as a long-term assistive neuroprosthesis. In this role, the function provided by NMES is not maintained once the stimulation is turned off, so NMES will need to be applied whenever the individual wants to perform movements or functions beyond their volitional ability. For individuals who have adapted to hemiplegia by using one arm for daily life, neuroprosthetic NMES interventions are most useful if they can enable them to perform bimanual tasks or functions that typically require a caregiver. In the lower extremities, weakened ankle dorsiflexion makes walking slow and unsafe, so an effective neuroprosthesis will increase stability and gait speed while reducing the risk of falls. Also, 40% of individuals cannot walk or require caregiver assistance for walking, so the ideal NMES neuroprosthetic effect for them would be independent walking.

NMES FUNDAMENTALS

Neuromuscular electrical stimulation activates the lower motor neurons and not the muscle fibers directly. Therefore, effective NMES systems can produce muscle contractions using a relatively small amount of electrical charge that does not cause discomfort. Stimulation waveforms typically consist of monophasic or biphasic current pulses, and muscle contraction strength is determined by pulse frequency, amplitude, and duration. Muscle contractions are produced through the application of electrical current to activate peripheral motor nerves that innervate a targeted muscle. A muscle contracts when the applied electrical current depolarizes the axonal membranes and thereby generates action potentials in the muscle's lower motor axons.[14] As long as the lower motor neurons are intact and the neurotransmitter release mechanisms and muscle tissue are healthy, which is usually the case after stroke, NMES can be used to produce muscle contractions. However, this usually excludes individuals with lower motor neuron damage (i.e., peripheral nerve injuries) and muscular dystrophies.

NMES Device Components

NMES devices typically consist of a stimulation controller unit that is connected to multiple electrodes, which are positioned near targeted muscles or nerves. The number of electrode channels refers to the number of independent stimulation waveforms that the stimulator can generate, each usually applied to different muscles or muscle groups. The stimulation control unit is usually an enclosure that houses a battery or wired power supply, a pulse generator (which outputs the waveforms), and manual controls or computer programs to set stimulation waveform pulse parameters such as frequency, amplitude, and duration. Both the stimulation controller and electrodes can be external or implanted.

External NMES

External (transcutaneous) electrodes are adhered to the skin surface and connected with an external stimulator control unit. These external NMES systems can be applied and removed as needed, but may not be able to stimulate nerves that are deeper and further from the skin surface without pain. Also, the large surface area of external NMES electrodes (relative to the nerves being stimulated) makes it difficult to selectively and independently activate multiple muscles that are in close proximity to one another.

Implanted NMES

Implanted NMES stimulators and/or electrodes may require surgery to set up, and have risks associated with the necessary procedures, but have several advantages over external NMES. They do not require donning or doffing of electrodes, which is inconvenient for frequent longterm use (i.e., neuroprosthetic applications) and for interventions that require many electrodes, or for individuals who do not have sufficient hand function to apply adhesive external electrodes. Also, implanted NMES is better able to elicit certain muscle functions activated by nerves that are difficult to selectively stimulate from the skin surface, such as the shoulder abduction and hip flexion.

Implanted electrodes can be placed intramuscularly, epimsially, or around peripheral nerves (Fig. 14.1). Epimysial and nerve electrodes need to be sutured into place, so they require surgical placement and are typically connected to implanted stimulator units. Intramuscular electrodes may be implanted by a minimally invasive surgical procedure or may be inserted through the skin into the muscle percutaneously and have wires that exit the skin to connect to an external stimulator. Percutaneous insertion allows intramuscular electrodes to be inserted and removed without surgery for temporary NMES applications.

Mechanisms of Action for NMES-Mediated Motor Relearning After Stroke

Mechanisms of action that facilitate motor relearning using NMES are not yet clear. The most likely factors include both peripheral effects that reverse muscle atrophy and/or central nervous system changes. It has been demonstrated that NMES increases the contractile force and fatigue resistance of targeted muscles,[15,16] increases muscle mass,[17] and converts fast-twitch fast-fatiguing type II muscle fibers to slow-twitch fatigue-resistant

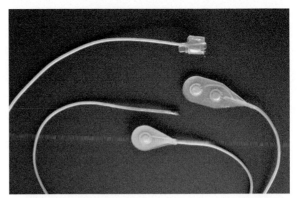

FIG. 14.1 Examples of implanted NMES electrodes include *(from top to bottom)* epimysial, intramuscular, epimysial EMG recording, and spiral nerve cuff. (From Cleveland FES Center; with permission.)

type I muscle fibers.[16] There is also evidence that movement intent synchronized with NMES and volitional effort can strengthen pre- and postsynaptic connections in anterior horn cells.[18] Specifically, transcranial magnetic stimulation studies showed that cortical excitability was increased when NMES was paired with volitional muscle contraction compared to NMES alone.[19] It is also hypothesized that the afferent proprioceptive and sensory feedback produced by NMES can cause longterm potentiation in the sensorimotor cortex.[20–23] Interventions that used volitional residual electromyographic (EMG) activity to trigger NMES to the same muscle demonstrated increased cortical metabolic activity (as seen in PET[24] and MRI[25]) and cortical perfusion compared to cyclic NMES that repeatedly stimulates without volitional effort (i.e., not EMG-triggered).

UPPER EXTREMITY NMES

Cyclic Stimulation

The most widely available NMES modality in commercial devices is repetitive cyclic stimulation of muscles to produce movement at a joint affected by paresis, such as wrist, elbow, and finger extension. Cyclic NMES devices like the Chattanooga Revolution Wireless Electrotherapy System (Fig. 14.2) and Empi 300PV (DJO Global Corp., Carlsbad, CA) stimulate on and off for a programmable duration. The timing of the on/off cycle is programmed by a therapist. The advantages of cyclic stimulation are that it (like all NMES modalities) can increase muscle strength and resistance to fatigue via peripheral mechanisms without requiring the patient to retain any residual volitional movement.[15,16] Its disadvantages are that it is not likely to promote central nervous system changes, possibly

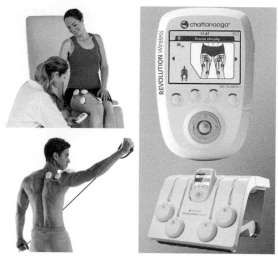

FIG. 14.2 DJO Global Corp. Chattanooga Revolution Wireless NMES stimulator uses wireless stimulators with integrated pulse generator and battery *(left)* that communicate wirelessly to a stimulation controller and display *(upper right)*. Components are charged on a docking station *(lower right)*. (From DJO Global Corp.; with permission.)

because it does not require individuals to exert volitional effort in synchrony with the stimulation. Also, cyclic stimulation is difficult to incorporate into task-specific therapy because the timing and intensity of the stimulation onset are preset and not modulated in real time as the task requires. This leads to passive movement where the individual does not actively attempt to move the paretic muscles being stimulated, which may not benefit motor relearning as much as active participation.[19]

EMG-, Switch-, and Sensor-Triggered Stimulation

In an effort to link or synchronize the patients' intentions to move with the movement elicited by stimulation, NMES triggered by EMG signals from the paretic limb,[20,21] external mechanical switches,[26,27] and inertial sensors (accelerometers and gyroscopes[28]) were developed. Devices such as Neuromove (Zynex Medical Corp., Lone Tree, CO) have EMG electrodes that can measure volitional activation of the targeted paretic muscle and only provides NMES when the patient's volitional EMG signal exceeds a programmable threshold. The limitation of EMG-triggered NMES is that it cannot be used very easily during task practice because the patient only controls the onset, but not the duration or intensity, of the stimulation. Additionally, EMG-triggered NMES relies upon volitional activation of the paretic

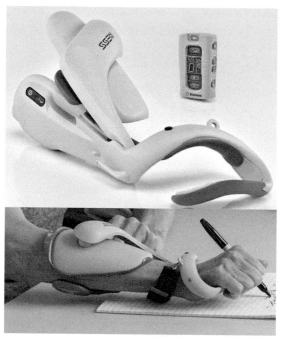

FIG. 14.3 Bioness Corp. H200 external button-triggered NMES device can stimulate wrist and finger extension and flexion. The H200 device has integrated batteries, pulse generator, and external skin electrodes. It is worn over the forearm and wrist and positioned so the electrodes are over finger and wrist extensors and flexors. Stimulation onset and intensity are controlled by buttons on a wireless remote. (From Bioness Corp.; with permission.)

limb, which can trigger spasticity or hypertonia that reduces the range of motion that NMES can provide.[29–32] Switch-triggered NMES devices, like the H200 (Bioness Corp., Valencia, CA), have buttons that are to be pressed by the therapist or by the patient's unaffected hand to stimulate finger extensors (Fig. 14.3). Sensor-triggered devices use body-worn sensors, such as accelerometers, to trigger stimulation so that it occurs in synchrony with desired movement. For example, a device for improving reaching triggers triceps stimulation when the patient succeeds in reaching some defined minimum distance (threshold) along a track.[33] The advantage of switch- and sensor-triggered modalities is that they allow NMES to be used during task practice because the user or therapist controls the timing of stimulation. Disadvantages are that both switch and EMG-triggered NMES use preset stimulation intensities that are difficult to integrate with upper limb movements and practice of complex skill-requiring activities of daily living. These limitations may have contributed to the findings that EMG-triggered NMES and cyclic NMES were no better at improving upper extremity function than controls receiving sub-motor threshold sensory stimulation.[34–36] Others compared conventional occupational therapy to switch-triggered NMES-assisted occupational therapy for 15 h over 2 weeks in 11 severely impaired individuals more than 12 months after stroke and reported improved gains in motor impairment (Fugl–Meyer Motor Assessment), but not hand function (Arm Motor Abilities Test[37]). For NMES to assist with complex tasks, knowledge of the individual's intent and precise control of NMES intensity to correct changes or errors is needed during movement execution.

Contralaterally Controlled Stimulation

Contralaterally controlled NMES devices are applied to individuals with hemiplegia to give individuals a means of proportionally controlling the intensity of stimulation to the paretic limb so that the NMES can assist with task practice. There are currently no commercial systems that do this, but research devices exist that synchronize NMES of the affected hand with movements or EMG signals from the unaffected upper extremity. The earliest NMES systems for upper extremities used a shoulder movement sensor on the unaffected side to proportionally control stimulation to finger extensor muscles on the forearm.[38,39] This allowed individuals with paresis to practice using their hands to practice everyday tasks. More recently, the Cleveland FES Center developed contralaterally controlled functional electrical stimulation (CCFES) that applies NMES to open the paretic finger extensors in synchrony with and proportional to volitional opening of the unaffected hand, as sensed by bend sensors in a glove worn on the unaffected hand (Fig. 14.4).[40,41] With CCFES, patients are instructed to try to open both hands at the same time; in this way, CCFES links the patient's movement intent to the intensity of stimulation to their affected hand. The advantage of proportional NMES is that it can assist during practice of complex everyday tasks. Randomized controlled trials of CCFES-mediated hand therapy for 12 weeks, 10 h per week, showed greater gains in hand dexterity (Box and Blocks Test) than cyclic NMES for individuals in subacute (less than 6 months)[42] and chronic (more than 6 months)[41,43] stages after stroke. A secondary analysis revealed that the greatest improvements in hand dexterity (Box and Blocks Test) and function (Arm Motor Abilities Test) were achieved by CCFES participants who were less than 2 years after stroke and moderately impaired (retained more than 10 deg volitional extension in the

wrist, thumb, and two other fingers) (Fig. 14.4). However, participants with severe impairment also experienced reduction in motor impairment (Upper Extremity Fugl–Meyer Assessment) from CCFES.

Implanted NMES Control

Control modalities for implanted NMES mirror those of external NMES, with switch triggering, EMG, and kinematic or inertial sensors. The main difference is that EMG, kinematic, and inertial sensors can also be implanted for more reliable sensing and to eliminate the need for the individual to don or doff electrodes and other instrumentation.[44] Also, implanted EMG electrodes may be more sensitive for sensing residual EMG and the sensing circuitry can be programmed to differentiate volitional muscle activity from the NMES stimulation artifacts.[45–47] This ability makes EMG-triggered NMES more accurate to the individual's intent and can even provide NMES proportional control based on volitional residual muscle contraction strength.

Present-day implantable upper extremity NMES systems are being developed. The first FDA-approved implanted NMES device, the Freehand System (NeuroControl Corp, Cleveland, OH) was available for spinal cord injury patients with tetraplegia between 1997 and 2002.[48] A 12-channel version of this system with two EMG-recording electrodes for stimulation control was trialed in one individual 4.8 years post stroke. It had positive neuroprosthetic effects on motor impairment and function. However, EMG control was not feasible because spasticity was triggered by volitional activation of the paretic limb; therefore, switch control was used.[49] Researchers at Case Western Reserve University are currently conducting FDA-monitored clinical trials of a networked neuroprosthesis implanted NMES technology that is modular and multifunctional (Fig. 14.5). It is designed to integrate a variety of upper and lower extremity functions across an individual's body.[50–52]

LOWER EXTREMITY NMES
Peroneal Nerve NMES for Foot Drop

There are three FDA-approved external NMES devices for foot drop: Odstock dropped-foot stimulator (Odstock Medical Ltd, Salisbury, United Kingdom), WalkAide (Innovative Neurotronics Corp., Reno, NV), and the L300 (Bioness Corp.). All three devices feature an external stimulator control unit and external electrodes mounted to an adjustable cuff worn around the lower leg. The cuff is positioned with one electrode over the peroneal nerve at the head of the fibula and

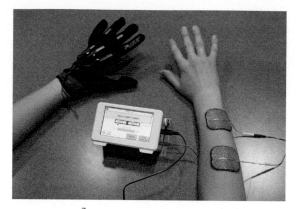

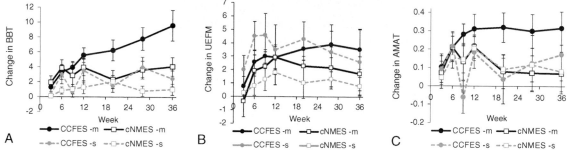

FIG. 14.4 *Top*: Cleveland FES Center Contralaterally Controlled Functional Electrical Stimulation (CCFES) is an investigational external NMES device that extends the paretic finger extensors synchronously with the opening of the unaffected hand. A kinematic sensor glove is worn on the unaffected *(left)* hand, which is connected to the stimulation control unit. This unit applies current to external surface electrodes placed on the finger extensors of the affected arm. A touchscreen interface is used to program the stimulator so the stimulated opening of the affected hand matches the opening of the unaffected hand. The device can also guide individuals using visuals and sound to perform hand opening and closing practice. *Bottom:* Outcomes of CCFES and cyclic NMES (cNMES) groups for participants less than 2 y post stroke (and more than 6 months post stroke). Change in **(A)** Box and Block Test (BBT), **(B)** upper extremity Fugl–Meyer (UEFM), and **(C)** Arm Motor Abilities Test (AMAT). *m*, moderate hand impairment at baseline; *s*, severe hand impairment at baseline. ((Top) From Cleveland FES Center; with permission. (Bottom) Data from Knutson JS, Harley MY, Hisel TZ, Hogan SD, Maloney MM, Chae J. Contralaterally controlled functional electrical stimulation for upper extremity hemiplegia: an early-phase randomized clinical trial in subacute stroke patients. *Neurorehabil Neural Repair.* 2012;26(3):239–246. https://doi.org/10.1177/1545968311419301; with permission.)

other over the tibialis anterior. Stimulation is triggered on the Odstock and L300 when a wireless heel switch in the shoe on the affected side detects heel lift. The WalkAide detects heel lift using a tilt sensor on the cuff below the knee. Stimulation of the peroneal nerve causes contraction of the tibialis anterior and consequent ankle dorsiflexion during the swing phase of gait.

Three large randomized clinical trials reported similar neuroprosthetic and therapeutic effects when comparing ankle foot orthoses (AFO) to peroneal nerve stimulators (PNS) in individuals beyond the subacute phase of stroke.[53–55] Sheffler examined therapeutic effects by randomizing 110 individuals (more than

3 months after stroke) to either 12 weeks of surface peroneal nerve stimulation or usual care (AFO or no device) and found that both groups improved significantly from baseline in Fugl–Meyer Motor Assessment of impairment, modified Emory Functional Ambulation Profile, and Stroke Specific Quality of Life questionnaire, but did not find significant differences between the intervention groups. Kluding and colleagues investigated a longer treatment of 40 weeks in 119 individuals (more than 3 months after stroke) and also found improvements from baseline, but no between-group differences. Bethoux and colleagues examined a shorter 6-week treatment in 399 individuals

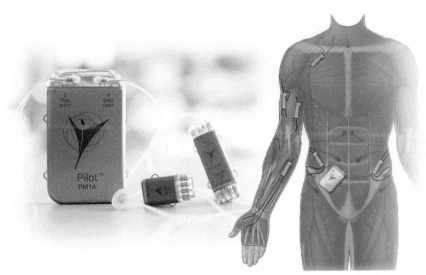

FIG. 14.5 Cleveland FES Center Networked Neural Prosthesis is a modular, fully implanted neuromuscular electrical stimulation system that is undergoing FDA-monitored trials. The command module on the left consists of an inductively rechargeable battery, programmable microcontroller, and wireless communications interface to an external programming device. The command module can be connected by wire to daisy chain many smaller, multifunction units, which can enclose sensors for measurement and pulse generators for stimulation. (From Cleveland FES Center; with permission.)

(more than 6 months after stroke) and found that both groups improved from baseline on the 10-Meter Walk Test, but there were no between-group differences in any outcomes (10-Meter Walk Test, Stroke Impact Scale, 6-Minute Walk Test, GaitRite Functional Ambulation Profile, Modified Emory Functional Ambulation Profile, Berg Balance Scale, Timed Up and Go, and Stroke-Specific Quality of Life). A fourth study examined 93 individuals less than 1 year after stroke using a cross-over design and also found similar effects from 6 weeks of treatment with either PNS or AFO.[56] Although both interventions produced similar improvements in functional mobility and walking speed across a wide range of dose and patient demographics, a majority of individuals surveyed preferred the stimulator because of easier comfort, donning, and doffing.[54,56]

Implanted NMES foot drop stimulators have received regulatory approval in Europe and are suitable for individuals who experience pain from external stimulators or difficulty effectively placing the electrodes. STIMuSTEP (FineTech Medical Ltd., Welwin Garden City, United Kingdom) and ActiGait (OttoBock, Duderstadt, Germany) both use nerve cuff electrodes that wrap around the peroneal nerve and are triggered by external heel switches. Use of ActiGait showed a neuroprosthetic effect of improved walking speed by 0.4 m/s

in 27 individuals with chronic stroke.[57] Individuals with chronic stroke using STIMuSTEP experienced a greater neuroprosthetic effect than those treated with usual care (AFO, orthopedic shoes, or no devices), but they did not experience lasting ability to dorsiflex their ankle without stimulation after using the device for 26 weeks.[58]

Multijoint NMES for Walking

In addition to ankle dorsiflexion, NMES can also produce knee flexion to elevate the leg during swing phase or knee extension for better standing ability. The L300 Plus (Bioness Corp.) has two pairs of bipolar electrodes, so it can stimulate knee flexion or extension in addition to ankle dorsiflexion (Fig. 14.6). A trial in 45 individuals showed that adding knee stimulation to peroneal knee flexion increased gait speed by a statistically significant (but not clinically significant) amount of 0.04 m/s.[59]

More severely impaired individuals may benefit from additional channels of NMES implanted in the lower extremities. Multichannel systems can compensate for impairment at multiple joints to stabilize stance and assist walking by appropriately coordinating stimulation to the hip, knee, and ankle muscles. When standing, stimulating knee and hip extensors together prevents buckling and improves standing stability.

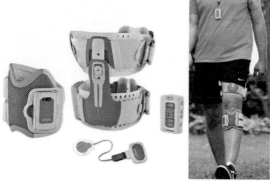

FIG. 14.6 Bioness Corp. L300 Plus is a heel switch-triggered lower extremity external NMES device that stimulates either knee extension or flexion (chosen by placing the electrodes over the hamstrings or quadriceps muscles) and ankle dorsiflexion using two separate stimulator cuffs. Both the knee and ankle cuffs have integrated batteries, pulse generators, and electrodes. The device can be triggered using a wireless remote or wireless heel switch that is placed in the wearer's shoe. (From Bioness Corp.; with permission.)

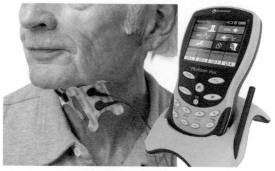

FIG. 14.7 DJO Global Corp. Chatanooga VitalStim Plus device for dysphagia rehabilitation. Surface NMES electrodes are placed over the infrahyoid muscles to contract it and depress the hyoid and require the individual to repeatedly swallow, which raises the hyoid against the resistance of the contracted muscles. (From DJO Global Corp; with permission.)

During the early swing phase of walking, stimulating hip flexors and ankle dorsiflexors together improves toe clearance and minimizes fall risk. During the push-off phase of walking, stimulating hip flexors, hip extensors, and plantar flexors together provides maximum forward force to improve walking speed. These patterns of stimulation can be delivered to the muscles in response to sequential button presses on a control unit where each button press produces a step. Alternatively, a single button press can produce continuous sequential stepping. Such systems are under development by researchers at the Cleveland VA Advanced Platform Technology Center and Cleveland FES Center. A case study of an individual with chronic poststroke hemiplegia experienced an increase in walking speed by over 0.4 m/s (over 4 times the clinically important difference of 0.1 m/s) using a fully implanted NMES to provide hip flexion, knee flexion and extension, and ankle flexion and extension.[60] Future systems will use joint angle or inertial sensors to coordinate and control stimulation that produces closed-loop walking function.

NMES FOR SWALLOWING

The problem of poststroke dysphagia was described in Chapter 4. Dysphagia treatments using NMES exist, but their effectiveness compared to conventional therapy and longterm effects still require additional examination, as large randomized controlled trials are

needed. VitalStim Plus (DJO Global Corp.) is a commercially available device designed for treating dysphagia based on the method of repetitive swallow training[61] against contracted infrahyoid muscles (Fig. 14.7). Surface electrodes are placed over the infrahyoid muscle (innervated by the ansa cervicalis and hypoglossal nerves) that produce muscle contraction, depress the hyoid, and provide resistance against effortful swallow to raise the hyoid. Continuous stimulation is initiated by pressing a button on the stimulator. The VitalStim Plus also has an EMG-triggered mode, so that hyoid resistance occurs only when volitional EMG from the infrahyoid exceeds a programmable threshold.

This type of training has only been tested in small controlled trials lasting up to 6 weeks for up to 30 min per day and treatment effects were similar to conventional care. Studies found that repetitive swallowing with NMES resulted in increased pharyngeal constriction, hyoid elevation, and related changes in cortical organization.[62,63] A recent metaanalyses of eight controlled trials also found swallow training with NMES to have more benefit than swallow training without NMES in terms of feeding status (foods that can be swallowed), video fluoroscopic swallowing measures, biomechanical measures of larynx excursion, and bolus velocity during swallowing.[64] However, the effects of swallow training with NMES were not significantly better than conventional swallow rehabilitation care (which can be a combination of oral motor exercise, diet modifications, compensatory maneuvers, pharyngeal swallowing exercises, and thermal stimulation via deep pharyngeal neuromuscular stimulation).

NMES for Shoulder Pain

Severity of arm motor impairment and mechanical instability are major contributors to hemiplegic shoulder pain and subluxation. External cyclic NMES has been used to treat shoulder subluxation by contracting the posterior deltoid and supraspinatus muscles in a repetitive fashion for up to 6 h per day for up to 6 weeks. According to a metaanalysis of 11 trials, external NMES improved shoulder subluxation when used early after stroke, but did not improve pain or motor function.[65] This is consistent with findings that conventional therapies improve biomechanics and subluxation, but hemiplegic shoulder pain can persist in 65% of individuals.[66] In addition to lack of effect on pain, clinical adoption of external NMES for the shoulder has also been limited because it is difficult to reliably place surface electrodes and to externally stimulate shoulder muscles without causing discomfort.[67]

Percutaneous NMES has shown promise for reducing hemiplegic shoulder pain with less discomfort than surface electrodes. This approach uses intramuscular electrodes to cyclically stimulate shoulder muscle contractions (posterior deltoid, middle deltoid, trapezius, and supraspinatus).[68] Unlike the external approach, implanted electrodes produce more reliable muscle contractions and bypass skin sensory receptors that are often the source of stimulation discomfort when stimulating large muscles like those at the shoulder. Several controlled studies of this approach reported a therapeutic effect on shoulder pain after treatment for 6 h per day for 6 weeks.[69-71] Pain was significantly reduced and maintained for over 12 months after electrodes were removed. The most likely responders were individuals less than 18 months post stroke.[71] This intervention has been commercialized as the SPRINT device (SPR Therapeutics Corp., Cleveland, OH), which recently received FDA clearance as a peripheral nerve stimulator for chronic pain. An optimized version of this approach that stimulates only the axillary nerve (causing contractions of the middle and posterior deltoid) for 3 weeks, 6 h per day, has been developed, and a randomized trial of 25 individuals with chronic shoulder pain after stroke showed significant decrease in reported pain compared to usual care of physical therapy (Fig. 14.8).[70]

NMES FOR SPASTICITY

Many studies have reported that applying NMES to affected muscles can reduce spasticity. There is evidence that this occurs because NMES activation of agonist muscles causes reciprocal inhibition of antagonist

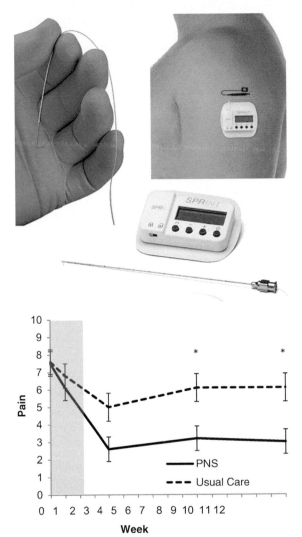

FIG. 14.8 (*Top*) SPRINT peripheral nerve stimulation system for hemiplegic shoulder pain uses a percutaneous electrode placed intramuscularly near the axillary nerve. The electrode lead exits the skin and is connected to the stimulator control unit, which is adhered to the skin of the upper arm. The control unit contains a pulse generator, control switches, and battery. (*Bottom*) Worst pain in the last week (Brief Pain Inventory Short Form question 3, where 0 is no pain and 10 is worst pain) reported by 25 participants with chronic hemiplegic shoulder pain (12 to usual care, 13 to SPRINT). After 3 weeks of treatment for 6 h per day (shaded region), the SPRINT group had significantly greater pain reductions at weeks 4, 10, and 16 than usual care. ((Top) From SPR Therapeutics Corp.; with permission. (Bottom) Data from Yu DT, Chae J, Walker ME, et al. Intramuscular neuromuscular electric stimulation for poststroke shoulder pain: a multicenter randomized clinical trial. *Arch Phys Med Rehabil*. 2004;85(5):695–704; with permission.)

muscles.[72,73] For instance, NMES to finger extensors may reduce tone in finger flexors and peroneal nerve stimulation can decrease tone in the calf muscles.

Researchers at Case Western Reserve University and MetroHealth Medical Center are developing high frequency and direct current electrical stimulation nerve block techniques to directly block hypertonia-producing signals from reaching the muscle and enable NMES to be more effective. However, this is still at the preclinical stage.[74]

ANALYSIS OF NMES FOR STROKE REHABILITATION

The first experiments with NMES for stroke rehabilitation occurred over 60 years ago.[75] Since then, NMES devices have become a familiar tool to stroke rehabilitation clinicians. Even though decades of research have explored its potential applications, enthusiasm for new NMES approaches is still very high. This could be reflective of the unsolved problems that still exist in NMES and neurorehabilitation. What follows is a strengths, weaknesses, opportunities, and threats (SWOT) analysis of NMES for stroke rehabilitation as we see them today.

Strengths

Despite advances in robotic and electromechanical technology, NMES still has major advantages in terms of portability and versatility. No means of external electromechanical movement matches NMES in terms of power-to-weight ratio, energy efficiency, and suitability for daily community use.[76] Because NMES relies on muscles as actuators, stimulation can produce a variety of functional physical movements, and yet run for days on lightweight rechargeable batteries. The portability makes NMES suitable for daily use in the home and community, which is increasingly important as cost-effectiveness becomes a focus of rehabilitation medicine. Implanted NMES systems have an added advantage of minimal setup and low cosmetic impact for daily use.

Therapeutically, NMES has the unique advantage that it strengthens and increases fatigue resistance of targeted muscles— even if the individual is passive.[15,16] Compared to passive external movement or nonuse, NMES produces muscle contractions that provide afferent signals back to the central nervous system that may enhance motor learning and reduce pain perception. The greatest benefit to impairment and function appear to be when movement intent is closely synchronized with NMES-produced movement, and individuals are treated less than 24 months after stroke.[43] Furthermore, NMES can provide severely motor-impaired individuals a significant neuroprosthetic effect for ankle dorsiflexion when their volitional ability is insufficient.

Weaknesses

Although NMES interventions in general have therapeutic effects compared to no intervention, the effects are frequently no better than conventional therapies in large controlled trials. Another major weakness is that the "active ingredients" and mechanisms of action responsible for the therapeutic effects remain poorly understood and difficult to study in large numbers. Such factors include the effects of dose, severity of impairment, and chronicity of stroke.

Other limiting factors on the efficacy of NMES interventions include muscle fatigue, discomfort, and inability to reliably activate target muscles.[14,15,67] With surface stimulation, some individuals experience pain before muscle contraction, or it is not possible to selectively contract targeted muscles without causing adjacent muscle contraction. Also, NMES cannot cause useful muscle contractions if there is severe hypertonia.[31] Conversely, NMES may not be effective if the muscle is denervated or has been injected with botulinum toxin to reduce spasticity. Furthermore, implanted NMES systems require surgery that can be expensive and lengthy, which increases clinical risks and recovery time. Complex implanted systems will require a specially trained interdisciplinary team of clinicians and engineers, which will likely limit the dissemination and availability of such NMES systems.

Opportunities

There is much active research to improve NMES human interface, control, and integration with synergistic interventions. Synchronization of movement intent with NMES may be possible with cortical signals[77–80] and more studies are investigating its therapeutic effects. There is also work on automatic calibration of electrode arrays to target desired muscles and make setup less time-consuming.

The field is also recognizing that multimodal interventions may be needed to address the complexity of motor relearning and that no single device or intervention can serve as an independent solution.[81] Specifically, NMES is being integrated with or compared against video games,[82] robotics,[78,83] transcranial brain stimulation,[84,85] and mirror therapy.[86]

For many of these new NMES efforts to progress, advances in stimulation control and a method to overcome hypertonia and spasticity are needed. There is early stage technology development of high frequency

NMES to inhibit spasticity so that NMES can be more effective and quickly reversed.[74] Currently, there are no fast-acting ways to relieve spasticity, and botulinum toxin is a contraindication for NMES. Furthermore, stimulation parameters in current NMES are usually preprogrammed through trial and error and executed in open loop fashion. In many devices, the stimulator transmits current to the electrodes with no feedback of whether the hand or leg is moving as intended. Unlike robotic devices, which have joint angle sensors on the actuating motors, it is difficult to sense joint positions or volitional effort during NMES use. However, methods to accurately sense joint angles and residual muscle activations are necessary for NMES interventions to make instant corrections to increase the likelihood of delivering intended movements and effects.

Threats

A challenge facing NMES therapeutic interventions (beyond demonstration of efficacy) is their ability to integrate into conventional care. Using external cyclic NMES as an example, which is the most familiar to rehabilitation clinicians, still faces barriers to adoption. Therapists are often treating more than one individual in a 1-h time slot and the extra effort to set up electrodes and stimulation parameters can limit their use. Additionally, cyclic stimulation is difficult to integrate with conventional movement practice; so, it needs to be used as an adjunct for a period of time. Therefore, unless therapeutic effects of NMES can justify the extra effort, clinical adoption of NMES interventions may be hindered by clinical time limitations.

For NMES interventions to be adopted by consumers and clinicians, the amount of benefit to motor relearning must be sufficient to justify the burden of device cost and setup/use. NMES interventions may require months of use to achieve therapeutic effects and can be permanent devices if implanted, but interventions for cognitive and communication impairments are also commonly necessary and may compete for the individual's time and resources. There is also very limited support from Medicare or private insurance for consumer purchase of NMES devices. Since motor impairment often reduces an individual's ability to work, paying out of pocket for devices not covered by insurance can create barriers to adoption.

A long-standing challenge for any motor relearning intervention (NMES included) is to be at least as effective as conventional occupational or physical therapy in large randomized control trials.[87] This is especially true for individuals with severe impairment, who do not tend to exhibit significant and lasting therapeutic effects after NMES-assisted training. Many interventions for stroke motor relearning benefit motor impairment, but not necessarily improve function or the ability of individuals to use their hands. Unlike pharmaceuticals or motor training techniques, NMES interventions require proprietary equipment in addition to clinician participation to deliver the therapy. Therefore, to be accepted by clinicians, NMES therapeutic advantages must be significant and not just comparable to conventional care. This goal faces the challenge of high heterogeneity in impairments, demographics, and pathophysiology that accompanies larger sample sizes.[88] In response, the National Center for Medical Rehabilitation Research in the United States has advocated for defining therapies' active ingredients and integrating them into multimodal therapies capable of maximum efficacy in diverse populations.[81] Therefore, as multimodal treatments are of greater focus, it is important for the field to better understand how NMES affects motor learning processes, so that it can be combined in a synergistic manner with other interventions.

CONCLUSION

In summary, clinically available NMES interventions have therapeutic efficacy and are recommended for use as adjuncts to and during (if possible) conventional occupational and physical therapy. Specifically, NMES assistance for arm, wrist, and finger extension and ankle dorsiflexion have the most clinical evidence of therapeutic and neuroprosthetic effects. There is evidence that individuals with moderate impairment less than 2 years post stroke receive the greatest therapeutic effects for upper extremity function and that synchronization of movement intent with NMES can yield greater effects. The NMES devices that are commercially available today do not employ control strategies that are driven by motor intent, but there is active research to develop devices that do. The effectiveness of NMES for swallowing training is still not clear, but it may improve outcomes for those with moderate impairment. Hemiplegic shoulder pain has been shown to improve markedly with NMES and multicenter trials are underway. Despite these successes, there are many who do not respond or are not yet suitable for NMES interventions. Therefore, there is still a need of NMES interventions for individuals who are severely impaired or have hypertonia and spasticity. Multichannel and modular implanted NMES systems are also needed to compensate for multiple impairments simultaneously. It is also important to seek a more precise understanding of motor learning mechanisms, so NMES can be successfully integrated with the continuum of care.

ACKNOWLEDGEMENT

The authors were supported in part by the Department of Veterans Affairs (grant I01RX002249), National Institute for Child Health and Human Development (National Center for Medical Rehabilitation Research grants R01HD068588 and R21HD088987), and Metro-Health Foundation.

REFERENCES

1. Benjamin EJ, Blaha MJ, Chiuve SE, et al. Heart disease and stroke statistics-2017 update: a report from the American Heart Association. *Circulation*. 2017;135(10):e146—e603. https://doi.org/10.1161/CIR.0000000000000485.

2. Lawrence ES, Coshall C, Dundas R, et al. Estimates of the prevalence of acute stroke impairments and disability in a multiethnic population. *Stroke*. 2001;32(6): 1279—1284.

3. Hendricks HT, van Limbeek J, Geurts AC, Zwarts MJ. Motor recovery after stroke: a systematic review of the literature. *Arch Phys Med Rehabil*. 2002;83(11): 1629—1637. https://doi.org/10.1053/apmr.2002.35473.

4. Beebe JA, Lang CE. Absence of a proximal to distal gradient of motor deficits in the upper extremity early after stroke. *Clin Neurophysiol*. 2008;119(9):2074—2085. https://doi.org/10.1016/j.clinph.2008.04.293.

5. Lang CE, Bland MD, Bailey RR, Schaefer SY, Birkenmeier RL. Assessment of upper extremity impairment, function, and activity after stroke: foundations for clinical decision making. *J Hand Ther*. 2013;26(2): 104—114. https://doi.org/10.1016/j.jht.2012.06.005.

6. Dewald JP, Pope PS, Given JD, Buchanan TS, Rymer WZ. Abnormal muscle coactivation patterns during isometric torque generation at the elbow and shoulder in hemiparetic subjects. *Brain J Neurol*. 1995;118(Pt 2):495—510.

7. Sommerfeld DK, Gripenstedt U, Welmer A-K. Spasticity after stroke: an overview of prevalence, test instruments, and treatments. *Am J Phys Med Rehabil*. 2012;91(9):814—820. https://doi.org/10.1097/PHM.0b013e31825f13a3.

8. Sullivan JE, Hedman LD. Sensory dysfunction following stroke: incidence, significance, examination, and intervention. *Top Stroke Rehabil*. 2008;15(3):200—217. https://doi.org/10.1310/tsr1503-200.

9. Chae J, Yang G, Park BK, Labatia I. Delay in initiation and termination of muscle contraction, motor impairment, and physical disability in upper limb hemiparesis. *Muscle Nerve*. 2002;25(4):568—575.

10. Chae J, Yang G, Park BK, Labatia I. Muscle weakness and cocontraction in upper limb hemiparesis: relationship to motor impairment and physical disability. *Neurorehabil Neural Repair*. 2002;16(3):241—248. https://doi.org/ 10.1177/154596830201600303.

11. Chae J, Labatia I, Yang G. Upper limb motor function in hemiparesis: concurrent validity of the arm motor ability test. *Am J Phys Med Rehabil*. 2003;82(1):1—8. https:// doi.org/10.1097/01.PHM.0000034950.95737.91.

12. Wolf SL, Lecraw DE, Barton LA, Jann BB. Forced use of hemiplegic upper extremities to reverse the effect of learned nonuse among chronic stroke and head-injured patients. *Exp Neurol*. 1989;104(2):125—132.

13. Lee RG, van Donkelaar P. Mechanisms underlying functional recovery following stroke. *Can J Neurol Sci J Can Sci Neurol*. 1995;22(4):257—263.

14. Mortimer JT, Bhadra N. Fundamentals of electrical stimulation. Philadelphia, PA. In: *Neuromodulation*; 2009: 109—121. https://www.clinicalkey.com/#!/content/book/ 3-s2.0-B9780123742483000124.

15. Peckham PH, Mortimer JT, Marsolais EB. Alteration in the force and fatigability of skeletal muscle in quadriplegic humans following exercise induced by chronic electrical stimulation. *Clin Orthop*. 1976;(114):326—333.

16. Gondin J, Brocca L, Bellinzona E, et al. Neuromuscular electrical stimulation training induces atypical adaptations of the human skeletal muscle phenotype: a functional and proteomic analysis. *J Appl Physiol (Bethesda MD) 1985*. 2011;110(2):433—450. https://doi.org/ 10.1152/japplphysiol.00914.2010.

17. Arija-Blázquez A, Ceruelo-Abajo S, Díaz-Merino MS, et al. Effects of electromyostimulation on muscle and bone in men with acute traumatic spinal cord injury: a randomized clinical trial. *J Spinal Cord Med*. 2014;37(3):299—309. https://doi.org/10.1179/2045772313Y.0000000142.

18. Rushton DN. Functional electrical stimulation and rehabilitation—an hypothesis. *Med Eng Phys*. 2003;25(1): 75—78.

19. Khaslavskaia S, Sinkjaer T. Motor cortex excitability following repetitive electrical stimulation of the common peroneal nerve depends on the voluntary drive. *Exp Brain Res*. 2005;162(4):497—502. https://doi.org/ 10.1007/s00221-004-2153-1.

20. Francisco G, Chae J, Chawla H, et al. Electromyogram-triggered neuromuscular stimulation for improving the arm function of acute stroke survivors: a randomized pilot study. *Arch Phys Med Rehabil*. 1998;79(5):570—575.

21. Fields RW. Electromyographically triggered electric muscle stimulation for chronic hemiplegia. *Arch Phys Med Rehabil*. 1987;68(7):407—414.

22. Cauraugh JH, Kim SB. Stroke motor recovery: active neuromuscular stimulation and repetitive practice schedules. *J Neurol Neurosurg Psychiatry*. 2003;74(11):1562—1566.

23. Liu H, Au-Yeung SSY. Corticomotor excitability effects of peripheral nerve electrical stimulation to the paretic arm in stroke. *Am J Phys Med Rehabil*. April 2017. https:// doi.org/10.1097/PHM.0000000000000748.

24. Hong IK, Choi JB, Lee JH. Cortical changes after mental imagery training combined with electromyography-triggered electrical stimulation in patients with chronic stroke. *Stroke*. 2012;43(9):2506—2509. https://doi.org/ 10.1161/STROKEAHA.112.663641.

25. Kimberley TJ, Lewis SM, Auerbach EJ, Dorsey LL, Lojovich JM, Carey JR. Electrical stimulation driving functional improvements and cortical changes in subjects with stroke. *Exp Brain Res*. 2004;154(14618287):450—460.

26. Thrasher TA, Zivanovic V, McIlroy W, Popovic MR. Rehabilitation of reaching and grasping function in severe hemiplegic patients using functional electrical stimulation therapy. *Neurorehabil Neural Repair.* 2008; 22(6):706–714. https://doi.org/10.1177/15459683083 17436.

27. Ring H, Rosenthal N. Controlled study of neuroprosthetic functional electrical stimulation in sub-acute post-stroke rehabilitation. *J Rehabil Med.* 2005;37(1):32–36. https:// doi.org/10.1000/16501970410035387.

28. Mann G, Taylor P, Lane R. Accelerometer-triggered electrical stimulation for reach and grasp in chronic stroke patients. *Neurorehabil Neural Repair.* 2011;25(8): 774–780. https://doi.org/10.1177/1545968310397200.

29. Lin C. The effects of ipsilateral forearm movement and contralateral hand grasp on the spastic hand opened by electrical stimulation. *Neurorehabil Neural Repair.* 2000;14(3):199–205. https://doi.org/10.1177/ 154596830001400305.

30. Makowski N, Knutson J, Chae J, Crago P. Interaction of poststroke voluntary effort and functional neuromuscular electrical stimulation. *J Rehabil Res Dev.* 2013;50(1):85–98.

31. Chae J, Hart R. Intramuscular hand neuroprosthesis for chronic stroke survivors. *Neurorehabil Neural Repair.* 2003;17(2):109–117. https://doi.org/10.1177/0888 439003017002005.

32. Hines AE, Crago PE, Billian C. Hand opening by electrical stimulation in patients with spastic hemiplegia. *IEEE Trans Rehabil Eng.* 1995;3(2):193–205. https://doi.org/10.1109/ 86.392368.

33. Hayward KS, Barker RN, Brauer SG, Lloyd D, Horsley SA, Carson RG. SMART Arm with outcome-triggered electrical stimulation: a pilot randomized clinical trial. *Top Stroke Rehabil.* 2013;20(4):289–298. https://doi.org/10.1310/ tsr2004-289.

34. Wilson RD, Page SJ, Delahanty M, et al. Upper-limb recovery after stroke: a randomized controlled trial comparing EMG-triggered, cyclic, and sensory electrical stimulation. *Neurorehabil Neural Repair.* 2016;30(10):978–987. https://doi.org/10.1177/1545968316650278.

35. de Kroon JR, IJzerman MJ. Electrical stimulation of the upper extremity in stroke: cyclic versus EMG-triggered stimulation. *Clin Rehabil.* 2008;22(8):690–697. https:// doi.org/10.1177/0269215508088984.

36. Boyaci A, Topuz O, Alkan H, et al. Comparison of the effectiveness of active and passive neuromuscular electrical stimulation of hemiplegic upper extremities: a randomized, controlled trial. *Int J Rehabil Res Int Z Für Rehabil Rev Int Rech Réadapt.* 2013;36(4):315–322. https://doi.org/10.1097/MRR.0b013e328360e541.

37. Kopp B, Kunkel A, Flor H, et al. The arm motor ability test: reliability, validity, and sensitivity to change of an instrument for assessing disabilities in activities of daily living. *Arch Phys Med Rehabil.* 1997;78(6):615–620. https:// doi.org/10.1016/S0003-9993(97)90427-5.

38. Rebersek S, Vodovnik L. Proportionally controlled functional electrical stimulation of hand. *Arch Phys Med Rehabil.* 1973;54(8):378–382.

39. Merletti R, Acimovic R, Grobelnik S, Cvilak G. Electrophysiological orthosis for the upper extremity in hemiplegia: feasibility study. *Arch Phys Med Rehabil.* 1975;56(12): 507–513.

40. Knutson JS, Harley MY, Hisel TZ, Chae J. Improving hand function in stroke survivors: a pilot study of contralaterally controlled functional electric stimulation in chronic hemiplegia. *Arch Phys Med Rehabil.* 2007;88(4):513–520. https://doi.org/10.1016/j.apmr.2007.01.003.

41. Knutson JS, Hisel TZ, Harley MY, Chae J. A novel functional electrical stimulation treatment for recovery of hand function in hemiplegia: 12-week pilot study. *Neurorehabil Neural Repair.* 2009;23(1):17–25. https:// doi.org/10.1177/1545968308317577.

42. Knutson JS, Harley MY, Hisel TZ, Hogan SD, Maloney MM, Chae J. Contralaterally controlled functional electrical stimulation for upper extremity hemiplegia: an early-phase randomized clinical trial in subacute stroke patients. *Neurorehabil Neural Repair.* 2012;26(3): 239–246. https://doi.org/10.1177/1545968311419301.

43. Knutson JS, Gunzler DD, Wilson RD, Chae J. Contralaterally controlled functional electrical stimulation improves hand dexterity in chronic hemiparesis. *Stroke.* January 2016. https://doi.org/10.1161/STROKEAHA.116. 013791.

44. Bhadra N, Peckham PH, Keith MW, et al. Implementation of an implantable joint-angle transducer. *J Rehabil Res Dev.* 2002;39(3):411–422.

45. Nikolić ZM, Popović DB, Stein RB, Kenwell Z. Instrumentation for ENG and EMG recordings in FES systems. *IEEE Trans Biomed Eng.* 1994;41(7):703–706. https://doi.org/ 10.1109/10.301739.

46. Memberg WD, Stage TG, Kirsch RF. A fully implanted intramuscular bipolar myoelectric signal recording electrode. *Neuromodulation J Int Neuromodulation Soc.* 2014;17(8): 794–799; discussion 799. https://doi.org/10.1111/ner. 12165.

47. Hart RL, Kilgore KL, Peckham PH. A comparison between control methods for implanted FES hand-grasp systems. *IEEE Trans Rehabil Eng Publ IEEE Eng Med Biol Soc.* 1998; 6(2):208–218.

48. Peckham PH, Keith MW, Kilgore KL, et al. Efficacy of an implanted neuroprosthesis for restoring hand grasp in tetraplegia: a multicenter study. *Arch Phys Med Rehabil.* 2001;82(10):1380–1388. https://doi.org/10.1053/ apmr.2001.25910.

49. Knutson JS, Chae J, Hart RL, et al. Implanted neuroprosthesis for assisting arm and hand function after stroke: a case study. *J Rehabil Res Dev.* 2012;49(10): 1505–1516.

50. Peckham PH, Kilgore KL. Challenges and opportunities in restoring function after paralysis. *IEEE Trans Biomed*

Eng. 2013;60(3):602—609. https://doi.org/10.1109/tbme.2013.2245128.

51. Kilgore KL, Peckham PH, Crish TJ, Smith B. Implantable networked neural system. http://www.google.com/patents/US7260436; August 2007.

52. Smith B, Crish TJ, Buckett JR, Kilgore KL, Peckham PH. *Development of an Implantable Networked Neuroprosthesis.* IEEE; 2005. https://doi.org/10.1109/cne.2005.1419657.

53. Bethoux F, Rogers HL, Nolan KJ, et al. Long-term follow-up to a randomized controlled trial comparing peroneal nerve functional electrical stimulation to an ankle foot orthosis for patients with chronic stroke. *Neurorehabil Neural Repair.* February 2015. https://doi.org/10.1177/1545968315570325.

54. Kluding PM, Dunning K, O'Dell MW, et al. Foot drop stimulation versus ankle foot orthosis after stroke: 30-week outcomes. *Stroke.* 2013;44(6):1660—1669. https://doi.org/10.1161/STROKEAHA.111.000334.

55. Sheffler LR, Taylor PN, Gunzler DD, Buurke JH, IJzerman MJ, Chae J. Randomized controlled trial of surface peroneal nerve stimulation for motor relearning in lower limb hemiparesis. *Arch Phys Med Rehabil.* 2013;94(6):1007—1014. https://doi.org/10.1016/j.apmr.2013.01.024.

56. Everaert DG, Stein RB, Abrams GM, et al. Effect of a foot-drop stimulator and ankle-foot orthosis on walking performance after stroke: a multicenter randomized controlled trial. *Neurorehabil Neural Repair.* 2013;27(7):579—591. https://doi.org/10.1177/1545968313481278.

57. Martin KD, Polanski WH, Schulz A-K, et al. Restoration of ankle movements with the ActiGait implantable drop foot stimulator: a safe and reliable treatment option for permanent central leg palsy. *J Neurosurg.* 2016;124(1):70—76. https://doi.org/10.3171/2014.12.jns142110.

58. Kottink AI, Hermens HJ, Nene AV, et al. A randomized controlled trial of an implantable 2-channel peroneal nerve stimulator on walking speed and activity in poststroke hemiplegia. *Arch Phys Med Rehabil.* 2007; 88(8):971—978. https://doi.org/10.1016/j.apmr.2007.05.002.

59. Springer S, Vatine J-J, Lipson R, Wolf A, Laufer Y. Effects of dual-channel functional electrical stimulation on gait performance in patients with hemiparesis. *Sci World J.* 2012; 2012:1—8. https://doi.org/10.1100/2012/530906.

60. Makowski NS, Kobetic R, Lombardo LM, et al. Improving walking with an implanted neuroprosthesis for hip, knee, and ankle control after stroke. *Am J Phys Med Rehabil.* 2016;95(12):880—888. https://doi.org/10.1097/phm.0000000000000533.

61. The evaluation and treatment of swallowing disorders. *Current Opinion in Otolaryngology & Head and Neck Surgery;* 1998. LWW. http://journals.lww.com/co-otolaryngology/Fulltext/1998/12000/The_evaluation_and_treatment_of_swallowing.8.aspx

62. Kiger M, Brown CS, Watkins L. Dysphagia management: an analysis of patient outcomes using VitalStim™ therapy compared to traditional swallow therapy. *Dysphagia.* 2006; 21(4):243—253. https://doi.org/10.1007/s00455-006-9056-1.

63. Shaw GY, Sechtem PR, Searl J, Keller K, Rawi TA, Dowdy E. Transcutaneous neuromuscular electrical stimulation (VitalStim) curative therapy for severe dysphagia: myth or reality? *Ann Otol Rhinol Laryngol.* 2007;116(1):36—44. https://doi.org/10.1177/000348940711600107.

64. Chen Y-W, Chang K-H, Chen H-C, Liang W-M, Wang Y-H, Lin Y-N. The effects of surface neuromuscular electrical stimulation on post-stroke dysphagia: a systemic review and meta-analysis. *Clin Rehabil.* 2016;30(1):24—35. https://doi.org/10.1177/0269215515571681.

65. Lee J-H, Baker LL, Johnson RE, Tilson JK. Effectiveness of neuromuscular electrical stimulation for management of shoulder subluxation post-stroke: a systematic review with meta-analysis. *Clin Rehabil.* March 2017. https://doi.org/10.1177/0269215517700696.

66. Lindgren I, Jonsson A-C, Norrving B, Lindgren A. Shoulder pain after stroke: a prospective population-based study. *Stroke.* 2006;38(2):343—348. https://doi.org/10.1161/01.str.0000254598.16739.4e.

67. Chae J, Hart R. Comparison of discomfort associated with surface and percutaneous intramuscular electrical stimulation for persons with chronic hemiplegia. *Am J Phys Med Rehabil.* 1998;77(6):516—522.

68. Yu DT, Chae J, Walker ME, et al. Intramuscular neuromuscular electric stimulation for poststroke shoulder pain: a multicenter randomized clinical trial. *Arch Phys Med Rehabil.* 2004;85(5):695—704.

69. Chae J, Yu DT, Walker ME, et al. Intramuscular electrical stimulation for hemiplegic shoulder pain. *Am J Phys Med Rehabil.* 2005;84(11):832—842. https://doi.org/10.1097/01.phm.0000184154.01880.72.

70. Wilson RD, Gunzler DD, Bennett ME, Chae J. Peripheral nerve stimulation compared with usual care for pain relief of hemiplegic shoulder pain. *Am J Phys Med Rehabil.* 2014;93(1):17—28. https://doi.org/10.1097/phm.0000000000000011.

71. Chae J, Ng A, Yu DT, et al. Intramuscular electrical stimulation for shoulder pain in hemiplegia: does time from stroke onset predict treatment success? *Neurorehabil Neural Repair.* 2007;21(6):561—567. https://doi.org/10.1177/1545968306298412.

72. Takeda K, Tanabe S, Koyama S, et al. Influence of transcutaneous electrical nerve stimulation conditions on disynaptic reciprocal Ia inhibition and presynaptic inhibition in healthy adults. *Somatosens Mot Res.* 2017;34(1):52—57. https://doi.org/10.1080/08990220.2017.1286311.

73. Day BL, Marsden CD, Obeso JA, Rothwell JC. Reciprocal inhibition between the muscles of the human forearm. *J Physiol.* 1984;349(1):519—534. https://doi.org/10.1113/jphysiol.1984.sp015171.

74. Kilgore KL, Bhadra N. Reversible nerve conduction block using kilohertz frequency alternating current. *Neuromodulation Technol Neural Interf.* 2013;17(3):242—255. https://doi.org/10.1111/ner.12100.

75. Liberson WT, Holmquest HJ, Scot D, Dow M. Functional electrotherapy: stimulation of the peroneal nerve synchronized with the swing phase of the gait of hemiplegic patients. *Arch Phys Med Rehabil.* 1961;42:101—105.

76. Maciejasz P, Eschweiler J, Gerlach-Hahn K, Jansen-Troy A, Leonhardt S. A survey on robotic devices for upper limb rehabilitation. *J NeuroEngineering Rehabil.* 2014;11(3). https://doi.org/10.1186/1743-0003-11-3.

77. Daly JJ, Cheng R, Rogers J, Litinas K, Hrovat K, Dohring M. Feasibility of a new application of noninvasive Brain Computer Interface (BCI): a case study of training for recovery of volitional motor control after stroke. *J Neurol Phys Ther JNPT.* 2009;33(4):203−211. https://doi.org/10.1097/NPT.0b013e3181c1fc0b

78. Looned R, Webb J, Xiao ZG, Menon C. Assisting drinking with an affordable BCI-controlled wearable robot and electrical stimulation: a preliminary investigation. *J Neuroengineering Rehabil.* 2014;11:51. https://doi.org/10.1186/1743-0003-11-51.

79. Young BM, Nigogosyan Z, Nair VA, et al. Case report: poststroke interventional BCI rehabilitation in an individual with preexisting sensorineural disability. *Front Neuroengineering.* 2014;7:18. https://doi.org/10.3389/fneng.2014.00018.

80. Ibáñez J, Monge-Pereira E, Molina-Rueda F, et al. Low latency estimation of motor intentions to assist reaching movements along multiple sessions in chronic stroke patients: a feasibility study. *Front Neurosci.* 2017;11:126. https://doi.org/10.3389/fnins.2017.00126.

81. Nitkin R. *Support for Clinical Trials at the National Center for Medical Rehabilitation Research and the NIH*; November 2014. http://www.asnr.com/files/NitkinHandouts.pdf.

82. Fu MJ, Curby A, Suder R, Chae J, Knutson JS. Contralaterally controlled functional electrical stimulation and hand therapy video games for cerebral palsy. *Neurorehabil Neural Repair.* 2016;30(2):NP1−NP44. https://doi.org/10.1177/1545968315625245.

83. McCabe J, Monkiewicz M, Holcomb J, Pundik S, Daly JJ. Comparison of robotics, functional electrical stimulation, and motor learning methods for treatment of persistent upper extremity dysfunction after stroke: a randomized controlled trial. *Arch Phys Med Rehabil.* November 2014. https://doi.org/10.1016/j.apmr.2014.10.022.

84. Koyama S, Tanabe S, Warashina H, et al. NMES with rTMS for moderate to severe dysfunction after stroke. *NeuroRehabilitation.* 2014;35(3):363−368. https://doi.org/10.3233/NRE-141127.

85. Satow T, Kawase T, Kitamura A, et al. Combination of transcranial direct current stimulation and neuromuscular electrical stimulation improves gait ability in a patient in chronic stage of stroke. *Case Rep Neurol.* 2016;8(1):39−46. https://doi.org/10.1159/000444167.

86. Schick T, Schlake H-P, Kallusky J, et al. Synergy effects of combined multichannel EMG-triggered electrical stimulation and mirror therapy in subacute stroke patients with severe or very severe arm/hand paresis. *Restor Neurol Neurosci.* 2017;35(3):319−332. https://doi.org/10.3233/RNN-160710.

87. Winstein C. *Translating the Science into Neurorehabilitation Practice: Challenges and Opportunities*; November 2014. http://www.asnr.com/files/ASNR_Viste%20Award_Winstein.pptx.pdf.

88. Muir KW. Heterogeneity of stroke pathophysiology and neuroprotective clinical trial design. *Stroke J Cereb Circ.* 2002;33(6):1545−1550.

CHAPTER 15

Returning to Work After Stroke

GUNILLA MARGARETA ERIKSSON, REG OT, PHD • ULLA JOHANSSON, PHD •
LENA VON KOCH, REG OT, PHD

INTRODUCTION

As a takeoff point for this chapter we will reveal the perspective we have as researchers in vocational rehabilitation for persons that have had a stroke. Vocational rehabilitation seeks ways to develop a "match" between the abilities and limitations of the person, the demands of the job, and the work environment.[1] In addition, concepts used in vocational rehabilitation will be outlined and some definitions will be provided. Concepts often used but with various definitions are *return-to-work* and *work ability/work disability*, and even the term *work* has been defined differently.

Work is defined by the international Classification of Functioning, Disability and Health (ICF) as "engaging in all aspects of work, as an occupation, trade, profession or other form of employment, for payment or when payment is not provided, as an employee, full time or part-time, or self-employed."[2] This framing of the concept of work differs from ways of using the term in which only paid employment is related to the success of returning to work after an illness/disability, or in regulations whether a person is entitled sickness benefits or other economic compensations. Work plays an essential role in peoples' lives, may be therapeutic, and has positive health effects for people with or without disabilities.[3,4] Not participating in working life has both social and personal economic consequences, as well as a negative impact on quality of life.[5]

Return-to-work is broadly used but with various meanings. Return-to-work, often abbreviated RTW, can mean the process of returning to work but also refers to an outcome of the process of vocational rehabilitation.[6] Furthermore, *working* or *not working* can be a state or a vocational outcome and a duration of or extent of disability to work due to impairment or disability.

In our perspective return-to-work is framed as a developing and dynamic process. Young and Wasiak, together with other return-to-work researchers, conceptualized return-to-work as a process[6,7]:

RTW is not merely a state; rather it is a multi-phase process, encompassing both a series of events, transitions, and phases as well as interaction with other individuals and the environment. The process begins at the onset of the work disability and concludes when a satisfactory long-term outcome has been achieved.

This framing indicates that the return-to-work process is complex, requires constructive collaboration between stakeholders, and an openness for new solutions. The return-to-work process has four phases: off work when the worker first experiences work disability, integration of work into daily life, work maintenance when work is resumed, and advancement.[7]

In this chapter, the process of return-to-work and how to enable collaboration between stakeholders over time to be able to succeed is the main content.

There are numerous definitions of *work ability* in the literature. Based on in-depth analyses of the concept, Lederer and coresearchers[8] defined work disability or work ability as follows: "Work (dis)ability is multidimensional and results from individual, organizational and societal conditions and is relational and dynamic in nature." Further, work disability is framed by Loisel as "occurring when a worker is unable to stay at work or return to work because of an injury or disease."[9] The conceptualization of work (dis)ability seems to have become more dynamic over time and consequently there is a need to consider several factors, that is, the accordance and balance between the individual's resources and the work demands, influencing work ability.[10] Work ability is described by Ilmarinen and colleagues as being made up of four components with different substance: (1) health and functional capacity which is the basis for work ability; (2) education, occupational skills, competence; (3) attitudes and motivation for work; and (4) content of work, work organization, work community, and management.[10] The work ability is influenced by how these components are maintained and support each other. This

Stroke Rehabilitation. https://doi.org/10.1016/B978-0-323-55381-0.00015-9

implies that other factors than just the individuals with reduced work ability are important to promote return-to-work.

> ### Main Message
>
> **Work** includes all aspects of work and employments or being self-employed, for payment or unpaid.
>
> **Return-to-work** is a complex, developing, and dynamic process that requires constructive collaboration between stakeholders and an openness for new solutions.
>
> **Work (dis)ability** results from individual, organizational, and societal conditions and is relational and dynamic in nature and occurs when a worker is unable to stay at work or return to work due to an injury or disease.

STROKE IN WORKING AGES
Incidence of Stroke Among People in the Working Ages

A major consequence of stroke is work disability.[11] The incidence of stroke among working-age adults is increasing[12,13] in Europe, and up to one-third of those having their first-ever stroke occur in persons <65 years of age,[14] though the number of people in working ages suffering a stroke varies between countries. In Sweden 20% are younger than 65 years, the general retirement age.[13] An estimated 6,400,000 Americans >20 years of age have had a stroke (extrapolated to 2006 using NCHS/NHANES 2003 to 2006 data). Overall stroke prevalence during this period was an estimated 2.9%. In the youngest age group (20–39 years of age) 0.3% men and 0.6% women had had a stroke. In the next age group (40–59 years) 1% men and 2.7% women had had a stroke.[15] Approximately 152,000 persons have a stroke each year in the UK.[16] Twenty-five percent of all strokes in the UK occur in people under 65 years of age.[17]

Proportions of People Not Returning to Work After Stroke

A systematic review conducted 2009 including 78 studies on social consequences of stroke for working-aged adults revealed that return-to-work varied widely across studies reviewed, as did the measurement time points.[17] The mean return-to-work rate across studies was 44%, but the average time point was not specified. Less than 50% of those under 65 years return-to-work in Sweden[18] and 69% of 25–59-year-old persons with stroke were unable to return-to-work in the UK.[19]

Further reintegration to work has not been perceived as successful after a mild stroke; in those who had returned to work almost half of them reported working slower, having problems concentrating while working, and being unable to do their jobs as well as previously.

About a third reported they were not able to keep organized.[20] More recent literature indicates similar numbers of not returning to work. In a Danish study 50% were self-supporting or job-seeking 1 year post stroke, while 11% had left the workforce permanently,[21] and 39% still were on sick absence. Further, in a Dutch study it was found that young persons with stroke (<50 years of age) had a 2–3 times higher risk of unemployment at a follow-up 8 years post stroke compared to their peers.[22]

> ### Main Message
>
> Approximately 40%–50% of those having stroke in working ages do not return to work.

PREDICTORS FOR RETURNING OR NOT RETURNING TO WORK AFTER STROKE

Predictive factors for return-to-work after stroke are independence in activities of daily living,[23] younger age, high education, and white-collar work.[24] Severe stroke is a predictor for not returning to work[25] as well as aphasia and attention dysfunction.[26,27] There are significantly lower return-to-work rates for persons with cognitive impairment and depression after stroke compared to those without these disabilities.[28] Poststroke fatigue appears to be a strong determinant for not returning to paid work[29] and was rated as the greatest barrier for those returning to work within the first year of stroke.[30] According to Alaszewski et al. 80% of the stroke survivors experience fatigue.[31] In a study conducted in Korea 60% returned to work at 6 months after stroke.[32] In the Korean study sex, age, educational level and comorbidity levels were independent factors related to return to work, that is, men returned to work to a higher extent and so did the younger group with fewer comorbidities. In a recent 6-year Swedish follow-up study of return-to-work after stroke, 75% worked 6 years after onset, and people continued to return-to-work until just 3 years post stroke, indicating that the return-to-work process is long. Dependency in everyday activities at discharge from hospital and being on sick-leave prior to stroke were significant risk factors for not returning to work.[33] In addition, there are a number of psychosocial and environmental factors that need to be taken into consideration for return-to-work, for example, number of working years remaining until retirement, type of occupation, and related needs, as these are issues that can influence the decision making. Furthermore, persons with stroke who are flexible, accept the consequences of their stroke, and are realistic in their goals appear more likely to return to work.[75]

> **Main Message**
>
> Predictors for *not returning to work* are severe stroke, cognitive impairment, depression, poststroke fatigue, dependency in activities of daily living, comorbidities, and being on sick-leave prior to stroke.
>   Predictors for *returning to work* are younger age, higher education level, and white-collar work.

SYSTEMS AND ORGANIZATIONS FOR RETURN-TO-WORK

The process of returning to work for persons with disabilities is complex, and there are numerous challenges due to legal, administrative, social, political, and cultural systems. The complexity in the process is captured by Loisel and colleagues in the Sherbrooke-model, where the importance of different stakeholders/actors involved in the process is identified.[34] The Sherbrooke model has the worker in the center and describes four systems affecting the work situation: the personal system—including social, emotional, cognitive, and physical levels, the healthcare system, the workplace system, and the compensation system. The actors in these systems have different responsibilities in the return-to-work process and the social context can influence how the actors fulfill their responsibility.

The systems involved in the return-to-work, healthcare, social services/compensation system, and workplace differ much between countries. The systems can be run by governmental or private agencies, paid for by insurance companies or/and the government, with various number of stakeholders involved with diverse responsibilities in the return-to-work process. For persons with stroke, the return-to-work process involves a complicated collaboration and navigating between persons with different duties due to the many stakeholders involved.[34,35]

In Sweden, for example, five stakeholders are involved in the vocational rehabilitation process. These are the individual and the employer, together with the three governmental agencies; Swedish Social

Insurance Agency, Swedish Public Employment Office, and Health Care who share the responsibility to support people on sickness absence in return-to-work. Swedish Social Insurance Agency main responsibility is to determine if an individual has the right to sick-leave compensation and to coordinate rehabilitation resources for persons in sickness absence with the aim of returning to the workforce. The employer has the main responsibility for taking measures that facilitate the return-to-work process at the workplace and for providing workplace-related adjustments according to the Swedish Working Environment Act. Swedish Public Employment Office ensures use of support options for persons that are unemployed or are at risk of unemployment. Healthcare providers are typically multidisciplinary teams specialized in medical rehabilitation, who are responsible mainly for medical treatment and rehabilitation related to the injury. Medical certificates issued by a physician are the basis for the Social Insurance Office decisions concerning eligibility for sickness benefit or sickness compensation. Healthcare is responsible for linking the rehabilitation with the actual workplace.

> **Main Message**
>
> The systems involved in the return-to-work: healthcare, social services/compensation system, and workplace differ much between countries. For persons with stroke, the return-to-work process involves a complex navigation and collaboration due to the many stakeholders involved.

REHABILITATION INTERVENTION FOR RETURN-TO-WORK
Current evidence-based knowledge of vocational rehabilitation for people with stroke

The support from employers and coworkers, factors related to the individual, the context of work, and the process for return-to-work are all important factors for a successful outcome.[36]

Interventions developed to promote return-to-work for all with work disabilities generally involve people at the workplace, an important arena for action.[36,37] In a systematic review of the evidence for return-to-work interventions after acquired brain injuries, including stroke, different components or combinations of components in interventions or rehabilitation programs were revealed.[37] The authors found that there was strong evidence that work-directed interventions, for example, adaptation of work tasks in combination with education and coaching, were associated with successful return-to-work after stroke. In the review, the authors also found indications for a positive outcome in the return-to-work process when providing work-directed interventions in combination with training of various skills as work-related and social skills including coping and emotional support. The review also underlined the significance of components in the programs such as early intervention, tailoring work and work-place adjustments, involvement of the employer, and work practice. Successful intervention for return-to-work is dependent on whether the individuals' former work and workplace was available and on a constructive cooperation with the employer.[37] Donker-Cools et al. also found that work-directed interventions, that is, addressing the work, the workplace, and involving the employer were proven to facilitate the return-to-work process for people with various diagnoses and were beneficial regardless of underlying cause to an acquired brain injury. These findings imply that a broader view on the choice of vocational rehabilitation programs can be recommended as will be described in the coming paragraphs, that is, both stroke-specific and traumatic brain injury-oriented rehabilitation programs will be included.

> ### Main Message
>
> Workplace and work-directed interventions are important for a successful return-to-work. Early contact with the workplace, tailoring work and workplace adjustments, involvement of the employer as well as coworkers, and work practice are important components in vocational rehabilitation programs.

Vocational Rehabilitation Intervention Programs

There are few vocational rehabilitation programs that are designed specifically for persons with stroke that have been evaluated.[37] In a review of vocational rehabilitation models for persons with traumatic brain injury, Tyerman divided the models into three main groups; (1) integrated or added vocational rehabilitation components; (2) programs adapted for persons with acquired brain injury, also known as a supported employment model or individual placement and support (IPS) model; (3) case coordination/resource facilitation models.[38]

There are few studies and limited evidence regarding the model with integrated or added vocational rehabilitation components or for the supported employment model used for persons with acquired

brain injury.[39] Fadyl et al. reported that the strongest evidence was found for the case coordination model. In this section of the chapter we will describe the content of three vocational rehabilitation programs from different contexts and cultures. The first two of these programs have been evaluated in randomized controlled trials and the third program was tested in a feasibility trial. They are all based on the case coordination model. Key components in this model are early intervention, a hospital-based vocational case coordinator who assists in developing a vocational plan, on-the-job assessments, coaching and support to the person with stroke, work adjustments, support and education to employers and colleagues, and regular follow-up at the workplace.

The programs that will be outlined are: (1) a workplace intervention program from South Africa, (2) a resource facilitation program for return-to-work and participation in home and community from the United States, (3) an early stroke-specific vocational rehabilitation program from the UK.

The Workplace Intervention Program

The 6-week program, administered by a physiotherapist and an occupational therapist, was tailored according to the stroke survivor's functioning and challenges at the workplace.[30] The program was initiated about 5 to 6 weeks after stroke onset and initiated the return-to-work process. All sessions except for the assessments took place at the workplace.

The stroke survivors were seen at the workplace once a week for a 1-h session.

Usual rehabilitation at the clinic continued alongside the return-to-work program. While participating in this vocational rehabilitation, the specific job requirements of the person with stroke were taken into consideration.

Outline of the Workplace Intervention Program

Week one: Assessment of work skills was performed including work modules identifying potential problems such as: visual discrimination; eye-hand coordination; form and spatial perception; manual dexterity; color discrimination; cognitive problems, and job-specific physical demand factors. Further a questionnaire was used to gain insight about the person's job skill discretion and job demands. The assessments provided a basis for formulating rehabilitation plans by gaining insight into the persons' skills in relation to job demands.

Week two: Interviews with the person with stroke and employer were performed separately to gain knowledge on perceived barriers and enablers of return-to-work. A meeting was arranged where the therapist, the person with stroke, and the employer together developed a plan to meet identified barriers and to strengthen the enablers. The workplace intervention plan did not, at this stage, mean that the employee should return to work immediately and the intervention was still part of the rehabilitation at the clinic.

Week three. Actions to reduce barriers identified during week two were implemented. A workplace visit with the person with stroke was carried out to show what he/she usually did at work and which work tasks that could be performed safely and which were now too demanding. The visit included vocational counseling/coaching; emotional support; work environment adaptation; advice on coping strategies to compensate for mobility and other activity limitations; and, management of fatigue. A social worker/psychologist/speech therapist was involved if necessary. A plan for possible work adaptations was discussed (e.g., working less hours at the beginning; individual tailoring of working hours; using technical aids; doing work tasks that demand less strength and mobility while recovering).

Weeks four, five, and six: The therapist monitored the progress, and made necessary adjustments according to the stroke survivor's and the employer's needs. The return-to-work intervention was performed at the workplace while the persons with stroke continued with their usual therapy at the clinic.

The Resource Facilitation Program

This program focusing on resource facilitation continued for 6 months.[40] The persons were eligible for the program if they had had their acquired brain injury less than a year ago. All persons with acquired brain injury were seen in an initial face-to-face evaluation and were assigned to one of two individuals who served as resource facilitators. The resource facilitators contacted the persons with stroke every 2 weeks. The services were provided in various settings and through telephone contact, including inpatient and outpatient neurorehabilitation clinics, at home, in the community, and at the work place. The focus of the intervention was to proactively engage the former employer of the person with acquired brain injury in a return-to-work plan. Strategies used to promote return-to-work were employer education, discussions on and development of return-to-work schedules, and utilization of job supports through both occupational therapists and employment specialists in collaboration with the state vocational rehabilitation agency.

The support to the persons with acquired brain injury varied and was individualized based on their needs directly or indirectly related to return-to-work. The support included, for example, arranging transportation, promoting access to mental health services, and assisting with access to a variety of state agency resources. The facilitators provided the persons with acquired brain injury approximately 10 h of intervention during the program. The facilitators had access to persons for supervision and clinical problem solving, and case conferences with a vocational rehabilitation counselor from the vocational rehabilitation state agency.

Early Stroke Specific Vocational Rehabilitation Program

This vocational rehabilitation program was run by an occupational therapist who worked in collaboration with rehabilitation staff on the stroke wards, neurological outpatient rehabilitation services, early supported discharge teams, community stroke services, vocational rehabilitation teams, and the employers, as well as other services and agencies.[41] The intervention usually started within the first 30 days post stroke. The program consisted of three phases: early intervention and work preparation, phased return-to-work, and sustaining work return, which included several different components that will be described in the following.

Early Intervention and Work Preparation

Early after stroke a conversation took place between the person with stroke and the occupational therapist about how to ensure that return to his/her work was something to consider. Assessment of impact of stroke on work ability was then conducted, as well as analysis of job demands. Involvement of family members and employers was initiated. Information, education, and provision of support to the person with stroke and the family were provided according to individual needs. Activities to prepare for returning to work were encouraged. Such activities, intended to be performed at home, could entail practicing physical, cognitive, or communication skills depending on consequences of the stroke and job demands. The therapist communicated with the workplace, had a case coordination role, and initiated contact with other services and sectors to ensure that the vocational rehabilitation was well coordinated without overlaps.

Phased Return-to-Work

The second phase included planning and implementing a phased return-to-work process. This could entail a workplace visit in which negotiations were held between the person with stroke and the employer about realistic timing of return-to-work and necessary workplace adjustments. The employer received information and education to increase the understanding of the impact of the stroke on the person with stroke and how this might influence the work ability.

Sustaining Work Return

In the third phase of the program when the person with stroke had returned to work the occupational therapist implemented regular workplace visits/reviews with the focus of sustaining work. Communication with the person who had returned to work and the employer regarding progress, need of modifications, and so on was carried out. The contact with the person with stroke and the workplace was sustained as long as there was a need and then gradually withdrawn.

> **Main Message**
>
> The key components in the case coordination model are early intervention, a hospital-based vocational case coordinator who assists in developing a vocational plan, on-the-job assessments, coaching and support, work adjustments, support and education to employers and colleagues, and regular follow-up at the workplace.

COORDINATOR

The advantage of a coordinator in return-to-work after stroke has been emphasized in several studies. A stroke coordinator may remediate the stakeholders' divergent perspectives and increase collaboration between them, supply information on the consequences of stroke, and how these could be dealt with in the work environment.[42,43]

A coordinator with specialist knowledge of stroke and work rehabilitation could also deliver guidelines for setting up vocational training[43] and be a valuable source of knowledge for the person with stroke, as well as other stakeholders in the return-to-work process.[44] In a recent study, the coordinator was seen as an authority, which had a role in improving communication between stakeholders and also being a lifeline to the person with stroke in a longterm process.[44]

Rehabilitation coordinators have been used in different contexts with different mandates. In Sweden, a development of the coordinator role has taken place during the last decade. However, this model in which a coordinator in medical rehabilitation has the specific

aim to improve collaboration among stakeholders during work-related rehabilitation has only been reported from Sweden. The work coordinator's work tasks/job assignments may differ according to the organization and general healthcare, or specialist clinics. The generalist coordinator usually has broad knowledge about many different areas while the specialist coordinator typically has deeper knowledge in specific areas. In rehabilitation after stroke, as well as after many other conditions, there is a need for specialist knowledge. Regardless, synchronized interventions are more cost-effective than interventions without collaboration according to a literature review by Caroll and coworkers.[45]

> **Main Message**
>
> In rehabilitation after stroke there is a need for a coordinator with specialist knowledge who can increase collaboration between stakeholders, supply information on the consequences of stroke, and how these could be dealt with in the work environment.

ASSESSMENTS USED IN THE RETURN-TO-WORK PROCESS

The return-to-work process takes place in the interaction of multiple systems and stakeholders and thereby considers biomedical, psychological, and social factors that can be described as a balance between personal resources and the work demands.[46] There is a consensus about work capacity being influenced by several factors. As introduced earlier, Ilmarinen describes four influencing components: (1) health and functional capacity, which is the basis for work ability; (2) education, occupational skills, competence; (3) attitudes and motivation for work; and (4) content of work, work organization, work community, and management.[10] Assessment used in the return-to-work process should therefore cover these areas. People who get medical rehabilitation interventions after their stroke often have their strengths and limitations (both physical and cognitive) evaluated by the rehabilitation team corresponding to the first component, that is, health and functional capacity. This information together with a mapping of the person's work history, that is, education, skills, and competence (corresponding to the second component) is valuable when initiating a plan for return-to-work. Moreover, the motivation for return-to-work and attitudes toward work, representing component number three, are fundamental for the return-to-work process. Having collected this information, a dialogue can start with the employer at the workplace about suitable work tasks, working hours, and need of environmental adjustments, that is, component four.

There is a need for adequate, valid, and reliable methods for assessing work ability, valuable for both the individual on sick-leave and for the society as a whole. Evaluation of persons' work ability is important for returning to work or sustaining work or finding a new job. Through sound and precise work assessments the person can be guided to suitable interventions using a minimum of rehabilitation resources.[47] Different assessments can be used in evaluation of work ability and environmental factors in relation to work covering the different components that together configure a person's work ability.

> **Main Message**
>
> Work capacity can be described as a balance between personal resources and the work demands. It is influenced by (1) health and functional capacity, which is the basis for work ability, (2) education, occupational skills, competence, (3) attitudes and motivation for work and (4) content of work, work organization, work community, and management. Assessments used in the return-to-work process should therefore cover these areas.

THE EXPERIENCE OF RETURN-TO-WORK OF PEOPLE WITH STROKE, THE MEANING OF WORK

The experiences of people with stroke of their return-to-work process have been reported in several interview studies. Work has been referred to as important to a person's identity and holds multiple meanings that are important for motivation.[3] Returning to work has also been equaled with being back to normal.[31] Even if it is common that return-to-work is a major goal after stroke in younger ages, the rehabilitation phase can generate mixed feelings, including both trust and fear for the future work-situation.[31,42,48] The insecurity of their future work-ability was sometimes a source of fear when they realized that one option was to be out of the labor market, being early retired. Other times they were hopeful, feeling confident when the work trial went well.[42]

Adaptations made to accomplish an acceptable work performance were experienced with mixed feelings if the person with stroke did not realize a need of such alterations.[42] Learning about consequences after stroke helped them to appreciate advices and strategies how to deal with those hindrances. The value of including the person with stroke in different decisions during the work rehabilitation phase was further underlined in a recent study. Being involved in the planning helped them follow and feel that they had a roadmap for return-to-work to guide them.[44]

People with stroke have revealed experiences of lack of support in the process of return-to-work including handling the consequences of stroke at work.[49] One main factor that was experienced as facilitating return-to-work for persons with stroke was a supportive employer[49] in combination with strong own motivation[50] and modifications at the work place.[42] In a meta-synthesis of qualitative studies exploring experiences of return-to-work after stroke, identification of strengths and weaknesses of the person and the employer's readiness to provide facilitation were found to affect the person's motivation for return-to-work and therefore crucial for success.[51] Schwarz and coworkers discussed similar aspects in their metasynthesis of qualitative studies aiming to identify hindrances and facilitators for return to work after stroke.[46] They found three basic principles; adaptiveness, purposefulness, and cooperativeness important to consider in rehabilitation strategies. Adaptiveness entails both the person with stroke being ready to adapt to his/her present work ability, as well as readiness and understanding at the workplace for adaptations needed. To find work and vocational rehabilitation purposeful was underlined as the driving force for the often demanding process of return-to-work. Successful return-to-work after stroke depends on cooperation between all involved stakeholders, which makes the process both more effective and clear.

> **Main Message**
>
> The vocational rehabilitation phase can generate mixed feelings, including both trust and fear for the future work-situation. Being involved in the planning for the return—to-work gave the person with stroke a roadmap, and learning about consequences after stroke helped them to appreciate advices and strategies how to deal with those hindrances. To experience work and vocational rehabilitation as meaningful was highlighted as the driving force for the many times demanding return-to-work process.

EXPERIENCES OF CO-WORKERS AND EMPLOYERS

Employers and coworkers face complex emotional and practical issues during the return-to-work process for people with stroke.[52] Through studies of return-to-work after other illness than stroke, an understanding of the co-workers important role in the social context of the work has grown. These studies underline the value of all workplace actors, especially coworkers, to be involved in planning for the return-to-work of a colleague, paying attention to different aspects of work, task related as well as social.[53,54] A main issue experienced by the employer and the co-workers of a person with stroke was the uncertainty how stroke had affected the work capacity of the employee.[52] This has been confirmed in an ongoing Swedish study. A recurring concern was not to put too much pressure on the person with stroke which may negatively affect the health. Advice and support from clinicians knowledgeable in rehabilitation of people with stroke were often welcomed as employers reported a lack of knowledge and experience of assisting people in return-to-work process, and the quality of support networks they access varies.[52] Close cooperation between the individual, health/rehabilitation professionals, and supportive employers was experienced as being of great importance for return-to-work. As work rehabilitation after stroke can last over long time, there is a need of extended support; sometimes, recurrent intervention over time are required.[43]

Main Message

Employers and co-workers have important roles in vocational rehabilitation. To support a colleague during the return-to-work process, they need information about the impact of stroke on work ability and advice for planning the rehabilitation.

REFERENCES

1. Waddell G, Burton AK, Kendall NAS. *Vocational Rehabilitation: What Works, for Whom, and when?* London: TSO; 2008.
2. International Classification of Functioning. *Disability and Health, ICF.* Geneva: World Health Organization; 2001.
3. Waddel G, Burton K. *Is Work Good for Your Health and Wellbeing?* United Kingdom: Department for Work and Pensions, The Stationary Office; 2006.
4. Coutu M-F, Coté D, Baril R. The work-disabled patient. In: Losiel P, Anema J, eds. *Handbook of Work Disability.* New York: Springer; 2014:15–29.
5. Naess H, Nyland K, Thomassen L, et al. Longterm outcome of cerebral infarction in young adults. *Acta Neurol Scand.* 2004;110:107–112.
6. Young AE, Roessler RT, Wasiak R, et al. A developmental conceptualization of return to work. *J Occup Rehabil.* 2005;15:557–568.
7. Wasiak R, Young A, Roessler R, et al. Measuring return to work. *J Occup Rehabil.* 2007;17:766–781.
8. Lederer V, Loisel P, Rivard M, et al. Exploration the diversity of conceptualizations of work (dis)ability: a scoping review of published definitions. *J Occup Rehabil.* 2014;24:242–267.
9. Loisel P, Anema JR, Feuerstein M, MacEachen E, Pransky G, Costa-Black K. *Handbook of Work Disability.* New York: Springer; 2014.
10. Ilmarinen V, Ilmarien J, Huuhtanen P, et al. Examining the factorial structure, measurement invariance and convergent and discriminent validity of a novel self-report measure of work ability: work ability – personal radar. *Ergonomics.* 2015;58:1445–1460.
11. Arwer HJ, Schults M, Meesters JJL, et al. Return to work 2-5 years after stroke: a cross sectional study in a hospital-based population. *J Occup Rehabil.* 2017;27:239–246.
12. Rolfs A, Fazekas F, Grittner U, et al. Acute cerebrovascular disease in the young: the stroke in young Fabry patients study. *Stroke.* 2013;44:340–349.
13. Rosengren A, Giang KW, Lappas G, et al. Twenty-four-year trends in the incidence of Ischemic stroke in Sweden from 1987 to 2010. *Stroke.* 2013;44:2388–2393.
14. The European Registers of Stroke (EROS) Investigators. Incidence of stroke in Europe at the beginning of the 21st century. *Stroke.* 2009;40:1557–1563.
15. Heart Disease and Stroke Statistics—2010 Update. A Report from the American Heart Association. *Circulation.* 2010;121:7. Available at: http://circ.ahajournals.org/.
16. Townsend N, Wickramasinghe K, Bhatnagar P, et al. *Coronary Heart Disease Statistics. A Compendium of Health Statistics. 2012 edition.* London: British Heart Foundation; 2012.
17. Daniel K, Wolfe CDA, Busch MA, et al. What are the social consequences of stroke in working aged adults? A systematic review. *Stroke.* 2009;40:431–440.
18. Riks-Stroke. *Ett år efter stroke. 1-årsuppföljniung 2009-livssituation, tillgodosedda behov och resultat av vårdens och omsorgens insatser.* [Eng: Riks-Stroke, the Swedish Stroke Register: 1-year follow-up 2009-lifesituation, fulfilled needs and results of health care services interventions]; 2010. Available at: http://www.riksstroke.org/wp-content/uploads/2014/05/RS-1-årsuppf.rapport-2010-års-data.pdf.
19. *Stroke Association State of the Nation: Stroke Statistics;* January 2015. Available at: https://www.stroke.org.uk/sites/default/files/stroke_statistics_2015.pdf.
20. Wolf TJ, Baum C, Connor LT. Changing face of stroke: implications for occupational therapy practice. *Am J Occup Ther.* 2009;63:621–625.
21. Larsen LP, Biering K, Johnsen SP, et al. Self-rated health and return to work after first-time stroke. *J Rehabil Med.* 2016;48:339–345.

22. Noortje AMM, Rutten-Jacobs L, Arntz R, et al. Long-term increased risk of unemployment after young stroke. A long-term follow-up study. *Neurology®*. 2014;83:1132–1138.
23. Donker-Cols B, Wind H, Frings-Dresen M. Prognostic factors of return to work after traumatic or non-traumatic acquired brain injury. *Disabil Rehabil*. 2016;38:733–741.
24. Treger J, Giaquinto S, Ring H. Return to work in stroke patients. *Disabil Rehabil*. 2007;29:1397–1403.
25. Wang Y-C, Kapellusch J, Garg A. Important factors influencing the return to work after stroke. *Work*. 2014;47:553–559.
26. Wozniak MA, Kitte S. Return to work after ischemic stroke: a methodological review. *Neuroepidemiology*. 2002;21:159–166.
27. Tanaka H, Toyonaga T, Hashimoto H. Functional and occupational characteristics predictive of a return to work within 18 months after stroke in Japan: implications for rehabilitation. *Int Arch Occup Environ Health*. 2014;87:445–453.
28. Fride Y, Adamit T, Maeir A, et al. What are the correlates of cognition and participation to return to work after first ever mild stroke? *Top Stroke Rehabil*. 2015;22:317–325.
29. Andersen G, Christensen D, Kirkewold M, et al. Post-stroke fatigue and return to work: a 2 year follow-up. *Acta Neurol Scand*. 2012;125, 248-25.
30. Ntsiea MV, Van Aswegen H, Lord S, et al. The effect of a workplace intervention programme on return to work after stroke: a randomized control trial. *Clin Rehabil*. 2015;29:663–673.
31. Alaszewski A, Alaszewski H, Potter J, et al. Working after stroke: survivors' experiences and perceptions of barriers to and facilitators of the return to paid employment. *Disabil Rehabil*. 2007;29:1858–1869.
32. Chang WH, Sohn MK, Lee J, et al. Return to work after stroke: the Kosco study. *J Rehabil Med*. 2016;48:273–279.
33. Westerlind E, Persson HC, Sunnerhagen KS. Return to work after a stroke in working age persons; a six-year follow up. *PLoS One*. 2017;12. e0169759.
34. Loisel P, Buchbinder R, Hazard R, et al. Prevention of work disability due to musculoskeletal disorders: the challenge of implementing evidence. *J Occup Rehabil*. 2005;15:507–524.
35. Young AE, Wasiak R, Roessler RT, et al. Return-to-work outcomes following work disability: stakeholder motivations, interests and concerns. *J Occup Rehabil*. 2005;15:543–556.
36. Ekberg K, Eklund M, Hensing G. *Återgång i arbete. Processer, bedömningar, åtgärder*. Lund: Studentlitteratur; 2015.
37. Donker-Cools B, Daams J, Wind H, et al. Effective return-to-work interventions after acquired brain injury: a systematic review. *Brain Injury*. 2016;30:113–131.
38. Tyerman A. Vocational rehabilitation after traumatic brain injury: models and services. *Neurorehabilitation*. 2012;31:51–62.
39. Fadyl K, McPherson K. Approaches to vocational rehabilitation after traumatic brain injury: a review of the evidence. *J Head Trauma Rehabil*. 2009;24:195–212.
40. Trexler L, Trexler L, Malec J, et al. Prospective randomized controlled trial of resource facilitation on community participation and vocational outcome following brain injury. *J Head Trauma Rehabil*. 2010;25:440–446.
41. Grant M. Developing, delivering and evaluating stroke specific vocational rehabilitation: a feasibility randomised controlled trial. *PhD thesis, University of Nottingham*; 2016. http://eprints.nottingham.ac.uk/35108/.
42. Vestling M, Ramel E, Iwarsson S. Thoughts and experiences from returning to work after stroke. *Work*. 2013;45:201–211.
43. Hellman T, Bergström E, Eriksson G, et al. Return to work after stroke – important factors shared and contrasted by five stakeholder groups. *Work*. 2016;55:901–911.
44. Öst-Nilsson A, Eriksson G, Johansson U, et al. Experiences of the return to work process after stroke while participating in a person-centered rehabilitation program. *Scan J Occup Ther*. 2016;11:1–8.
45. Carroll C, Rick J, Pilgrim H, et al. Workplace involvement improves return to work rates among employees with back pain on long-term sick leave: a systematic review of the effectiveness and cost-effectiveness of interventions. *Disabil Rehabil*. 2010;32:607–621.
46. Schwarz B, Claros-Salinas D, Streibelt M. Meta-synthesis of qualitative research on facilitators and barriers of return to work after stroke. *J Occup Rehabil*. 2017. https://doi.org/10.1007/s10926-017-9713-2.
47. Sandkvist J. *Medical Dissertation, No. 1009. Development and Evaluation of Validity and Utility of the Instrument Assessment of Work Performance (AWP)*. Sweden: Linköping University; 2007.
48. Hartke J, Trierweiler R, Bode R. Critical factors related to return to work after stroke: a qualitative study. *Top Stroke Rehabil*. 2011;18:341–351.
49. KH WYC, Byers K, et al. Barriers and facilitators of return to work for individuals with strokes: perspectives of the stroke survivor, vocational specialist, and employer. *Top Stroke Rehabil*. 2011;18:325–340.
50. Gilworth G, Phil M, Cert A, et al. Personal experiences of returning to work following stroke: an exploratory study. *Work*. 2009;34:95–103.
51. Frostad Liaset I, Lorås H. Perceived factors in return to work after acquired brain injury: a qualitative meta-synthesis. *Scan J Occup Ther*. 2016;23:446–457.
52. Coole C, Radford K, Grant M, et al. Returning to work after stroke: perspectives of employer stakeholders, a qualitative study. *J Occup Rehabil*. 2013;23:406–418.
53. Tjulin Å, Maceachen E, Edvardsson Stiwne E, et al. The social interaction of return to work explored from co-workers experience. *Disabil Rehabil*. 2011;33:21–22.
54. Dunstan D, MacEachen E. Bearing the brunt: co-workers' experiences of work reintegration processes. *J Occup Rehabil*. 2013;23:44–54.

CHAPTER 16

Driving Rehabilitation

ABIODUN AKINWUNTAN, PHD, MPH, MBA • HANNES DEVOS, PHD

INTRODUCTION

Driving is a complex and multidimensional task that requires seamless and timely integration of many motor, visual, and cognitive skills to adequately react to many transient events in a highly dynamic environment.[1] In spite of the complexity of driving and the skillset required to drive safely on public roads, the ability to drive in the highly motorized world of today is considered a right rather than a privilege.[2,3] Inability to drive has been associated with reduced physical activities, social status, economic wellbeing, and depression.[3–5] Loss of driving privileges, particularly among individuals with debilitating medical conditions, can also lead to poor health outcomes, increased healthcare costs, and decreased access to care.[4,5] While it can be expected that survivors of a severe stroke will not contemplate returning to driving, it is typical for survivors of moderate or mild stroke to consider returning to driving.[6] In this chapter, we will focus on opportunities that are available to stroke survivors who wish to retrain their driving-related skills and improve their chances of resuming safe driving on public roads.

In this chapter:

1. Some of the different methods of retraining driving skills in stroke survivors reported in the literature will be examined and a summary of their findings will be described.
2. Common models of driving that have been proposed to deconstruct the complexity of driving will be examined.
3. Paradigms underlying different training approaches will be discussed.
4. An example of a structured training program will be presented.
5. Possibilities for vehicle modification and adaptive equipment will be discussed.
6. Alternatives to driving resumption will be presented.
7. A summary of the chapter and most important take-home messages will be presented.

DRIVING TRAINING METHODS

Only a few studies have been reported on attempts to retrain driving-related skills of stroke survivors. The attempts involved the use of one of five different methods of training, which included (1) paper-and-pencil, (2) computerized-video, (3) Dynavision (Dynavision International LLC, West Chester, Ohio), (4) simulator, and (5) on-road training.

Paper-and-Pencil-Based Driving Training

Paper-and-pencil-based training is one of the earliest forms of intervention to improve driving performance of individuals who survive a brain injury.[7] Given that the driving performance of some brain damaged persons is directly related to the extent of impairment observed during a paper-and-pencil-based evaluation of driving-related skills, it is hoped that benefits from the training program will generalize to improvements in impaired motor, visual, and cognitive skills necessary to return safe driving. The perceptual evaluation is made up of tests such as the picture completion, picture arrangement, and block design tests that have been assumed to measure visuo-perceptual problems. Other tests are symbol digit modalities test, trail making tests, short memory test, and the letter cancellation test, all of which require intact visual scanning skills. The training activities, which are modified to appear driving-related, are comprised of target cancellation and pathfinding tasks, pattern visualization and identification tasks, visual line tracing and pattern matching tasks, and analysis of construction designs on pages of paper. The benefits of the paper-and-pencil training program were investigated in a study that included five stroke survivors who were between 5 and 85 months post onset of stroke. Each survivor received 8–10 h of individualized paper-and-pencil-based perceptual training for 5–9 sessions.[7] Participants' performance on the perceptual evaluation and on a practical on-road test after training showed significant improvements in

Stroke Rehabilitation. https://doi.org/10.1016/B978-0-323-55381-0.00016-0

comparison to performance on the same evaluation and road test before training. Improvement in perceptual skills accounted for 53% of the variance of the difference observed before and after training. Specific driving skills such as gap acceptance, car positioning, visual observation, lane tracking, and speed control improved after training.

Computerized Video-Based Driving Training

In a recent randomized controlled trial,[8] Mazer and colleagues evaluated the effect of a visual attention training program using a computerized visual attention analyzer on driving after stroke. Ninety-seven stroke survivors (<6 months post stroke onset) were randomly allocated to either an experimental or a control group. The experimental group received visual information processing and attention training on the visual attention analyzer. The control group received visuo-perceptual training of driving-related skills using ordinary computer software. Both training instruments were touch screen-based and were of equal sizes to create similar experience across both groups. Irrespective of group allocation, each participant received 20 sessions of training, which lasted 30–60 min per session at a rate of 2–4 sessions per week. All participants performed a battery of visuo-perceptual evaluations and a useful field of view test that measured percentage reduction in field of view before and after training. Additionally, participants performed a "daily attention test" and an on-road driving evaluation post training. Before performing the posttraining evaluations however, all participants received 4 sessions training on use of the original or modified accelerator pedal, brake pedal, and steering wheel in a simulator to avoid extremely poor performance in the on-road test. The pass or fail outcome after the on-road test were compared to those of a historical cohort of stroke survivors who received no driving-related training or rehabilitation. Results revealed that performance by the experimental and control participants did not differ at posttraining for the on-road test, visuo-perceptual evaluations, and the "daily attention" test. The rate of success in the road test was also not significantly different between the study participants and those from the historical cohort. However, there was significant difference between groups in the outcome of the useful field of view test post training in favor of the experimental group that received training on the instrument and tasks of the test.

Dynavision-Based Driving Training

The use of Dynavision (Dynavision International LLC, West Chester, Ohio) to retrain the driving ability stroke survivors was reported by Klavora et al.[9] The Dynavision apparatus, which can be used to retrain and assess peripheral visual attention and scanning, among other tasks, is a wall-mounted board (1.2 m^2) containing 64 small buttons arranged in a pattern of five nested rings (see Fig. 16.1). Target buttons are either randomly illuminated and extinguished during apparatus-paced tasks or the button remains illuminated until it is manually pressed during the self-paced tasks. For the peripheral visual attention training task, a person is asked to fix his or her central vision on a point while using peripheral vision to locate the illuminated button. The user is free to shift his head and eyes to locate the illuminated button in the scanning task. Moderate benefit from the training program was presented in a study that included 10 stroke survivors who were between 6 and 17 months post stroke and who trained using the Dynavision for 20 min per session, 3 sessions a week, over 6 weeks.[9] Performances on the Dynavision tasks, with the exception of choice visual reaction time and anticipation time, significantly improved from pre-to posttraining. Six out of 10 who participated in the study passed an on-road test post training. The findings of a more recent study by Crotty and George,[10] however, failed to show the benefits of retraining the driving-related skills of stroke survivors using the Dynavision apparatus. In the study,[10] which included 26 stroke survivors who were at least 1 month

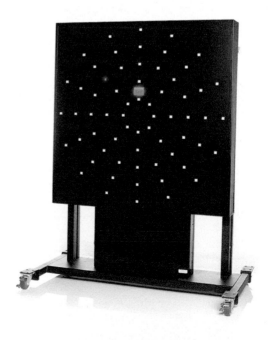

FIG. 16.1 A Dynavision system.

post stroke, 13 randomly allocated to the experimental group received 3 sessions per week training as described in the equipment manual[11] for 6 weeks on the Dynavision. The other 13 participants (controls) were placed on a wait list for 6 weeks. Experimental participants did not show better performance than controls in any of the outcome measures, which included an on-road test, response speed, visual scanning, and self-efficacy.

Simulator-Based Driving Training

Kent and colleagues[12] reported the first use of a simulator to retrain impaired driving-related skills in a population that included 44 stroke survivors. Not only was the description of the simulator excluded, detailed content and duration of the training program were not provided. The training included becoming familiar with laws regarding disabled driving, ability to read traffic signs, and a modified version of an official new driver licensing evaluation. When possible, training also involved driving a vehicle around the training ground, then to residential areas, and eventually to complex freeways. Forty-one of the 44 stroke survivors who participated in the study received certificates that allowed them to resume driving based on performances in a written test and road test after training.

A more advanced driving simulator-based training program was reported by Cimolino and Balkovec.[13] The driving simulator consisted of driver seats with all necessary operational parts of a car such as accelerator and brake pedals, steering wheel, left-turn indicator lever, and horn. Training was conducted by instructing an individual on driving through series of driving-related films displayed on a computer screen attached to the simulator. Trainees responded naturally to visual and audio cues from the films by pressing the accelerator pedal to increase speed, braking to reduce speed and stop, turning the steering wheel in curves, and to avoid accidents. Errors in accelerating, speeding, braking, and steering were automatically registered in a computer connected to the simulator. In the study, which included 41 stroke survivors who were between 4 and 8 months poststroke onset, participants received between 3 and 8 sessions of training which lasted between 2 and 7 h in the driving simulator. Results of performance in the driving simulator tasks after completion of training revealed moderate benefits from the program. Twenty-five out of 37 stroke survivors who completed the training program demonstrated satisfactory driving skills during an on-road test and were recommended to an official authority to be considered for a driver's license. Follow-up of

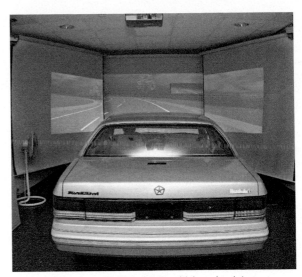

FIG. 16.2 A high-fidelity driving simulator.

participants at the licensing office showed that 21 out of the 25 stroke patients were licensed to resume driving (Fig. 16.2).

With the advent of more realistic fidelity of the simulated traffic environments, traffic, situations, graphic images, and improving flexibilities of the programing languages, the use of driving simulators to retrain the driving skills of stroke survivors is more common. In a study that included 83 survivors of a first-ever mild or moderate stroke, who were less than 75 years old, and between 6 and 9 weeks post stroke, 42 experimental participants received structured training in a high-fidelity driving simulator (*full description of the training is provided later in this chapter*).[14] Forty-one controls also received structured paper-and-pencil-based driving-related cognitive training. Each participant, irrespective of group membership, received 15 h of training over a period of 6 weeks in addition to standard rehabilitation. Significantly more experimental participants (73%) than controls (42%) who were officially evaluated for their driving ability about 3 months after completion of training succeeded and were legally allowed to resume driving. The simulator-based program was found to be better at retraining divided and selective attentions skills, anticipation of traffic events, perception of traffic signs, making a left turn at intersections, visual behavior and communication, and overall quality of traffic participation than the paper-and-pencil-based program.[15,16] Participants who received simulator-based driving training were three times the odds more likely to pass the official driving evaluation in comparison to those who received the paper-and-pencil-based training.[17] The report of a 5-year follow-up study of participants in the randomized controlled trial showed that 18 of 30 (60%) stroke survivors who received the simulator-based program versus 15 of the 31 (48%) who received the paper-and-pencil-based training still passed the official driving evaluation.[17]

The potential benefits from simulator-based driving training was also reported in a more recent randomized controlled study in which 23 stroke survivors were randomized into an experimental group and 22 survivors into a control group.[18] While the control group received no intervention, the experimental group received simulator-based training that was conducted in 60-min sessions, at 2 sessions per week over 8 weeks. Although the training protocol was standardized, individual programs were modified to address each experimental participant's deficits. Following completion of training, 86% of participants with moderate stroke-related deficits who were trained in the driving simulator passed an on-road test while only 17% in the control group passed the same on-road test. There were no differences for those with severe impairments.

On-Road Driving Training

On-road driving evaluation is still considered the gold standard of the determination of an individual's driving ability. Typically, the process of determining the driving ability of novice drivers involves an off-road assessment of vision and knowledge of driving rules along with a practical on-road assessment. Naturally, it is logical to assume that the best way to retrain driving after a mild stroke is to put survivors behind the wheel, in a real car, and during real traffic. Quigley and DeLisa[19] evaluated the effect of on-road driving training in 23 left-sided and 27 right-sided brain lesion stroke survivors who were at least 6 months post onset of stroke. For survivors who were judged as capable of benefiting from training based on the outcome of an extensive pre-driving evaluation, instructions were first given in a classroom before proceeding to the on-road driving training. The on-road training always started in a parking lot where familiarity with the brake pedal, accelerator pedal, and steering control were trained. Training continued in residential areas with low traffic before progressing to freeway driving. The on-road training program was completed in 6–13 sessions after which participants were immediately referred to perform an official written and driving test. Seventeen out of 23 (74%) of left-sided lesion and 14 out of 27 (52%) right-sided lesion survivors passed the official driving assessment. However, issues such as continuous drifting

to one side of the road in survivors with unilateral neglect, confusion while driving in cluttered traffic, and abrupt stopping prompted suspension of the training in 9 survivors with right-sided lesion. A study that involved 34 first-ever stroke survivors,[20] who performed a comprehensive driving evaluation that included a driving test, examined the benefit of on-road training of stroke survivors. Thirteen of the 15 stroke survivors who had initially failed an on-road test eventually passed the test after 6–12 h of on-road driving training. However, authors doubt if the on-road training program led to improvement in driving function, since there were no associated improvements in any visuo-cognitive functions. The authors surmised that the passage of time, awareness of driving difficulties, or familiarization with the test process led to passing the driving test the second time.

COMMON MODELS OF DRIVING

Many methods of retraining impaired driving-related skills in stroke survivors have been attempted with low to moderately high benefits, and with moderate generalization to on-road driving performance. As mentioned earlier, driving is a complex and dynamic activity involving timely and simultaneous interaction of multiple skills. An insight into the multiple constructs underlying driving is needed to better appreciate why the rehabilitation of driving may be very challenging.

Several models have been proposed to deconstruct the multidimensionality and complexity of driving. A few of the models are commonly cited in the literature. Summala[21] proposed the *motivational model* in which the risk level involved in any driving situation is said to be dependent on the extent of motor, visual, and cognitive resources allocated. The model postulates that driving is a transient and situation-specific activity that is self-paced, and that a driver selects the amount of risk that he or she is willing to take. The limitation of this model is that it is too focused on what the driver does in traffic situations (risk acceptance) rather than on the multiple factors that influence driving.[22]

Another commonly cited model is the *information-processing model*[23] in which it is assumed that driving occurs in a sequence of stages. A proper *perception* of the traffic situation is needed to make an appropriate *decision* on what to do, which is then followed by *selecting a response* and finally *executing* the decided action. The limitation of the model is the lack of incorporation of the motivational or emotional components of driving.[24] The *cybernetic model* of driving was proposed by Galski et al.[25] It consists of three programs: a general driving program (GDP), a specific driving program (SDP), and a resident diagnostic program (RDP). The GDP is "an expert system that is required to apply road knowledge and operating principles in routine situations, yet maintain the capacity to adapt to new situations with the use of acquired or available information." The GDP uses previous knowledge about driving obtained from education and experience to initiate and direct all current driving-related activities. It also has an executive component that kicks into action as soon as a person decides to drive. The executive function includes activating necessary scanning and attention mechanisms while continuously calculating and processing all driving-related information. The SDP takes information such as destination, distance, time of day, weather, and vehicle, as well as driver condition, into consideration to come up with a plan. The plan is usually specific to the particular driving activity. The RDP uses information obtained from the GDP and the SDP to continuously provide warnings on the potential dangers during each drive activity.

One of the most common models cited in the literature is the model that was proposed by Michon,[24] who described driving as involving three hierarchical levels of cognitive processing namely: operational, tactical, and strategic. The operational level involves driving activities such as stepping on the accelerator and brake pedals, and controlling the steering in response to different traffic situations. Activities at the operational level are highly time-dependent and need to be precise to maintain safety while driving. The tactical level involves the drivers' perceptions and reactions to traffic situations such as speed adaptation, gap acceptance during overtaking, driving through intersections, lane maintenance, and joining the traffic stream. Activities performed at the tactical level are not as time-sensitive as the operational level activities. There is no real-time pressure involved in the strategic level activities. Such activities include planning, the conscious decision to drive, choice of time to drive, and route planning prior to actively entering the vehicle to commence driving.

The skill-based, rule-based, and knowledge-based behaviors during driving were proposed by Rasmussen.[26] The skill-based behavior involves the use of automated sequences that ensure smooth driving processes such as pressing on the gas pedal to increase speed and braking to reduce speed. Rule-based behavior refers to use of common driving rules that are not necessarily written traffic rules. For instance, changing of gear and slowing down when approaching and turning at an intersection. Knowledge-based behavior occurs in situations during which no known driving rule is applicable except personal driving experiences. An example is the knowledge that driving during snow or in heavy fog creates higher accident risks.

In a recent study,[1] we proposed a "top-down" or "bottom-up" model that was developed based on the knowledge gained from the other models described above, and from extensive personal experience with the assessment and rehabilitation of individuals with neurologic conditions, including stroke. Fig. 16.3 tries to show the complexity and interactivity of the multiple factors involved in driving. In unfamiliar situations, recruitment of the appropriate higher-order skills such as planning, decision-making, and judgment to adjust safety buffers (e.g., speed, following distance, lane choice) and to reduce errors is a conscious "top-down" activity. The speed at which any decision is made in the "top-down" mode is dependent on the driver's intelligence, experience, and personality. While the reliance on stored memory of the driving route and usual traffic demand is minimal to nonexistent, it is high on paying attention and accurate perception of the traffic situation. In familiar and unchallenging situations such as driving through a very familiar route, driving is primarily a "bottom-up" activity that requires very little attention and becomes almost automated (a proceduralized, overlearned task performance). The age, personality, experience, disease, fatigue level, and sobriety of the driver also play important roles in the extent to which "top-down" or "bottom-up" control is activated.

PARADIGMS UNDERLYING DIFFERENT TRAINING APPROACHES

Retraining of driving-related motor, visual, and cognitive skills capable of significantly improving the real-life driving ability of stroke survivors has yet to reach its full potential primarily because studies found in the literature have not convincingly demonstrated the benefits from the different training methods discussed above. In the pencil-and-paper-based and Dynavision-based training methods, the training focuses on improving performance in the individual motor, visual, and cognitive skills (restorative training) with the hope that the trainee will be able to use the skills interactively during driving. Cognitive rehabilitation literature suggests that retraining individuals in neurocognitive skills may improve some fundamental elements of cognition, such as attention and visual scanning; however, to activate the iterative loop of perceptual and cognitive input that can lead to behavioral output, the context of

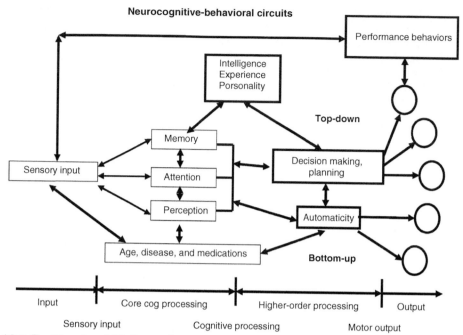

FIG. 16.3 The "Top-down" "Bottom-up" model of driving based on the interaction of basic and higher-order abilities in driving performance.

training needs to be somewhat similar to the actual performance of the activity. In the computerized video-based, simulator-based, and on-road training methods, the focus is on exposing survivors to different driving situations with the hope that such exposure will lead to improvement of the impaired driving-related skills, or compensation for impaired higher-order visuo-cognitive skills (compensatory training) in dynamic and realistic driving situations. Conversely, contextual training of complex driving skills may contribute to more generalized benefits because this approach elicits more natural and reality-based experiences.[27] Restorative and compensatory processes are not mutually exclusive but are interactive and mutually reinforcing.[27] The realistic environment afforded by interactive driving simulator or by on-road training offer ideal platforms for such integrative retraining. The safety implications of exposing trainees to hazardous situations needed to retrain driving-related high-order executive functions should be considered. Driving simulators may be a more appealing instrument to retrain driving skills of stroke survivors at higher risk for injury. Not only do driving simulators enable the possibility of incorporating the knowledge gained from the driving models presented above into the rehabilitation process, it can incorporate features of visual perception,

memory, attention, and directed search in a driving-relevant context.[28] Simulator-based evaluation also enables trainers to retrain and evaluate driving behaviors during near-realistic driving experiences. Although the fidelity of simulation scenarios is constantly improving, currently available systems generate photorealistic images that can nonetheless closely match the actual on-road experience.[29] Other simulator features, such as instant replay, can provide the driver with immediate feedback, which may improve outcomes.[26] Although the issue of "simulator sickness" (feelings of dizziness and nausea), linked to a disjuncture between the simulator's visual cues of movement and the subject's kinesthetic cues of being stationary, remains an issue with some simulators, better mitigation strategies have greatly reduced the frequency and severity of simulation sickness.

AN EXAMPLE OF A STRUCTURED SIMULATOR-BASED TRAINING PROGRAM

Studies have shown that an average of 10 h of training is sufficient to retrain the impaired driving-related skills in most survivors of a mild or moderate stroke. Some mild cases might only require between 5 and 9 h of training to achieve maximum benefits, while some moderate cases might require 11 or more hours of training. Our simulator-based driving training typically lasts 1 h per session, 2−3 sessions per week, over 5 weeks. During each training session, participants' driving skills, especially those they had difficulties with during the pre-training road test, are retrained using an interaction between both restorative and compensatory strategies. Knowledge of performance, knowledge of results, and feedback are provided as necessary during training sessions. Summary feedback is provided at the end of each session.

Two 8.5-mile (A & B) and six 3.5-mile (1−6) scenarios simulating regular day-to-day traffic, but specifically developed to retrain major driving skills and major visuo-cognitive skills required for driving skills, are incorporated throughout the retraining program (see Table 16.1).

Vehicle Modification and Adaptive Equipment

In many cases, stroke survivors require some vehicle modifications to optimize the possibility to resume safe driving on public roads. Commonly prescribed modifications include conversion of the gas pedal to the left, attachment of a spinner knob to the steering wheel, extension or crossover of turn signal lever, and addition of extra mirrors such as a panoramic mirror (blind spot mirror) to improve the field of view. Use of adaptive equipment can also make driving easier for stroke survivors. The most commonly prescribed adaptive equipment are different types of hand controls (e.g., push/pull; push/twist; push/rock; and push/right-angle) that enable the driver to operate the gas pedal and/or brake pedal using the driver's hand in place of the driver's foot. Vehicle modification and adaptive

TABLE 16.1
An Example of a Structured Simulator-Based Training Program

THE DRIVING SKILL AND VISUO-COGNITIVE SKILLS TRAINED IN EACH SCENARIO

Scenario	Driving Skill	Visuo-Cognitive Skills Trained
A (8.5 miles)	All required skills	Integration of all driving-related skills
1 (3.5 miles)	Lane maintenance	Spatial awareness, motor control
2 (3.5 miles)	Adherence to speed limit	Visual scanning and memory
3 (3.5 miles)	Keeping safe distance (gap)	Simple and complex reaction time
4 (3.5 miles)	Checking blind spot	Visual search and memory
5 (3.5 miles)	Hazard detection and avoidance	Divided attention, executive function, and reaction time
6 (3.5 miles)	Executing left and right turns	Executive function and reaction time

THE SCHEDULE AND ACTIVITIES OF EACH TRAINING SESSION

Sessions	Activities
1	10 min discussion, 40 min driving through scenario **A**, 10 min feedback
2	10 min discussion, 40 min driving through scenario **1**, 10 min feedback
3	10 min discussion, 40 min driving through scenario **2**, 10 min feedback
4	10 min discussion, 40 min driving through scenario **3**, 10 min feedback
5	10 min discussion, 40 min driving through scenario **1−3**, 10 min feedback
6	10 min discussion, 40 min driving through scenario **4**, 10 min feedback
7	10 min discussion, 40 min driving through scenario **5**, 10 min feedback
8	10 min discussion, 40 min driving through scenario **6**, 10 min feedback
9	10 min discussion, 40 min driving through scenario **4−6**, 10 min feedback
10	10 min discussion, 40 min driving through scenario **A**, 10 min feedback

Note: During each session, trainee repeats the scenario until proficiency is achieved.

equipment are typically prescribed by a driving rehabilitation specialist and installed by a trained mobility equipment dealer with expertise in vehicle modifications for individuals with disabilities.

Alternative to Driving Resumption

Common alternatives to driving resumption by stroke survivors include being driven by someone else, use of public transportation, use of commercial transportation services, and, where available, scheduling transportation from social support services. Although the technology is still in development and not currently available, the emergence of driverless cars may offer another possible alternative to self-driving that will be available to stroke survivors in the future.

SUMMARY AND TAKE-HOME MESSAGES

- In the highly motorized world of today, driving is a very important activity.
- Driving is a complex and dynamic activity that involves timely and simultaneous interaction of motor, sensory, cognitive, and visual skills.
- These skills are commonly affected after stroke and compromise the ability of survivors to resume driving.
- Five different methods have been employed at different times to help stroke survivors resume safe driving with moderate success.
- Considering the safety implications of on-road driving training, driving simulators seem to offer the best method to retrain driving in a safe, repeatable, and naturalistic way.
- The appropriate vehicle modification and adaptive equipment can further improve the ease and success of return to safe driving for stroke survivors.

REFERENCES

1. Akinwuntan AE, Wachtel J, Rosen P. Driving simulation for evaluation and rehabilitation of driving after stroke. *J Stroke Cerebrovasc Dis.* 2012;21(6):478−486.
2. Collia DV, Sharp J, Giesbrecht L. The 2001 National Household Travel Survey: a look into the travel patterns of older Americans. *J Saf Res.* 2003;34:461−470.
3. Marottoli RA. Consequences of driving cessation: decreased out-of-home activities. *J Gerontol Sci Soc Sci.* 2000;55:334−340.
4. Fonda SJ, Wallace RB, Herzog AR. Changes in driving and worsening depressive symptoms among older adults. *J Gerontol Sci Soc Sci.* 2001;56:343−351.
5. Marottoli RA, Mendes de Leon CF, Glass TA, et al. Driving cessation and increased depressive symptom: prospective evidence from the New Haven EPESE. *J Am Geriatr Soc.* 1997;4:202−206.
6. Akinwuntan AE, Devos H, Verheyden G, et al. Confirmation of the accuracy of a short battery to predict fitness-to-drive of stroke survivors without severe deficits. *J Rehabil Med.* 2007;39(9):698−702.
7. Sivak M, Hill CS, Henson DL, Butler BP, Silber SM, Olson PL. Improved driving performance following perceptual training in persons with brain damage. *Arch Phys Med Rehabil.* 1984;65:163−167.
8. Mazer BL, Sofer S, Korner-Bitensky N, Gelinas I, Hanley J, Wood-Dauphinee S. Effectiveness of a visual attention retraining program on the driving performance of clients with stroke. *Arch Phys Med Rehabil.* 2003;84:541−550.
9. Klavora P, Gaskovski KM, Forsyth RD, Heslegrave RJ, Young M, Quinn RP. The effects of dynavision rehabilitation on behind-the-wheel and selected psychomotor abilities of persons after stroke. *Am J Occup Ther.* 1995;49: 534−542.
10. Crotty M, George S. Retraining visual processing skills to improve driving ability after stroke. *Arch Phys Med Rehabil.* 2009;90(12):2096−2102.
11. Dynavision International LLC. Dynavision D2 operators manual Rev. 9. https://dynavisioninternational.com/wpInt/wp-content/uploads/2013/10/dynavisiond2-operators-manual-march11-2012-rev9.pdf; March 11, 2012.
12. Kent H, Sheridan J, Wasko E, June C. A driver training program for the disabled. *Arch Phys Med Rehabil.* 1979;60: 273−276.
13. Cimolino N, Balkovec D. The contribution of a driving simulator in the driving evaluation of stroke and disabled adolescent clients. *Can J Occup Ther.* 1988;55:119−125.
14. Akinwuntan AE, DeWeerdt W, Feys H, et al. Effect of simulator training on the driving ability of stroke patients: a randomized controlled trial (RCT). *Neurology.* 2005; 65(6):843−850.
15. Akinwuntan AE, Devos H, Verheyden G, et al. Retraining moderately impaired stroke survivors in driving-related visual attention skills. *Top Stroke Rehabil.* 2010;17: 328−336.
16. Devos H, Akinwuntan AE, Nieuwboer A, et al. Comparison of two driving retraining programs on on-road performance in mildly impaired stroke survivors. *Neurorehabil Neural Repair.* 2009;23(7):699−705.
17. Devos H, Akinwuntan AE, Nieuwboer A, et al. Effect of simulator training on driving after stroke: a 5 year follow-up of a randomized trial. *Neurorehabil Neural Repair.* 2010;24(9):843−850.
18. Mazer B, Gelinas I, Duquette J, Vanier M, Rainville C, Chilingaryan G. A randomized clinical trial to determine effectiveness of driving simulator retraining on the driving performance of clients with neurological impairment. *Br J Occup Ther.* 2015;78(6):369−376.

19. Quigley FL, DeLisa JA. Assessing the driving potentials of cerebral vascular accident patients. *Am J Occup Ther.* 1983;37:474−478.

20. Soderstrom ST, Pettersson RP, Leppert J. Prediction of driving ability after stroke and the effect of behind-the-wheel training. *Scand J Psychol.* 2006;47:419−429.

21. Summala H. Modeling driving behavior: a pessimistic prediction? In: Evans L, Schwing R, eds. *Human Behavior and Traffic Safety.* New York: Plenum Press; 1985.

22. Molen HH, van der Bottıcher AM. A hierarchical risk model for traffic participants. *Ergonomics.* 1988;31: 537−555.

23. Wickens CD. *Engineering Psychology and Human Performance.* New York: Harper Collins; 1992.

24. Michon JA. A critical view of driver behavior models: what do we know, what should we do? In: Evans L, Schwing R, eds. *Human Behavior and Traffic Safety.* New York: Plenum Press; 1985.

25. Galski T, Bruno RI, Ehle HT. Driving after cerebral damage: a model with implications for evaluation. *Am J Occup Ther.* 1992;46:324−332.

26. Rasmussen J. The definition of human error and a taxonomy for technical system design. In: Rasmussen J, Duncan K, Leplat J, eds. *New Technology and Human Error.* Chichester, UK: Wiley; 1987.

27. Michel JA, Mateer CA. Attention rehabilitation following stroke and traumatic brain injury: a review. *Eur Medicophys.* 2006;42:59−67.

28. Wachtel JA. Applications of appropriate simulator technology for driver training, licensing and assessment. In: Gale AG, ed. Vision in Vehicles. Vol V [Amsterdam]; 1996.

29. Rosen PN, Wachtel J. Driving assessment in the clinical setting: utility for testing and treatment. *Adv Transp Stud.* 2004:91−96 [special issue].

CHAPTER 17

Rehabilitation Robotics for Stroke

SCOTT BARBUTO, MD, PHD • JOEL STEIN, MD

REHABILITATION ROBOTICS FOR STROKE

The field of rehabilitation robotics started in 1989 with the development of a robot designed to provide shoulder and elbow therapy. Although slow to start, the field has grown rapidly since the mid-1990s, and the number of therapeutic rehabilitation robots has expanded dramatically during the past two decades. This growth may reflect a growing emphasis on therapies that can facilitate and enhance exercise therapy intended to promote motor recovery after stroke.[1]

DEFINITION OF A ROBOT

The difference between robots and electronic devices can be nuanced. The *Oxford English Dictionary* defines a robot as:

1. A machine that can perform a complicated series of tasks automatically.
2. A machine that is made to look like a human and that can do some things that a human can do.[2]

The first definition is too broad, and simple electromechanical devices such as a kitchen aid or continuous passive motion (CPM) machine could be considered robots. The second definition is also problematic as rehabilitation robots are not designed to resemble humans, but rather are specialized devices that vary in size, shape, and complexity and share an increasing level of sophistication. A more appropriate definition for a robot comes from The Robot Institute of America, which defines a robot as:

1. A programmable, multi-functional manipulator designed to move material, parts, or specialized devices through variable programmed motions for the performance of a variety of tasks.[3]

Thus, a robot is defined by its capability of movement with various levels of autonomy.[4]

BENEFITS OF ROBOTICS IN REHABILITATION

The incorporation of robots into stroke rehabilitation has two major rationales: (1) to serve as a labor-saving device allowing greater amounts of rehabilitation therapy without requiring additional personnel, and/or (2) to provide therapy that is superior to conventional therapy (i.e., exercise treatments under the direct supervision of occupational and physical therapists) in promotion of motor recovery. Existing evidence finds that robot-assisted therapy had similar or modest benefits relative to conventional therapy.[5] However, as new robotic devices become more sophisticated and the optimal timing, duration, and dosing of stroke therapy is better elucidated, superior outcomes with robotic therapy may be achieved. Robots have the theoretical advantage of delivering exercise in a more consistent fashion, with more precise control over the parameters of exercises, including movement pattern, number of repetitions, and forces exerted by the robot on the patient.

The use of robotics has been proposed as a labor-saving approach in stroke rehabilitation. Demand for stroke rehabilitation continues to rise as the population ages and life expectancy continues to increase. At present, there are almost 800,000 new strokes a year in the United States with millions of stroke survivors.[6] Robot-guided exercise can, in principle, substitute for a portion of exercise now provided under direct guidance of a therapist. Models for incorporating robotics into stroke rehabilitation include: (1) having a single therapist provide supervision to several patients using robot-assisted therapy, (2) having a patient work at home with a robot with remote supervision of a therapist, or (3) having a patient work independently with the robot device with periodic review and adjustment from trained personnel.[7] Although these models are proposed, most robotic therapy currently is performed under direct supervision in an institutional setting. As robots become easier to use and more devices designed for home use are developed, this paradigm may shift, and robots may help meet the demand for stroke rehabilitation.

Another potential, but as of yet unrealized, benefit of incorporating robotic therapy into stroke rehabilitation would be cost savings. In the United States, Japan, and western Europe, there has been a steady decrease in the cost of technology-based devices, while labor costs continue to rise.[8] Thus, substantial cost savings might be achievable by having one supervising therapist monitoring multiple patients using robot-assisted therapy. Current reimbursement models, however, do not support this "group" robotic therapy, as only the directly human supervised portions of therapy are recognized as billable. The economics of home robot use remains challenging due to the costly nature of these devices at present. Large randomized clinical trials showing clear benefit of robot-assisted therapy over conventional therapy would be needed before insurance companies are likely to reimburse the cost of home-based robots.

Another proposed benefit of robotic therapy might be the improvement of stroke patients' adherence to exercise programs. Typically, formal stroke rehabilitation under the supervision of a therapist is relatively short-term, followed by instruction of the patient in a long-term home exercise program. Compliance is often limited, however, due perhaps to limited functional gains, lack of motivation, boredom while performing exercises, or concern about performing exercises incorrectly without guidance. Robotic devices can monitor patient compliance and provide reports back to clinicians, adding accountability. In addition, robots can be programmed to make repetitive exercise more interesting and enjoyable by integrating computer-based video games into robotic training.

Rehabilitation robots are also important research tools. Highly repetitive, task-specific exercise training has been shown to induce neuroplastic changes in the brain with improved motor abilities and enhanced functional performance in stroke patients.[9,10] Despite this, the optimal timing, duration, and dosing of rehabilitation after stroke remains uncertain. Users of some upper limb robotic devices can make approximately 1000 movements in an hour-long session compared with an average of 33 movements reported in inpatient rehabilitation occupational therapy sessions.[11] Moreover, robotic therapy is highly consistent from patient to patient and session to session, avoiding the variability occurring with human-delivered

rehabilitation. Thus, rehabilitation robots provide a platform to determine the best way to rehabilitate after stroke.

CATEGORIES OF REHABILITATION ROBOTICS

There are numerous ways in which rehabilitation robots can be categorized. For this chapter, rehabilitation robots will be divided into two main categories: workstation and wearable robots. Workstation robots are designed mainly for exercise training whereas wearable robots are devices that most easily adapt to potential functional orthoses. Robots which typically mount on wheelchairs to aid in activities of daily living will also be discussed.

Workstation Robots—Upper Extremity

Several research groups have tested the effects of robotic therapy for poststroke upper-limb motor recovery. Robots in these clinical studies vary greatly in complexity from unimanual single-joint devices to bimanual ones with multiple degrees of freedom.

The MIT-Manus robot, now commercialized (inMotion Arm, Bionik, Inc., Toronto, Canada), is one of the best studied robots to date. It has two degrees of freedom that provide shoulder and elbow exercises in the horizontal plane where the patient's forearm and hand are attached to the robot with a splint (Fig. 17.1A and B). This robot has three main modes: active assist, resistive exercise, and passive mode, in which neither assistance nor resistance are provided. With the active assist mode, patients with profound weakness, including those who are not candidates for constraint-induced movement therapy due to the severity of their paresis, can successfully undergo exercise training. Furthermore, an algorithm has been developed for this mode that alters the amount of assistance provided by the robot based on the patient's performance.[12] In all modes, subjects attempt to move the robotic arm guided by simple games displayed on a computer screen.

A trial with the MIT-Manus robot randomized 96 patients within 1 month of stroke to either 1 h of active assistive exercises 5 times per week for 5 weeks, or to the control group where subjects received sham exercises (passive mode) with the robot once a week.[13–16] All patients received conventional therapy (usual care) in addition to the robotic therapy. Results indicated that the robot treated group had significantly greater improvement in motor impairment measured on the Motor Status Scale (MSS) and the Medical Research

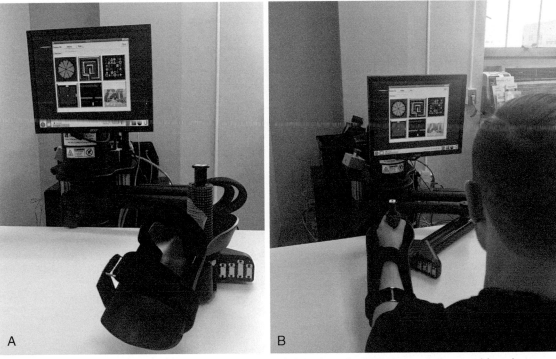

FIG. 17.1 **(A** and **B)** InMotion Shoulder-Elbow robot based on the MIT-Manus design provides planar exercises for the upper limb involving shoulder and elbow movements.

Council Motor Power Scale (MRC) for shoulder and elbow motor function. These improvements were maintained at 3-year follow-up.[17]

Two other randomized controlled trials used this device for patients within 1 month post stroke (subacute). In the first study, control subjects received twelve 40-min sessions of occupational therapy whereas the treatment group received the same amount of robotic therapy. Once again, both groups were treated with the standard 3 h a day of poststroke rehabilitation therapy during inpatient rehabilitation. Of the 20 patients tested, both groups had similar MSS, Functional Independence Measures (FIM), and Fugl—Meyer Assessment Scale scores upon discharge.[18] In the other study, the treatment group received 30 sessions of robotic therapy versus the control group which received 30 sessions of the same duration of conventional therapy. In this study of 53 patients, Modified Ashworth Scale-Shoulder (MAS-S), Modified Ashworth Scale-Elbow (MAS-E), and passive range of motion-shoulder/elbow all showed significant improvement in the robotic group compared to the control group. Fugl—Meyer and Motricity index improved significantly in both

groups, but no statistical difference was found between the groups.[19]

The MIT-Manus has also been studied in patients at least 6 months post stroke (chronic). In one study, 42 subjects received either active assistive or progressive resistive reaching training for 1-h sessions, 3 times per week for 6 weeks. Baseline testing served as a control procedure to ensure that patient's motor impairments were stable before treatment. Subjects in both the active assistive and the progressive resistive groups demonstrated significant gains in Fugl—Meyer, MSS, and MRC scores post treatment that persisted when measured at 4-month follow-up evaluations.[20] Other studies have found similar results.[21—24] However, in a small study where the control group received occupational therapy of the same duration as the robotic therapy, Fugl—Meyer scores improved in both groups, and no statistical difference was seen.[25]

In the studies discussed above, the benefits of the MIT-Manus were seen primarily in shoulder and elbow movements, rather than at the wrist. This is consistent with the design of the device, which provides exercises for the shoulder and elbow while the wrist and hand are immobilized in the splint that attaches to the robot. The magnitude of the motor impairment improvement for MIT-Manus therapy has been modest (slightly greater than a three point increase in Fugl—Meyer scores in most studies) and appears to be close to the minimal clinically significant difference.[18–20] Further studies are needed to determine which subgroups of patients would benefit the most from robotic therapy with the MIT-Manus.

Robots that work in conjunction with the MIT-Manus have been developed. One such device allows patients to perform wrist flexion and extension exercises, as well as radial and ulnar deviation exercises (Fig. 17.2A—C). Another device provides a way to perform grip and release exercises. A reaching robot can be positioned to provide upward reaching movements at the shoulder and elbow. A clinical trial combining the MIT-Manus with these three other robots was published in 2010.[26] One hundred and

twenty-seven patients with moderate to severe upper limb impairment from strokes that occurred at least 6 months prior were recruited. Patients were assigned to one of three groups: intensive robotic therapy, intensive comparison therapy mimicking robot-delivered exercises, or usual care group. Intensive robotic and comparison therapy consisted of thirty-six 1-h sessions over a 12-week period. Robotic therapy was divided into four 3-week modules: (1) planar shoulder-elbow training, (2) antigravity shoulder and hand-grasp training, (3) wrist training, and (4) integrative training, where all robots were used simultaneously. Results indicated that robot-assisted therapy significantly improved the Fugl—Meyer score and the time on the Wolf Motor Function Test as compared to the usual care group, but not compared to the intensive therapy group. Furthermore, the magnitude of the motor function gains observed (3.87 increase in Fugl—Meyer score) was comparable to other studies in which the

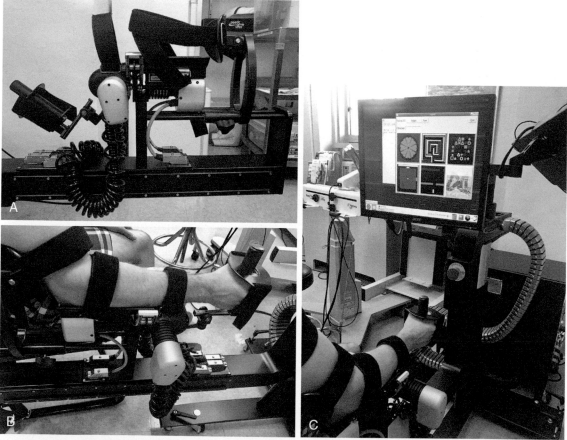

FIG. 17.2 **(A–C)** InMotion Wrist robot allows patients to perform wrist flexion and extension exercises in addition to radial and ulnar deviation exercises.

MIT-Manus shoulder-elbow robot was used alone, raising questions about the impact of the other three training robots on stroke recovery.[26] Studies still need to be conducted to determine the best way to incorporate training on multiple robotic devices. Whether training should be done with one device at a time in sequence or interspersed training sessions using these devices simultaneously to promote coordination of movements is still debated.

In 2006, the Neuro-Rehabilitation-Robot (NeReBot) (Padua University, Padua, Italy) was introduced. The NeReBot is a three degrees of freedom robotic device for the upper limb with direct-drive wire actuation. Three nylon cables are used to suspend and move the patient's forearm, which is attached to the robot via a rigid splint. Like the MIT-Manus, the NeReBot allows for exercises at the shoulder and elbow, but the patients can perform these exercises in 3D trajectories. Other advantages of the NeReBot is that it is easily movable to hospital rooms, can be used in both supine and sitting positions, and is likely to be less expensive than more rigid robotic devices, although it is not currently commercially available.[27]

In the initial pilot study, 20 patients who had strokes within 1 month were randomly assigned to either exposure to robotic device without training or to additional sensorimotor robotic training (4 h per week) for 4 weeks. Results indicated that the robotic group had 5.3 point greater gains on Fugl—Meyer scores than the control group, and these gains were maintained at 3 month follow-up.[28] In a follow-up study, 35 patients less than 1 week post stroke were randomized to either early robotic training (4 h per week) for 5 weeks or control group that received robotic therapy to the unimpaired upper limb for 30 min a day, twice a week. The robotic group showed significant gains in motor recovery as measured by Fugl—Meyer shoulder and elbow score (4.8 increase) and FIM motor scores (32.6 gain). These gains were sustained at 3 and 8-month follow-up.[29,30]

In 2014, the group conducted another trial with 30 patients who had a stroke within 15 days. All participants received 120 min of rehabilitation, 5 days a week for 5 weeks. The robotic group received standard therapy for 65% of this time and robotic training for 35% whereas the control group did not receive robotic training. No statistical difference was seen between groups as measured by Fugl—Meyer, Box and Block, and FIM tests.[31]

One of the drawbacks to many upper limb robotic systems is that these devices' heavy weight significantly alters the inertia of the natural arm. A novel lightweight Cable-driven Arm Exoskeleton (CAREX), which is similar in some aspects to the NeReBot, has been developed to address this problem. Instead of rigid links and joints, CAREX uses light-weight cuffs and tensioned cables, decreasing the weight by approximately one-tenth that of conventional robotic devices. Preliminary studies show that the assistance force applied by CAREX helps healthy and stroke subjects follow a desired path more accurately. More complete studies are being conducted to determine the benefit in stroke patients.[32]

Another limitation of early generation stroke rehabilitation robots was the limited hand capabilities. Some of the newer robots, however, have the ability to provide individualized training for each finger. Unlike the first generation robots which showed improvement specific to the shoulder and elbow, data from hand robotic therapy indicates that gains in motor impairment may generalize to the entire arm. For example, preliminary data from a study by Krebs et al. indicated that training the distal before the proximal upper extremity led to twice as much carryover effect to the proximal segment than training in the reverse order.[33]

The Amadeo Robot (Tyromotion, Graz, Austria) has five degrees of freedom and provides the motion of one or all five fingers. Each finger has a small permanent magnet attached to its distal tip with an adhesive bandage. These magnets in turn adhere via magnetic forces to magnetic targets on the robot, providing a strong attachment that releases if excessive forces should occur. The wrist is secured in a splint using a strap (Fig. 17.3A—C). In a randomized-controlled trial, 20 patients who had a stroke within 30 days received twenty 40-min sessions of robot-assisted hand therapy or the same amount of occupational therapy, in addition to usual care. Statistically significant improvements in both the robot and control groups were seen in Fugl—Meyer, Box and Block, Motricity index, and MCR scores. No statistical difference was seen between groups, however.[34]

In contrast to the robots described above which primarily focus on one movement type, other robots have been designed to train multiple joint movements at the same time. The ReoGo (Motorika, Caesarea, Israel) is a robotic device that allows 3-dimensional movements and exercises to be performed with forearm, wrist, or handgrip support. In a noncontrolled pilot study, patients with chronic stroke benefited from the utilization of the ReoGo.[35,36] In 2016, a prospective, open, blinded end point, randomized clinical trial was conducted on 60 subjects with mild to moderate hemiplegia 4—8 weeks post stroke. Subjects received standard therapy

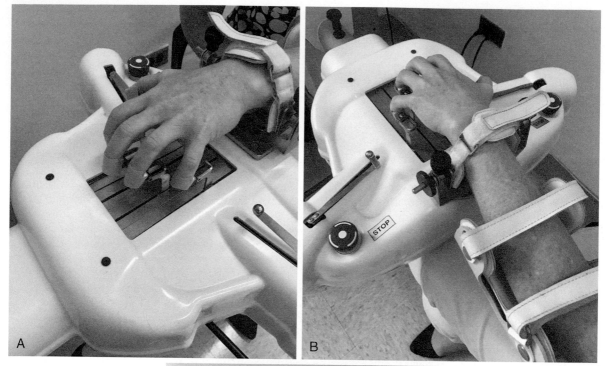

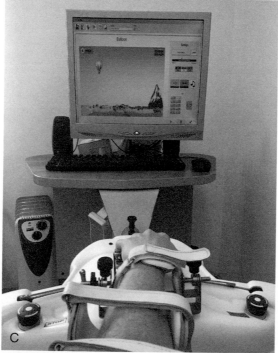

FIG. 17.3 **(A–C)** The Amadeo Robot has five degrees of freedom and provides the motion of one or all five fingers. Each finger has a small magnet attached to its distal tip with an adhesive bandage that adheres to magnetic targets on the robot.

plus either 40 min of robotic therapy using ReoGo or self-guided therapy daily for 6 weeks. Results indicated that the robotic therapy group had significantly improved Fugl—Meyer shoulder-elbow assessment (average of 2.9 point increase) and flexor synergy (average of 2.2 point increase) compared to the control group, whereas Wolf Motor Function Test scores were not significantly different. Of note, robotic therapy in low functioning patients (baseline Fugl—Meyer Assessment < 30 and Wolf Motor Function Test ≥ 120) had more significant improvements in Fugl—Meyer Assessment (4.4 point increase) than the self-guided therapy group. Thus, lower functioning subjects may benefit more from robotic therapy than higher functioning subjects, but future research still needs to be conducted to further support this conclusion.[37]

The ARMin robot (now commercialized as the Armeo Power, Hocoma) uses an exoskeleton workstation design that allows large ranges of motion in three dimensions. It has seven degrees of freedom and supports movements of the shoulder, arm, and handgrip (Fig. 17.4A and B). In a randomized controlled study of 73 patients with chronic stroke, patients received either 45 min of robotic therapy three times a week for 8 weeks or conventional therapy of the same duration. The primary outcome was change in score on Fugl—Meyer shoulder and elbow. Results indicated that the robotic therapy group improved by a mean of 0.78 points more than the conventional therapy group with statistical significance ($P = .041$)

achieved, but this difference is not clinically meaningful.[38]

Bimanual robotic therapy, where the nonparetic arm helps guide paretic arm movement, has also been studied. The mirror image movement enabler (MIME) robot is a six degrees of freedom robot that can administer four distinct modes of upper-limb reaching exercise in three dimensions. The four modes are passive, active assistive, active constrained, and bimanual mode where the robot assists the paretic limb's movements as necessary to mirror the less impaired limb.

In a 2002 study, 27 patients with chronic stroke were randomized to either MIME robotic therapy for twenty-four 60-min sessions over 2 months or to the same duration of conventional therapy. Subjects in the robotic group repeatedly practiced 12 reaching movements in 4 directions and at 3 vertical levels, receiving identical proportions of robot-guided passive and bimanual exercise and variable amounts of active assistive and active constrained exercise based on ability. The conventional therapy group received exercise designed to facilitate progression from mass upper limb movements to more isolated ones in the context of functional task performance. Results revealed that the robotic therapy group significantly improved more than the control group on Fugl—Meyer shoulder and elbow assessment, upper limb strength measures, and free-reach distance. Statistical significance for Fugl—Meyer scores was no longer evident at the 6-month follow-up evaluations, however.[39]

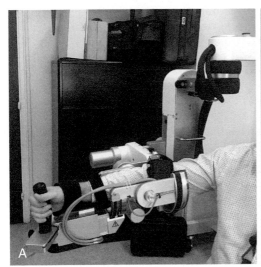 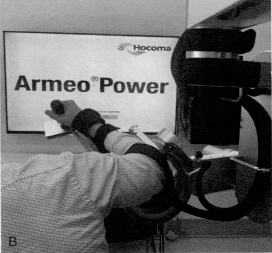

FIG. 17.4 **(A** and **B)** The Armeo Power uses an exoskeleton workstation design that allows large ranges of motion in three dimensions. It has seven degrees of freedom and supports movements of the shoulder, arm, and handgrip.

A randomized control trial of a commercially available bimanual robot, Bi-Manu-Track (Reha-Stim, Berlin), was reported in 2012. Twenty patients with chronic stroke were randomized to either robotic arm trainer, which enabled bilateral mirror-like movement cycles of forearm pronation-supination and wrist flexion-extension, or to conventional therapy. Each group received a total of 90—105 min of therapy a day, 5 days a week for 4 weeks. The robot group significantly increased motor function, as accessed by Fugl—Meyer, and bilateral arm coordination, as accessed by ABILHAND questionnaire, as compared to dose-matched controls.[40]

Dosing and Timing of Robotic Therapy

Research has shown that poststroke recovery is most rapid within the first 3 months from the stroke event. There is other evidence from animal studies that excessive exercise of the paretic limb within the first days of the stroke can result in more severe brain damage.[41] The best time to initiate robotic therapy still needs to be determined. Robotic therapy has been used during the acute, subacute, and chronic phases of stroke. Most data have indicated a benefit to robotic therapy during all three phases; however, the benefits are comparable to conventional therapy. It appears that continuation of therapy beyond shortterm rehabilitation may be useful, given that even chronic stroke patients improve when undergoing either conventional or robotic therapy. Robotic therapy may play a role in this regard as it can increase compliance by providing accountability and making therapy more enjoyable by incorporating computer-based games into repetitive therapy.

Determination of how much robotic therapy to perform is also still under investigation. In the 2003 study with MIT-Manus, subjects performed up to 18,000 point-to-point movements over the trial and significant impairment level gains were seen.[20] A study conducted with the Assisted Rehabilitation and Measure (ARM) guide, designed to administer active assistive reaching practice in three dimensions, had the opposite results. In this study, seven subjects received twenty-four 1-h robotic therapy sessions over the course of 8 weeks. In each session, only about 65 movement attempts were conducted, making the total for the study about 1560 movements. Results indicated no improvement in free-reaching distance and the control group had better performance times in measured functional activities.[42] To further this point, a study by Hesse and colleagues compared Bi-Manu-Track robotic training to EMG-initiated electrical stimulation of the

paretic upper limb in chronic stroke patients. Subjects receiving robotic training showed significantly larger improvements in Fugl—Meyer motor scores, and the authors speculated the reason for the different outcomes was that the robotic training group received a 10-fold increase in the number of repetitions compared to the EMG group.[43] Thus, there are suggestions that achieving higher numbers of repetitions is important for stroke recovery, but further studies are needed.

Workstation Robots—Lower Extremity

Robots for lower limb are primarily used to facilitate partial body-weight supported treadmill gait training (BWST). BWST consists of unloading the weight of a subject suspended above a treadmill while a therapist manually assists the patient to step, shift weight, and maintain appropriate gait patterns. Several initial studies reported improved gait performance after BWST post stroke,[44] Parkinson disease,[45] and cerebral palsy.[46] However, a large clinical trial in 2011 found no benefit to BWST after stroke, slowing the enthusiasm to develop new robots to enhance gait training.[47]

The electrical gait trainer (EGT) was one of the first robotics developed for gait training. EGT resembles an elliptical machine and consists of two foot-plates positioned on two bars, two rockers, and two cranks. The footplates symmetrically generate the stance and swing phases as the feet are always in contact with the platform. A harness suspends the patient above the footplates to provide for variable unweighting during training.

EGT was compared to conventional BWST in a randomized control study in 30 subacute stroke patients who required assistance for ambulation at baseline.[48] Subjects received either 4 weeks of EGT with 2 weeks of BWST at weeks 3 and 4 (EGT group) or 4 weeks of BWST with 2 weeks of EGT at weeks 3 and 4 (control group). All patients received 15—20 min of gait training with either BWST or EGT in addition to conventional therapy for 6 weeks. Results indicated that both groups had gains in functional ambulation category (FAC), gait velocity, and Rivermead Motor Assessment scores. The EGT group had comparatively higher FAC scores, but this advantage was no longer evident at 6 month follow-up.[48] The study also concluded that the patients were able to use EGT without therapist assistance at the end of the trial, but still required one therapist for BWST.

In another trial, EGT plus conventional therapy was compared to conventional therapy alone in 155 subacute subjects.[49] The EGT group showed greater improvement in gait and ADL measures than the control group over the course of a 4-week protocol. Improved gait ability was maintained at the 6-month follow-up, though the difference in ADL ability was no longer apparent.

A 2016 study tried to determine the effect of EGT compared to dose matched controls in 106 subacute stroke patients that were all nonambulatory at baseline. Both the EGT and control group received 45 min of physiotherapy 6 times per week for 8 weeks. Of the 45 minutes, the EGT group received 20 min of EGT training and 5 min of conventional stance/gait training without EGT. The control group received 25 min of conventional stance/gait training instead of EGT. Results indicated similar results between the two groups, and a statistical difference was not achieved when measuring FAC, Barthel index, and gait speed.[50]

The driven gait orthosis (DGO) or Lokomat (Hocoma, Switzerland) is a lower limb robot automated for gait training. DGO has hip and knee motors in an exoskeletal leg brace suspended over a treadmill. The motors are controlled by a computer and generate physiologically correct gait patterns. There is some evidence that DGO may require less effort to operate than BWST and treadmill walking,[51] although there are conflicting reports.[52]

Results studying DGO in stroke patients have been variable. In a 2016 study, 18 patients with chronic stroke were randomized to either DGO or treadmill gait training. Each group completed twenty 1-h sessions over 4 weeks. Gait speed, cadence, step length, Berg Balance Scale (BBS) score were all significantly higher in the DGO group when compared to the treadmill training group.[53] In a 2015 study, 30 patients were randomized to either DGO training or conventional therapy for 3.5 h per week for a total of 8 weeks. Patients were then followed for 36 weeks to compare effects of training. Although all patients showed gains in walking speed and lower limb strength, there were no significant differences between the two groups at any time during the study.[54] Thus, more research needs to be conducted to determine the benefit of DGO in stroke.

A Cochrane review of 23 trials involving 999 participants showed that robotic training combined with conventional therapy might improve recovery of independent walking in poststroke patients. The most benefit was seen in patients who used robotic training within the first 3 months of stroke and those who were unable to walk prior to use. The review concluded that the frequency, duration, and timing of robotic training still need to be researched further.[55]

The AnkleBot (Interactive Motion Technologies, Watertown, MA) is a two degrees of freedom robot that functions as a powered ankle-foot orthosis that is semiwearable, but is tethered to power source and controllers. It has the ability to control and assist with ankle dorsiflexion, plantarflexion, inversion, and eversion. In a 2014 study, 34 subacute stroke patients were randomized to training with AnkleBot or to passive manual stretching. Both groups received the same duration of treatment, and at the end of the study, the AnkleBot group had significantly longer paretic step lengths and improved ankle control than did the control group.[56] Similar results were found in earlier studies.[57]

Other robotic devices, the Active Leg Exoskeletons (ALEX and ALEXII), have innovative feedback interfaces and were designed to study human training. ALEX is a workstation device that straps to a patient walking on a treadmill at the trunk, thigh, and calf. These attachments allow flexibility during walking. The orthosis has joint encoders that record movements of the trunk, hip, leg, and ankle. In order to provide feedback to the user, a virtual tunnel is created around the desired foot trajectory that is dependent on the subject's size, age, and walking speed.[7] The controller can then prescribe force to help the subject stay on the desired foot path.[58–60] Trials still need to be conducted with these devices to determine if they have benefit in gait training of stroke patients.

Wearable Robots

Wearable robots are exoskeletal robots or powered orthoses that can provide therapeutic exercise and/or serve to compensate for chronic weakness. The main advantage to wearable robots is the ability to move therapy outside of the clinic and use the device in multiple environments including the patient's home.

A small pilot study of a powered wearable elbow brace (Myomo, Inc., Boston, MA) that uses surface EMG signals to control the amount of force provided found stroke survivors were capable of using the device for exercise training.[61] In 2013, 16 chronic stroke patients were randomized to training sessions with or without the Myomo device. The results indicated that both groups were equally efficacious.[62]

Another wearable robot includes the AlterG Bionic Leg (AlterG, Fremont, CA). This unilateral powered knee brace uses a combination of sensors to determine the user's intended action and can infer whether the user is walking, ascending/descending stairs, or transferring from sit to stand. It then provides assistance to the user to achieve the best movement type to perform that activity. Twenty-four ambulatory patients with chronic stroke were enrolled in a study and randomized to

18 h of therapy with or without AlterG. No significant difference was seen between the two groups in terms of function at the completion of training or the 3-month follow-up visit .[63]

The ReWalk (Argo Medical Technologies, Ltd., Yokneam Ilit, Israel), Ekso (Ekso Bionics, Richmond, CA), and Indego (Parker Hannifin, Cleveland, OH) are all bilateral wearable powered long-leg braces that have been developed mostly for individuals with paraplegia rather than stroke. Some have proposed that certain stroke survivors may benefit from such devices, but these benefits have not yet been demonstrated and would likely pertain only to certain subpopulations of stroke survivors.[64]

Disadvantages of Wearable Robots

Wearable robots main advantage over workstation robots is their ability to function in multiple environments. This is also a drawback, however, as the robots must function in less controlled environments and may expose the user to unanticipated risk because of situations that arise beyond the intended activities of the robot. The possibility of being forced into anatomically dangerous positions is also more likely with wearable robots than workstation ones. Wearable robots require proper fit and donning and doffing. Improper positioning of the robot either due to slippage from improper fit or from poor donning could lead to injuries, as the axis of rotation may no longer be aligned with the target joint.

An ideal wearable robot would have a lightweight, portable power supply and an actuator that was as unobtrusive as possible. These technical issues remain a work in progress. Heavy external battery packs are needed for many wearable robots to provide sufficient power. Actuators that are small, lightweight, durable, and generate sufficient force remain under development. The use of surface or implantable EMG signals and neural prostheses capable of capturing brain activity are both under exploration.[65,66]

Limitations of Workstation Robots

Both workstation and wearable robots are used predominately for therapeutic exercise. The main limitation of workstation robots is that these robots are designed for very specific types of exercise and are limited in their degrees of freedom motion. For example, the MIT-Manus robots provide only two degrees of freedom and are designed only to provide reaching type exercises for the shoulder and elbow. Even the MIME robot that has six degrees of freedom does not provide robotic training for the wrist or

hand. A strategy to overcome this limitation is to combine the use of multiple robots that provide different exercises, similar to circuit training in a gym. The clinical impact of this approach is still being evaluated.[67]

The development of training algorithms for robot-aided exercise remains in early stages. Due to their programmable nature, there is no inherent limit to the ways in which robot-assisted exercise can be designed. Questions remain regarding the complexity of exercises, the most effective duration and frequency of training, the benefits of resistive training, and many other issues.[68,69]

Overall, published research on workstation robots use after stroke is encouraging, but has not demonstrated superiority over conventional treatment therapies. Differences in robot design and training algorithms makes it difficult to compare studies and likely account for variable results. Further research needs to be conducted to expand the scope of robot-aided exercise training and explore the best training modules and algorithms.

Robots for ADL Assistance

Computer-based technologic aids have been used to improve communication, assist with powered mobility, and help in performing ADLs. Appropriately designed robotic devices may be useful in manipulating objects in the environment that the user is incapable of handling independently.

The iARM robot (Exact Dynamics, Didam, the Netherlands) and the JACO (Kinova, Inc., Montreal, Canada) are robotic arms that mount on a power wheelchair. These robots are controlled by a joystick, keypad, or sip-and-puff interface and can be used to pick up objects, open refrigerators and remove items, and more. The iARM robot is potentially useful for individuals with large brainstem strokes with bilateral weakness, as well as nonstroke conditions such as spinal cord injuries, limb deficiencies, and neuromuscular conditions.

This type of robot arm has a substantial number of degrees of freedom, but accomplishing functional tasks can be slow and difficult. However, the psychological benefits of improved ability to manipulate one's own environment appear considerable and are supported by a few reports.[70,71] An economic analysis suggested potential saving achieved through reduced caregiver hours.[72] New control mechanisms, including brain-computer interfaces, are being studied in an effort to integrate these devices more closely with the central nervous system.[73]

Limitations of ADL Robots

Although a great tool to improve the functionality of patients, technical issues with ADL robots arise due to the absence of sensory feedback. Objects can be grasped too hard or not hard enough. These robotic arms are also slow and difficult to use, requiring patience, good perceptual skills, and intact cognitive abilities to master. Furthermore, fine motor control tasks, such as writing, or those that require two hands, are not feasible with the current robots.

Cost is also a major limitation to the use of ADL robots. For example, the JACO robot arm costs more than $35,000, a price that places the device outside the affordable range for most patients. Unlike some exercise robots, which may be used for a limited period of time, ADL robots are intended for long-term use in a home-setting.

CONCLUSION

Stroke rehabilitation robots are undergoing a phase of rapid development and testing and are likely to start appearing in clinical settings more regularly within the next few years. Robots designed to perform specialized tasks are likely to remain the core of stroke rehabilitation technology as developing general-purpose rehabilitation devices is extraordinarily complex. Cost consideration and reimbursement issues are likely to grow in importance as the cost/benefit ratio of incorporating robotics into stroke rehabilitation is debated.

REFERENCES

1. Hermano IK, Dipietro L, Levy-Tzedek S, et al. A paradigm shift for rehabilitation robotics. *IEEE Eng Med Biol Mag.* 2008;27:61—70.
2. http://www.oxfordlearnersdictionaries.com/definition/american_english/robot.
3. Xie M. *Fundamental of Robotic: Linking Perception to Action.* Singapore: World Scientific; 2003.
4. Morone G, Paolucci S, Cherubini A, et al. Robot-assisted gait training for stroke patients: current state of the art and perspectives of robotics. *Neuropsychiatric Dis Treat.* 2017;13:1303—1311.
5. Chang WH, Kim YH. Robot-assisted therapy in stroke rehabilitation. *J Stroke.* 2013;15:174—181.
6. Center of Disease Control and Prevention. Available: https://www.cdc.gov/stroke/facts.htm.
7. Stein J, Bishop L, Agrawal SK, Fasoli SE, Igo Krebs H, Hogan N. Robots in stroke rehabilitation. *Stroke Recovery Rehabil.* 2015;2:359—373.
8. Wagner TH, Lo CA, Peduzzi P, et al. An economic analysis of robot-assisted therapy for long-term upper limb impairment after stroke. *Stroke.* 2011;42:2630—2632.
9. Stein J. Robotics in rehabilitation: technology as destiny. *Am J Phys Med Rehabil.* 2012;91.
10. Liepert J, Bauder H, Wolfgang HR, et al. Treatment-induced cortical reorganization after stroke in humans. *Stroke.* 2000;31:1210—1216.
11. Lang CE, Macdonald JR, Reisman DS, et al. Observation of amounts of movement practice provided during stroke rehabilitation. *Arch Phys Med Rehabil.* 2009;90:1692—1698.
12. Krebs HI, Palazzolo JJ, Dipietro L, et al. Rehabilitation robotics: performance-based progressive robot-assisted therapy. *Am J Phys Med Rehabil.* 2003;15:7—20.
13. Aisen FL, Krebs HI, Hogan N, et al. The effect of robot-assisted therapy and rehabilitative training on motor recovery following stroke. *Arch Neurol.* 1997;54:443—446.
14. Volpe BT, Krebs HI, Hogan N, et al. A novel approach to stroke rehabilitation: robot-aided sensorimotor stimulation. *Neurology.* 2000;54:1938—1944.
15. Krebs HI, Volpe BT, Ferraro M, et al. Robot-aided neurorehabilitation: from evidence-based to science-based rehabilitation. *Top Stroke Rehabil.* 2002;8:54—70.
16. Volpe BT, Krebs HI, Hogan NI, et al. Robot-aided sensorimotor training in stroke rehabilitation a realistic option? *Curr Opin Neurol.* 2001;14:745—752.
17. Volpe BT, Krebs HI, Hogan N, et al. Robot training enhanced motor outcome in patients with stroke maintained over 3 years. *Neurology.* 1999;53:1874—1876.
18. Rabadi M, Galgano M, Lynch D, Akerman M, Lesser M, Volpe B. A pilot study of activity-based therapy in the arm motor recovery post stroke: a randomized controlled trial. *Clin Rehabil.* 2008;22:1071—1082.
19. Sale P, Franceschini M, Mazzoleni S, Palma E, Agosti M, Posteraro F. Effects of upper limb robot-assisted therapy on motor recovery in subacute stroke patients. *J NeuroEng Rehabil.* 2014;11:104.
20. Fasoli SE, Krebs HI, Stein J, et al. Effects of robotic therapy on motor impairment and recovery in chronic stroke. *Arch Phys Med Rehabil.* 2003;84:477—482.
21. Ferraro M, Palazzolo JJ, Krol J, et al. Robot-aided sensorimotor arm training improves outcomes in patients with chronic stroke. *Neurology.* 2003;61:1604—1607.
22. Finley MA, Fasoli SE, Dipietro L, et al. Short duration upper extremity robotic therapy in stroke patients with severe upper extremity impairment. *VA J Rehabil Res Devel.* 2005;42:683—692.
23. Daly J, Hogan N, Perepezko E, et al. Response to upper limb robotics and functional neuromuscular stimulation following stroke. *VA J Rehabil Res Devel.* 2005;42:723—736.
24. MacClellan LR, Bradham DD, Whitall J, et al. Robotic upper extremity neuro-rehabilitation in chronic stroke patients. *VA J Rehabil Res Devel.* 2005;42:717—722.
25. Volpe BT, Lynch D, Rykman-Berland A, et al. Intensive sensorimotor arm training mediated by therapist or robot improves hemiparesis in patients with chronic stroke. *Neurorehabil Neural Repair.* 2008;22:305—310.

26. Lo AC, Guarino PD, Richards LG, et al. Robot-assisted therapy for long-term upper-limb impairment after stroke. *N Engl J Med.* 2010;362:1772–1783.

27. Masiero S, Armani M, Rosati G. Upper-limb robot-assisted therapy in rehabilitation of acute stroke patients: focused review and results of new randomized controlled trial. *J Rehabil Res Dev.* 2011;48:355–366.

28. Masiero S, Celia A, Armani M, Rosati G. A novel device in rehabilitation of post-stroke hemiplegic upper limbs. *Aging Clin Exp Res.* 2006;18:531–535.

29. Masiero S, Celia RG, Armani M. Robotic-assisted rehabilitation of the upper limb after acute stroke. *Arch Phys Med Rehabil.* 2007;88:142–149.

30. Rosati G, Gallina P, Masiero S. Design, implementation and clinical tests of a wire-based robot for neurorehabilitation. *IEEE Trans Neural Syst Rehabil Eng.* 2007;15:560–569.

31. Masiero S, Armani M, Ferlini G, Rosati G, Rossi A. Randomized trial of a robotic assistive device for the upper extremity during early inpatient stroke rehabilitation. *Neurorehabil Neural Repair.* 2014;28:377–386.

32. Mao Y, Jin X, Gera Dutta G, Scholz JP, Agrawal SK. Human movement training with cable driven arm exoskeleton (CAREX). *IEEE Trans Neural Syst Rehabil Eng.* 2015;23:84–92.

33. Krebs HI, Volpe BT, Williams D, et al. Robot-aided neurorehabilitation: a robot for wrist rehabilitation. *IEEE Trans Neural Syst Rehabil Eng.* 2007;15:327–335.

34. Sale P, Mazzoleni S, Lombardi V, et al. Recovery of hand function with robot-assisted therapy in acute stroke: a randomized controlled trial. *Int J Rehabil Res.* 2014;37:236–242.

35. Bovolenta F, Goldoni M, Clerici P, et al. Robot therapy for functional recovery of the upper limbs: a pilot study on patients after stroke. *J Rehabil Med.* 2009;41:971–975.

36. Bovolenta F, Sale P, Dall'Armi V, Clerici P, Franceschini M. Robot-aided therapy for upper limbs in patients with stroke-related lesions. Brief report of a clinical experience. *J Neuroeng Rehabil.* 2011;8:18.

37. Takahashi K, Domen K, Sakamoto T, et al. Efficacy of upper extremity robotic therapy in subacute poststroke hemiplegia. *Stroke.* 2016;47:1385–1388.

38. Klamroth-Marganska V, Blanco J, Campen K, et al. Three-dimensional, task-specific robot therapy of the arm after stroke: a multicenter, parallel-group randomized trial. *Lancet Neuro.* 2014;13:159–166.

39. Lum PS, Burgar CG, Shor PC, et al. Robot-assisted movement training compared with conventional therapy techniques for the rehabilitation of upper-limb motor function after stroke. *Arch Phys Med Rehabil.* 2002;83:952–959.

40. Liao WW, Wu CY, Hsieh YW, Lin KC, Chang WY. Effects of robot-assisted upper limb rehabilitation on daily function and real-world arm activity in patients with chronic stroke: a randomized controlled trial. *Clin Rehabil.* 2012;26:111–120.

41. Krakauer JW, Carmichael ST, Corbett D, Wittenberg GF. Getting neurorehabilitation right: what wan be learned from animal models? *Neurorehabil Neural Repair.* 2012;26:923–931.

42. Kahn LE, Zygman ML, Rymer WZ, Reinkensmeyer DJ. *Effect of Robot-assisted and Unassisted Exercise on Functional Reaching in Chronic Hemiparesis.* Conference Proceedings of the 23rd Annual International Conference of the IEEE Engineering in Medicine and Biology Society. Istanbul. 2001, 4(4132).

43. Hesse S, Werner C, Pohl M, et al. Computerized arm training improves the motor control of the severely affected arm after stroke: a single-blinded randomized trial in two centers. *Stroke.* 2005;36:915–920.

44. Sullivan KJ, Knowlton BJ, Dobkin BH. Step training with body weight support: effect of treadmill speed and practice paradigms poststroke locomotor recovery. *Arch Phys Med Rehabil.* 2002;83:683–691.

45. Miyai I, Fujimoto Y, Ueda Y, et al. Treadmill training with body weight support: its effect on Parkinson's disease. *Arch Phys Med Rehabil.* 2000;81:849–852.

46. Schindl MR, Forstner C, Kern H, Hesse S. Treadmill training with partial body weight support in nonambulatory patients with cerebral palsy. *Arch Phys Med Rehabil.* 2000;81:301–306.

47. Duncan PW, Sullivan KJ, Behrman AL, et al. Body weight supported treadmill rehabilitation after stroke. *N Eng J Med.* 2011;364:2026–2036.

48. Werner C, Von Frankenberg S, Treig T, et al. Treadmill training with partial body weight support and an electromechanical gait trainer for restoration of gait in subacute stroke patients: a randomized controlled study. *Stroke.* 2002;33:2895–2901.

49. Pohl M, Werner C, Holzgraefe M, et al. Repetitive locomotor training and physiotherapy improve walking and basic activities of daily living after stroke: a single-blind, randomized multicenter trial. *Clin Rehabil.* 2007;21:17–27.

50. Chua J, Culpan J, Menon E. Efficacy of an electromechanical gait trainer poststroke in Singapore: a randomized controlled trial. *Arch Phys Med Rehabil.* 2016;97:683–690.

51. Israel JF, Campbell DD, Kahn JH, Hornby TG. Metabolic costs and muscle activity patterns during robotic and therapist-assisted treadmill walking in individuals with incomplete spinal cord injury. *Phys Ther.* 2006;86:1466–1478.

52. Hidler JM, Wall AE. Alterations in muscle activation patterns during robotic-assisted walking. *Clin Biomech.* 2005;20:184–193.

53. Bang DH, Shin WS. Effects of robot-assisted gait training on spatiotemporal gait parameters and balance in patients with chronic stroke: a randomized controlled pilot trial. *NeuroRehabilitation.* 2016;38:343–349.

54. Van Nunen MP, Gerrits KH, Konijnenbelt M, Janssen TW, de Haan A. Recovery of walking ability using a robotic device in subacute stroke patients: a randomized controlled study. *Disabil Rehabil Assist Technol.* 2015;10:141–148.

55. Mehrholz J, Elsner B, Werner C, Kugler J, Pohl M. Electro-mechanical assisted training for walking after stroke. *Cochrane Database Syst Rev.* 2013;7. CD006185.

56. Forrester LW, Roy A, Krywonis A, Kehs G, Krebs HI, Macko RF. Modular ankle robotics training in early sub-acute stroke: a randomized controlled pilot study. *Neurore-habil Neural Repair.* 2014;28:678—687.

57. Forrester LW, Roy A, Krebs HI, Macko RF. Ankle training with a robotic device improves hemiparetic gait after stroke. *Neurorehabil Neural Repair.* 2011;25:369—377.

58. Banala SK, Kim SH, Agrawal SK, Scholz JP. Robot assisted gait training with active leg exoskeleton (ALEX). *IEEE Trans Neural Syst Rehabil Eng.* 2009;17:2—8.

59. Stegall P, Winfree K, Zanotto D, Agrawal SK. Rehabilita-tion exoskeleton design and the effect of anterior lunge degree-of-freedom. *IEEE Trans Robot.* 2013;29:838—846.

60. Kao PC, Srivastava S, Agrawal SK, Scholz JP. Effects of ro-botic performance-based error-augmentation versus error-reduction training on the gait pattern of healthy individuals. *Gait Posture.* 2013;37:113—120.

61. Stein J, Narendran K, McBean J, et al. EMG-controlled exoskeletal upper limb powered orthosis for exercise training post-stroke. *Am J Phys Med Rehabil.* 2007;86: 255—261.

62. Page SJ, Hill V, White S. Portable upper extremity robotics is as efficacious as upper extremity rehabilitative therapy: a randomized controlled pilot trial. *Clin Rehabil.* 2013;27: 494—503.

63. Stein J, Bishop L, Stein DJ, Wong CK. Gait training with a robotic leg brace after stroke: a randomized controlled pi-lot study. *Am J Phys Med Rehabil.* 2004;93:987—994.

64. Sales P, Franceschini M, Waldner A, Hesse S. Use of the robot assisted gait therapy in rehabilitation of patients with stroke and spinal cord injury. *Eur J Phys Rehabil Med.* 2012;48:111—121.

65. Kuiken TA, Dumanian GA, Lipschutz RD, et al. The use of targeted muscle reinnervation for improved myoelectric prosthesis control in a bilateral shoulder disarticulation amputee. *Prosthet Orthot Int.* 2004;28: 245—253.

66. Friehs GM, Zerris VA, Ojakangas CL, et al. Brain-machine and brain-computer interfaces. *Stroke.* 2004;35: 2702—2705.

67. Bustamante Valles K, Montes S, Madrigal J, et al. Technology-assisted stroke rehabilitation in Mexico: a pi-lot randomized trial comparing traditional therapy to cir-cuit training in a robot/technology-assisted therapy gym. *J Neuroeng Rehabil.* 2016;13:83.

68. Fasoli SE, Krebs HI, Hogan N. Robotic technology and stroke rehabilitation: translating research into practice. *Top Stroke Rehabil.* 2004;11:11—19.

69. Poli P, Morone G, Rosati G, Masiero S. Robotic technolo-gies and rehabilitation: new tools for stroke patients' therapy. *Biomed Res Int.* 2013;2013:153872. https:// doi.org/10.1155/2013/153872.

70. Bach JR, Zeelenberg AP, Winter C. Wheelchair-mounted robot manipulators. Long term use by patients with Duchenne muscular dystrophy. *Am J Phy Med Rehabil.* 1990;69:55—59.

71. Hammel JM, Van der Loos HF, Perkash I. Evaluation of a vocational robot with a quadriplegic employee. *Arch Phys Med Rehabil.* 1992;73:683—693.

72. Maheu V, Frappier J, Archambault PS, Routhier F. Evalua-tion of the JACO robotic arm: clinico-economic study for powered wheelchair users with upper-extremity disabilities. *IEEE Int Conf Rehabil Robot.* 2011;2011: 5975397. https://doi.org/10.1109/ICORR.2011.5975397.

73. Brose SW, Weber DJ, Salatin BA, et al. The role of assistive robotics in the lives of persons with disability. *Am J Phys Med Rehabil.* 2010;89:509—521.

CHAPTER 18

Efficacy of Noninvasive Brain Stimulation for Motor Rehabilitation After Stroke

DAVID A. CUNNINGHAM, PHD • YIN-LIANG LIN, PHD •
KELSEY A. POTTER–BAKER, PHD • JAYME S. KNUTSON, PHD •
ELA B. PLOW, PHD, PT

Stroke is a leading cause of longterm adult disability, where 60%–80% of survivors experience neurological impairments often affecting motor function.[1,2] The goal of current therapy practice is to enable patients to reach their maximum functional potential. One of the challenges to optimum recovery is the reduced number of therapy sessions patients receive due to shortened lengths of stay and limited insurance coverage for ongoing therapy. Therefore, there is a need for new therapy approaches that accelerate recovery within the constraints of time permitted for outpatient clinical therapy, as well as enhance the degree of functional recovery.

NONINVASIVE BRAIN STIMULATION: REPETITIVE TRANSCRANIAL MAGNETIC STIMULATION AND TRANSCRANIAL DIRECT CURRENT STIMULATION

A possible strategy to accelerate and enhance rehabilitative gains involves augmenting mechanisms of neuroplasticity that underlie rehabilitation-related recovery with the use of noninvasive brain stimulation (NIBS). NIBS has been approved by the U.S. Food and Drug Administration for the treatment of depression and anxiety in the clinical setting. Studies are underway to determine whether using NIBS to promote motor recovery in the stroke population can provide a similar efficacy. Two emerging means of applying NIBS are repetitive transcranial magnetic stimulation and transcranial direct current stimulation.

Repetitive transcranial magnetic stimulation (rTMS) (Fig. 18.1) operates on the principle of electromagnetic induction using an insulated coiled wire placed on the scalp. The coil produces a brief and strong alternating current that induces a perpendicular spatially focused magnetic field. The magnetic field induces current, which passes unimpeded through the skull, resulting in depolarization or hyperpolarization of neurons in superficial cortices, depending on the frequency of stimulation.[3] The mechanism of rTMS is thought to induce N-methyl-D-aspartate (NMDA) receptor-dependent long-term potentiation (LTP) or depression (LTD). If the stimulation pulses are applied at frequencies ≥ 5 Hz (considered "high" frequency in this context), it is thought to increase synaptic strength (LTP) and therefore increase corticospinal excitability. Corticospinal excitability in this context is measured as the magnitude of electromyographic (EMG) signal recorded in target muscles in response to single-pulse TMS applied over the corresponding contralateral motor area of the brain. If the rTMS pulses are applied at frequencies ≤ 1 Hz (considered "low" frequency) it is thought to decrease synaptic efficacy (LTD) and therefore reduce corticospinal excitability.[4] The typical dose of rTMS is anywhere from 10 to 30 min where rTMS is applied immediately prior to physical/occupational therapy. High-frequency protocols are generally applied in shorter periods of rTMS separated by periods of no stimulation. Low frequency protocols are administered in one continuous train.

Transcranial direct current stimulation (tDCS) (Fig. 18.2) adopts a different approach to stimulating the brain by applying direct, rather than alternating, current to targeted regions of the brain. Using a constant current stimulator, surface electrodes (usually saline-soaked sponges) deliver low-levels of direct current (0–4 mA) to the scalp and create changes in

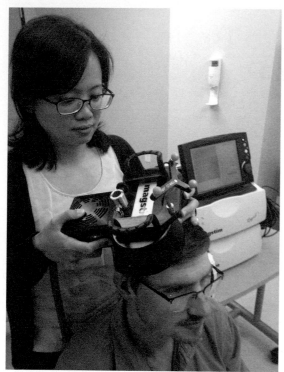

FIG. 18.1 Repetitive transcranial magnetic stimulation (rTMS).

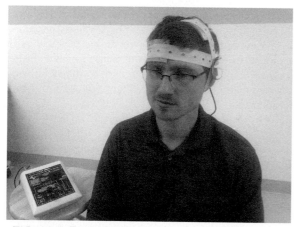

FIG. 18.2 Transcranial direct current stimulation (tDCS).

corticospinal excitability.[5] In context to stroke motor rehabilitation, anode and cathode electrodes (5 × 7 sq. cm sponges) are most commonly placed over the primary motor cortex and over the supraorbital area contralateral to the hemisphere being stimulated. tDCS has also been used to modulate both hemispheres

concurrently such that electrodes are placed on homologous primary motor cortices.[6] Depending on the direction of current flow, superficial membrane potentials can either be depolarized or hyperpolarized. Anodal tDCS depolarizes membrane potentials and is therefore considered excitatory, similar to high frequency rTMS, while cathodal tDCS hyperpolarizes membrane potentials and is considered inhibitory, similar to low frequency rTMS.[7] The typical dose of tDCS is anywhere from 20 to 30 min at a time with breaks and ranges from 1 to 2 mA in intensity. Advantages of tDCS over rTMS are that it does not require expensive equipment, and it can be easily applied concurrently with physical/occupational therapy. While the exact mechanisms of tDCS are unclear,[4] based on pharmacological studies,[8,9] tDCS likely upregulates receptors that contribute to increased synaptic strength with anodal tDCS, or downregulates synaptic strength with cathodal tDCS. In this way, tDCS modulates the membrane potentials and therefore the spontaneous firing rate of the neurons. It has been postulated that lasting aftereffects of tDCS may reflect LTP-like and LTD-like plasticity, similar to rTMS.[4]

SAFETY CONSIDERATIONS

Safety guidelines have been published for applying NIBS, including rTMS and tDCS, to the stroke population.[10–13] Some of the more common side effects of rTMS are local transient pain and discomfort (39%), sleepiness, and mild headaches (28%), most of which subside immediately following stimulation. Headaches, however, may occasionally persist and can be treated with an oral analgesic. A rare but acute adverse effect of rTMS is seizures. The majority of seizure cases occurred prior to the safety guidelines reported by Wassermann in 1998.[11] In order to mitigate the risk of seizure in patients with stroke, it is important to consider the patient's history of seizure, as well as use of any drugs and substances that may lower the seizure threshold. Given the large number of subjects and patients that have undergone rTMS over the past two decades, the risk of seizure in participants is considered low. The guidelines established by Wassermann (1998) as well as those by Rossi and colleagues (2009) regarding intensity, frequency, and duration of stimulation should be followed.

tDCS has been considered safer than rTMS because there have not been any incidence of seizure with the use of the device.[12,13] Some of the more common side effects include moderate fatigue (35%), transient mild headaches (11.8%), and tingling in the area of stimulation.[14] This often results in temporary itchiness and/or redness of the skin. As recently as 2016, Bikson and colleagues[12] report that based on 33,000 sessions of tDCS they found no evidence for irreversible injury produced by stimulation sessions that are ≤40 min in duration using a stimulation intensity of ≤4 mA.

NONINVASIVE BRAIN STIMULATION APPLICATION FOR THE STROKE BRAIN

NIBS for upper limb rehabilitation after stroke is applied based on maladaptive neuronal plasticity that occurs following the stroke. Studies have shown that the increased activation of the nonlesioned hemisphere produces abnormally high interhemispheric inhibition of the primary motor cortex of the lesioned hemisphere. This is commonly referred to as the "interhemispheric competition model" (Fig. 18.3). According to this model, paresis originates from loss of corticospinal

output to the paretic upper limb, but it persists due to interhemispheric imbalances. The nonlesioned hemisphere excessively inhibits the lesioned hemisphere, which has lost its reciprocal inhibitory input to the nonlesioned hemisphere.[15–17] As patients rely on using the nonparetic upper limb to compensate for failures in using the paretic upper limb, interhemispheric competition intensifies.[18] Output from the lesioned hemisphere weakens further, while excitability and inhibition imposed from the nonlesioned hemisphere continues to rise,[16] which further reduces the output of the lesioned hemisphere in addition to what is due to anatomical damage. In accordance with the interhemispheric competition model, present-day NIBS approaches aim to facilitate excitability of the lesioned hemisphere and suppress excitability of the nonlesioned hemisphere during, or prior to, physical/occupational therapy to enhance rehabilitative outcomes. Towards this end, multiple research groups

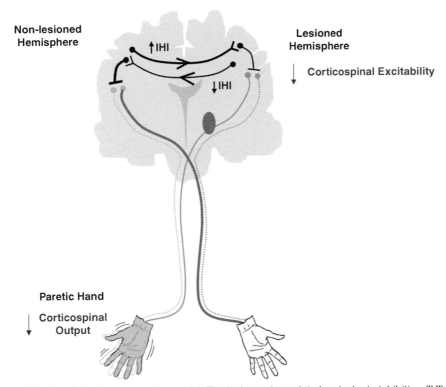

FIG. 18.3 Interhemispheric competition model. The lesion reduces interhemispheric inhibition (IHI) exerted by the effect of the nonlesioned hemisphere. In turn, the disinhibited nonlesioned hemisphere generates exaggerated inhibition on the lesioned hemisphere, which reduces excitability and corticospinal output to the paretic limb. Dark circle represents the lesion. (Figure adapted from Cunningham DA, Potter-Baker KA, Knutson JS, Sankarasubramanian V, Machado AG, Plow EB. Tailoring brain stimulation to the nature of rehabilitative therapies in stroke: a conceptual framework based on their unique mechanisms of recovery. *Phys Med Rehabil Clin N Am.* 2015;26(4):759–774. https://doi.org/10.1016/j.pmr.2015.07.001.)

have sought to either increase the excitability of the lesioned hemisphere with high-frequency rTMS or anodal tDCS or to inhibit the nonlesioned hemisphere with low-frequency rTMS or cathodal tDCS (Fig. 18.4) (For a review, please refer to Hoyer and Celnik[19] or Sandrini and Cohen[20]). In either hemisphere, the most common target is the primary motor cortex (M1) because it offers the maximum corticospinal output to the upper extremity, and evidence suggests its adaptive plasticity is intimately associated with paretic upper limb recovery.[21-23]

EFFICACY OF NONINVASIVE BRAIN STIMULATION TO IMPROVE MOTOR FUNCTION IN PATIENTS WITH STROKE

Early evidence of NIBS to directly and/or indirectly excite M1 and promote upper limb motor function recovery has shown promise. For example, Conforto and colleagues[24] demonstrated in 30 patients with acute/subacute stroke that inhibitory stimulation to the nonlesioned hemisphere (duration: 25 min) prior to therapy (10−60 min sessions) improved impairment scores by 12.3% compared to 5.5% in patients who

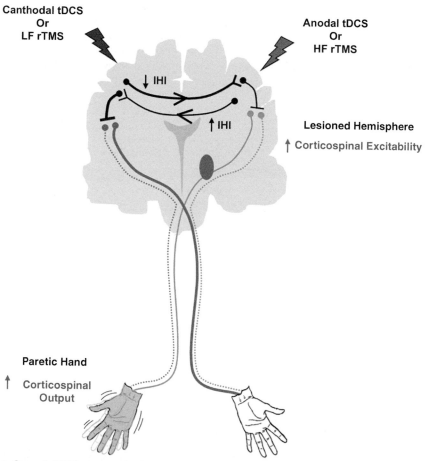

FIG. 18.4 Current NIBS approach. Anodal tDCS or high-frequency (HF) rTMS targets the lesioned hemisphere to increase the excitability of the lesioned hemisphere and the corticospinal output to the paretic hand. Cathodal tDCS or low-frequency (LF) rTMS is applied to the nonlesioned hemisphere to reduce the inhibition imposed on the lesioned hemisphere. Dark circle represents the lesion. (Figure adapted from Cunningham DA, Potter-Baker KA, Knutson JS, Sankarasubramanian V, Machado AG, Plow EB. Tailoring brain stimulation to the nature of rehabilitative therapies in stroke: a conceptual framework based on their unique mechanisms of recovery. *Phys Med Rehabil Clin N Am.* 2015;26(4):759−774. https://doi.org/10.1016/j.pmr. 2015.07.001.)

received sham stimulation. Additionally, Lindenberg and colleagues[6] reported in a sample of 10 chronic stroke patients that when inhibitory tDCS is applied to the nonlesioned hemisphere and anodal tDCS is applied to the lesioned hemisphere simultaneously (30 min) during therapy (five 60-min sessions), patients improved impairment scores by 20.7% compared to 3.2% in patients who received sham stimulation.

However, larger clinical trials and metaanalyses have failed to demonstrate benefits of pairing NIBS with physical and occupational therapies.[25-31] Hesse and colleagues[26] showed that with 96 patients with acute stroke, regardless of the stimulation montage, that is, inhibitory stimulation to the nonlesioned hemisphere or excitatory stimulation to the lesioned hemisphere (duration: 20 min) showed no advantage to rehabilitation (400 repetitions each of 2 bilateral movements on a robotic device) as all groups improved to the same degree when compared to sham stimulation. Likewise, Talelli and colleagues[29] showed in 41 patients with chronic stroke that neither montage (duration: 40–200 s) demonstrated an advantage over sham stimulation when combined with rehabilitation. Overall, there is not enough evidence to support that a combination of NIBS and traditional therapy can produce greater effect sizes than physical/occupational therapy of the upper limb alone.[32-34] For example, Hao and colleagues[34] included 19 clinical trials with a total of 588 participants and concluded that current evidence does not support the routine use of rTMS for the treatment of motor recovery for stroke. Likewise, Elsner and colleagues[32] included 32 studies with a total of 748 participants and concluded that there is limited evidence to support the use of tDCS for improving activities of daily living for patients with stroke.

FACTORS AFFECTING EFFICACY OF NONINVASIVE BRAIN STIMULATION TO IMPROVE MOTOR FUNCTION IN PATIENTS WITH STROKE

The discrepancy between studies (Tables 18.1 and 18.2)[31] and the failed metaanalyses for the efficacy of NIBS and motor recovery may be due to the heterogeneity of stroke chronicity and severity included in many studies. The heterogeneity of stroke can vary from the time since stroke, which offers differing mechanisms of neuroplasticity such that some NIBS montages may be more beneficial than others at different times post stroke. Also, patients often have a wide range of damage such that the lesioned hemisphere may be more

damaged in some and less in others. Ultimately, the general severity of stroke may result in differing neuroplasticity and NIBS montages should be applied to target the individual's unique potential residual mechanisms of recovery. Lastly, a stroke can occur in a variety of locations, and there is evidence to suggest that NIBS has different effects depending on whether a patient has a cortical or subcortical stroke. The following sections will briefly describe subpopulations of patients with stroke and various montages that may benefit each patient, whether it is based on the timing, severity, or location of stroke.

TIME SINCE STROKE

NIBS has been shown to provide benefit as an add-on to existing physical/occupational therapy anywhere from the first month since stroke well into the chronic phase of recovery (>6 months) (for a review, please refer to Lüdemann-Podubeck and colleagues[35]). For example, Khedr and colleagues[36] applied inhibitory rTMS to the nonlesioned hemisphere in 24 patients (12 active, 12 sham) who were within 1 month of stroke for five 15-min sessions and demonstrated an 18% improvement in functional outcomes over sham stimulation. Furthermore, they reported a 33% improvement at 3-month follow-up when compared to the sham stimulation group. Likewise, Takeuchi and colleagues[37] applied inhibitory rTMS to the nonlesioned hemisphere for 25 min prior to 15 min of motor training in 40 patients (20 active, 20 sham) who were more than 6 months post stroke and demonstrated a 19% improvement in functional outcomes over sham stimulation.

Despite the positive findings of smaller studies that included participants with homogenous poststroke chronicity, studies that enroll participants over a wide range of chronicity have generally diminished effect sizes, and in some cases negative outcomes are reported. For example, Seniow and colleagues[28] applied inhibitory stimulation to the nonlesioned hemisphere in 40 patients (20 active, 20 sham) who were less than 3 months post stroke for fifteen 45-min sessions. On average, they demonstrated that sham stimulation improved general motor function by 10% over the active stimulation group. Likewise, Etoh and colleagues[38] applied inhibitory stimulation to the nonlesioned hemisphere in 18 patients (9 active, 9 sham) who were 5–60 months post stroke for ten 40-min sessions. On average they reported that sham stimulation improved general motor function by 14% over the active stimulation group.

TABLE 18.1
Studies Discussing the Positive Effects of Brain Stimulation as an Add-On in Rehabilitation (Plow et al.[31])

Study	Final Target	Type of Stimulation	Study Design	Frequency/Duration of Training	Paired/Training Rehabilitation	Findings/Remarks
Bolognini and others (2011)	M1	tDCS, upregulating the lesioned hemisphere while downregulating the nonlesioned hemisphere	Randomized, sham controlled in chronic (N = 14)	10 sessions	Constraint induced movement therapy	Stimulation improves paretic hand function, strength, and its perceived use presumably by upregulating the lesioned hemisphere M1 and reducing callosal inhibition from the nonlesioned hemisphere
Chang and others (2010)	M1	rTMS, upregulating the lesioned hemisphere	Longitudinal, pseudorandomized, sham controlled in subacute (N = 28)	10 sessions over 2 weeks	Motor practice: reaching and grasping	All improved, but stimulation generated additional benefit over long term
Conforto and others (2012)	M1	rTMS, downregulating the nonlesioned hemisphere	Randomized, sham controlled in acute to subacute (N = 30)	10 sessions over 2 weeks	Customary rehabilitation	Tasks related to daily living; strength improved in patients receiving stimulation as add-on
Edwards and others (2009)	M1	tDCS, upregulating the lesioned hemisphere	Preliminary in chronic (N = 6)	1 session	Robotic training	Functional improvement not witnessed, although excitability of the lesioned hemisphere M1 was upregulated and sustained with robotic training
Kakuda and others (2011)	M1	rTMS, downregulating the nonlesioned hemisphere	Single-group design, multicenter for chronic stroke (N = 204); no control group	22 sessions over 15 days	Offline 2-h occupational therapy	Motor function improved; effects significant despite short duration of constraint-induced therapy; lack of control group expressed as limitation

Study	Region	Intervention	Design	Sessions	Task	Outcome
Khedr and others (2005)	M1	rTMS, upregulating the lesioned hemisphere	Randomized, sham controlled in acute (N = 52)	10 sessions	Standard physical therapy	Stimulation, as add-on, alleviated functional disability and improved independence more than rehabilitation potentially by aiding the lesioned hemisphere excitability, although effect not significant versus sham
Kim and others (2006)	M1	rTMS, upregulating the lesioned hemisphere	Randomized, sham controlled, crossover in chronic (N = 15)	Single session each	Offline motor sequence learning	Stimulation as add-on to motor sequence training improved accuracy and movement time versus training alone; excitability of the lesioned hemisphere M1 was upregulated in association with accuracy
Lefebvre and others (2014)	M1	tDCS, upregulating ipsilesional while downregulating contralesional	Randomized, sham controlled, crossover in chronic (N = 18)	Single session each	Online motor skill learning involving tracking	Add-on stimulation benefited skill, efficiency, and retention versus learning alone
Lindenberg and others (2010); Lindenberg and others (2012b)	M1	Upregulating the lesioned hemisphere while downregulating the nonlesioned hemisphere	Single-group design for chronic stroke (N = 10)	5 daily sessions (early training) followed by another 5 (late training)	Online physical and occupational therapy	Stimulation as add-on benefited rehabilitative outcomes more in early than late training; related study (2010) shows fMRI activation of the lesioned hemisphere M1 increased with stimulation

Continued

TABLE 18.1
Studies Discussing the Positive Effects of Brain Stimulation as an Add-On in Rehabilitation (Plow et al.[31])—cont'd

Study	Final Target	Type of Stimulation	Study Design	Frequency/Duration of Training	Paired/Training Rehabilitation	Findings/Remarks
Nair and others (2011)	M1	tDCS, downregulating the nonlesioned hemisphere	Randomized, sham controlled in chronic (N = 14)	5 daily sessions	Online occupational therapy	Stimulation conferred advantage to rehabilitation, improving range and upper limb function; stimulation associated with reduced fMRI intensity of activation in the nonlesioned hemisphere M1
Ochi and others (2013)	M1	tDCS, upregulating the lesioned hemisphere in one group and downregulating the nonlesioned hemisphere in another	Randomized, controlled, crossover design in chronic with moderate to severe paresis (N = 18)	5 daily sessions each, with 2-d interval crossover	Robotic training involving forearm rotation and wrist flexion/extension	Limited although similar improvement for hand function and its perceived use in both groups; spasticity alleviated with the nonlesioned hemisphere stimulation, more so in right hemispheric stroke
Sasaki and others (2013)	M1	rTMS, upregulating in one group and downregulating the nonlesioned hemisphere in another	Randomized, sham controlled; early after stroke (N = 27)	5 daily sessions	Offline conventional rehabilitation	Both types of stimulation were effective in improving strength and tapping frequency; although differences between stimulation groups were not significant; benefits of upregulating the lesioned hemisphere M1 outweighed those versus sham

Study	Target	Intervention	Study design	Duration	Training	Findings
Takeuchi and others (2012)	M1	rTMS, upregulating the lesioned hemisphere in one group and downregulating the nonlesioned hemisphere in another; both offered concurrently in third group	Randomized, controlled (N = 27)	single session	Offline pinch training	Downregulating the nonlesioned hemisphere M1, and its combination with upregulating the lesioned hemisphere, improves motor training; downregulating the nonlesioned hemisphere causes bimanual coordination to deteriorate, but its combination with upregulating M1 prevents such deterioration
Wu and others (2013)	M1	tDCS, downregulating the lesioned hemisphere to reduce spasticity	Randomized, sham controlled (N = 45)	5 sessions/week × 4 week	Offline physical therapy	Stimulation significantly improved tone, motor function, and activities of daily living
Zimerman and others (2012)	M1	tDCS, downregulating the nonlesioned hemisphere	Randomized, sham controlled, crossover; subcortical well recovered (N = 12)	Single session each	Online motor sequence learning	Downregulating the nonlesioned hemisphere M1 facilitates early learning and retention; effects associated with upregulating intracortical excitability of the lesioned hemisphere

TABLE 18.2
Studies Discussing the Variable Success of Brain Stimulation as an Add-On in Rehabilitation

Study	Final Target	Type of Stimulation	Study Design	Frequency/Duration of Training	Paired/Training Rehabilitation	Findings/Remarks
Ackerley and others (2010)	M1	rTMS, upregulating lesioned while downregulating the nonlesioned hemisphere	Randomized, sham controlled, crossover in chronic (N = 10)	Single session each	Precision grip	Upregulating the lesioned hemisphere M1 before training effective; downregulating the nonlesioned hemisphere ineffective at upregulating excitability of the lesioned hemisphere and instead reduced function
Emara and others (2009)	M1	rTMS, upregulating the lesioned hemisphere in one group and downregulating the nonlesioned hemisphere in another	Randomized, sham controlled in acute (N = 60)	10 sessions over 2 weeks	Physical therapy	Improvement in select patients; affecting the nonlesioned hemisphere M1 failed to benefit individuals with cortical lesions, while affecting the lesioned hemisphere M1 directly benefited those with cortical or noncortical lesions consistently; no improvement in those with total anterior circulation stroke or ones with no residual arm function
Hesse and others (2011)	M1	tDCS, upregulating the lesioned hemisphere in one group and downregulating the nonlesioned hemisphere in another	Randomized, sham controlled, multicenter in acute–subacute who were severe (N = 96)	5 sessions/week × 6 weeks	Online bilateral robot training, offline physical and occupational therapy	All improved but no advantage of stimulation; majority had large infarct with cortical–subcortical or predominantly cortical damage; most showed no evoked response in paretic limb, confirming lack of viable corticospinal tracts from the lesioned hemisphere M1; when only subcortical analyzed, benefit of downregulating the nonlesioned hemisphere tended to be significant

Malcolm and others (2007)	M1	rTMS, upregulating the lesioned hemisphere	Randomized, sham controlled in chronic (N = 20)	10 consecutive weekday sessions plus home exercises	Offline constraint-induced movement therapy	Although stimulating the lesioned hemisphere M1 upregulated its excitability, it failed to translate to advantage in motor function; no added advantage for group receiving stimulation in rehabilitation
Pomeroy and others (2007)	M1	rTMS, downregulating the lesioned hemisphere	Randomized, placebo controlled, 4-group design; early after stroke (N = 24)	8 daily sessions	Offline voluntary muscle contraction or placebo	No additional advantage of stimulation for function, although stimulation as add-on to voluntary movement upregulated the lesioned hemisphere excitability
Seniow and others (2012)	M1	rTMS, downregulating the nonlesioned hemisphere	Randomized, sham controlled in moderate impairment (N = 40)	5 daily sessions × 3 weeks	Offline physical therapy	Both groups improved significantly, but there was no greater advantage of additive stimulation
Talelli and others (2012)	M1	rTMS, upregulating the lesioned hemisphere in one and downregulating the nonlesioned hemisphere in another	Semirandomized, controlled in chronic with mild to moderate impairment (N = 41)	10 sessions	Offline physical therapy	All patients improved, but addition of stimulation did not augment improvements

The smaller effect size, and in some cases negative results, may be due to the differing neurophysiology at the various times since stroke onset. Within the first hours following stroke, signaling of the excitatory neurotransmitter glutamate is excitotoxic and will contribute to cell death; however, there is an increase signaling of the inhibitory neurotransmitter GABA which serves to counteract the toxicity of glutamate.[39] Studies have shown that the GABA-mediated inhibition is necessary in the first days following stroke in order to limit an expansion of the infarct size. However, the beneficial effects of GABA-mediated inhibition become detrimental over time and ultimately prevent motor recovery, while the initial detrimental effects of glutamate become beneficial and promote longterm potentiation during recovery (weeks to months).[40] Additionally, in the early phase of stroke, studies have observed that there is a general increase in activation of the nonlesioned hemisphere, and this is thought to support residual motor function and recovery during the first couple of weeks, especially in those with severe motor deficits at the onset of stroke.[41] However, over time, the prolonged activation of the nonlesioned hemisphere into the chronic phase of stroke (>3–6 months) may eventually have a negative impact on the lesioned hemisphere through tonic inhibition imposed on the hypoactive lesioned hemisphere, previously described as the interhemispheric competition model.[15–18]

Based on the poststroke time course of neuroplasticity, there is reason to suggest that one NIBS montage may be more beneficial than the other depending on the time since stroke. For example, suppressing corticospinal excitability of the nonlesioned hemisphere during the early phase of stroke may negate the nonlesioned hemisphere's support of residual motor function, where suppressing the nonlesioned hemisphere into the chronic phase of stroke may aid in reducing its excessive inhibition upon the lesioned hemisphere. In fact, Lüdemann-Podubeck and colleagues[35] reported that there is more evidence to support excitatory stimulation to the lesioned hemisphere during the early phase of stroke (i.e., enhance glutamatergic benefits in the lesioned hemisphere) and inhibitory stimulation to the nonlesioned hemisphere is more beneficial during the chronic phase of stroke (i.e., suppress interhemispheric competition originating from the nonlesioned hemisphere). Still, these suggestions are based on observation of the literature; there has not been a study that has described the differential effectiveness of NIBS on motor recovery of the paretic upper limb depending on the time since stroke. Future work systematically determining which NIBS approach depending on the time since stroke is required.

SEVERITY OF IMPAIRMENT

Of the 60%–80% of patients with chronic stroke that experience motor deficit of the upper limb, 15%–30% are permanently disabled and 20% require institutionalized care due to severe paralysis.[42] The overall severity of stroke may be attributed to the amount of damage that occurred to the underlying white matter within the corticospinal tract.[43–46] Thus, patients with severe motor impairments often do not have adequate residual corticospinal pathways that can be excited in the lesioned hemisphere with NIBS. In fact, when severe and sometimes moderately impaired patients are included in studies that use the previously described conventional stimulation approaches in accordance with poststroke maladaptive plasticity, there is often little to no benefit for those patients.[26,28,47,48] The differences in the effectiveness of brain stimulation may result from variation in neuroplasticity and reorganization among the patients with different levels of severity.

Contrary to the view of the interhemispheric competition model, influence of the nonlesioned hemisphere upon the paretic upper limb may vary depending on the degree of cortical/subcortical damage and the resulting impairment. Several studies have demonstrated the importance of the nonlesioned hemisphere in motor recovery, especially in patients with moderate or severe impairment. For example, clinical evidence has demonstrated that a second stroke in the nonlesioned hemisphere affects the primary paretic upper limb function.[49,50] Moreover, virtual lesion techniques that allow for transient disruption of activity of underlying cortical regions suggest that suppressing activity of the nonlesioned hemisphere induces delay in reaction time of the paretic upper limb,[51,52] especially in patients with moderate to severe impairment.[53] Therefore, the role of the nonlesioned hemisphere may be more supportive for movement of the paretic upper limb in patients who experience severe damage and impairment than what was originally believed.

A popular hypothesis that has helped explained the role of the nonlesioned hemisphere and how it may contribute to upper limb motor recovery is the bimodal balance-recovery model proposed by Di Pino and colleagues.[54] The model links the patterns of reorganization following stroke to the extent of damage to the lesioned hemisphere and pathways. For example, when the damage is mild, the lesioned hemisphere mainly contributes to recovery and the nonlesioned hemisphere contributes to upper limb paresis, as proposed by the interhemispheric competition model. However, if the damage is severe, the residual lesioned pathways cannot support the recovery, and therefore the nonlesioned hemisphere may take the primary role in recovery of paretic upper limb function via uncrossed ipsilateral pathways devoted to the paretic upper limb.[51,54-57]

Based on the bimodal balance-recovery model, patients with moderate to severe impairment fail to improve with brain stimulation[26,28,47,48] because the cortical areas supporting their recovery differ from those targeted with the previously described conventional approaches. Specifically, while patients with moderate to severe impairment rely on the nonlesioned hemisphere for recovery, the conventional approach to brain stimulation facilitates the excitability of lesioned hemisphere instead, or even suppresses the excitability of the nonlesioned hemisphere. Therefore, instead of the conventional approaches, patients with moderate to severe impairment may need stimulation approaches that are delivered to facilitate the excitability of areas in the nonlesioned hemisphere. A recent study by Sankarasubramanian and colleagues (2017) revealed that patients with moderate to severe impairment can achieve immediate improvement in paretic upper limb movement with a single session of stimulation delivered to facilitate the excitability of the dorsal premotor cortex in the nonlesioned hemisphere even when they fail to achieve much improvement with the conventional approach.[56] Future work is still needed to investigate the longterm effect of facilitatory stimulation over the nonlesioned hemisphere to improve paretic upper limb function in patients with moderate to severe impairment.

Due to various patterns of reorganization following stroke, Di Pino and colleagues[54] and others[31,56-60] suggest that instead of a "one size fits all" approach, it is important to stratify patients with stroke and apply tailored approaches to brain stimulation. Therefore, several studies have tried to identify the characteristics of the responders to the conventional approaches[61-63] based on demographic factors, genotypes, function and impairment, response to TMS, and corticospinal tract integrity. In addition, Sankarasubramanian and colleagues[56] also defined a cutoff on measures of impairment and corticospinal tract integrity to categorize patients with stroke as responders to two types of brain stimulation, inhibition of nonlesioned primary cortex or facilitation of the nonlesioned premotor cortex. These studies generally confirm the concepts of

bimodal balance-recovery model that only patients with mild impairment and damage benefit from the conventional approaches. Therefore, more studies are still needed to focus on patients with moderate to severe impairment.

STROKE LESION LOCATION AND ITS RELATION TO STIMULATION TARGETS

Stroke lesion location is highly heterogeneous.[64] Heterogeneity exists given that any vessel within the highly vascularized central nervous system can produce a stroke. The most common artery involved in a stroke lesion is the middle cerebral artery (MCA). An MCA stroke typically results in subcortical damage to the internal capsule, basal ganglia, putamen, and caudate nucleus,[65] although damage to cortical areas can occur depending on the origin of the occlusion. Other arteries such as the posterior cerebral (PCA) and anterior cerebral arteries (ACA) can also become occluded resulting in cortical or subcortical damage.

The location of the stroke lesion in the brain has been shown to directly affect baseline motor function and immediate recovery after stroke. For example, Bentley and colleagues (2014) demonstrated that the lesion location is significantly related to functional recovery during the first week post stroke. Bentley noted that subjects showing the highest amount of recovery were those with a lesion to the cortical superficial left fronto-temporal lobe.[64] Others have found that individuals with a subcortical stroke have more disability as shown by a lower modified Rankin scale score.[66] In general, though, retrospective analyses have shown that individuals with a cortical stroke are less impaired and more likely to recover movement of the paretic upper limb in comparison to those with subcortical or mixed (cortical and subcortical) strokes.[67-69]

More importantly, evidence has begun to emerge that individuals with a cortical stroke demonstrate different mechanisms of recovery that may influence their response to adjunctive technologies like NIBS.[70] Ameli and colleagues (2009) have previously demonstrated that following one session of excitatory rTMS over the lesioned hemisphere, patients with subcortical stroke improved finger and hand tapping speed up to 19% over sham stimulation. Patients with cortical stroke demonstrated no improvement following active stimulation when compared to sham stimulation.[71] The authors were able to demonstrate that one factor that influenced the benefit of excitatory rTMS to the lesioned hemisphere is the amount of neural activity of the lesioned primary motor cortex at baseline. They postulated that the amount of neural activity might be determined whether cortical areas are involved or not. In another experiment, Thickbroom and colleagues[72] aimed to identify how the excitability of the nonlesioned hemisphere differed between individuals with a cortical and mixed stroke. Thickbroom and colleagues found that the excitability of the nonlesioned hemisphere was positively related to functional impairment; however, such relationships were only observed with subjects with a subcortical stroke. Thus, it was concluded that individuals with the most impairment following a subcortical stroke have a hyperexcitable nonlesioned hemisphere As a result; it is hypothesized that due to the mechanisms of recovery, only individuals with severe impairment following a subcortical stroke will likely respond to NIBS paradigms targeting the nonlesioned hemisphere. Future work aiming to regulate the excitability of the nonlesioned hemisphere would therefore likely produce a greater effect size if only severely impaired subjects with a subcortical stroke were enrolled.

Although a few studies in humans indicate that individuals with cortical stroke may not respond as favorably to NIBS compared to subcortical strokes, majority of the work is being tested in an animal model. For example, using a rat stroke model, Boychuk and colleagues (2015) determined how infarct location influenced motor recovery following rehabilitation paired with cortical electrical stimulation.[73] Rats were given either an MCA stroke resulting in a mixed stroke with damage to the frontal cortex and striatum or a subcortical stroke targeting the thalamus and internal capsule. A subset of rats in each lesion group received either cortical stimulation and rehabilitation or rehabilitation only for 20 days. The authors found that rats with a mixed stroke responded more favorably to cortical stimulation combined with rehabilitation as shown by improvements in motor function and cortical excitability. Although seemingly contradictory to clinical studies, as rats with cortical lesions experienced improved motor function with electrical stimulation, one caveat of Boychuk's findings is the nature of the cortical and subcortical stroke. First, the rats with mixed stroke may not have had extensive cortical damage by nature of the mixed stroke such that electrical stimulation was able to influence baseline cortical activation, as previously suggested by Ameli and colleagues.[71] Second, the subcortical stroke targeted the internal capsule. The internal capsule encompasses the corticospinal tract, that is, the primary efferent motor pathway. Boychuk's study highlights an important finding that the extent of the subcortical stroke may

also influence the efficacy of NIBS. As such, damage to the internal capsule results in poor prognosis for patients with stroke[43–45,59] such that they have limited neuronal capacity to propagate signals originating from the cortex to the lower motor neurons within the spinal cord.

Boychuk's findings highlight a critical issue that will need to be addressed in the field of stroke rehabilitation: Will the NIBS location need to change based on the location of the stroke lesion? fMRI studies suggest that such fluidity in NIBS placement may be required. Work by Luft and colleagues[70] have shown that individuals with a cortical and subcortical stroke have unique patterns of brain activation during paretic hand movement. For individuals with a subcortical stroke, movement of the paretic hand resulted in activation of the contralateral motor cortex, ipsilateral cerebellum, bilateral SMA, and perisylvian regions. In contrast, individuals with a cortical lesion only recruited the ipsilateral postcentral, mesial regions and areas at the rim of the stroke cavity. Further, it was found that overall brain activation in individuals with a cortical stroke was reduced compared to healthy controls, while those with a subcortical stroke had more activation. Taken collectively, this suggests and builds upon the notion that individuals with a subcortical lesion may respond more favorably to NIBS purely based on motor circuitry that is utilized for paretic upper limb movement. In contrast, based on the earlier described mechanisms, stimulation paradigms aiming to improve motor function in cortical strokes may need to target subcortical areas that are spared. For example, the use of a TMS cone-type coil that has the ability to induce electrical fields deeper in the cortical tissue may be more ideal when trying to improve motor recovery in an individual with a cortical stroke.

SUMMARY

In summary, NIBS is an emerging stroke rehabilitation modality that is intended to accelerate and enhance the effects of physical and occupational therapy. Much work remains to be done to determine optimum dosing and delivery methods and the ideal patient types. Despite promising early studies, larger clinical trials and metaanalyses have shown somewhat limited effect of NIBS to accelerate and enhance rehabilitative outcomes for patients with stroke. Hence, its use remains investigational for stroke rehabilitation. To get the best outcome from NIBS, models of stroke recovery and neuroplasticity suggest that the method of NIBS delivery must be adjusted based on time post stroke,

stroke severity, and lesion location. Therefore, research is underway to determine how to tailor NIBS delivery based on these patient characteristics.

REFERENCES

1. Broeks JG, Lankhorst GJ, Rumping K, Prevo AJ. The long-term outcome of arm function after stroke: results of a follow-up study. *Disabil Rehabil.* 1999;21(8):357–364.

2. Wilkinson PR, Wolfe CD, Warburton FG, et al. A long-term follow-up of stroke patients. *Stroke J Cerebral Circ.* 1997;28(3):507–512.

3. Terao Y, Ugawa Y. Basic mechanisms of TMS. *J Clin Neurophysiol.* 2002;19(4):322–343.

4. Dayan E, Censor N, Buch ER, Sandrini M, Cohen LG. Noninvasive brain stimulation: from physiology to network dynamics and back. *Nat Neurosci.* 2013;16(7):838–844. https://doi.org/10.1038/nn.3422.

5. Wagner T, Fregni F, Fecteau S, Grodzinsky A, Zahn M, Pascual-Leone A. Transcranial direct current stimulation: a computer-based human model study. *NeuroImage.* 2007;35(3):1113–1124. https://doi.org/10.1016/j.neuroimage.2007.01.027.

6. Lindenberg R, Renga V, Zhu LL, Nair D, Schlaug G. Bihemispheric brain stimulation facilitates motor recovery in chronic stroke patients. *Neurology.* 2010;75(24):2176–2184. https://doi.org/10.1212/WNL.0b013e318202013a.

7. Purpura DP, McMurtry JG. Intracellular activities and evoked potential changes during polarization of motor cortex. *J Neurophysiol.* 1965;28:166–185.

8. Nitsche MA, Liebetanz D, Schlitterlau A, et al. GABAergic modulation of DC stimulation-induced motor cortex excitability shifts in humans. *Eur J Neurosci.* 2004;19(10):2720–2726. https://doi.org/10.1111/j.0953-816X.2004.03398.x.

9. Nitsche MA, Fricke K, Henschke U, et al. Pharmacological modulation of cortical excitability shifts induced by transcranial direct current stimulation in humans. *J Physiol.* 2003;553(Pt 1):293–301. https://doi.org/10.1113/jphysiol.2003.049916.

10. Rossi S, Hallett M, Rossini PM, Pascual-Leone A. Safety, ethical considerations, and application guidelines for the use of transcranial magnetic stimulation in clinical practice and research. *Clin Neurophysiol.* 2009;120(12):2008–2039. https://doi.org/10.1016/j.clinph.2009.08.016. pii:S1388-2457(09)00519-7.

11. Wassermann EM. Risk and safety of repetitive transcranial magnetic stimulation: report and suggested guidelines from the International Workshop on the safety of repetitive transcranial magnetic stimulation, June 5–7, 1996. *Electroencephalogr Clin Neurophysiol.* 1998;108(1):1–16.

12. Bikson M, Grossman P, Thomas C, et al. Safety of transcranial direct current stimulation: evidence based update 2016. *Brain Stimul.* 2016;9(5):641–661. https://doi.org/10.1016/j.brs.2016.06.004.

13. Nitsche MA, Liebetanz D, Antal A, Lang N, Tergau F, Paulus W. Modulation of cortical excitability by weak direct current stimulation–technical, safety and functional aspects. *Suppl Clin Neurophysiol.* 2003;56:255–276.

14. Dhaliwal SK, Meek BP, Modirrousta MM. Non-invasive brain stimulation for the treatment of symptoms following traumatic brain injury. *Front Psychiatry.* 2015;6:119. https://doi.org/10.3389/fpsyt.2015.00119.

15. Nowak DA, Grefkes C, Ameli M, Fink GR. Interhemispheric competition after stroke: brain stimulation to enhance recovery of function of the affected hand. *Neurorehabil Neural Repair.* 2009;23(7):641–656. https://doi.org/10.1177/1545968309336661.

16. Murase N, Duque J, Mazzocchio R, Cohen LG. Influence of interhemispheric interactions on motor function in chronic stroke. *Ann Neurol.* 2004;55(3):400–409. https://doi.org/10.1002/ana.10848.

17. Duque J, Hummel F, Celnik P, Murase N, Mazzocchio R, Cohen LG. Transcallosal inhibition in chronic subcortical stroke. *NeuroImage.* 2005;28(4):940–946. https://doi.org/10.1016/j.neuroimage.2005.06.033. pii:S1053-8119(05)00480-5.

18. Avanzino L, Bassolino M, Pozzo T, Bove M. Use-dependent hemispheric balance. *J Neurosci.* 2011;31(9):3423–3428. https://doi.org/10.1523/JNEUROSCI.4893-10.2011.

19. Hoyer EH, Celnik PA. Understanding and enhancing motor recovery after stroke using transcranial magnetic stimulation. *Restor Neurology Neuroscience.* 2011;29(6):395–409. https://doi.org/10.3233/RNN-2011-0611.

20. Sandrini M, Cohen LG. Noninvasive brain stimulation in neurorehabilitation. *Handb Clinical Neurol.* 2013;116:499–524. https://doi.org/10.1016/B978-0-444-53497-2.00040-1.

21. Adkins-Muir DL, Jones TA. Cortical electrical stimulation combined with rehabilitative training: enhanced functional recovery and dendritic plasticity following focal cortical ischemia in rats. *Neurol Res.* 2003;25(8):780–788.

22. Plautz EJ, Milliken GW, Nudo RJ. Effects of repetitive motor training on movement representations in adult squirrel monkeys: role of use versus learning. *Neurobiol Learn Mem.* 2000;74(1):27–55.

23. Bolognini N, Pascual-Leone A, Fregni F. Using non-invasive brain stimulation to augment motor training-induced plasticity. *J Neuroeng Rehabil.* 2009;6:8. https://doi.org/10.1186/1743-0003-6-8.

24. Conforto AB, Anjos SM, Saposnik G, et al. Transcranial magnetic stimulation in mild to severe hemiparesis early after stroke: a proof of principle and novel approach to improve motor function. *J Neurol.* 2012;259(7):1399–1405. https://doi.org/10.1007/s00415-011-6364-7.

25. Plow EB, Carey JR, Nudo RJ, Pascual-Leone A. Invasive cortical stimulation to promote recovery of function after stroke: a critical appraisal. *Stroke.* 2009;40(5):1926–1931. https://doi.org/10.1161/STROKEAHA.108.540823.

26. Hesse S, Waldner A, Mehrholz J, Tomelleri C, Pohl M, Werner C. Combined transcranial direct current stimulation and robot-assisted arm training in subacute stroke patients: an exploratory, randomized multicenter trial. *Neurorehabil Neural Repair.* 2011;25(9):838–846. https://doi.org/10.1177/1545968311413906.

27. Malcolm MP, Triggs WJ, Light KE, et al. Repetitive transcranial magnetic stimulation as an adjunct to constraint-induced therapy: an exploratory randomized controlled trial. *Am J Phys Med Rehabil Assoc Acad Physiatrists.* 2007;86(9):707–715. https://doi.org/10.1097/PHM.0b013e31813e0de0.

28. Seniow J, Bilik M, Lesniak M, Waldowski K, Iwanski S, Czlonkowska A. Transcranial magnetic stimulation combined with physiotherapy in rehabilitation of poststroke hemiparesis: a randomized, double-blind, placebo-controlled study. *Neurorehabil Neural Repair.* 2012;26(9):1072–1079. https://doi.org/10.1177/1545968312445635.

29. Talelli P, Wallace A, Dileone M, et al. Theta burst stimulation in the rehabilitation of the upper limb: a semirandomized, placebo-controlled trial in chronic stroke patients. *Neurorehabil Neural Repair.* 2012;26(8):976–987. https://doi.org/10.1177/1545968312437940.

30. Tomasevic L, Zito G, Pasqualetti P, et al. Cortico-muscular coherence as an index of fatigue in multiple sclerosis. *Mult Sclerosis.* 2013;19(3):334–343. https://doi.org/10.1177/1352458512452921.

31. Plow EB, Cunningham DA, Varnerin N, Machado A. Rethinking stimulation of the brain in stroke rehabilitation: why higher motor areas might be better alternatives for patients with greater impairments. *Neurosci Rev J Bring Neurobiol Neurol Psychiatry.* 2014. https://doi.org/10.1177/1073858414537381.

32. Elsner B, Kugler J, Pohl M, Mehrholz J. Transcranial direct current stimulation (tDCS) for improving function and activities of daily living in patients after stroke. *Cochrane Database Syst Rev.* 2013;(11):CD009645. https://doi.org/10.1002/14651858.CD009645.pub2.

33. Hsu WY, Cheng CH, Liao KK, Lee IH, Lin YY. Effects of repetitive transcranial magnetic stimulation on motor functions in patients with stroke: a meta-analysis. *Stroke.* 2012;43(7):1849–1857. https://doi.org/10.1161/STROKEAHA.111.649756.

34. Hao Z, Wang D, Zeng Y, Liu M. Repetitive transcranial magnetic stimulation for improving function after stroke. *Cochrane Database Syst Rev.* 2013;(5):CD008862. https://doi.org/10.1002/14651858.CD008862.pub2.

35. Ludemann-Podubecka J, Bosl K, Nowak DA. Repetitive transcranial magnetic stimulation for motor recovery of the upper limb after stroke. *Prog Brain Res.* 2015;218:281–311. https://doi.org/10.1016/bs.pbr.2014.12.001.

36. Khedr EM, Abdel-Fadeil MR, Farghali A, Qaid M. Role of 1 and 3 Hz repetitive transcranial magnetic stimulation on motor function recovery after acute ischaemic stroke. *Eur J Neurol.* 2009;16(12):1323–1330. https://doi.org/10.1111/j.1468-1331.2009.02746.x.

37. Takeuchi N, Tada T, Toshima M, Chuma T, Matsuo Y, Ikoma K. Inhibition of the unaffected motor cortex by 1 Hz repetitive transcranial magnetic stimulation enhances motor performance and training effect of the paretic hand in patients with chronic stroke. *J Rehabil Med.* 2008;40(4):298–303. https://doi.org/10.2340/16501977-0181.

38. Etoh S, Noma T, Ikeda K, et al. Effects of repetitive trascranial magnetic stimulation on repetitive facilitation exercises of the hemiplegic hand in chronic stroke patients. *J Rehabil Med.* 2013;45(9):843–847. https://doi.org/10.2340/16501977-1175.

39. Moskowitz MA, Lo EH, Iadecola C. The science of stroke: mechanisms in search of treatments. *Neuron.* 2010;67(2):181–198. https://doi.org/10.1016/j.neuron.2010.07.002.

40. Carmichael ST. Brain excitability in stroke: the yin and yang of stroke progression. *Arch Neurol.* 2012;69(2):161–167. https://doi.org/10.1001/archneurol.2011.1175.

41. Rehme AK, Fink GR, von Cramon DY, Grefkes C. The role of the contralesional motor cortex for motor recovery in the early days after stroke assessed with longitudinal FMRI. *Cereb Cortex.* 2011;21(4):756–768. https://doi.org/10.1093/cercor/bhq140.

42. Lloyd-Jones D, Adams RJ, Brown TM, et al. Heart disease and stroke statistics–2010 update: a report from the American Heart Association. *Circulation.* 2010;121(7):e46–e215. https://doi.org/10.1161/CIRCULATIONAHA.109.192667.

43. Lindenberg R, Zhu LL, Ruber T, Schlaug G. Predicting functional motor potential in chronic stroke patients using diffusion tensor imaging. *Hum Brain Mapping.* 2012;33(5):1040–1051. https://doi.org/10.1002/hbm.21266.

44. Cunningham DA, Machado A, Janini D, et al. The assessment of inter-hemispheric imbalance using imaging and non-invasive brain stimulation in patients with chronic stroke. *Arch Phys Med Rehabil.* 2014. https://doi.org/10.1016/j.apmr.2014.07.419.

45. Stinear CM, Barber PA, Smale PR, Coxon JP, Fleming MK, Byblow WD. Functional potential in chronic stroke patients depends on corticospinal tract integrity. *Brain.* 2007;130(Pt 1):170–180. https://doi.org/10.1093/brain/awl333.

46. Ward NS, Newton JM, Swayne OB, et al. Motor system activation after subcortical stroke depends on corticospinal system integrity. *Brain.* 2006;129(Pt 3):809–819. https://doi.org/10.1093/brain/awl002.

47. Bradnam LV, Stinear CM, Barber PA, Byblow WD. Contralesional hemisphere control of the proximal paretic upper limb following stroke. *Cereb Cortex.* 2012;22(11):2662–2671. https://doi.org/10.1093/cercor/bhr344.

48. Ackerley SJ, Stinear CM, Barber PA, Byblow WD. Combining theta burst stimulation with training after subcortical stroke. *Stroke.* 2010;41(7):1568–1572. https://doi.org/10.1161/STROKEAHA.110.583278.

49. Yamamoto S, Takasawa M, Kajiyama K, Baron JC, Yamaguchi T. Deterioration of hemiparesis after recurrent stroke in the unaffected hemisphere: three further cases with possible interpretation. *Cerebrovasc Dis.* 2007;23(1):35–39. https://doi.org/10.1159/000095756.

50. Song YM, Lee JY, Park JM, Yoon BW, Roh JK. Ipsilateral hemiparesis caused by a corona radiata infarct after a previous stroke on the opposite side. *Arch Neurol.* 2005;62(5):809−811. https://doi.org/10.1001/archneur.62.5.809.

51. Johansen-Berg H, Rushworth MF, Bogdanovic MD, Kischka U, Wimalaratna S, Matthews PM. The role of ipsilateral premotor cortex in hand movement after stroke. *Proc Natl Acad Sci USA.* 2002;99(22):14518−14523. https://doi.org/10.1073/pnas.222536799.

52. Lotze M, Markert J, Sauseng P, Hoppe J, Plewnia C, Gerloff C. The role of multiple contralesional motor areas for complex hand movements after internal capsular lesion. *J Neurosci.* 2006;26(22):6096−6102. https://doi.org/10.1523/jneurosci.4564-05.2006.

53. Mohapatra S, Harrington R, Chan E, Dromerick AW, Breceda EY, Harris-Love M. Role of contralesional hemisphere in paretic arm reaching in patients with severe arm paresis due to stroke: a preliminary report. *Neurosci Lett.* 2016;617:52−58. https://doi.org/10.1016/j.neulet.2016.02.004.

54. Di Pino G, Pellegrino G, Assenza G, et al. Modulation of brain plasticity in stroke: a novel model for neurorehabilitation. *Nat Rev Neurol.* 2014;10(10):597−608. https://doi.org/10.1038/nrneurol.2014.162.

55. Bestmann S, Swayne O, Blankenburg F, et al. The role of contralesional dorsal premotor cortex after stroke as studied with concurrent TMS-fMRI. *J Neurosci.* 2010;30(36):11926−11937. https://doi.org/10.1523/jneurosci.5642-09.2010.

56. Sankarasubramanian V, Machado AG, Conforto AB, et al. Inhibition versus facilitation of contralesional motor cortices in stroke: deriving a model to tailor brain stimulation. *Clin Neurophysiol.* 2017;128(6):892−902. https://doi.org/10.1016/j.clinph.2017.03.030.

57. Cunningham DA, Potter-Baker KA, Knutson JS, Sankarasubramanian V, Machado AG, Plow EB. Tailoring brain stimulation to the nature of rehabilitative therapies in stroke: a conceptual framework based on their unique mechanisms of recovery. *Phys Med Rehabil Clin N Am.* 2015;26(4):759−774. https://doi.org/10.1016/j.pmr.2015.07.001.

58. Bradnam LV, Stinear CM, Byblow WD. Ipsilateral motor pathways after stroke: implications for non-invasive brain stimulation. *Front Hum Neurosci.* 2013;7:184. https://doi.org/10.3389/fnhum.2013.00184.

59. Stinear CM, Barber PA, Petoe M, Anwar S, Byblow WD. The PREP algorithm predicts potential for upper limb recovery after stroke. *Brain.* 2012;135(Pt 8):2527−2535. https://doi.org/10.1093/brain/aws146.

60. Cunningham DA, Varnerin N, Machado A, et al. Stimulation targeting higher motor areas in stroke rehabilitation: a proof-of-concept, randomized, double-blinded placebo-controlled study of effectiveness and underlying mechanisms. *Restor Neurol Neurosci.* 2015;33(6):911−926. https://doi.org/10.3233/RNN-150574.

61. Carey JR, Deng H, Gillick BT, et al. Serial treatments of primed low-frequency rTMS in stroke: characteristics of responders vs. nonresponders. *Restor Neurol Neurosci.* 2014;32(2):323−335. https://doi.org/10.3233/RNN-130358.

62. Lee JH, Kim SB, Lee KW, Kim MA, Lee SJ, Choi SJ. Factors associated with upper extremity motor recovery after repetitive transcranial magnetic stimulation in stroke patients. *Ann Rehabil Med.* 2015;39(2):268−276. https://doi.org/10.5535/arm.2015.39.2.268.

63. Chang WH, Uhm KE, Shin YI, Pascual-Leone A, Kim YH. Factors influencing the response to high-frequency repetitive transcranial magnetic stimulation in patients with subacute stroke. *Restor Neurol Neurosci.* 2016;34(5):747−755. https://doi.org/10.3233/rnn-150634.

64. Bentley P, Kumar G, Rinne P, et al. Lesion locations influencing baseline severity and early recovery in ischaemic stroke. *Eur J Neurol.* 2014;21(9):1226−1232. https://doi.org/10.1111/ene.12464.

65. Buffon F, Molko N, Herve D, et al. Longitudinal diffusion changes in cerebral hemispheres after MCA infarcts. *J Cerebral Blood Flow Metab.* 2005;25(5):641−650. https://doi.org/10.1038/sj.jcbfm.9600054.

66. Cheng B, Forkert ND, Zavaglia M, et al. Influence of stroke infarct location on functional outcome measured by the modified rankin scale. *Stroke.* 2014;45(6):1695−1702. https://doi.org/10.1161/STROKEAHA.114.005152.

67. FdNAP S, Reding MJ. Effect of lesion location on upper limb motor recovery after stroke. *Stroke.* 2001;32(1):107−112. https://doi.org/10.1161/01.str.32.1.107.

68. Chen CL, Tang FT, Chen HC, Chung CY, Wong MK. Brain lesion size and location: effects on motor recovery and functional outcome in stroke patients. *Arch Phys Med Rehabil.* 2000;81(4):447−452. https://doi.org/10.1053/mr.2000.3837.

69. Burke Quinlan E, Dodakian L, See J, et al. Neural function, injury, and stroke subtype predict treatment gains after stroke. *Ann Neurol.* 2015;77(1):132−145. https://doi.org/10.1002/ana.24309.

70. Luft AR, Waller S, Forrester L, et al. Lesion location alters brain activation in chronically impaired stroke survivors. *NeuroImage.* 2004;21(3):924−935. https://doi.org/10.1016/j.neuroimage.2003.10.026.

71. Ameli M, Grefkes C, Kemper F, et al. Differential effects of high-frequency repetitive transcranial magnetic stimulation over ipsilesional primary motor cortex in cortical and subcortical middle cerebral artery stroke. *Ann Neurol.* 2009;66(3):298−309. https://doi.org/10.1002/ana.21725.

72. Thickbroom GW, Cortes M, Rykman A, et al. Stroke subtype and motor impairment influence contralesional excitability. *Neurology.* 2015;85(6):517−520. https://doi.org/10.1212/WNL.0000000000001828.

73. Boychuk JA, Schwerin SC, Thomas N, et al. Enhanced motor recovery after stroke with combined cortical stimulation and rehabilitative training is dependent on infarct location. *Neurorehabil Neural Repair.* 2015. https://doi.org/10.1177/1545968315624979.

CHAPTER 19

Children and Stroke

LAINIE K. HOLMAN, MD

The developmental variability of children requires special considerations for treatment, rehabilitation, and outcome expectations after stroke. An earlier age of onset has ramifications medically, economically, and socially which are not seen in adults. Considerations include lost productivity for the family as well as the patient, with costs accumulating over a lifespan,[1] as well as a potentially longer period of treatment and rehabilitation. Motor, sensory, and cognitive effects differ in children, as they are in the process of gaining new skills, not only in reestablishing those previously acquired.

A cornerstone of pediatric care for all children is the timely, age-appropriate provision of *anticipatory guidance*, a framework for caregivers to understand and navigate typical childhood development, not just physical, but psychological and social. In well-child visits, reminders, education, and information provided before the next milestone in development is reached help smooth transitions and ensure support and structure for the child. This concept can and should be expanded and customized for children with the sequelae of neurologic insult, as well as for those with other chronic conditions.

Rehabilitation for children after stroke requires both relearning already accomplished milestones, but also new learning and development. The composition of the pediatric rehabilitation team expands to include education, behavior, and development specialists who can help individualize not just the treatment but the anticipatory guidance for the needs of the particular child. Unlike for most adults, the school environment becomes a crucial component of the child's recovery and reentry to the community.[2] Also unique to children is the transition from the classroom to adulthood, a stage which must be carefully considered as principles of rehabilitation widen to include vocation and legal and financial questions.

DEFINITION

Stroke in children is commonly divided by age of onset, with those occurring before 28 days of life considered perinatal, and those after day 28 pediatric. Perinatal stroke can be further classified as fetal and neonatal. These commonly are an etiology of cerebral palsy, fall under the discussion of such, and are beyond the scope of this chapter. For purposes of this text, pediatric stroke is defined as after 28 days of life.

EPIDEMIOLOGY/RISK

Incidence estimates vary widely between 1.2 per 100,000 person years to as high as 13 per 100,000 person years[3] but is generally regarded to be stable.[4] There is a bimodal age distribution, highest before 1 year of age, then falling and increasing again in adolescence. Risk is higher for black children than for white, even accounting for sickle cell disease, and higher for boys than for girls.[3] These statistics must be considered with the knowledge that some number goes undiagnosed, partially due to relative rarity.[5]

ETIOLOGY

As in adults, etiology is defined as acute ischemic stroke (AIS), due to emboli, vasoconstriction, or inadequate perfusion, and hemorrhagic, due most often to ruptured vascular malformations (Table 19.1).[6] However, children have a broader set of risk factors than adults[7] reflected in the fact that only half of strokes in children are ischemic.[8]

Arteriopathy is thought to be present in 40%−80% of AIS.[9] The understanding of transient arteriopathy is evolving, but may be associated with infection or the inflammatory response to infection.[10,11] Certain infections such as varicella zoster virus (VZV) and herpes simplex virus (HSV) have been seen to cause arteriopathy.[12] Noninflammatory arteriopathies such as moyamoya and fibromuscular dysplasias are also a consideration in children, as they can lead to arterial dissection. Similar noninflammatory arteriopathies may also be seen in the setting of other diseases or syndromes, and should all be considered in the evaluation of childhood AIS.

Stroke Rehabilitation. https://doi.org/10.1016/B978-0-323-55381-0.00019-6

TABLE 19.1

Summary of the Various Causes and Risk Factors for Childhood Acute Ischemic Stroke

Arteriopathies
    Focal or transient cerebral arteriopathy
    Craniocervical arterial dissection
    Fibromuscular dysplasia
    Moyamoya disease
    Primary CNS angiitis

Cardiac disease
    Congenital heart disease
    Cardiomyopathy
    Arrhythmia
    Catheterization/surgery
    ECMO

Inherited thrombophilia
    Protein C, S, Antithrombin deficiency
    Factor V Leiden
    Prothrombin G20210A
    MTHFR C677T
    Lipoprotein(a) elevations

Acquired thrombophilia
    Antiphospholipid syndrome
    Drug-induced thrombophilia (i.e., asparaginase)

Sickle cell disease

Malignancy

Congenital vascular syndromes

Inborn errors of metabolism
    Mitochondrial disorders
    Fabry Disease

Rheumatologic disease
    Systemic lupus erythematosus
    Systemic vasculitis (i.e., Takayasu arteritis, Churg Strauss)

From Felling; have permission.

Childhood cancer and its treatments, particularly cranial irradiation therapy (CRT), carry a risk for stroke. While the exact mechanism remains somewhat unclear, it is known to be dose-dependent. The additional comorbidities of hypertension and diabetes mellitus in children who have had CRT increase stroke risk significantly.[13] Leukemia can also lead to a hypercoagulable state.[14–16]

Cardiac disease, both structural and physiologic, is a risk factor for pediatric stroke. Congenital heart disease has an incidence of about 8/1000 live births, and is present in more than half of AIS in the International Pediatric Stroke Registry.[17] Cyanotic lesions can cause polycythemia and anemia, increasing the risk for thrombosis. Additionally, many cardiac disorders in children carry with them the need for procedures such as catheterization and surgery, and support such as extracorporeal membrane oxygenation (ECMO), which all increase risk for stroke.

Sickle cell disease (SCD) has historically been a major contributor to pediatric AIS, but the incidence has decreased with the use of chronic transfusion therapy.[18] Prior to this, 11% of children with SCD had a stroke before age 20. In SCD, ischemic stroke is more common than hemorrhagic, which is more prevalent in adolescence.[19] Transcranial doppler screening (TCD) can be used to detect children with SCD who are at risk for stroke.

Hemorrhagic stroke in children is caused most often by ruptured vascular malformations, of which arteriovenous malformations (AVMs) are most common. AVMs represent 40% of hemorrhagic stroke and can be associated with various syndromes such as neurofibromatosis and Sturge–Weber. Pediatric aneurysms are larger than in adults, and are sometimes the underlying cause for a hemorrhagic stroke.

Other risk factors of note are trauma, substance use, metabolic disorders, and vasculitis.[20]

COMPLICATIONS

About 70% of children with stroke in the Canadian Pediatric Ischemic Stroke Registry had residual neurologic deficits. Ramifications from the various residual deficits can lead to functional impairment for children.[21] The functional impairments can limit children in mobility, cognition, behavior, nutrition and growth, sensation, and language. More often, there is a challenging combination of several impairments. In spite of the fact that pediatric stroke is relatively rare, the functional limitations and changed ability to reach new milestones may persist over several decades, magnifying the personal, social, and economic costs in all realms.[21–23]

Mobility

Motor recovery is related to lesion size and age at onset and does not follow a linear pattern in children.[24] Some mobility milestones may have lain ahead of the child at the time of the injury, and so often the child is not "relearning" a motor pattern, but encountering it for the first time with an impaired processing ability. In addition to motor planning, functional mobility recovery is frequently limited by spasticity, weakness, cognitive deficits, visuospatial changes, and musculoskeletal issues such as contracture and hip subluxation.

Spasticity complicates motor and functional recovery from stroke in children as it does in adults. Spasticity combined with relative immobility leads to joint contracture, and joint contracture can beget skin breakdown, positioning, and seating difficulties. In addition to mobility, spasticity also commonly affects sleep in children, potentially worsening behaviors, learning, and school performance.

The mainstay of spasticity management and contracture preventions is the same as for adults: regular, sustained stretching. Stretching in children can be more difficult to accomplish than for adults, as they are often resistant to being restrained or held in place for any length of time. Strategies can include positioning while doing a favorite activity, which now most often involves screen time. While parents must seek to limit screen time for children to reasonable durations, the time allowed can be combined with long-leg sitting, standing on an incline board, or static or dynamic splinting.[25]

When spasticity is significant, early static splinting is crucial, and first involves accordance and motivation on the part of the child's caregivers. The most frequently used static splints are ankle-foot-orthoses (AFOs), either solid-ankle, or articulated with a stretching strap for nighttime wear, and soft knee immobilizers. Knee immobilizers are often more readily accepted if worn on alternating legs on alternating nights. Serial casting for increased dorsiflexion range of motion alone or in conjunction with botulinum toxin therapy is often used with good results.[26–28] Risks include pain from overstretching and skin breakdown; however, with weekly cast changes, these can be mitigated.

Dynamic splinting often becomes a question, especially when introducing an AFO for the hemiparetic child. Typically an articulated AFO with a plantarflexion stop is used for an ambulatory child with increased tone but active dorsiflexion. All lower limb orthoses must be custom designed keeping in mind growth of the child, ambulation status, potential sensory issues, weight, and safety. Children's shoes are difficult to fit over AFOs, but there are an increasing number of brands being manufactured.

Often, in long-standing hemiparesis, a leg-length discrepancy will evolve over time. This can be managed by adding height to the shoe or to an orthosis. Exact measures may be made radiographically, if necessary. Such a discrepancy rarely requires surgical intervention (Fig. 19.1A and B).

While there are few studies of pharmacologic treatments for spasticity in childhood stroke, it is treated much the same as spasticity due to other neurologic causes such as cerebral palsy, and we may extrapolate from those. Particular pediatric considerations for treatment include weight-based dosing for antispasticity medications, the lack of pediatric efficacy trials, and

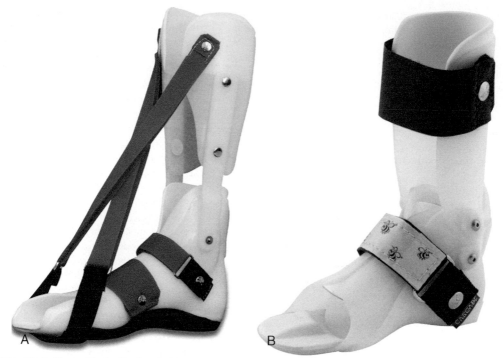

FIG. 19.1 The ankle foot orthosis (AFO) on the left may be used for stretching. At left, an AFO with free dorsiflexion and a plantarflexion stop. (Photo with permission of Cascade)

acceptance of drug form. Additionally, comorbidities such as epilepsy and cognitive deficits must be considered.

The most commonly used medication, baclofen, a GABA agonist, crosses the blood—brain barrier and can have cognitive side effects such as confusion and sedation.[29] For enteral administration, it is manufactured in tablet form only, making dosing in children challenging, as some do not/will not swallow tablets. In clinical practice, crushing the tablets and administering them in a small amount of food such as applesauce or yogurt can circumvent this issue. An extemporaneous preparation is often made using crushed tablets, but the dosing can be unreliable due to the nature of the suspension, resulting in over- or underdosing in some cases. Enteral baclofen is typically tapered up over a period of several days to weeks in hopes of lessening the sedative effect. Baclofen is typically used with caution in children with epilepsy; however, the role for seizure potentiation remains controversial.[30,31]

Intrathecal administration of baclofen may be used in children who weigh more than 15 kg, avoiding many of the side effects of enteral use, and most patients have decreased spasticity and improved comfort.[32] Intrathecal administration can be associated with complications such as infection which must be considered when weighing interventions. Both routes of baclofen administration carry a small but significant risk of withdrawal.[33]

Tizanidine, an α2 adrenergic agonist is frequently used in children and adolescents. It has a similar side effect profile to baclofen: sedation and depression, but also sometimes nausea, and rarely, hepatotoxicity.[34] In pediatric clinical practice, transaminase levels are typically followed every 6 months during tizanidine therapy.

Dantrolene, which inhibits the release of calcium at the sarcoplasmic reticulum, is sometimes used, as it is prepared as a true suspension, but likewise requires laboratory surveillance. Side effects include nausea, vomiting, diarrhea, and hepatotoxicity. In clinical practice, liver function tests are typically monitored as with tizanidine.

Botulinum toxin was first FDA-approved for adult strabismus and blepharospasm, and was initially used in cerebral palsy in the 1980s. Since then it has been approved by the FDA for use in the lower limbs of children aged over 2 years. Botulinum toxin A is the form most often used in clinical practice, likely due to a longer duration of action. It is particularly useful in cases of very focal spasticity, as is the case in hemispheric ischemic stroke. Most scientific evidence seems to support the safety and efficacy of botulinum toxin use in children.[35] Side effects include discomfort at the injection site, weakness, bleeding, infection, effects on unintended musculature, and respiratory depression. However, the largest barrier to using botulinum toxin in children is their near-universal unwillingness to believe that the injections are for their benefit, and worth the discomfort (see Table 19.2).

Selective dorsal rhizotomy is a surgical procedure for spasticity management most typically used in school-aged children with diplegic cerebral palsy, but is increasingly considered for management of spasticity with other etiologies and patterns. The procedure involves ablation of selected sensory afferents to interrupt the signaling loop to decrease tone and improve gross motor function. Success in cerebral palsy is predicated on judicious patient selection, and it has not been extensively studied in hemiparetic children or specifically in pediatric stroke.[36-38]

When the neurologic lesion significantly impairs mobility, hip growth and development can be affected. Hip dysplasia in children with cerebral palsy is more common in quadriparesis than in hemiparesis, and while there are no large studies of hip subluxation in pediatric stroke, one can be convinced that periodic monitoring of the hips of any young child with spasticity and decreased mobility is warranted.[39] Both hip subluxation and unavoidable contractures may be evaluated by an orthopedic surgeon for further management.

Dysphagia

As in adults, dysphagia is common, but may be complicated by an acquired aversion to food or oral textures, and to behaviors surrounding food that are not strictly a result of oral-motor dysfunction. If self-feeding had not been premorbidly accomplished, it must be undertaken with potential new deficits in consideration. If self-feeding was well established before the stroke, it must be reintroduced. As in adults, a bedside swallowing evaluation and imaging are the mainstays of diagnosis and basis for recommendations. Growth and changing nutritional needs are also special considerations in children, whose protein and calorie intake are crucial for development. Approximately, 15%−50% of children who have had a stroke are deficient in essential fatty acids; iron; selenium; zinc; vitamins C, D, and E.[40] Growth charts must be consistently monitored, and early intervention sought for growth failure or malnutrition.

Cognitive

Cognitive impairment is present in about half of pediatric stroke survivors[2] and due to the nature of childhood development may not be initially observable, that is, until the child is near to taking on more complex tasks. Notable findings include below-average full-scale IQ with performance IQ more affected than verbal IQ.[41] Attention and executive function seem to be particularly vulnerable after stroke, though all domains can be affected. Visuospatial deficits are described, but sometimes difficult to qualify, and likely lesion-specific.[42] It is important to include surveillance for these potential problems in therapy and in neuropsychological testing.

Language impairment in children is particularly notable, as compensatory plasticity for the right hemisphere to manage language reorganization is present. The window for most hemispheric remodeling is thought to be between ages two−five years, but increasingly seems to be < 2.[43]

Epilepsy, which occurs in 15%−30% of children after stroke, can also complicate intellectual function and recovery.[21] Acute seizures around the stroke ictus are associated with increased risk for later epilepsy.[44] Epilepsy can have deleterious effects on cognition, attention, and executive function and therefore on quality of life in children who have had a stroke.[45,46] Executive functioning affects social functioning, which can negatively affect school performance during a period when the child is relying on the school environment to be a setting for rehabilitation.[47]

Similarly, behavioral and emotional problems are also common after stroke and can be manifest as mood disorders, anxiety, and aggression, complicating recovery, and especially school reentry.[2]

While there is no established protocol for neuropsychological testing after pediatric stroke, in clinical practice, it is often repeated about every 2−3 years in order to best inform the child's individual education plan (IEP). Testing should include IQ, memory, attention, executive function, visuospatial skills, processing speed, behavior, and social skills. The testing should be shared with the child's caregivers (and the child as appropriate) and with the school in the formal individual educational program planning meeting and throughout the year as needed.

THERAPIES

Most children over age three receive therapy services in both school and outpatient settings. Therapy in the school environment is typically geared toward integrated therapy and educational goals, that is,

TABLE 19.2
Medications Used to Treat Spasticity in Children

Drug	Mechanism of Action	Side Effects and Precautions	Pharmacology and Dosing
Baclofen	• Binds to receptors (GABA) in the spinal cord to inhibit reflexes that lead to increased tone • Also binds to receptors in the brain leading to sedation	• Sedation, confusion, nausea, dizziness, muscle weakness, hypotonia, ataxia, and paresthesias • Can cause loss of seizure control • Withdrawal can produce seizures, rebound hypertonia, fever, and death	• Rapidly absorbed after oral dosing, mean half-life of 3.5 h • Excreted mainly through the kidney • Dosing: in children start 2.5–5 mg/d, increase to 30 mg/d (in children 2–7 years of age) or 60 mg/d (in children 8 years of age and older)
Diazepam	Facilitates postsynaptic binding of a neurotransmitter (GABA) in the brain stem, reticular formation and spinal cord to inhibit reflexes that lead to increased tone	• Central nervous system depression causing sedation, decreased motor coordination, impaired attention and memory • Overdoses and withdrawal both occur • The sedative effect generally limits use to severely involved children	• Well absorbed after oral dosing, mean half-life 20–80 h • Metabolized mainly in the liver • In children, doses range from 0.12 to 0.8 mg/kg/d in divided doses
Clonidine	Alpha2 agonist. Acts in both the brain and spinal cord to enhance presynaptic inhibition of reflexes that lead to increased tone	• Bradycardia, hypotension, dry mouth, drowsiness, dizziness, constipation, and depression • These side effects are common and cause half of patients to discontinue the medication	• Well absorbed after oral dosing, mean half-life is 5–19 h • Half is metabolized in liver and half is excreted by kidney • Start with 0.05 mg bid, titrate up until side effects limit tolerance • May use patch
Tizanidine	• Alpha2 agonist • Acts in both the brain and spinal cord to enhance presynaptic inhibition of reflexes that lead to increased tone	Dry mouth, sedation, dizziness, visual hallucinations, elevated liver enzymes, insomnia, and muscle weakness	• Well absorbed after oral dosing, half-life 2.5 h • Extensive first pass metabolism in liver • Start with 2 mg at bedtime and increase until side effects limit tolerance, maximum 36 mg/d
Dantrolene sodium	• Works directly on the muscle to decrease muscle force produced during contraction • Little effect on smooth and cardiac muscles	• Most important side effect is hepatotoxicity (2%), which may be severe • Liver function tests must be monitored monthly, initially, and then several times per year • Other side effects are mild sedation, dizziness, diarrhea, and paresthesias	• Oral dose is approximately 70% absorbed in small intestine, half-life is 15 hours • Mostly metabolized in the liver • Pediatric doses range from 0.5 mg/kg bid up to a maximum of 3 mg/kg bid

From Green. Have permission.

handwriting, note-taking, visual and sensory processing, cognition, communication, and mobility in the classroom and associated areas. Adaptive gym or recreation should be, and is often included. School-based therapies fall under the control of the IEP and goals are reevaluated annually. Children younger than three in the United States typically qualify for inclusion in early intervention programs and frequently receive ongoing therapies in both home and outpatient settings through programs administered by the states. At age three, children most often transition to a combination of school and outpatient therapies depending on their needs. It is crucial to manage this first transition without losing preschoolers to follow-up. Pitfalls and considerations are the family's ability to navigate the school system, finding a school equipped for and interested in the education of a child with a disability, adapted mobility for the child in the classroom, and transportation to and from school.

Occupational therapy is typically ongoing, in both the school and outpatient settings, due to the needs of the child to continually master new tasks. Constraint Induced Movement Therapy (CIMT) has been found to be safe and effective in children with hemiparetic cerebral palsy[48,49] and is a commonly used method in childhood stroke as well. A modified or "baby" CIMT is used for children under two, ultimately directed by parents.[50,51] Some studies have found the addition of repetitive transcranial stimulation to CIMT to enhance functional gains.[52,53] Robot-assisted therapy is increasingly considered as an adjunct to conventional methods, as it is easily adapted for the pediatric patient, in terms of customizing gaming-based feedback.[54,55] Regardless, all methods continue to focus on the acquisition or refinement of age-appropriate activities of daily living, and on modifying the home or school surroundings to foster independence.

Physical therapy for these children focuses most often on gait, strengthening, and motor planning with always an eye toward both the home and school environment. Motor learning practices are best geared toward functional independence. As with upper-limb therapy, robotics is used in physical therapy. The most common example is with a gait-driven orthosis such as the Lokomat (Fig. 19.2).[54] The trajectory of the use of technology in the rehabilitation of the pediatric stroke patient leads most certainly to the use of virtual reality to augment the therapeutic environment, but these interventions are in preliminary stages.

In the school setting, physical therapy often focuses on safety, for example in a crowded hallway, or how

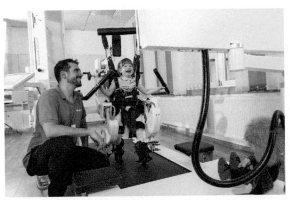

FIG. 19.2 Robot-assisted therapy (photo courtesy of Hocoma).

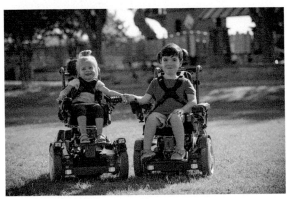

FIG. 19.3 Custom powered mobility. (Photo-Permobil).

to carry textbooks and materials in the most efficient manner. Many schools are accessible only by stairs, an unfortunate carried-over barrier to independent mobility, and this can be a focus of school therapy. Manual wheelchairs may be considered for not only nonambulatory children, but for those with accomplished short-distance walking to safely and efficiently maneuver longer community distances, such as school trips. Powered mobility should be considered and pursued at the first indication, if the child's caregivers have the home and transportation resources and substructure to accommodate a power wheelchair (Fig. 19.3).

Equine-assisted therapies such as therapeutic riding (TR) and hippotherapy (HT) (Fig. 19.4) are activities often used for children. Therapeutic riding is defined as the modified or adapted sport, providing therapy in a recreational and leisure environment, with often the added benefit of being outdoors and with other

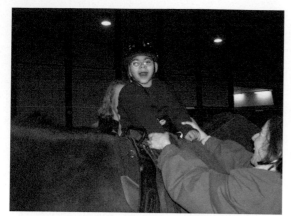

FIG. 19.4 A patient participating in hippotherapy.

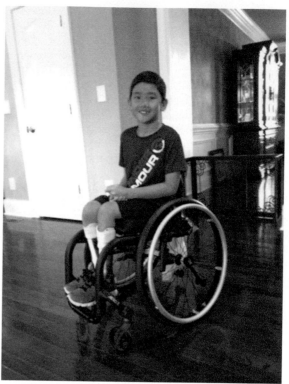

FIG. 19.5 Custom ultralightweight wheelchair. (Photo: Permobil).

children. HT is physical therapy using the movement of the horse to address impairments in balance, core strength, posture, and function. Both can have positive benefits for coordination, endurance, flexibility, and overall strength[56] and in clinical practice, are wildly popular and well-attended.

Also different from adults are considerations for equipment, as children who are thriving outgrow equipment nearly as fast as it can be provided. Wheelchairs (Fig. 19.5) are a particular pediatric concern; both Medicaid and most managed care organizations will fund only one form of wheeled mobility every 5 years. This requires the physiatrist to consider and incorporate the next 5 years of not only growth, but also intellectual and social development. Mobility needs must be seen in light of their caregivers' ability to manage devices or equipment provided. As always, equipment must be custom designed and provided for the individual patient's needs.

Ongoing speech therapy is often needed for not only articulation and oral-motor skills but for higher-level cognitive deficits that are sometimes not apparent until an older age when the child is confronted by increasing complexity.[53] A focus on executive function, memory, and attention may be necessary throughout the school years, even when school-based PT and OT are no longer needed. In children who do not have fully effective verbal communication, an augmented communication plan should be pursued at the earliest possible opportunity. Both simple and complex strategies are available to children who have had a stroke to develop functional communication at home and in their communities (Fig. 19.6A and B). Ideally, augmented communication strategies can be supported in both the outpatient and school environments.

An often overlooked aspect of pediatric rehabilitation is adaptive sports and recreation. Exercise, team interaction, competition, triumph, and failure are a significant part of the life of a child. Every effort should be made to include the pediatric patient with stroke sequelae in community recreation, exercise, and socialization.[57] Many communities now have inclusive sports programs ranging from archery to rock climbing, and many online resources are available (Fig. 19.7). In the event there is no program in the community, often there is an unaffiliated but interested coach, teacher, or trainer who would adapt their sport or team. In the absence of that, many parents become the best founders of such programs.

SCHOOL

The work of a child is also school, and so another difference in the approach to pediatric stroke rehabilitation is the school setting, a crucial piece for both substitution and restoration of function.[2] As the recovery is typically lengthy, the child after stroke is necessarily reintegrated into the school environment while still mastering a new baseline, placing novel demands on the child and

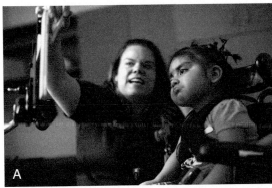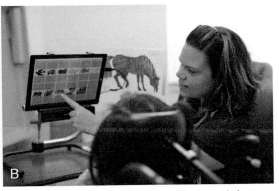

FIG. 19.6 Patient and therapist using communication device. (Photo credit Russell Lee Photography).

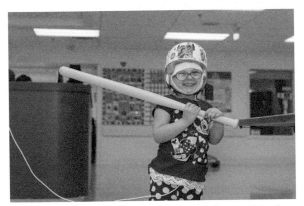

FIG. 19.7 Most sports can be adapted to allow participation.

her caregivers and educators. School settings vary in willingness and capacity to contribute fully to a child's recovery, and strategies to support, enhance, and engage the school system are integral to optimal rehabilitation.[53,58]

Building on civil rights precedent in *Brown v. Board of Education,* The Individuals with Disabilities Education Act (IDEA) is an United States legislation enacted in 1990 (amended 1997 and 2004) with the goal of ensuring that children with disabilities have access to a Free Appropriate Public Education (FAPE) that is customized to their individual needs. It has six elements, one of which establishes the Individualized Education Program (IEP; part B of IDEA), a program specifying the services to be provided based on assessment of the student's performance. This is expected to be provided in the Least Restrictive Environment (LRE) possible.[59] There are also monitoring parameters to ensure proportionality based on race and ethnicity in special education.[60]

The IEP is designed by a team of school-based professionals in consultation with parents and outside rehabilitation specialists, and is arguably the most important support for the ongoing needs of children with disabilities of all etiologies. It must contain specific goals along with accommodations and modifications needed to provide FAPE. It can include issues such as how standardized testing will be handled, how the child will be able to access school activities, what modifications will be made in the physical environment, and adaptations for activities such as physical education.

Often school districts have advocates for children with disabilities and their families who can help navigate the IEP process. Parents are permitted by IDEA to have a representative participate in the creation of the IEP. IDEA requires prior written notice from the school to the parents for any changes that are to be made. The law provides a specific framework for grievances and dispute resolution in cases of noncompliance.

The rehabilitation team can support the child in this system by ensuring access to appropriate neuropsychologic testing, providing custom equipment in good repair, encouraging dialogue regarding behavioral strategies, and continuing support for the caregivers to facilitate carryover from home to school and back.

TRANSITION

Another aspect particular to pediatric rehabilitation is the need to help facilitate the transition to adulthood. Multiple considerations are in order, not only the potential transition to other healthcare providers in the adult medical community, but transition from school to vocation, or from school to college. It can also involve supports to transition from one living situation to another, hopefully a more independent one. There is often necessarily a change in caregivers as others age, sometimes posing legal questions of guardianship and powers-of-attorney with regard to finances and health decisions. It should ideally involve proactive provider-initiated discussions in these dimensions, keeping in mind autonomy and confidentiality in the provider-patient relationship. Like all aspects of rehabilitation, this is best addressed with a team approach inclusive of caregivers and the young adult and effective communication between all parties.[61-63]

CONCLUSION

The rehabilitation of children with stroke shares a number of similarities with that of adults; spasticity management, bracing, therapies, and equipment prescription. But most importantly, it employs the team-driven care model and the long-view of incremental changes designed to improve global function both at home and in the larger community. Commonalities include not only individual interventions, but research, environmental modifications, technologies, and policy-making intercessions for improving the lives of all people with disabilities.

Pediatric stroke rehabilitation differs from that of adults in some important ways as well: the length of the potential treatment and lifetime consequences, the need for new skill acquisition, the importance of activities in the school setting, and a complex transition to adulthood. It is crucial for the rehabilitation team to evaluate the child and family periodically and to return to the individualized anticipatory guidance framework to ensure that global aspects of development are supported, and that age-appropriate interventions are accessible. It is necessary to maintain open communication with the school system, and to be aware of transitions in the classroom and IEP, ideally before they occur. At stake is the potential of the child to master the skills needed for full participation in the social, cultural, and economic community. Vigilance is required in the pursuit of removing barriers to inclusion for all people in education, in recreation, and in vocation.

REFERENCES

1. Ellis C, McGrattan K, Mauldin P, Ovbiagele B. Costs of pediatric stroke care in the United States: a systematic and contemporary review. *Expert Rev Pharmacoecon Outcomes Res.* 2014;14(5):643–650.
2. Greenham M, Anderson V, Mackay MT. Improving cognitive outcomes for pediatric stroke. *Curr Opin Neurol.* 2017;30(2):127–132.
3. Fullerton HJ, Wu YW, Zhao S, Johnston SC. Risk of stroke in children: ethnic and gender disparities. *Neurology.* 2003;61(2):189–194.
4. Kleindorfer D, Khoury J, Kissela B, et al. Temporal trends in the incidence and case fatality of stroke in children and adolescents. *J Child Neurol.* 2006;21(5):415–418.
5. Braun KP, Kappelle LJ, Kirkham FJ, Deveber G. Diagnostic pitfalls in paediatric ischaemic stroke. *Dev Med Child Neurol.* 2006;48(12):985–990.
6. Broderick J, Talbot GT, Prenger E, Leach A, Brott T. Stroke in children within a major metropolitan area: the surprising importance of intracerebral hemorrhage. *J Child Neurol.* 1993;8(3):250–255.
7. Riela AR, Roach ES. Etiology of stroke in children. *J Child Neurol.* 1993;8(3):201–220.
8. Carvalho KS, Garg BP. Arterial strokes in children. *Neurol Clin.* 2002;20(4):1079–1100, vii.
9. Mackay MT, Wiznitzer M, Benedict SL, et al. Arterial ischemic stroke risk factors: the international pediatric stroke study. *Ann Neurol.* 2011;69(1):130–140.
10. Wintermark M, Hills NK, deVeber GA, et al. Arteriopathy diagnosis in childhood arterial ischemic stroke: results of the vascular effects of infection in pediatric stroke study. *Stroke.* 2014;45(12):3597–3605.
11. Fullerton HJ, Wintermark M, Hills NK, et al. Risk of recurrent arterial ischemic stroke in childhood: a prospective international study. *Stroke.* 2016;47(1):53–59.
12. Askalan R, Laughlin S, Mayank S, et al. Chickenpox and stroke in childhood: a study of frequency and causation. *Stroke.* 2001;32(6):1257–1262.
13. Mueller S, Fullerton HJ, Stratton K, et al. Radiation, atherosclerotic risk factors, and stroke risk in survivors of pediatric cancer: a report from the childhood cancer survivor study. *Int J Radiat Oncol Biol Phys.* 2013;86(4):649–655.
14. Bowers DC. Strokes among childhood brain tumor survivors. *Cancer Treat Res.* 2009;150:145–153.
15. Bowers DC, Mulne AF, Reisch JS, et al. Nonperioperative strokes in children with central nervous system tumors. *Cancer.* 2002;94(4):1094–1101.
16. Campen CJ, Kranick SM, Kasner SE, et al. Cranial irradiation increases risk of stroke in pediatric brain tumor survivors. *Stroke.* 2012;43(11):3035–3040.
17. Felling RJ, Sun LR, Maxwell EC, Goldenberg N, Bernard T. Pediatric arterial ischemic stroke: epidemiology, risk factors, and management. *Blood Cells Mol Dis.* 2017; Sep;67:23–33. https://doi.org/10.1016/j.bcmd.2017.03.003. Epub 2017 Mar 7. Review. PMID: 28336156.
18. Adams RJ. TCD in sickle cell disease: an important and useful test. *Pediatr Radiol.* 2005;35(3):229–234.
19. Ohene-Frempong K, Weiner SJ, Sleeper LA, et al. Cerebrovascular accidents in sickle cell disease: rates and risk factors. *Blood.* 1998;91(1):288–294.
20. Tsze DS, Valente JH. Pediatric stroke: a review. *Emerg Med Int.* 2011;2011. https://doi.org/10.1155/2011/734506.

21. deVeber GA, Kirton A, Booth FA, et al. Epidemiology and outcomes of arterial ischemic stroke in children: the canadian pediatric ischemic stroke registry. *Pediatr Neurol.* 2017;69:58–70.

22. Gordon AL, Anderson V, Ditchfield M, et al. Factors associated with six-month outcome of pediatric stroke. *Int J Stroke.* 2015;10(7):1068–1073.

23. Westmacott R, Askalan R, MacGregor D, Anderson P, Deveber G. Cognitive outcome following unilateral arterial ischaemic stroke in childhood: effects of age at stroke and lesion location. *Dev Med Child Neurol.* 2010;52(4):386–393.

24. Cooper AN, Anderson V, Hearps S, et al. Trajectories of motor recovery in the first year after pediatric arterial ischemic stroke. *Pediatrics.* 2017; Aug;140(2). pii: e20163870. https://doi.org/10.1542/peds.2016–3870. Epub 2017 Jul 14.

25. Council on Communications and Media. Media use in school-aged children and adolescents. *Pediatrics.* 2016; 138(5). https://doi.org/10.1542/peds.2016-2592.

26. Dai AI, Demiryurek AT. Serial casting as an adjunct to botulinum toxin type A treatment in children with cerebral palsy and spastic paraparesis with scissoring of the lower extremities. *J Child Neurol.* 2017;32(7):671–675.

27. Dursun N, Gokbel T, Akarsu M, Dursun E. Randomized controlled trial on effectiveness of intermittent serial casting on spastic equinus foot in children with cerebral palsy after botulinum toxin-A treatment. *Am J Phys Med Rehabil.* 2017;96(4):221–225.

28. Gough M. Serial casting in cerebral palsy: panacea, placebo, or peril? *Dev Med Child Neurol.* 2007;49(10):725.

29. Katz RT, Rymer WZ. Spastic hypertonia: mechanisms and measurement. *Arch Phys Med Rehabil.* 1989;70(2):144–155.

30. De Rinaldis M, Losito L, Gennaro L, Trabacca A. Long-term oral baclofen treatment in a child with cerebral palsy: electroencephalographic changes and clinical adverse effects. *J Child Neurol.* 2010;25(10):1272–1274.

31. Hansel DE, Hansel CR, Shindle MK, et al. Oral baclofen in cerebral palsy: possible seizure potentiation? *Pediatr Neurol.* 2003;29(3):203–206.

32. Rawicki B. Treatment of cerebral origin spasticity with continuous intrathecal baclofen delivered via an implantable pump: long-term follow-up review of 18 patients. *J Neurosurg.* 1999;91(5):733–736.

33. Verrotti A, Greco R, Spalice A, Chiarelli F, Iannetti P. Pharmacotherapy of spasticity in children with cerebral palsy. *Pediatr Neurol.* 2006;34(1):1–6.

34. Gracies JM, Nance P, Elovic E, McGuire J, Simpson DM. Traditional pharmacological treatments for spasticity. part II: general and regional treatments. *Muscle Nerve Suppl.* 1997;6:S92–S120.

35. Quality Standards Subcommittee of the American Academy of Neurology and the Practice Committee of the Child Neurology Society, Delgado MR, Hirtz D, et al. Practice parameter: pharmacologic treatment of spasticity in children and adolescents with cerebral palsy (an evidence-based review): report of the quality standards subcommittee of the American academy of neurology and the practice committee of the child neurology society. *Neurology.* 2010;74(4):336–343.

36. Dudley RW, Parolin M, Gagnon B, et al. Long-term functional benefits of selective dorsal rhizotomy for spastic cerebral palsy. *J Neurosurg Pediatr.* 2013;12(2):142–150.

37. Gump WC, Mutchnick IS, Moriarty TM. Selective dorsal rhizotomy for spasticity not associated with cerebral palsy: Reconsideration of surgical inclusion criteria. *Neurosurg Focus.* 2013;35(5):E6.

38. Steinbok P. Selective dorsal rhizotomy for spastic cerebral palsy: a review. *Childs Nerv Syst.* 2007;23(9):981–990.

39. Givon U. Management of the spastic hip in cerebral palsy. *Curr Opin Pediatr.* 2017;29(1):65–69.

40. Marchand V, Motil KJ. NASPGHAN Committee on Nutrition. Nutrition support for neurologically impaired children: a clinical report of the north American society for pediatric gastroenterology, hepatology, and nutrition. *J Pediatr Gastroenterol Nutr.* 2006;43(1):123–135.

41. Christerson S, Stromberg B. Stroke in Swedish children II: long-term outcome. *Acta Paediatr.* 2010;99(11): 1650–1656.

42. Paul B, Appelbaum M, Carapetian S, et al. Face and location processing in children with early unilateral brain injury. *Brain Cogn.* 2014;88:6–13.

43. Lidzba K, Kupper H, Kluger G, Staudt M. The time window for successful right-hemispheric language reorganization in children. *Eur J Paediatr Neurol.* 2017; Sep;21(5):715–721. https://doi.org/10.1016/j.ejpn.2017.06.001. Epub 2017 Jun 12.

44. Billinghurst LL, Beslow LA, Abend NS, et al. Incidence and predictors of epilepsy after pediatric arterial ischemic stroke. *Neurology.* 2017;88(7):630–637.

45. Kim EH, Ko TS. Cognitive impairment in childhood onset epilepsy: up-to-date information about its causes. *Korean J Pediatr.* 2016;59(4):155–164.

46. Reuner G, Kadish NE, Doering JH, Balke D, Schubert-Bast S. Attention and executive functions in the early course of pediatric epilepsy. *Epilepsy Behav.* 2016;60:42–49.

47. Schraegle WA, Titus JB. Executive function and health-related quality of life in pediatric epilepsy. *Epilepsy Behav.* 2016;62:20–26.

48. Chen HC, Chen CL, Kang LJ, Wu CY, Chen FC, Hong WH. Improvement of upper extremity motor control and function after home-based constraint induced therapy in children with unilateral cerebral palsy: immediate and long-term effects. *Arch Phys Med Rehabil.* 2014;95(8): 1423–1432.

49. Chen YP, Pope S, Tyler D, Warren GL. Effectiveness of constraint-induced movement therapy on upper-extremity function in children with cerebral palsy: a systematic review and meta-analysis of randomized controlled trials. *Clin Rehabil.* 2014;28(10):939–953.

50. Coker P, Lebkicher C, Harris L, Snape J. The effects of constraint-induced movement therapy for a child less than one year of age. *NeuroRehabilitation.* 2009;24(3):199–208.

51. Nordstrand L, Holmefur M, Kits A, Eliasson AC. Improvements in bimanual hand function after baby-CIMT in two-year old children with unilateral cerebral palsy: a retrospective study. *Res Dev Disabil.* 2015;41–42: 86–93.

52. Kirton A, Andersen J, Herrero M, et al. Brain stimulation and constraint for perinatal stroke hemiparesis: the PLAS-TIC CHAMPS trial. *Neurology*. 2016;86(18):1659–1667.

53. Hebert D, Lindsay MP, McIntyre A, et al. Canadian stroke best practice recommendations: stroke rehabilitation practice guidelines, update 2015. *Int J Stroke*. 2016;11(4):459–484.

54. Fasoli SE, Ladenheim B, Mast J, Krebs HI. New horizons for robot-assisted therapy in pediatrics. *Am J Phys Med Rehabil*. 2012;91(11 suppl 3):S280–S289.

55. Beretta E, Cesareo A, Biffi E, Schafer C, Galbiati S, Strazzer S. A comparative study among constraint, robot-aided standard therapies upper limb rehabilitation children acquired brain injury. *J Healthc Eng*. 2018; Mar; 14.

56. Stergiou A, Tzoufi M, Ntzani E, Varvarousis D, Beris A, Ploumis A. Therapeutic effects of horseback riding interventions: a systematic review and meta-analysis. *Am J Phys Med Rehabil*. 2017; Oct;96(10):717–725. https://doi.org/10.1097/PHM.0000000000000726.

57. Shikako-Thomas K, Majnemer A, Law M, Lach L. Determinants of participation in leisure activities in children and youth with cerebral palsy: systematic review. *Phys Occup Ther Pediatr*. 2008;28(2):155–169.

58. Hawks C, Jordan LC, Gindville M, Ichord RN, Licht DJ, Beslow LA. Educational placement after pediatric intracerebral hemorrhage. *Pediatr Neurol*. 2016;61:46–50.

59. USC03. *Individuals with Disabilities Education Act*. 1990: 33.

60. Strassfeld NM. The future of IDEA: monitoring disproportionate representation of minority students in special education and intentional discrimination claims. *Case W Res L Rev*. 2016;67:1121.

61. Bjorquist E, Nordmark E, Hallstrom I. Living in transition - experiences of health and well-being and the needs of adolescents with cerebral palsy. *Child Care Health Dev*. 2015; 41(2):258–265.

62. Bagatell N, Chan D, Rauch KK, Thorpe D. "Thrust into adulthood": transition experiences of young adults with cerebral palsy. *Disabil Health J*. 2017;10(1):80–86.

63. Burns F, Stewart R, Reddihough D, Scheinberg A, Ooi K, Graham HK. The cerebral palsy transition clinic: administrative chore, clinical responsibility, or opportunity for audit and clinical research? *J Children's Orthopaedics*. 2014;8(3):203–213.

CHAPTER 20

Promoting Healthy Behaviors in Stroke Survivors

MATTHEW A. PLOW, PHD • JULIA CHANG, RN, BSN, SCRN, PHD

In the pursuit of limiting the consequences of a stroke, it is important that stroke survivors receive support to engage in healthy behaviors. Several common problems experienced by stroke survivors, including depression, mobility problems, and secondary strokes, can be addressed by encouraging engagement in healthy behaviors. Stroke survivors who engage in physical activity, maintain a healthy diet, and take medications as prescribed can improve participation in meaningful life roles and can reduce cardiovascular risk factors, such as obesity, high blood pressure, and diabetes.[1–5] Routinely maintaining engagement in healthy behaviors can also reduce the utilization of healthcare services, decrease the need to take medications, and enhance the outcomes of healthcare services.[3,6–10] Thus, there are personal and societal benefits from supporting stroke survivors to engage in healthy behaviors.

Unfortunately, stroke survivors often face many personal and societal barriers to engaging in healthy behaviors, particularly due to stroke-related impairments interacting with an unsupportive physical and social environment.[11,12] Mobility impairments, cognitive deficits, and mood disorders are common problems experienced by stroke survivors.[3] These common health problems often interact with environmental barriers, such as inaccessible buildings and services, that decrease motivation and ability of stroke survivors to engage in healthy behaviors. Furthermore, healthcare providers often face competing demands on their time, which is not conducive to the teaching of skills that can facilitate behavior change.[13,14] Nonetheless, healthcare providers can play a pivotal role in supporting stroke survivors to engage in healthy behaviors that promote quality of life and reduce cardiovascular risks.

The effectiveness of many healthcare interventions depends on the patient's motivation and ability to make behavior changes.[15] Physicians, pharmacists, rehabilitation professionals, nurses, psychologists, and social workers, all deliver interventions to bring about behavior changes in stroke survivors. Indeed, a patient who does not change his or her behavior to follow treatment recommendation will be more likely to have worse outcomes.[13,16] For example, patients who do not change their behaviors to take medications as prescribed or do not engage in a rehabilitation program at an adequate frequency and intensity may be less likely to experience health benefits. Fortunately, there are now several studies in stroke survivors that have identified intervention strategies that can be used in healthcare settings to promote healthy behaviors.

The objective of this chapter is to provide healthcare providers with pragmatic strategies for supporting stroke survivors to engage in physical activity, eat healthy, and take medications as prescribed (i.e., medication adherence). We decided to focus on these three behaviors because of their importance in promoting quality of life and reducing secondary stroke risks. To accomplish the objective of this chapter, we will review observational studies in stroke survivors that have identified facilitators and barriers for engaging in physical activity, healthy eating habits, and taking medication as prescribed. We will also review clinical trials and meta-analyses of behavior change interventions. At the end of the chapter, we will focus on describing behavior change strategies that can be implemented in clinical practice. We will draw upon behavior change theory and lessons learned in our research to describe strategies that can be used in clinical practice to promote healthy behaviors in stroke survivors.

PHYSICAL ACTIVITY

Physical activity is defined as any bodily movement produced by skeletal muscle contraction that results in a substantially greater expenditure of energy compared to resting levels.[17] Physical activity can be described in

Stroke Rehabilitation. https://doi.org/10.1016/B978-0-323-55381-0.00020-2

terms of intensity, frequency, duration, and type. Exercise and rehabilitation programs are specific types of physical activity that are planned and have the specific goal of improving or maintaining health, function, and/or fitness. Both lifestyle physical activity programs, such as pedometer-based walking programs, and rehabilitation programs, such as therapeutic exercise programs, have been documented to have several health benefits in stroke survivors.[2,5,13,18−20] In this section, we will focus on describing studies that have practical implications for promoting engagement in physical activity, exercise, and/or rehabilitation programs. We refer readers to guidelines from the American Heart Association[2,13] and recommendations from the American College of Sports Medicine[21] for details on how to prescribe physical activity, exercise, and rehabilitation programs. Although this chapter does not focus on how to prescribe these programs, we note that these programs will likely not be adhered to if they do not account for the preferences and impairments specific to each stroke survivor.

Despite the benefits of physical activity and exercise, inactivity is a prevalent problem after a stroke. A recent study, using data from the National Health and Nutrition Examination Survey (NHANES), showed that stroke survivors engaged in less moderate (46.1% vs. 54.7%) and vigorous (9.1% vs. 19.6%) physical activity compared to adults without stroke.[22] Stroke survivors were less likely to report engagement in household chores, jogging, and recreational activities, but reported similar amounts of engagement in swimming activities and walking compared to adults without stroke. Stroke survivors were also more likely to report increased engagement in sedentary behaviors like watching TV. The findings of the NHANES study are consistent with a systematic review of the literature conducted by English et al.[23] They included 26 studies (n = 983) in their review, which indicated that stroke survivors consistently engaged in less than half the amount of walking as compared to age-matched controls. Because of the high rates of inactivity in stroke survivors, it is important to understand both facilitator and barriers to physical activity and exercise in stroke survivors.[23]

Research indicates that stroke survivors have facilitators and barriers to physical activity and exercise that are similar to the general population, but also have unique facilitators and barriers that are due to stroke impairments and comorbid conditions. In a 2014 systematic review of facilitators and barriers to engagement in physical activity, Nicholson et al.[24] identified six relevant qualitative and/or quantitative studies. The most commonly reported barriers were lack of motivation,

environmental barriers, health concerns, and stroke impairments. Environmental barriers included access to service, transportation, and cost. In a study of 83 stroke survivors, Rimmer et al.[12] reported the five most common barriers in rank order: (1) cost of the program (61%), (2) lack of awareness of a fitness center in the area (57%), (3) no means of transportation to a fitness center (57%), (4) no knowledge of how to exercise (46%), and (5) no knowledge of where to exercise (44%). Several of these barriers could be addressed by making stroke survivors aware of resources in their community and providing education on how to safely engage in physical activity and/or exercise in their home.

In the review article by Nicholson et al.,[24] the most commonly reported facilitators were social support and the desire to perform daily activities. They found several studies that showed meeting with peers in a group exercise class increased motivation to engage in physical activity. Stroke survivors were also motivated to engage in physical activity because of a desire to stay independent and carry out daily activities. A few studies in their report indicated that stroke survivors perceived that rehabilitation services were a strong motivator to encourage physical activity. However, it was noted that these services often ended abruptly, which resulted in a return to more sedentary behaviors.

Self-efficacy or perceived confidence in ability to engage in physical activity may also facilitate engagement in physical activity. Several studies have documented strong associations between self-efficacy and engagement in physical activity.[25] Furthermore, interventions targeting self-efficacy may promote physical activity in stroke survivors.[26] At the end of this chapter, we will provide specific strategies that healthcare providers can implement to promote self-efficacy in stroke survivors.

There have been several randomized clinical trials of physical activity and/or exercise interventions in stroke survivors. In a systematic review of physical activity interventions in stroke survivors by Morris et al.,[27] 11 studies with 1704 participants were identified. The authors classified the interventions into two types: individualized, tailored counseling with or without supervised exercise and supervised exercise with advice. Three intervention studies of tailored counseling showed significant improvements in promoting physical activity after 12 months. Two studies of supervised exercise without counseling showed improvements in step counts at 3 months, but improvements were not maintained. The authors concluded from their review that there was "some evidence that tailored counseling alone or with tailored supervised exercise improves long-term physical activity participation and functional exercise capacity after stroke better than does tailored supervised exercise with general advice only." Thus, prescribing tailored home exercise programs that incorporate behavior change strategies may be effective in promoting engagement in physical activity and exercise.

Recently, there has been a growing recognition on the importance of including behavior change strategies in physical activity, exercise, and rehabilitation interventions in stroke survivors.[2,13,27] Green et al.[28] found in a randomized controlled trial of 200 participants with stroke that motivational interviewing was effective in advancing participants' stage of readiness to engage in physical activity. Motivational interviewing is a tailored counseling approach that helps participants recognize what is most important to them to foster intrinsic motivation to promote behavior change. Harrington et al.[29] found in a randomized controlled trial of 243 stroke survivors that a supervised exercise program plus educational counseling was cost effective in promoting physical function. The counseling focused on promoting the utilization of community resources and enlisting social support. A promising ongoing clinical trial conducted by Mansfield et al.[30] is evaluating a theory-based behavior change intervention to promote physical activity in stroke survivors. The intervention will be implemented as part of routine care and includes promoting self-management skills (goal-setting and problem solving), increasing self-efficacy, discussing the benefits of exercise, addressing barriers, utilizing community resources, and prescribing a tailored exercise program.

NUTRITION AND WEIGHT MANAGEMENT

Compared to research on physical activity, there has been substantially less research on nutrition and weight management in stroke survivors. We do know that adults with disabilities are two to four times more likely to be obese compared to adults without disabilities.[31–33] Furthermore, obesity can initiate and accelerate a cycle of preventable functional declines, that is, obesity can exacerbate mobility impairments and symptoms, as well as increase the likelihood of other comorbid conditions, such as diabetes and cardiovascular disease, all of which can make it more difficult to engage in healthy behaviors.[34–37] Thus, there is a need to optimize energy balance in stroke survivors to avoid and disrupt the cycle of preventable functional declines. Similar to the section on physical activity, this section will focus on facilitators and barriers to

weight management and healthy eating rather than focus on specific nutritional guidelines for stroke survivors. The American Stroke Association can be a resource for learning about nutritional guidelines for stroke survivors.[3]

A complicating factor in promoting energy balance and weight management in stroke survivors is that interventions should ideally target multiple behaviors (e.g., nutrition, physical activity, and sleep). However, observational studies of stroke survivors have typically focused on single healthy behaviors.[38] Thus, few studies have addressed questions pertinent to promoting multiple behaviors. For example, fundamental questions remain about the linkages between healthy behaviors and how perceptions about one behavior may shape perceptions about another behavior. This lack of knowledge has translated into developing interventions that are ineffective in stroke survivors. Lager et al.[38] concluded from a systematic review and meta-analysis that interventions in stroke survivors that target multiple behaviors and/or multiple cardiovascular risk factors (e.g., obesity, high blood pressure, smoking, and alcohol abuse) are largely ineffective or inconclusive in changing multiple behaviors and reducing cardiovascular risks.

In a mixed method study of 25 stroke survivors,[39] we examined the relationships between stroke impairments and physical activity, sleep, and nutrition, as well as the relationships between physical activity, sleep, and nutrition. We found statistically significant and moderate correlations between hand function and healthy eating habits ($r = 0.45$), sleep disturbances and limitations in activities of daily living ($r = -0.55$), body mass index (BMI) and limitations in activities of daily living ($r = -0.49$), sleep disturbances and physical activity ($r = -0.48$), sleep disturbances and BMI ($r = 0.48$), and physical activity and BMI ($r = -0.45$). We concluded that promoting multiple health behaviors in stroke survivors should include addressing sleep disturbances, activity limitations, self-image, and negative emotions (i.e., depression and anxiety).

Because of the limited research on promoting multiple behaviors specific to stroke survivors, the remaining part of this section will focus on observational studies of nutritional behaviors in stroke survivors. We will also review studies of nutrition and weight management interventions in people with disabilities. We note that most studies of nutrition in stroke survivors have focused on addressing eating difficulties, issues of dysphagia, and examining when feeding tubes are appropriate, which is outside the scope of this chapter.

Research has documented that poor nutritional status is a prevalent problem in stroke survivors. Poor nutritional status, such as obesity and malnutrition, is related to muscle wasting, functional limitations, restrictions in social roles, fatigue, and poor quality of life in stroke survivors.[40–44] In a study of 279 stroke survivors, Vahlberg et al.[41] found that about one-third of participants had nutritional disorders, that is, obesity, sarcopenia, or risk for malnutrition. Specifically, 22% of participants were obese, 14% were at risk for malnutrition, and 28% were at high risk for disability. They found that mobility impairments significantly increased the risk of experiencing malnutrition. Other researchers have also found that upper-extremity mobility impairments and dysphagia are related to difficulties with eating and unhealthy eating habits.[39,45,46]

Difficulties with eating may be a barrier to selecting healthy foods and can interfere with social activities.[39,44,47] Stroke survivors with eating difficulties may avoid social situations with friends and family because of being embarrassed to eat in front of other people. Difficulties with preparing foods can also result in the selection of highly processed foods or going to fastfood restaurants. In our mixed methods study,[39] several stroke survivors described prioritizing unhealthy foods because they perceived that unhealthy foods were easier to prepare. Consistent with the general population, mood disorders, such as depression, may also be associated with loss of appetite and malnutrition in stroke survivors. Also consistent with the general population, stroke survivors often express frustration because they receive conflicting advice on what constitutes a healthy diet.[39] Possible strategies to help stroke survivors overcome these barriers are to provide education on critically reviewing information, foster healthy coping skills to manage emotions, and encourage the enlistment of social support. Because stroke survivors may be reliant on family members or caregivers for grocery shopping and cooking, it is critical to include them in interventions that have the goal of changing nutritional behaviors.

In a systematic review of nutritional and weight management interventions in adults with mobility impairing neurologic and musculoskeletal conditions,[48] we identified 25 empirically tested behavior change interventions that included a total of only 44 stroke survivors. The most common behavior change strategies employed in the interventions were presenting instructive information (n = 25 interventions), followed by self-monitoring of behavior (n = 21 interventions), modeling or demonstrating the behavior (n = 13 interventions), presenting feedback about performance (n = 13 interventions), problem solving/barrier identification (n = 12 interventions), self-monitoring of outcomes (n = 10 interventions), and restructuring the environment (n = 9 interventions). Rimmer et al.[49] found in 102 participants with physical disabilities that a telephone-based weight management program supported with a web-based remote coaching tool was effective in promoting weight loss. The intervention focused on teaching participants to set realistic goals, encouraging positive changes in easily achievable increments, and providing tailored feedback. In another study by Rimmer et al.,[50] specific to stroke survivors (n = 35) who were predominantly African-American, it was found that a shortterm health promotion intervention significantly reduced total cholesterol and weight, as well as increased cardiovascular fitness, strength, flexibility, and ability to manage self-care needs. The intervention focused on providing education on nutrition and exercise, as well as teaching coping skills to reduce stress and teaching communication skills to facilitate a supportive home environment to eat healthy.

MEDICATION ADHERENCE

Medication adherence can be defined as the extent to which a person's behavior for taking medications corresponds with the agreed recommendations from a healthcare provider.[51] Depending on etiology, stroke survivors can be prescribed antithrombotic, blood pressure-lowering, and lipid-lowering medications. Each of these medications can reduce the risk of secondary strokes by 16%–45% and in combination may reduce the risk of a secondary stroke by as much as 80%.[1] Thus, it is important to promote medication adherence in stroke survivors. However, it is estimated that over 50% of stroke survivors stop taking medications as prescribed 1–2 years after their stroke.[52] Rates of adherence may be affected by the types of medications prescribed. For example, adherence to anticoagulant medications is typically less than the adherence to antiplatelet medications.[53]

Because of the high rates of nonadherence in stroke survivors, a substantial amount of research has been conducted to understand the facilitators and barriers to medication adherence. There have also been several randomized controlled trials of interventions designed to promote medication adherence in stroke survivors.[54] Similar to research on physical activity and exercise, a multitude of personal and environmental factors can influence medication adherence in stroke survivors. A clear message from existing research on medication adherence in stroke survivors is that it is simply not enough to just write a prescription for medications. To promote medication adherence, healthcare providers must take the time to understand the personal circumstances of their patients.

Stroke survivors have similar medication adherence rates to patients with other longterm chronic conditions.[55] In a recent metaanalysis of medication adherence rates, AlShaikh et al.[57] identified 29 studies that included 69,137 participants with stroke or transient ischemic attack. They reported the nonadherence medication rate to secondary preventative mediations was 30.9% (95% CI 26.8%—35.3%). Although the authors reported that many studies identified factors associated with adherence, such as age, disability, and polypharmacy, none of the factors were significant in the meta-analysis. This suggests that medication adherence is complex and that heterogeneity in the research designs and research samples may influence associations. In a 1-year cohort study of 21,077 stroke survivors from the Swedish Stroke Register, Glader et al.[56] found that nonadherence rates increased dramatically with the first 2 years after the stroke. During the first 4 months after discharge from the hospital, the proportion of stroke survivors adhering to medications ranged from 95.5% for antihypertensive medications to 89.1% for warfarin. However, the proportion of stroke survivors who adhered to medications at discharge substantially declined over the first 2 years to reach 74.2% for antihypertensive medications, 56.1% for statins, 63.7% for antiplatelet medications, and 45.0% for warfarin. Clearly, behavior change strategies need to be implemented to promote medication adherence in stroke survivors.

Studies on facilitators and barriers to medication adherence may provide some indications as to which behavior change strategies should be prioritized and implemented in clinical practice. In the systematic review conducted by AlShaikh et al.,[52] common factors reported to be associated with medication adherence included concerns about treatment, lack of support with medication intake, polypharmacy, increased disability, and having more severe stroke. Chamber et al.[57] conducted a qualitative study that compared stroke survivors who had high medication adherence to stroke survivors who had low medication adherence. Two main themes were identified: importance of establishing habits and enlistment of social support from family and healthcare providers. Stroke survivors who had high medication adherence understood the consequences of nonadherence and believed the benefits of taking the medication outweighed the risks of taking

the medications. Stroke survivors who had low medication adherence described forgetting to take their medications or intentionally not wanting to take the medication because of perceived risks or not believing in the benefits of the medications. They also frequently reported receiving limited support from healthcare providers. These finding were consistent with a qualitative study by Bauler et al.[58] They found that concern about taking too many medications was also a common reason for nonadherence. Together, these studies indicate that healthcare providers can play an important role in promoting medication adherence by providing education that describes the benefits of taking the medication and addresses concern about risks.

Several studies have also identified demographic, mental health, and psychologic characteristics as being associated with medication adherence in stroke survivors. In an interesting study by Kronish et al.,[59] it was found in 535 stroke survivors and adults with transient ischemic attacks that 18% of them likely had posttraumatic stress disorder (PTSD). Stroke survivors with PTSD were three time more likely to be nonadherent to taking medications even after controlling for depression. In a study by O'Carroll et al.,[60] it was found in 180 stroke survivors that younger age, concerns about medications, reduced cognitive function, and low perceived benefit of medications were associated with low medication adherence. Other studies have identified emotions (e.g., depression), costs, difficulties with swallowing, low trust in their physician, perceptions of discrimination from healthcare services, and difficulty accessing healthcare services are associated with low medication adherence.[61—64]

In spite of the array of factors that can influence medication adherence in stroke survivors, interventions have been effective in promoting medication adherence. In a systematic review of randomized controlled trials of medication adherence interventions, Wessol et al.[54] identified 18 studies that included 10,292 stroke survivors from the years of 2009—15. Significant improvements in medication adherence were reported in 5 out of the 18 studies. Interventions were described as using a cognitive behavioral approach or an educational-based approach. Behavior change strategies in the interventions included promoting self-efficacy and social support, using text messages, teaching self-management skills, and creating detailed intentions on when patients would take medications. In a recent systematic review and meta-analysis of self-management interventions in stroke survivor, AlShaikh et al.[65] confirmed that self-management interventions were effective in promoting medication adherence in stroke survivors. Self-management interventions typically focus on teaching skills such as resource utilization, problem-solving, emotional management, and promoting self-efficacy. Targeting these self-management skills are consistent with observational studies described above that identified facilitators and barriers to medication adherence.

There are also examples of effective medication adherence interventions that were brief and low-cost, which may be feasible to implement within clinical practices. O'Carroll et al.[66] conducted a pilot randomized controlled trial in 62 stroke survivors to examine the effects of a tailored intervention that was only two sessions. The intervention consisted of developing a plan that linked the participants' environment to a medication-taking routine and addressing any misconceptions about the medications. The intervention significantly improved medication adherence, that is, the intervention resulted in 10% more doses taken as prescribed. Kamal et al.[67] found in randomized controlled trails of 200 stroke survivors that text message can significantly improve medication adherence and diastolic blood pressure. The text messages were based on behavior change theory and consisted of messages that were tailored to participants' risk profile and their current prescription of medications. There are now several commercially available mobile apps that can provide text message reminders to promote medication adherence. Some of the key features of these apps are promoting self-monitoring, encouraging habit formations, providing education, and delivering reminders.

BEHAVIOR CHANGE STRATEGIES

This section will describe behavior change strategies that healthcare providers can use to promote behavior change. We will first review two behavior change theories that are commonly used in guiding the design of behavior change interventions: (1) Social Cognitive Theory and (2) Transtheoretical Model. We will then discuss the following behavior change strategies that can be used in clinical practice: (1) encouraging goal-setting and self-monitoring, (2) identifying barriers and providing feedback, and (3) reshaping social environment.

SOCIAL COGNITIVE THEORY

Social cognitive theory is one of the most commonly used behavior change theories. The central premise of social cognitive theory is reciprocal determinism, which is the interaction of person, environment, and behavior.[68,69] Person, environment, and behavior

continuously interact. A person's behavior is shaped by observing the people around them and their perceptions of the environment. A person's behavior is influenced by their capabilities or knowledge, positive and negative reinforcements, self-control (e.g., setting and meeting goals), perceived outcomes of performing behaviors and the values placed on those outcomes, and self-efficacy (i.e., confidence in overcoming barriers).[70] Thus, a person that does not know how to engage in the behavior, does not value the outcomes associated with engaging in the behavior, or is not confident that they will be able to overcome barriers is likely not to engage in the behavior. Fortunately, all of these factors can potentially be modified by healthcare providers. Healthcare providers can provide education on how to perform the behavior, teach skills in self-control (e.g., goal-setting and self-monitoring), influence perceptions about the behavior (e.g., encouraging positive reinforcement), and build confidence in overcoming barriers (e.g., increasing self-efficacy).

Self-efficacy has consistently been shown to influence behaviors in stroke survivors.[26] Social cognitive theory outlines four ways to improve self-efficacy: (1) mastery experiences, (2) vicarious experiences (i.e., social modeling), (3) social persuasion, and (4) states of emotions and physiology.[71] Healthcare providers can provide mastery experiences by encouraging patients to practice the behavior, ensuring that the patient has small successes in engaging in the behavior (i.e., start simple and progress in difficulty), and providing feedback on progress. Healthcare providers can facilitate vicarious experiences by encouraging patients to attend support groups, having them interact with other patients (e.g., group education), and describing success stories of patients engaging in the behavior. Social persuasion and states of emotions can both be addressed by providing education, for example, providing pamphlets on the benefits of exercising or medications, teaching the differences between fatigue felt after exercise and fatigue caused by the stroke, and addressing feelings of depression and/or anxiety. Table 20.1 provides details on implementing behavior strategies consistent with social cognitive theory.

TRANSTHEORETICAL MODEL

Another commonly used model to change behavior is the transtheoretical model.[72] The transtheoretical model provides a framework for categorizing individuals' readiness to change their behavior. Important concepts in the transtheoretical model include stages of change, self-efficacy, and processes of change. The five stages of change are precontemplation, contemplation,

TABLE 20.1
Behavior Changes Strategies Consistent With Social Cognitive Theory

Concept	Description	Behavior Change Strategy
Reciprocal determinism	Interaction between environment, person, and behavior	Address both personal and environmental factors to change behavior
Self-efficacy	Confidence in overcoming barriers to perform a specific behavior	Provide opportunities for mastery experiences, social modeling, verbal persuasion, and learning about emotions
Expectations	Outcomes that are expected	Teach about benefits
Expectancies	Outcomes that are valued	Provide feedback and have patients' evaluate what they value
Self-control	Ability to achieve goal	Set SMART goals and encourage self-monitoring and problem-solving
Reinforcements	Response to engaging in behavior	Provide positive feedback and encourage self-reward when goals are met

preparation, action, and maintenance. These stages reflect behavioral intentions and the temporal process from not considering engaging in a particular behavior to routine engagement. Self-efficacy and processes of change are the activities and cognitions that people use to progress through the stages.[73] A potential implication of this model is that healthcare providers can use it to tailor behavior change interventions, as well as prioritize which behaviors to target for change. For example, healthcare providers may choose to prioritize only those behaviors in which the patient is ready to change. Patients that are in the action stage, for example, may be more receptive to messages that promote self-efficacy and encourage the use of processes of change (e.g., enlistment of social support).[74] Table 20.2 provides details on implementing behavior change strategies consistent with the transtheoretical model.

ENCOURAGING GOAL-SETTING AND SELF-MONITORING

Perhaps one of the simplest yet most effective strategies to promote behavior change is encouraging goal-setting and self-monitoring.[75] Providing participants with worksheets can encourage them to set SMART goals, that is, specific, measurable, achievable, relevant, and time-bound. It is important that patients are encouraged to set detailed goals that require some effort to complete, but are also not too challenging. Locke and

Latham[76] have shown that goals that are sufficiently challenging and outcomes that are valued will direct attention toward goal-relevant activities and away from irrelevant activities, and helps foster intrinsic motivation to stay committed to the goal. Once a treatment or intervention plan is decided upon between the patient and healthcare provider, the healthcare provider can follow-up with questions that encourage the patient to create detailed intention for engaging in the behavior. For example, asking the patient when, where, and how they will engage in the behavior and then asking them to write down their goals and plans for achieving them. It is important that the healthcare provider convey that this is a collaborative effort and that they are not placing judgment on the patient.

Once goals have been set, it is important to encourage the patient to self-monitor progress in meeting the goal. Having patients self-monitor their behaviors helps to promote self-awareness and reflect upon their actions. We have found that both mobile health applications (mHealth apps) and paper diaries can be effective in helping patients self-monitor their behaviors. In randomized controlled trials, we found that both commercially available mHealth apps and paper diaries are significantly more effective in promoting behavior change compared to not tracking behaviors at all. However, there were no significant differences between using a paper diary and mHealth app. Thus, patients should be encouraged to track behaviors based on their preference for using a mHealth app or paper

TABLE 20.2
Behavior Changes Strategies Consistent With Transtheoretical Model

Concept	Description	Behavior Change Strategy
Stages of change	The process from not considering engaging in behavior to routine engagement Five stages: 1. Precontemplation 2. Contemplation 3. Preparation 4. Action 5. Maintenance	• Prioritize healthy behaviors that the patient is willing to change • In contemplation stage, emphasize benefits of engagement • In action stage, encourage self-efficacy and goal-setting, and provide details on how to engage in behavior • In maintenance stage, provide feedback on outcomes and prevent relapses
Process of change	Strategies used to progress through the stages	Both cognitive strategies, such as consciousness raising and self-reevaluation, and behavioral strategies, such as goal-setting, self-monitoring, and reminders, should be implemented
Decision balance	Ratio of benefits to disadvantages	Address misconceptions about benefits and risks

dairy. Anecdotally, we have found that patients who are successful in making longterm behavior changes consistently track their behaviors even years after making the change.

IDENTIFYING BARRIERS AND PROVIDING FEEDBACK

Identifying barriers and providing feedback are also important strategies in promoting behavior change. Patients can be asked to rate their confidence level in achieving a goal after it has been set. For example, on a scale of 1 to 10, how confident are you that you will be able to achieve the goal? If the patient response is less than 7, follow-up questions should occur about what barriers they anticipate encountering. A worksheet can be provided to help patients' problem-solve potential solutions or can be discussed during the clinical visit if time permits. Problem-solving can be approached in a systematic way by defining the barriers, generating solutions for overcoming the barrier (i.e., brainstorming), evaluating the pros and cons of each possible solution, and then selecting and implementing the solution. It is important to emphasize that changing behaviors will be a trial-and-error process and that setbacks should be expected, but that it is important not to give up.

With the increased emphasis on collecting patient-reported outcomes during clinical visits, it is important

that patients be provided with feedback about the outcomes that are collected. Similarly, if patients are asked to change behaviors and set goals, it is important that healthcare providers provide feedback about their progress. Briefly reviewing their tracking records or simply asking about their engagement in the behavior can show the patient that the behavior is important. Providing feedback can also help create accountability, which may be very effective in changing behaviors. Helping patients make connections between the behavior they engage in and the health outcomes they are experiencing can also be very motivating for the patient to maintain engagement. Alternatively, addressing concerns about the behaviors not producing the desired outcome is also very important. This could include changing treatment recommendations, adjusting goals, and having the patient reflect upon whether they are truly engaging in the behaviors as recommended. Again, it is important that feedback occur with empathy and not be judgmental, otherwise the patient may become resentful.

RESHAPING THE PHYSICAL AND SOCIAL ENVIRONMENT

The physical and social environment in which the behavior occurs is paramount in influencing whether behavior change persists. Although a healthcare

TABLE 20.3
Rearranging Physical and Social Environment to Support Healthy Behaviors

Concept	Description	Behavior Change Strategy
Ergonomics of physical environment	Designing and arranging the environment to make it easier to engage in healthy behavior	• Help the patient make connections between their behavior and environment • Help patient identify inefficient work spaces
Social support	Perceptions or experiences of having others who care for you	• Encourage patient to bring family and friends • Provide suggestions to family and friends about how to support engagement, such as reminders • Emphasize the importance of having emotional support, tangible support, informational support, and appraisal support
System thinking	Understanding of the linkages and interactions between the tasks that comprise the entirety of the behavior	Task analysis: encourage patient to think about the steps for engaging in the behavior and how that behavior is influenced by the surrounding social and physical environment

provider may have limited influence over changing administrative policy, insurance reimbursement, or the physical environment in which the patient lives, there are steps that healthcare providers can take to help patients reshape their environment so that it is more conducive to behavior change. Too often, patients are taught to relay on willpower and self-control to make behavior changes. This often results in failures and frustrations. Helping patients rearrange their environments can reduce reliance on willpower and make it easier to engage in the desired behavior. We conclude this chapter with Table 20.3, which describes some specific behavior change strategies that can be used to help patient rearrange their physical and social environment.

REFERENCES

1. Hackam DG, Spence JD. Combining multiple approaches for the secondary prevention of vascular events after stroke: a quantitative modeling study. *Stroke.* 2007; 38(6):1881−1885.
2. Billinger SA, Arena R, Bernhardt J, et al. Physical activity and exercise recommendations for stroke survivors: a statement for healthcare professionals from the American Heart Association/American Stroke Association. *Stroke.* 2014;45(8):2532−2553.
3. Kernan WN, Ovbiagele B, Black HR, et al. Guidelines for the prevention of stroke in patients with stroke and transient ischemic attack: a guideline for healthcare professionals from the American Heart Association/American Stroke Association. *Stroke.* 2014;45(7):2160−2236.
4. Barclay-Goddard R, Ripat J, Mayo NE. Developing a model of participation post-stroke: a mixed-methods approach. *Qual Life Res.* 2012;21(3):417−426.
5. Obembe AO, Eng JJ. Rehabilitation interventions for improving social participation after stroke: a systematic review and meta-analysis. *Neurorehabil Neural Repair.* 2016;30(4):384−392.
6. Carlson SA, Fulton JE, Pratt M, Yang Z, Adams EK. Inadequate physical activity and health care expenditures in the United States. *Prog Cardiovasc Dis.* 2015;57(4):315−323.
7. Brady TA. meta-analysis of health status, health behaviors, and health care utilization outcomes of the chronic disease self-management program. *Prev Chronic Dis.* 2013;10: 120112.
8. Hibbard JH, Greene J. What the evidence shows about patient activation: better health outcomes and care experiences; fewer data on costs. *Health Aff (Millwood).* 2013; 32(2):207−214.
9. Milani RV, Lavie CJ. Health care 2020: reengineering health care delivery to combat chronic disease. *Am J Med.* 2015;128(4):337−343.
10. Iuga AO, McGuire MJ. Adherence and health care costs. *Risk Manage Healthcare Policy.* 2014;7:35−44.

11. Rimmer JH, Rowland JL. Health promotion for people with disabilities: implications for empowering the person and promoting disability-friendly environments. *Am J Lifestyle Med.* 2008;2(5):409−420.

12. Rimmer JH, Wang E, Smith D. Barriers associated with exercise and community access for individuals with stroke. *J Rehabil Res Dev.* 2008;45(2):315−322.

13. Winstein CJ, Stein J, Arena R, et al. Guidelines for adult stroke rehabilitation and recovery: a guideline for healthcare professionals from the American Heart Association/American Stroke Association. *Stroke.* 2016;47(6): e98−e169.

14. Bauer UE, Briss PA, Goodman RA, Bowman BA. Prevention of chronic disease in the 21st century: elimination of the leading preventable causes of premature death and disability in the USA. *Lancet.* 2014;384(9937): 45−52.

15. Martin LR, Haskard-Zolnierek KB, DiMatteo MR. *Health Behavior Change and Treatment Adherence: Evidence-based Guidelines for Improving Healthcare.* USA: Oxford University Press; 2010.

16. Spring B, Ockene JK, Gidding SS, et al. Better population health through behavior change in adults a call to action. *Circulation.* 2013;128(19):2169−2176.

17. Bouchard C, Shephard RJ. *Physical Activity, Fitness, and Health: International Proceedings and Consensus Statement.* Champaign, IL: Human Kinetics Publishers; 1994.

18. Stretton CM, Mudge S, Kayes NM, McPherson KM. Interventions to improve real-world walking after stroke: a systematic review and meta-analysis. *Clin Rehabil.* 2017; 31(3):310−318.

19. Deijle IA, Van Schaik SM, Van Wegen EE, Weinstein HC, Kwakkel G, Van den Berg-Vos RM. Lifestyle interventions to prevent cardiovascular events after stroke and transient ischemic attack: systematic review and meta-analysis. *Stroke.* 2017;48(1):174−179.

20. Wattchow KA, McDonnell MN, Hillier SL. Rehabilitation interventions for upper limb function in the first four weeks following stroke: a systematic review and meta-analysis of the evidence. *Arch Phys Med Rehabil.* 2018;99(2):367−382. https://doi.org/10.1016/j.apmr.2017.06.014. Epub 2017 Jul 20.

21. Moore G, Durstine JL, Painter P, Medicine ACoS. ACSM's Exercise Management for Persons with Chronic Diseases and Disabilities, 4E. *Human Kinetics.* 2016:235−247.

22. Butler EN, Evenson KR. Prevalence of physical activity and sedentary behavior among stroke survivors in the United States. *Top Stroke Rehabil.* 2014;21(3):246−255.

23. English C, Manns PJ, Tucak C, Bernhardt J. Physical activity and sedentary behaviors in people with stroke living in the community: a systematic review. *Phys Ther.* 2014;94(2): 185−196.

24. Nicholson S, Sniehotta FF, van Wijck F, et al. A systematic review of perceived barriers and motivators to physical activity after stroke. *Int J Stroke.* 2013;8(5):357−364.

25. Ashford S, Edmunds J, French DP. What is the best way to change self-efficacy to promote lifestyle and recreational

physical activity? A systematic review with meta-analysis. *Br J Health Psychol.* 2010;15(2):265−288.

26. Jones F, Riazi A. Self-efficacy and self-management after stroke: a systematic review. *Disabil Rehabil.* 2011;33(10): 797−810.

27. Morris JH, Macgillivray S, McFarlane S. Interventions to promote long-term participation in physical activity after stroke: a systematic review of the literature. *Arch Phys Med Rehabil.* 2014;95(5):956−967.

28. Green T, Haley E, Eliasziw M, Hoyte K. Education in stroke prevention: efficacy of an educational counselling intervention to increase knowledge in stroke survivors. *Can J Neurosci Nurs.* 2007;29(2):13−20.

29. Harrington R, Taylor G, Hollinghurst S, Reed M, Kay H, Wood VA. A community-based exercise and education scheme for stroke survivors: a randomized controlled trial and economic evaluation. *Clin Rehabil.* 2010;24(1):3−15.

30. Mansfield A, Brooks D, Tang A, et al. Promoting Optimal Physical Exercise for Life (PROPEL): aerobic exercise and self-management early after stroke to increase daily physical activity-study protocol for a stepped-wedge randomised trial. *BMJ Open.* 2017;7(6):e015843.

31. Liou TH, Pi-Sunyer FX, Laferrere B. Physical disability and obesity. *Nutr Rev.* 2005;63(10):321−331.

32. Rimmer JH, Wang E. Obesity prevalence among a group of Chicago residents with disabilities. *Arch Phys Med Rehabil.* 2005;86(7):1461−1464.

33. Weil E, Wachterman M, McCarthy EP, et al. Obesity among adults with disabling conditions. *JAMA.* 2002;288(10): 1265−1268.

34. Vincent HK, Vincent KR, Lamb KM. Obesity and mobility disability in the older adult. *Obes Rev.* 2010;11(8): 568−579.

35. Rimmer JH. Exercise and physical activity in persons aging with a physical disability. *Phys Med Rehabil Clin N Am.* 2005;16(1):41−56.

36. Gariepy G, Wang J, Lesage A, Schmitz N. The interaction of obesity and psychological distress on disability. *Soc Psychiatry Psychiatr Epidemiol.* 2010;45(5):531−540.

37. Must A, Spadano J, Coakley EH, Field AE, Colditz G, Dietz WH. The disease burden associated with overweight and obesity. *JAMA.* 1999;282(16):1523−1529.

38. Lager KE, Mistri AK, Khunti K, Haunton VJ, Sett AK, Wilson AD. Interventions for improving modifiable risk factor control in the secondary prevention of stroke. *Cochrane Database Syst Rev.* 2014;5:CD009103.

39. Plow M, Moore SM, Sajatovic M, Katzan I. A mixed methods study of multiple health behaviors among individuals with stroke. *PeerJ.* 2017;5:e3210.

40. Westergren A. Nutrition and its relation to mealtime preparation, eating, fatigue and mood among stroke survivors after discharge from hospital-a pilot study. *Open Nursing J.* 2008;2:15.

41. Vahlberg B, Zetterberg L, Lindmark B, Hellstrom K, Cederholm T. Functional performance, nutritional status, and body composition in ambulant community-dwelling individuals 1-3 years after suffering from a

cerebral infarction or intracerebral bleeding. *BMC Geriatr.* 2016;16:48.

42. Adams J. An exploration of nutrition and eating disabilities in relation to quality of life at 6 months post-stroke. *Nurs Older People.* 2004;16(6):40.

43. Perry L, McLaren S. An exploration of nutrition and eating disabilities in relation to quality of life at 6 months post-stroke. *Health Soc Care Community.* 2004;12(4):288–297.

44. Klinke ME, Hafsteinsdottir TB, Thorsteinsson B, Jonsdottir H. Living at home with eating difficulties following stroke: a phenomenological study of younger people's experiences. *J Clin Nurs.* 2014;23(1–2):250–260.

45. Corrigan ML, Escuro AA, Celestin J, Kirby DF. Nutrition in the stroke patient. *Nutr Clin Pract.* 2011;26(3):242–252.

46. Foley NC, Martin RE, Salter KL, Teasell RW. A review of the relationship between dysphagia and malnutrition following stroke. *J Rehabil Med.* 2009;41(9):707–713.

47. Bailey RR. Promoting physical activity and nutrition in people with stroke. *Am J Occup Ther.* 2017;71(5): 7105360010p7105360011–7105360010p7105360015.

48. Plow MA, Moore S, Husni ME, Kirwan JP. A systematic review of behavioural techniques used in nutrition and weight loss interventions among adults with mobility-impairing neurological and musculoskeletal conditions. *Obes Rev.* 2014;15(12):945–956.

49. Rimmer JH, Wang E, Pellegrini CA, Lullo C, Gerber BS. Telehealth weight management intervention for adults with physical disabilities: a randomized controlled trial. *Am J Phys Med Rehabil.* 2013;92(12):1084–1094.

50. Rimmer JH, Braunschweig C, Silverman K, Riley B, Creviston T, Nicola T. Effects of a short-term health promotion intervention for a predominantly African-American group of stroke survivors. *Am J Prev Med.* 2000; 18(4):332–338.

51. Sabaté E. *Adherence to Long-term Therapies: Evidence for Action.* World Health Organization; 2003.

52. AlShaikh SA, Quinn T, Dunn W, Walters M, Dawson J. Predictive factors of non-adherence to secondary preventative medication after stroke or transient ischaemic attack: a systematic review and meta-analyses. *Eur Stroke J.* 2016;1(2): 65–75.

53. Wang Y, Wu D, Wang Y, Ma R, Wang C, Zhao W. A survey on adherence to secondary ischemic stroke prevention. *Neurol Res.* 2006;28(1):16–20.

54. Wessol JL, Russell CL, Cheng AL. A systematic review of randomized controlled trials of medication adherence interventions in adult stroke survivors. *J Neurosci Nurs.* 2017;49(2):120–133.

55. Nunes V, Neilson J, O'flynn N, et al. Clinical guidelines and evidence review for medicines adherence: involving patients in decisions about prescribed medicines and supporting adherence. *Lond Natl Collab Centre Prim Care R Coll Gen Pract.* 2009;364.

56. Glader E-L, Sjölander M, Eriksson M, Lundberg M. Persistent use of secondary preventive drugs declines rapidly during the first 2 years after stroke. *Stroke.* 2010;41(2): 397–401.

57. Chambers JA, O'Carroll RE, Hamilton B, et al. Adherence to medication in stroke survivors: a qualitative comparison of low and high adherers. *Br J Health Psychol.* 2011;16(3): 592–609.

58. Bauler S, Jacquin-Courtois S, Haesebaert J, et al. Barriers and facilitators for medication adherence in stroke patients: a qualitative study conducted in French neurological rehabilitation units. *Eur Neurol.* 2014;72(5–6): 262–270.

59. Kronish IM, Edmondson D, Goldfinger JZ, Fei K, Horowitz CR. Posttraumatic stress disorder and adherence to medications in survivors of strokes and transient ischemic attacks. *Stroke.* 2012;43(8):2192–2197.

60. O'Carroll R, Whittaker J, Hamilton B, Johnston M, Sudlow C, Dennis M. Predictors of adherence to secondary preventive medication in stroke patients. *Ann Behav Med.* 2011;41(3):383–390.

61. Crayton E, Fahey M, Ashworth M, Besser SJ, Weinman J, Wright AJ. Psychological determinants of medication adherence in stroke survivors: a systematic review of observational studies. *Ann Behav Med.* 2017;51(6):833–845. https://doi.org/10.1007/s12160-017-9906-0.

62. Levine DA, Morgenstern LB, Langa KM, Piette JD, Rogers MA, Karve SJ. Recent trends in cost-related medication nonadherence among stroke survivors in the United States. *Ann Neurol.* 2013;73(2):180–188.

63. Jamison J, Sutton S, Mant J, Simoni A. Barriers and facilitators to adherence to secondary stroke prevention medications after stroke: analysis of survivors and caregivers views from an online stroke forum. *BMJ Open.* 2017; 7(7):e016814.

64. Kronish IM, Diefenbach MA, Edmondson DE, Phillips LA, Fei K, Horowitz CR. Key barriers to medication adherence in survivors of strokes and transient ischemic attacks. *J Gen Intern Med.* 2013;28(5):675–682.

65. Al AlShaikh S, Quinn T, Dunn W, Walters M, Dawson J. Multimodal interventions to enhance adherence to secondary preventive medication after stroke: a systematic review and meta-analyses. *Cardiovasc Ther.* 2016;34(2): 85–93.

66. O'Carroll RE, Chambers JA, Dennis M, Sudlow C, Johnston M. Improving adherence to medication in stroke survivors: a pilot randomised controlled trial. *Ann Behav Med.* 2013;46(3):358–368.

67. Kamal AK, Shaikh Q, Pasha O, et al. A randomized controlled behavioral intervention trial to improve medication adherence in adult stroke patients with prescription tailored Short Messaging Service (SMS)-SMS4Stroke study. *BMC Neurol.* 2015;15:212.

68. Bandura A. *Social Foundations of Thought and Action: A Social Cognitive Theory.* Englewood Cliffs (NJ): Prentice-Hall; 1986.

69. Bandura A. Human agency in social cognitive theory. *Am Psychol.* 1989;44(9):1175–1184.

70. Bandura A. Social cognitive theory of self-regulation. *Organ Behav Hum Decis process.* 1991;50(2).

71. Bandura A. *Self-efficacy: The Exercise of Control*. New York: W.H. Freeman; 1997.

72. Prochaska J, Redding C, Evers K. The transtheoretical model and stages of change. In: Glanz K, Rimer BK, Viswanath K, eds. *Health Behavior and Health Education: Theory, Research, and Practice*. 4th ed. San Francisco, CA: Jossey-Bass; 2008;552:xxxiii.

73. Prochaska JO, DiClemente CC. Stages of change in the modification of problem behaviors. *Prog Behav Modif*. 1992;28:183−218.

74. Marcus BH, Dubbert PM, Forsyth LH, et al. Physical activity behavior change: issues in adoption and maintenance. *Health Psychol*. 2000;19(suppl 1):32−41.

75. Harkin B, Webb TL, Chang BP, et al. *Does Monitoring Goal Progress Promote Goal Attainment? A Meta-analysis of the Experimental Evidence*. American Psychological Association; 2016.

76. Locke EA, Latham GP. Building a practically useful theory of goal setting and task motivation. A 35-year odyssey. *Am Psychol*. 2002;57(9):705−717.

Index

Note: Page numbers followed by "f" indicate figures, "t" indicate tables, "b" indicate boxes.

Printed in the United States
By Bookmasters